READER'S DIGEST

GOOD HEALTH FACT BOOK

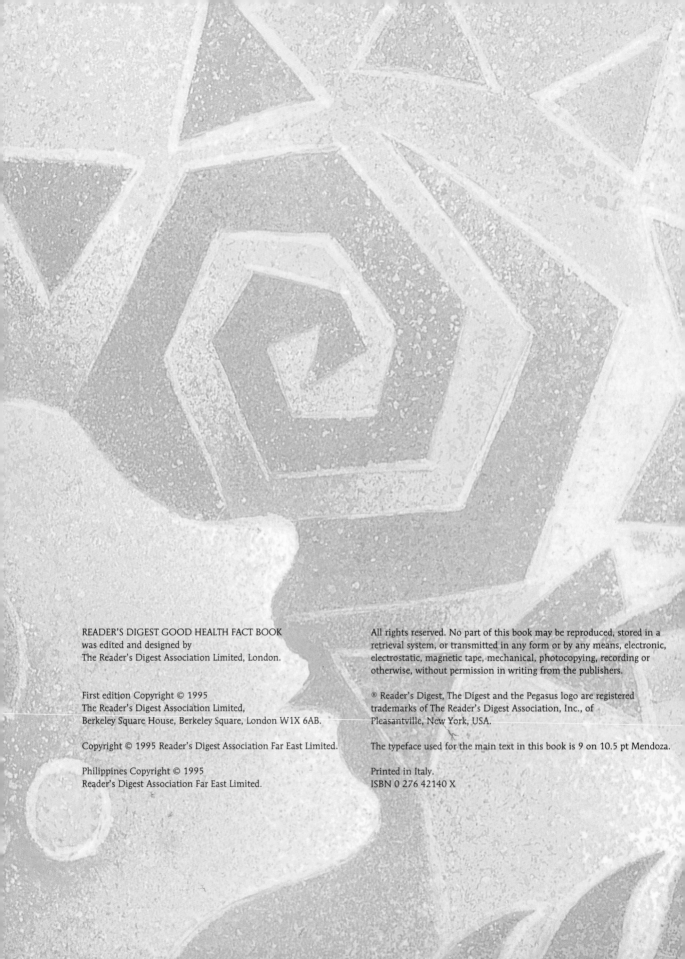

READER'S DIGEST GOOD HEALTH FACT BOOK
was edited and designed by
The Reader's Digest Association Limited, London.

First edition Copyright © 1995
The Reader's Digest Association Limited,
Berkeley Square House, Berkeley Square, London W1X 6AB.

Copyright © 1995 Reader's Digest Association Far East Limited.

Philippines Copyright © 1995
Reader's Digest Association Far East Limited.

The typeface used for the main text in this book is 9 on 10.5 pt Mendoza.

Printed in Italy.
ISBN 0 276 42140 X

READER'S DIGEST
GOOD HEALTH FACT BOOK

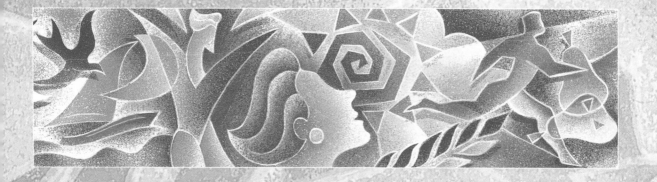

Published by The Reader's Digest Association Limited
LONDON · NEW YORK · SYDNEY · CAPE TOWN · MONTREAL

Editor Justine Scott-Macnab
Art Editor Iain Stuart
Consultant Editor Dr James Cox, MB, BS, FRCGP, MICGP, General Practitioner

CONTRIBUTORS

The publishers wish to express their thanks to the following people for their contributions to this book.

Writers and Consultants

Graham Barnby, BDS, DGDP, RCS
General Dental Practitioner

Dr D E Bateman, MA, MB, BChir, MRCP, MD
Consultant Neurologist, Royal United Hospital, Bath

Anita Bean, BSc
Nutrition and Fitness Consultant

Dr G C J Bennett, MB, FRCP
Senior Lecturer, Department of Health Care of the Elderly, Royal London Hospital

Dr Ron Behrens, MD, MRCP
Consultant Physician, Hospital for Tropical Diseases, UCL

Dr M Benson, MD, FRCP
Consultant Chest Physician, The Oxford Radcliffe Hospital

Jeffrey Boyling, MSc, BPhty, MCSP, MErgS

Dr Gary Brooke, MD, MRCP
Senior Registrar, The Archway Sexual Health Clinic

Jenny Brown, MCSP, DipTP
St George's Healthcare Trust

Robbi Campbell, MA, PGDip
Chair of Counselling in Medical Settings, British Association for Counselling

Dr Catherine Cassell, BSc, MA
Senior Lecturer in Organisation, Sheffield Hallam University

Anne Charlish

Dr Ed Charlton, FRCA
Consultant in Pain Management and Anaesthesia, The Royal Victoria Infirmary, Newcastle-upon-Tyne

Julia Cole, Cert Mt Rel
Counsellor and Psychosexual Therapist for Relate

Sue Couling, BSc, MSc, CChem, MRSC

Dr Hazel Curtis, MD, MRCP
Consultant Community Paediatrician, Torbay Hospital, Torquay

Dr R J Donaldson, OBE, CStJ, FFPuM, DPM
Consultant, Royal Society of Public Health

Della Duncan
Fitness Consultant

Dr Pamela Ewan, MB, MRCP, MRCPath
Hon Consultant in Allergy and Clinical Immunology, Medical Research Council

Dr D Fleming, MB, ChB, DRCOG, PhD
Director Birmingham Research Unit, The Royal College of General Practitioners

Dr Godfrey Fowler, OBE, BM, FRCGP, DCM, DRCOG
Clinical Reader in General Practice, University of Oxford, Department of Public Health and Primary Care

Dr John Frain, MB, ChB, DCH
General Practitioner

Professor C George, CSc, MD, FRCP
Professor of Clinical Pharmacology, University of Southampton

Dr Paul Goddard, BSc, MBBF, MD, DMRD, FRCR
Consultant Radiologist, Bristol Royal infirmary

Fran Godfrey
Advice Sister, Marie Stopes International

Dr Elizabeth M Graham, FRCP, DO, FRCOphth
Consultant Medical Ophthalmologist, St Thomas's Hospital, London

Professor Chris Ham, BA, MPhil, PhD
Professor of Health Policy and Management, University of Birmingham

Dr R Heatley, MD, FRCP
Consultant Physician, St James's University Hospital, Leeds

Professor S Hilton, MBBS, MD
Professor of General Practice and Primary Care, St George's Hospital, London

Professor James Horne, BSc, MSc, PhD, DSc, FIBiol, FBPSF
Professor of Psychophysiology University of Loughborough

Dr Judith Irving, MBBS

Dr Andrew MacDonald, MA (Oxon), MRCS, LRCP
General Practitioner

Dr Ann MacGregor, MBBS, DFFP
Registrar City of London Migraine Clinic

Professor David Mant, MB, ChB, MSc, MRCGP, MFPH
Professor of Primary Care Epidemiology, University of Southampton

Dr Sheena Meredith, MB, BS, LRCP, MRCS

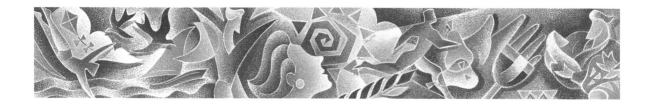

Maria Morris, BSc

Claire Nash

Dr David Peters, MB, CLB, DRCOG, MFHom, MRO
Centre for Community Care and Primary Health, London

Niamh Rice, BSc, SRD
Consultant Nutritionist and Dietician

Cynthia Robinson, BSc
Consultant Nutritionist

Dr C Shepherd, MB, BS
Medical Adviser to Myalgic Encephalomyelitis Association

Dr Karol Sikora, MB, BChir, PhD, FRCR, FRCP
Professor of Clinical Oncology, Hammersmith Hospital, London

Mrs Alex Smith
Teacher and Tutor for the National Childbirth Trust

Professor Lewis Smith, BSc, PhD, MRCPath
Institute for Environment and Health, University of Leicester

Helen Spence, BA

Myriam Thomson
Fitness Consultant

Dr Steve Tuckwell
Head of Supply Quality and Regulation, Wessex Water

Mark Wheeler
Health and Safety Executive

Richard Walker, BSc, PhD, PGCE

Professor Clyde Williams, BSc, MSc, PhD, MIBiol, C Biol
Professor of Sports Science, University of Loughborough

Jim Williams
British Red Cross

Janet Wilson, MD, FRCS
Otolaryngologist,,
Glasgow Royal Infirmary

Moira Wood, DPodM, MChS, SRCh
Podiatrist,
London Foot Hospital and School of Podiatric Medicine

Pat Young, BA (Hons), MA

Illustrators

Ian Atkinson	Grizelda Holderness *Represented by Jacqui Figgis*
Louise Brierley *Represented by CIA*	Laura Knight *Represented by CIA*
Chloë Cheese *Represented by CIA*	Pavel Kostal
Haydn Cornner *Represented by CIA*	Malcolm McGregor
Christopher Corr *Represented by Jacqui Figgis*	Alan Nanson
	Clare Petherick
Marion Deuchars	Precision Illustration
Carolyn Gowdy	Llewellyn Thomas
Lara Harwood	

MAPS
Raymond Turvey

Photography

EXERCISE PHOTOGRAPHER
Clive Arrowsmith

EXERCISE MODELS

Alexandra	Alan Jones
Sue Bradshaw	Gail McKenna
Tim Bradshaw	Parris Mitchell
Don Day	Tiffany Suchard

FOOD PHOTOGRAPHER
Jason Shenai

HOME ECONOMIST
Joyce Harrison

STYLIST
Sue Leighton

STILL LIFE PHOTOGRAPHER
Monique Le Luhandre

A further list of people and organisations who assisted in the preparation of this book appears on page 480.

CONTENTS

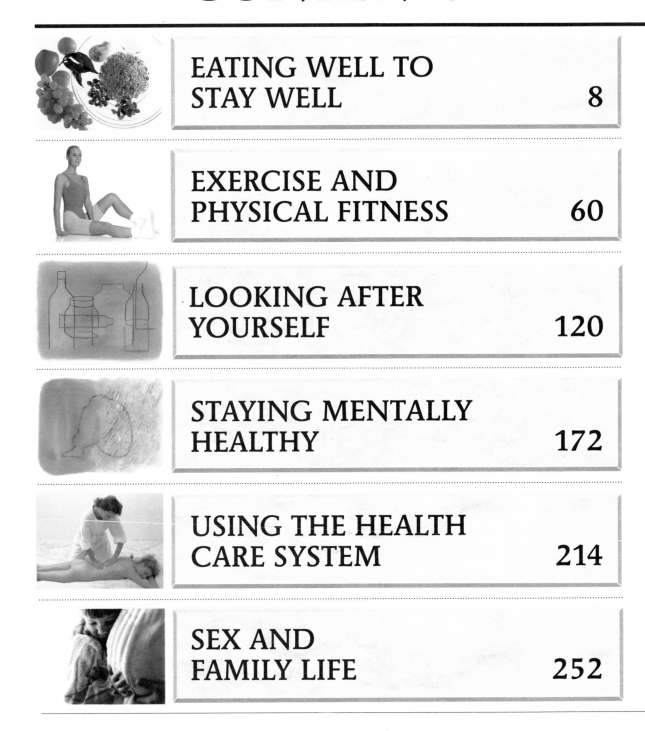

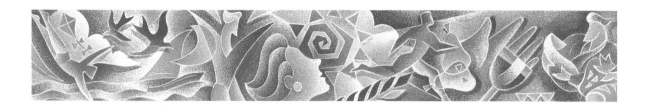

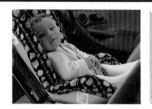
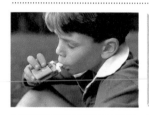
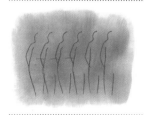
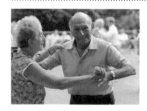
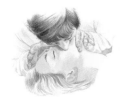

EATING WELL TO STAY WELL

With every meal you eat and every item of food you buy, you are making decisions that affect your health and wellbeing. Eating habits are learned early in life, but it is never too late to change them, and the results can pay off dramatically in terms of better health, vitality and longer life.

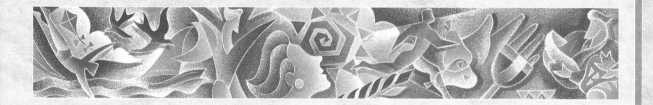

Are you eating too much fat?

Fat is an essential part of the diet. Yet eating too much of it – especially of highly saturated animal and dairy fats – appears to be a major factor in many illnesses.

The following questions are designed to help you to rate your own fat-eating habits. Tick the boxes that most closely reflect your diet and check your score.

1 How often do you eat fried food?

a) Most days. ☐
b) Once or twice a week. ☐
c) Occasionally or never. ☐

2 Which would you be most likely to order in an Italian restaurant?

a) Pizza with cheese and salami. ☐
b) Meat or chicken in a cream sauce. ☐
c) Pasta with tomato sauce and salad. ☐

3 What type of milk do you drink?

a) Whole milk. ☐
b) Semi-skimmed milk. ☐
c) Skimmed milk or soya milk. ☐

4 How often do you eat red meat, including meat in sandwiches?

a) About once a day or more. ☐
b) A few times a week. ☐
c) Occasionally or not at all. ☐

5 Which would you prefer as a dessert?

a) Apple pie with double cream. ☐
b) Fruit salad and ice cream. ☐
c) Piece of fresh fruit. ☐

6 Which group includes more of your favourite sandwich fillings?

a) Cream cheese, Cheddar, Brie, peanut butter, sausage, egg mayonnaise. ☐
b) Cold meat, chicken, tuna, salmon. ☐
c) Salad, cottage cheese, marmite. ☐

7 Which potato topping would you be more likely to choose?

a) Cheddar cheese and butter. ☐
b) Sour cream. ☐
c) Cottage cheese, yoghurt or fromage frais. ☐

8 Which of the following is closest to your average breakfast?

a) Fried eggs and bacon. ☐
b) Toast with butter or margarine. ☐
c) Cereal and fruit. ☐

9 How would you cook bacon, chops, sausages or other fattier meats?

a) Fried. ☐
b) Grilled. ☐
c) Don't eat fatty meats. ☐

10 How do you like your vegetables?

a) Roasted and served with butter, or topped with a rich cheese sauce. ☐
b) Microwaved, boiled or steamed with a little butter or olive oil as a dressing. ☐
c) Microwaved, boiled or steamed and served plain. ☐

SCORING

Award yourself 0 for each (a) answer, 1 for each (b) and 2 for each (c). Add up your score.

15-20: Your total fat consumption is probably about right, but remember that the kind of fat you eat matters, as well as the amount. For further information on this, see pages 36-37.

9-14: Your fat intake may be a little high, and this could make some health problems more likely in later life. A few small changes could make all the difference – and you won't have to give up all your favourite foods. If you want to try, start with the simple measures suggested on page 38.

8 or less: You seem to be eating a great deal of fat. Consider re-examining your diet as a whole and replacing high-fat items such as fried foods, cakes and pastries with more grains, pulses and vegetables. See pages 35-39 for an explanation of the risks and information on eating less fat.

Planning a healthy diet

NUTRITION IN A NUTSHELL

A lot of the advice I read about having a healthy diet is complicated and off-putting. Isn't there a simple way to eat properly?

Despite the endless torrents of nutritional advice in the Press, it is not necessary to give up all the foods you enjoy and plan your meals like a military campaign in order to ensure a good diet. In fact, the basic principles of healthy eating are simple.

● Eat a good variety of different foods every day to make sure that you get all the nutrients your body needs.
● Eat plenty of starchy foods, such as bread, potatoes and cereals, including pasta and rice – especially wholegrain varieties.
● Try to have five portions (or more) of fruit and vegetables a day. Include some pulses, such as lentils, baked beans or split peas.
● Go easy on fats and fatty foods, particularly those high in saturates, such as butter, hard margarine, fatty meat and meat products, crisps and fried foods. Choose instead lean meat, fish and dairy products with a lower fat content, such as cottage cheese and skimmed or semi-skimmed milk.
● Be sparing with salt and sugar, and with foods that contain large quantities of added salt or sugar. Highly salted foods include smoked products, savoury snacks such as peanuts and crisps, processed meat products and some breakfast cereals. Watch out for sugar in drinks, breakfast cereals, yoghurt and processed foods, as well as sweets, cakes and biscuits.
● Go easy on alcohol – know your limits (see page 155).
● Don't go to extremes by following fad diets or crash weight-loss programmes. Eat the right amount of food to maintain a healthy weight (see page 154).

CHOOSING MEALS OR SNACKS

I like nibbling snacks throughout the day but my husband insists that full meals are better. Who is right?

Both of you. Choose whichever way of eating suits you best and, provided that you eat the right foods, your diet will be healthy. Eating small, frequent snacks provides a constant supply of energy and nutrients, and can be especially suitable for very active people and those with a busy schedule. People who have medical conditions such as diabetes or stomach ulcers, or those troubled by indigestion, may find that the little-and-often approach suits their condition better. In addition, it is better for people who suffer from uncomfortable bloating after large servings of high-fibre foods. Small, regular snacks also help to maintain steady blood-sugar levels, preventing energy dips and hunger pangs.

On the other hand, there is a danger of simply eating more food this way. *What* you eat is of course more important than *when* you eat, and full meals make it easier to plan and keep track of your diet. If you nibble, choose healthy snacks and not crisps and biscuits. Don't forget the social side of food, either – shared sit-down meals are one of life's great pleasures.

BENEFITS OF BREAKFAST

My teenage daughter won't eat breakfast, a meal I have always believed to be the most important of the day. Does it matter?

Provided she makes up the nutrients at other times of the day, missing breakfast should not damage your daughter's health. But it

What is food?

Like air and water, food is one of the primary resources our bodies need in order to function. It provides:

● **Energy** – to move, stay warm, grow and repair tissue, and perform hundreds of bodily activities.
● **Nutrients** – substances needed for making body tissues and chemicals and performing chemical reactions. Carbohydrate, protein and lipids (fats and oils) – macronutrients – are needed in large amounts and also supply energy. Vitamins and minerals – micronutrients – are needed in much smaller quantities, but are equally important.
● **Fibre** – essential to keep the digestive tract in good order.

Starting the day well A nourishing breakfast gets children off to a good start in the playground and the classroom. Adults, too, show improved performance if they eat in the morning, whatever sort of day lies ahead.

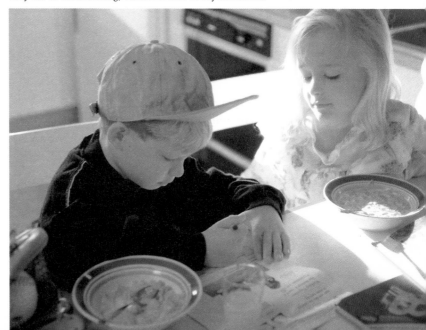

could possibly affect schoolwork. According to research done in the United States, by late morning breakfast-eaters are performing both physical and mental tasks more efficiently, and showing faster reaction times, than those who skip the meal. The body uses food as its fuel supply for energy, but the supply ceases during the night. If it is not replenished until lunch, you are essentially running on an empty tank all morning.

Try to find out why your daughter is avoiding breakfast. Is she put off by the thought of a large meal eaten in a rush, or is she trying to lose weight? In either case, a light breakfast of low-fat yoghurt and fresh fruit, or breakfast cereal and fruit juice, will be much better than no food at all. If she is in too much of a hurry in the mornings, try sending her off with a packed, homemade sandwich and some fruit.

EDUCATING CHILDREN

How can I teach my children good eating habits that will last?

The future eating habits of children depend largely on the example set by parents and schools. If hectic schedules force you and your family to snatch snacks, rather than sit at a table and enjoy food and conversation, then your children will tend to adopt similar habits. Try to put the following points into practice – they will encourage a healthier attitude in the children towards eating:

● Try to get as many members of the family as possible to sit down together at a table for their meals whenever practical.

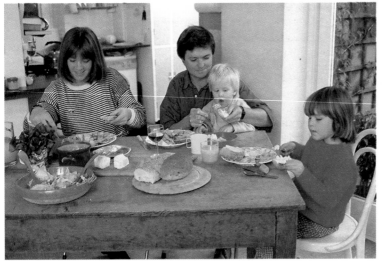

A time to relax Set an example to your children by sitting down with all the family whenever possible at mealtimes, and by not hurrying meals.

● Family mealtimes should always be relaxed – keep any disputes for another time.
● Avoid eating food when rushed or under stress. This can lead to indigestion or heartburn which can make you feel uncomfortable or unwell.
● Serve meals at regular times so that children do not have to go too long without food. Long delays between meals are one of the main reasons for a child turning to unhealthy snacks.
● Keep nutritious snacks in the house rather than sweets and biscuits.
● Don't use food as a bribe or as a substitute for attention.
● Encourage children to help plan meals and prepare food for the meals you are cooking. Good habits learned early will last a child a lifetime.
● If you prepare a packed lunch for school, give your children sandwiches, cheese and fruit, rather than high-fat pies, crisps, cakes or sweets.
● If your children have school lunches, try to find out what sort of options are presented and teach them the best choices.

CAUTION Don't give whole nuts to children who are under the age of five – they could easily choke.

ADAPTING RECIPES

I want to give my family a healthy diet, but they insist I go on making their old favourites. Are there any subtle changes I can make that won't cause a riot?

You are quite right to be concerned: traditional dishes often fall far short of modern standards of healthy eating.

Even so, it is quite possible to cook healthily and still produce delicious family meals. Start by adapting your recipes to suit the new ideas about fat, salt and sugar – you can find tips on how to do this for each one of these on pages 20, 38 and 40 respectively.

Provide lots of rice, pasta, bread and potatoes, and serve every meal with a large mixed salad or vegetables. Try giving your family brown rice and wholemeal bread instead of refined white products, and encourage those with larger appetites to eat more bread or potatoes with the main course, rather than filling up on a high-fat sugary dessert. Look for lower-fat and reduced sugar products when shopping – they often taste just the same as less healthy versions.

Finally, you can improve the nutritional value of meals by using healthier cooking techniques. Instead of frying your food, try grilling, boiling, baking, stir-frying, poaching and steaming. If you have a microwave oven, use it, especially for vegetables.

Here's how this might work in practice: instead of battered fish and deep-fried chips, try serving grilled fish with reduced-fat oven chips and salad or vegetables. If you make spaghetti bolognese, dry-fry the mince then pour off any surplus fat and add plenty of chopped vegetables to the sauce. And if burgers are a family favourite, buy the leanest type you can, or make your own from lean mince. Serve with a wholemeal bun and a large helping of salad.

WHAT'S BEST FOR A BABY

When I had my children, everyone admired chubby babies. But now I'm told that fat babies tend to become fat adults. Is baby fat really bad?

Chubby babies should not be thought of as unhealthy. Babies need a good start in life and if they are very slender can lose weight rapidly if they have an attack of diarrhoea or stop eating owing to illness. As with adults, of course, some babies naturally carry more weight than others. One of the reasons parents are encouraged to take babies to regular clinics is for weight monitoring. Any serious deviation from the normal range can be picked up early and steps taken to diagnose and correct the problem.

A considerable amount of research has gone into trying to find out if fat babies are more likely to become fat adults, but so far the results have been largely inconclusive. Some adults may be genetically predisposed to putting on weight, but if they adopt an unhealthy diet high in both fat and sugar then they can expect to gain weight much more quickly than if consuming a diet rich in high-fibre starches, fruit and vegetables. And if parents eat an unhealthy diet, children will inevitably learn to do the same.

Parents with heavily overweight babies or young children should discuss the problem with baby clinic staff or with their family doctor. Moderate chubbiness, however, is no cause for concern at all and usually disappears quite naturally as soon as the infant becomes an active toddler.

Unlike most adults, babies need to gain weight, so a low-fat, high-fibre diet is not suitable. Even after weaning, they continue to need the high fat content of breast or formula milk until about the age of one. After that, full-cream cow's milk can be given.

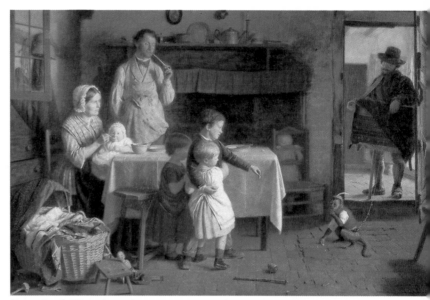

Bouncing babies The 19th-century painting *The Foreign Guest,* by Frederick Daniel Hardy, illustrates the infant chubbiness so admired in an age of high child mortality. A little excess fat is still considered perfectly healthy for babies.

EATING WELL ON A BUDGET

Is it possible to eat a healthy diet without spending a lot of money on food?

Eating healthily need not be expensive. With some of the most nutritious foods being among the cheapest, it is a case of choosing wisely, planning your meals in advance and basing your meals on a good variety of inexpensive foods. Here are some guidelines.

● Make bread, pasta, rice, potatoes or noodles the central part of your meal.
● Substitute beans and lentils for some, or all, of the meat in casseroles, stews, soups and curries – you will reduce the fat content as well as the cost.
● Buy fruit and vegetables in season and look for cheaper local produce.
● Instead of buying expensive prepared meals, cook larger quantities of food and freeze in portions.
● Make filling soups from vegetables and leftovers. Add pulses or potatoes to make them more substantial, and herbs and spices for flavour.
● For a quick, nutritious meal, try a baked potato and a topping such as baked beans, cottage cheese, tuna or sweetcorn.
● Instead of buying sauces, liquidise leftover vegetables, tomato puree and herbs.
● If you like desserts, use low-fat milk to make healthy, economical dishes such as rice pudding, custard and semolina.

WHAT DOES A HEALTHY DIET LOOK LIKE?

A good diet is a varied and interesting one – but not an expensive or difficult one. It is based on generous amounts of filling, energy-rich foods such as bread, rice, pasta and potatoes; and also plenty of fresh fruit and vegetables. For protein, choose lean meat, poultry, fish, game, eggs, pulses and lower-fat dairy products. Cheese and nuts also provide good protein but are higher in fat, so eat in small amounts. Use butter, margarine and other hard fats sparingly, substituting vegetable oils whenever you can. Sugar and products made with it, and added salt are not a necessary part of the diet – eat in moderation only.

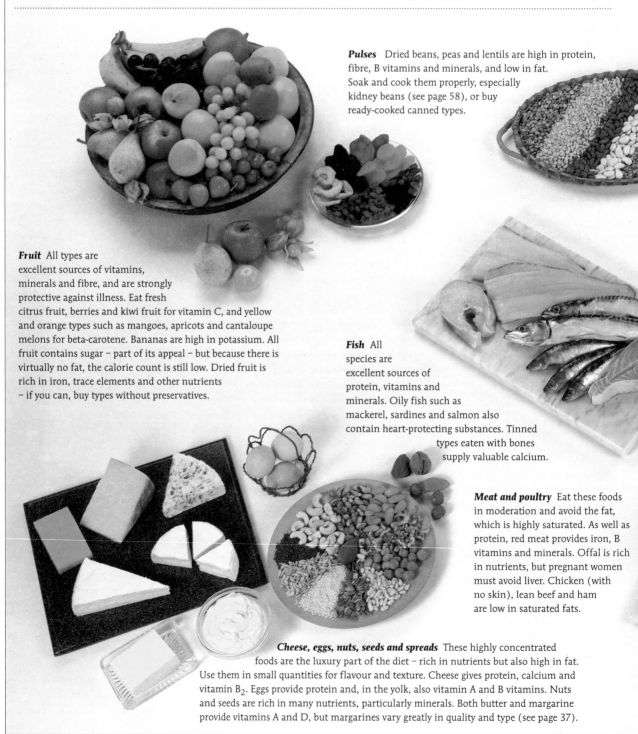

Pulses Dried beans, peas and lentils are high in protein, fibre, B vitamins and minerals, and low in fat. Soak and cook them properly, especially kidney beans (see page 58), or buy ready-cooked canned types.

Fruit All types are excellent sources of vitamins, minerals and fibre, and are strongly protective against illness. Eat fresh citrus fruit, berries and kiwi fruit for vitamin C, and yellow and orange types such as mangoes, apricots and cantaloupe melons for beta-carotene. Bananas are high in potassium. All fruit contains sugar – part of its appeal – but because there is virtually no fat, the calorie count is still low. Dried fruit is rich in iron, trace elements and other nutrients – if you can, buy types without preservatives.

Fish All species are excellent sources of protein, vitamins and minerals. Oily fish such as mackerel, sardines and salmon also contain heart-protecting substances. Tinned types eaten with bones supply valuable calcium.

Meat and poultry Eat these foods in moderation and avoid the fat, which is highly saturated. As well as protein, red meat provides iron, B vitamins and minerals. Offal is rich in nutrients, but pregnant women must avoid liver. Chicken (with no skin), lean beef and ham are low in saturated fats.

Cheese, eggs, nuts, seeds and spreads These highly concentrated foods are the luxury part of the diet – rich in nutrients but also high in fat. Use them in small quantities for flavour and texture. Cheese gives protein, calcium and vitamin B_2. Eggs provide protein and, in the yolk, also vitamin A and B vitamins. Nuts and seeds are rich in many nutrients, particularly minerals. Both butter and margarine provide vitamins A and D, but margarines vary greatly in quality and type (see page 37).

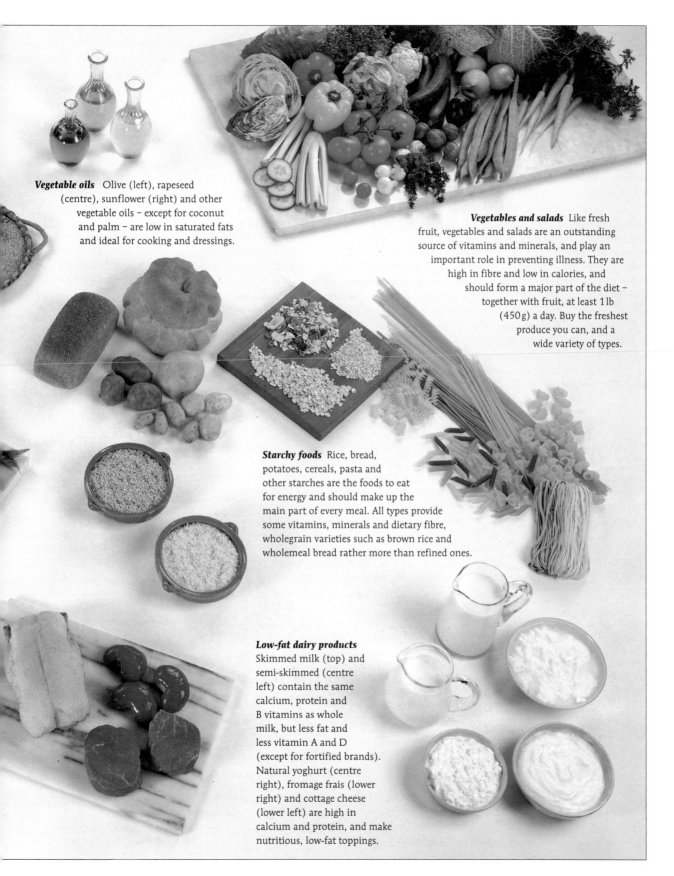

Vegetable oils Olive (left), rapeseed (centre), sunflower (right) and other vegetable oils – except for coconut and palm – are low in saturated fats and ideal for cooking and dressings.

Vegetables and salads Like fresh fruit, vegetables and salads are an outstanding source of vitamins and minerals, and play an important role in preventing illness. They are high in fibre and low in calories, and should form a major part of the diet – together with fruit, at least 1 lb (450 g) a day. Buy the freshest produce you can, and a wide variety of types.

Starchy foods Rice, bread, potatoes, cereals, pasta and other starches are the foods to eat for energy and should make up the main part of every meal. All types provide some vitamins, minerals and dietary fibre, wholegrain varieties such as brown rice and wholemeal bread rather more than refined ones.

Low-fat dairy products Skimmed milk (top) and semi-skimmed (centre left) contain the same calcium, protein and B vitamins as whole milk, but less fat and less vitamin A and D (except for fortified brands). Natural yoghurt (centre right), fromage frais (lower right) and cottage cheese (lower left) are high in calcium and protein, and make nutritious, low-fat toppings.

Eating for energy

CARBOHYDRATE POWER

You hear so much about carbohydrates these days. What exactly are they and what is so good about them?

There are three main types of carbohydrates – sugars, starches and fibre – and all play an essential role in good nutrition. Starches and sugars are both high in energy value, while fibre keeps the gut healthy and helps to regulate digestion (see pages 21–22). Chemically, all carbohydrates are composed of atoms of carbon, hydrogen and oxygen in various different arrangements.

The most basic carbohydrates are sugars, also called 'simple' carbohydrates. This group includes glucose and fructose (sugars found in fruit, vegetables and honey), lactose (in milk), maltose (in sprouting grains) and also sucrose (table sugar). Eaten in the form of whole foods such as fruit and milk, they provide valuable vitamins, minerals and fibre as well as energy. Purer and more concentrated forms such as table sugar and honey, are less nutritious and easier to over-indulge in.

Starches and fibre – 'complex' carbohydrates – consist of long chains of sugar molecules bonded together. They are found in many plant foods, particularly so-called staples such as rice, wheat, oats and potatoes. Starches, like sugars, are broken down and absorbed in the intestine. Fibre, on the other hand, although acted on by bacteria, has little nutritional value since few by-products enter the bloodstream. Nevertheless, it still plays a vital physiological role in keeping the digestive tract healthy.

SUGAR OR STARCH?

Is it true that sugary foods give you a quick burst of energy while starchy ones keep you going for longer?

It is not quite so simple. While it used to be thought that the small size of sugar molecules allowed them to be digested very quickly, while larger starch molecules took longer. It now seems that the situation is more complex and that the rate of digestion depends on many other factors as well, such as which foods are eaten at the time, how much fibre they contain, and which other nutrients are present. After digestion, both starches and sugars enter the bloodstream as simple sugars raising your blood glucose level. The glucose is transported around the body and used as a fuel to power activity in the muscles, organs and cells. Any extra glucose not needed immediately is stored in the muscles or liver as glycogen, or is converted into body fat.

Once all the glucose has been used, the blood sugar level drops, actually to below normal, before righting itself once again. When eaten on their own, some carbohydrates – refined sugars and starches in particular – can raise your blood sugar level far more than others, so giving a quick energy boost. Unfortunately, the higher carbohydrate makes your blood sugar rise at first, the lower it will fall later – so the temporary boost you get from a sugary drink, for example, won't last. In fact, some people end up feeling less energetic soon afterwards. It is also possible to develop sugar cravings and to fall into a cycle of blood sugar peaks and troughs. On the other hand, if you eat regular meals or have your carbohydrates in the form of a sandwich or a piece of fruit, your blood sugar level will not rise so much at the time nor fall so far afterwards.

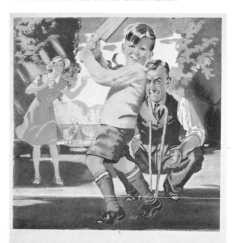

POTATOES
feed without fattening and give you *ENERGY*

Promoting the potato Inexpensive, filling, versatile and nutritious, potatoes have plenty of virtues to advertise. Government campaigns in the 1990s still urge us to eat more of them.

TWO TYPES OF SUGAR

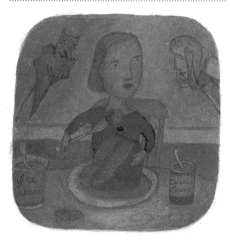

Why do people often suggest that sugar is unhealthy? Surely it's a natural food?

You do not actually need to eat sugar at all, but it makes food palatable and, in its natural state, comes in forms that provide vitamins, minerals and fibre as well. The main dangers are not really to do with sugar itself but with the way in which people tend to get it – all too often not as part of whole foods such as fruit, but in more refined forms such as granulated sugar and other products that are made from it.

There are three main reasons for avoiding large amounts of refined sugar and sugary products such as biscuits and cakes. Firstly, since refined sugar is high in calories but contains no fibre (and sugary foods such as sweets very little) to make you feel full, it is easy to take in more calories than you need – leading to weight gain. And as a corollary, the more of your calories you get from sweetened foods with low vitamin and mineral content, the fewer you will be getting from more nutritious foods – so you could start to miss out important nutrients.

Secondly, refined sugars can damage your teeth by promoting mouth acid. Sugar is particularly damaging when taken in solution, with acidic substances or at a time when you are not eating as well – precisely the conditions that apply to, say, a sweetened lime drink taken between meals.

Finally, refined sugar is very often combined with large quantities of fat in products such as biscuits, cakes, ice cream and sweets. The fat not only pushes up the calorie content considerably, but is often high in saturates, which is bad for the arteries.

So, no, sugar in itself is not the problem, But the way we eat it very often is. Small amounts of refined sugar do not harm, but it is important to stay aware of how much you are getting, and what you are getting with it. (See also panel on page 20.)

IS HONEY HEALTHIER?

I've always assumed that honey is a healthy substitute for sugar because it's sold in health shops, but is it really?

Sadly, no. Honey is a mixture of glucose and fructose, which are both types of sugar. Like ordinary sugar, it is absorbed fairly rapidly into the bloodstream and has a similar effect on your body. In spite of its healthy image, honey contains only traces of vitamins and minerals, so apart from providing calories it makes a negligible contribution to diet.

Weight for weight, honey contains fewer Calories (288 per 3½ oz (100 g)) than sugar (394 per 3½ oz (100 g)) since one quarter of its weight is water. What is more, it tastes sweeter than sugar, so you may need to use less if substituting for sugar in recipes. It is worth knowing that one tablespooon of honey weighs more than one tablespoon of sugar since it is denser – so substituting by volume (rather than weight) for sugar will in fact give you more calories.

One alternative you may want to try is fructose, or fruit sugar, sold in chemists and supermarkets. It has the same calorie count as sugar but is sweeter so you use less.

BREAKFAST CEREALS

Breakfast cereals have a reputation for being healthy, but do they live up to it?

All breakfast cereals are a good source of energy-giving carbohydrates, and many have also been fortified with extra vitamins and minerals, particularly iron. The main factors to consider when making your choice are the cereal's sugar, salt and fibre content. If possible, choose varieties with little or no added sugar and avoid very sweet, sugar-coated varieties. Try not to sprinkle sugar on your cereal either, and, if you can, discourage children from doing so. Add chopped fresh fruit instead or sprinkle a few raisins on top.

Salt or sodium content is displayed on the label of most cereals and it is worth comparing varieties – some processed brands contain a surprisingly large amount.

The fibre content also varies. Muesli and wholegrain or bran cereals are generally very good sources of fibre, but some more refined cereals contain almost none. Oat bran is

Sugar by other names

Don't be fooled into thinking that because you cannot see sugar listed among the ingredients of a food it is not there. The modern food industry uses many different types of sugar and manufacturers often identify them by their specific chemical names – not always recognisable to the general public as sugar in one form or another. So, if you are trying to cut down on added sugars get in to the habit of looking for any of these: sucrose, lactose, maltose, fructose, honey, molasses, glucose, dextrose, corn syrup and invert syrup. Whenever you see one of these, you are looking at the same basic ingredient – sugar.

used in some cereals and can help to reduce cholesterol. Again, reading labels will soon reveal the pros and cons of different brands.

Another way of controlling what's in your cereal is to buy plain oat or wheat flakes and add your own extras – it can be cheaper too.

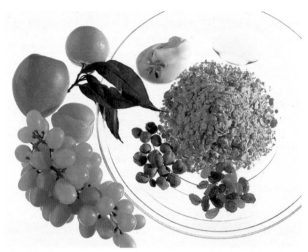

Muesli mixture You can make your own healthy breakfast from rolled oats or other cereal flakes, fresh or dried fruit, and nuts.

What's in a sweetener?

Three artificial sweeteners are currently widely used in Britain.

● **Aspartame** is made from amino acids, and is about 200 times sweeter than sugar. It is widely sold as Canderel and NutraSweet.

● **Acesulfame-K** is synthesised from sulphur and nitrogen, and is about 200 times sweeter than sugar. It is often blended with aspartame.

● **Saccharin** is derived from petroleum products and is about 400 times as sweet as sugar. After experiments on rats, fears were raised about a possible cancer risk in the 1970s, but research has so far failed to reveal any significant dangers to humans.

ARE THESE SWEETENERS SAFE?

More and more foods seem to contain artificial sweeteners these days. How safe are they – and can they really help slimmers to lose weight?

You are quite right. Many of the foods that you pick up in the supermarket now contain artificial sweeteners – and not just the obvious ones such as confectionery or low sugar and diet products. Sweeteners are now also found in some brands of crisps, sauces, canned beans and even in chewing gum.

There are two types of artificial sweeteners: 'intense' sweeteners and 'bulk' or granulated sweeteners. Intense sweeteners such as aspartame, acesulfame-K and saccharin are used in very tiny quantities in many low-calorie food products. Bulk sweeteners such as sorbitol and mannitol are mainly used in 'tooth friendly' sweets and diabetic food.

Sweeteners have to undergo extensive testing before they can be sold commercially, and the general consensus of opinion is that they are safe. An official body known as the Committee on Toxicity (COT) has set an Acceptable Daily Intake (ADI) for sweeteners – that is, an amount believed to be safe on the basis of current knowledge. However, ADIs are based on animal research and are difficult to use in practice, the best advice for consumers is to check the ingredients list on the label – though this will not tell you how much is used – and to vary your sweeteners to reduce the risk of exceeding the ADI for any one type.

Opinion remains divided about whether sweeteners can really help anyone to lose weight. There is a theory that some people gain *more* weight because low-sugar products do not satisfy the body's need for calories, and so appetite increases, but this has not been proven. It is important to remember that foods containing artificial sweeteners may still be high in fat, and fat contains more than twice as many calories, weight for weight, as sugar does. Overall, there is little evidence that sweeteners do much to help with weight loss or weight control.

EATING A MIXED-UP MEAL

My friend says that you shouldn't mix starches and proteins in the same meal. Is there any evidence to back up this theory?

Your friend's advice is derived from an idea developed by a doctor, William Hay, in 1929, that has recently resurfaced in several books promoting the so-called Hay Diet or food combining theory. Essentially, the theory is based on the idea that because protein stimulates acid production in the stomach, it can interfere with the digestion of carbohydrates – which need a more alkaline medium.

As a result, Hay believed, eating a mixed meal led to poorer digestion and absorption of both protein and carbohydrate, causing unpleasant symptoms such as bloating, flatulence, heartburn, indigestion and a general lack of energy. Our knowledge of nutrition has increased substantially since the 1920s and no evidence has been found to back up Hay's theory. Most experts now agree that human digestion is ideally adapted to coping with any combination of foods eaten at the same time. Indeed, the body naturally provides both acid (in the stomach) and alkali (in the small intestine) for digestion.

Furthermore, foods rich in complex carbohydrates, such as bread, rice and pulses, *also* often provide considerable quantities of protein, so it would be impossible to follow your friend's advice without excluding these valuable foods – a dangerous step to take, and almost impossible if you are vegetarian.

It is therefore surprising that this diet has gained popularity recently, mainly as a slimming method. Any weight loss that does occur is far more likely to be the result of reduced calorie intake than to any special method of food combining.

CHOOSING YOUR DAILY BREAD – GETTING THE BEST FROM A STAPLE FOOD

Since mankind first learned to cultivate, grind and cook grains, bread has been a staple food. Some sort of bread – basically milled grain mixed to a dough with water and baked – is eaten in almost every part of the world. Bread comes in a huge variety of types – risen or flat; wheat, corn or rye; enriched with fat or made only with water; refined or full of fibre from the whole grain. Most supermarkets now keep an excellent range of different breads. Here are some tips on how to choose among them.

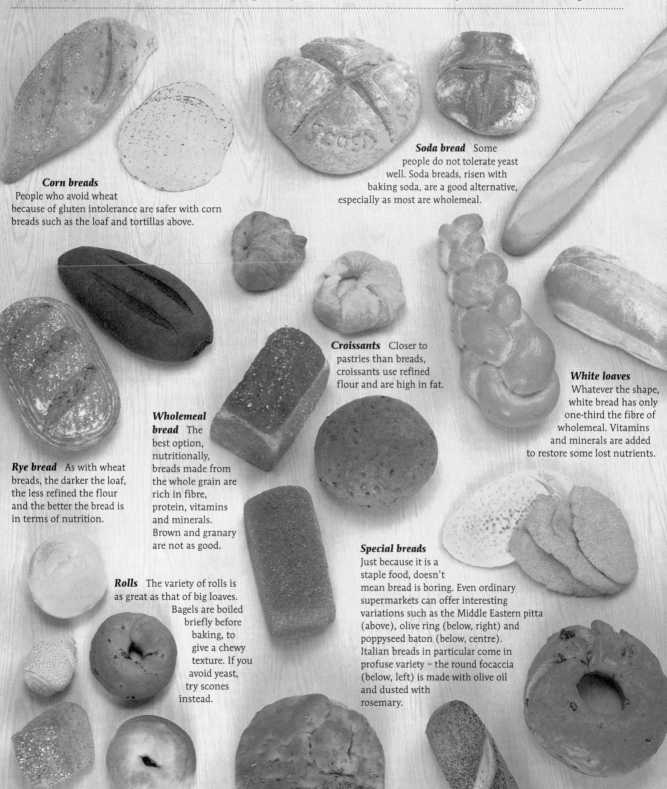

Corn breads People who avoid wheat because of gluten intolerance are safer with corn breads such as the loaf and tortillas above.

Soda bread Some people do not tolerate yeast well. Soda breads, risen with baking soda, are a good alternative, especially as most are wholemeal.

Croissants Closer to pastries than breads, croissants use refined flour and are high in fat.

White loaves Whatever the shape, white bread has only one-third the fibre of wholemeal. Vitamins and minerals are added to restore some lost nutrients.

Wholemeal bread The best option, nutritionally, breads made from the whole grain are rich in fibre, protein, vitamins and minerals. Brown and granary are not as good.

Rye bread As with wheat breads, the darker the loaf, the less refined the flour and the better the bread is in terms of nutrition.

Rolls The variety of rolls is as great as that of big loaves. Bagels are boiled briefly before baking, to give a chewy texture. If you avoid yeast, try scones instead.

Special breads Just because it is a staple food, doesn't mean bread is boring. Even ordinary supermarkets can offer interesting variations such as the Middle Eastern pitta (above), olive ring (below, right) and poppyseed baton (below, centre). Italian breads in particular come in profuse variety – the round focaccia (below, left) is made with olive oil and dusted with rosemary.

SHOULD YOU CUT DOWN ON SUGAR?

Nutritionists distinguish two types of sugar – so-called intrinsic sugars, which are contained within the cell walls of plants, and extrinsic sugars that are not. Intrinsic sugars are a natural, healthy part of the diet. They occur primarily in fruit, grains and sweet-tasting vegetables such as beetroot and carrots. Because they come packaged with fibre, there is a limit to how much of them you can eat. They also come together with valuable amounts of vitamins and minerals.

Extrinsic sugars are another matter. This group includes not just refined sugar products such as table sugar, syrup and glucose, but also honey, molasses, malt and the sugar in milk. The sugar in fruit juice is extrinsic, too, since the fruit cells are ruptured in juicing. Jams and other products sweetened with concentrated fruit juice may not have had any sugar added to them but they can still be very high in extrinsic sugar from the juice – nutritionally, it amounts to the same thing. You can get far more calories, and far faster, from honey, table sugar, syrup, jam, concentrated juice or sweetened products than you can from whole apples, bread or carrots. Extrinsic sugars are also more likely to attack your teeth, and most of us would do well to cut down. One exception is milk sugar (lactose), which does not damage teeth. Nutritionists refer to NMEs (non-milk extrinsic sugars) in order to distinguish only the types likely to be harmful to teeth, where there is good reason to cut down – not the case with lactose.

There is no need, however, to become obsessed with avoiding all NMEs. If the added sugar in products such as baked beans makes a basically healthy food more palatable to you, don't worry – the effect is negligible. Where sugar really starts to matter is with the kind of snacks shown below.

Key to sugar: whole cubes represent 4 g sugar, half cubes 2 g.

ADDED SUGAR

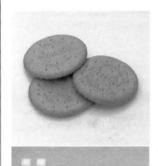

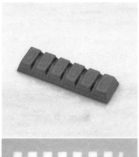

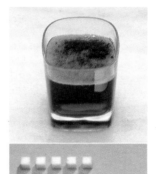

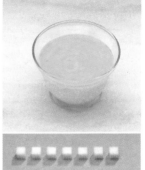

3 digestive biscuits
Not too much sugar, but a high fat content pushes up the calorie count.

Chocolate bar (1³/₄ oz/50 g)
Extremely high in both sugar and fat, but not as bad for teeth as boiled sweets.

Cola (7 fl oz/200 ml)
A fast way to get a lot of sugar. Dangerous for teeth, too, especially between meals.

Fruit yoghurt (small pot)
Not quite as healthy as it looks – the sugar content is exceptionally high.

NATURAL SUGAR

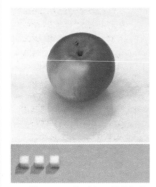

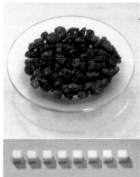

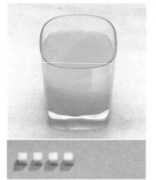

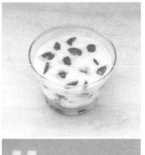

Medium apple (4 oz/120 g)
Moderate intrinsic sugar with fibre and vitamins, and safe for teeth – an ideal snack.

Raisins (1³/₄ oz/50 g)
Concentrated intrinsic sugar – eat sparingly if you are watching your weight.

Orange juice (7 fl oz/200 ml)
Natural sugar, but extrinsic. Whole fruit is better for teeth and higher in fibre.

Plain yoghurt (²/₃ pot) with fresh fruit (2 oz/60 g)
Moderate sugar content, and it won't harm teeth.

Getting enough fibre

WHAT FIBRE DOES

What exactly is 'dietary fibre' and why is it supposed to be so good for you?

The term dietary fibre does not refer to any single substance but rather to all the edible but largely indigestible parts of plant foods such as grains, fruits, vegetables and pulses. Technically, these substances are known as non-starch polysaccharides, or NSPs, and you may see this on some packaging.

Fibre is broken down in the gut but has negligible nutritive value – that is, it does not provide useful amounts of calories, protein, fat, vitamins or minerals. Even so, it is an essential part of a healthy diet. It keeps the digestive tract functioning properly and has been shown to play a part in preventing some serious diseases. And since fibre provides bulk and a feeling of fullness without excess calories, it can also help to control weight. Eating too little may result in constipation – which in turn can lead to piles – and other intestinal disorders. A low-fibre diet also tends to be high in refined carbohydrates and fats, promoting weight gain and, depending on the type of fat, heart disease.

Fibre is measured in grammes (g) (1oz= 30g) and nutritionists recommend an average daily intake of 18g, obtained from bread, cereals, fruit, vegetables and pulses. This is equivalent to about 12 slices of wholemeal bread or, more realistically, a bowl of muesli (3g), two slices of wholemeal bread (3g), two apples (5g), two helpings of vegetables (4g) and a medium jacket potato with skin (3g). Most people currently eat only about two-thirds the fibre they need.

SOLUBLE AND INSOLUBLE FIBRE

I have heard that there are two types of fibre – soluble and insoluble. What is the difference? Are they both necessary?

You are quite right about the two types of fibre and, yes, in their own way, each is necessary for good health. Soluble fibre – the type found in oat bran, leafy vegetables and fruits – can help to lower blood cholesterol, while insoluble fibre – found in pulses and wholegrains such as wholewheat and brown rice – promotes a healthy digestion preventing constipation and other bowel problems.

Neither soluble nor insoluble fibre is completely digested but both are broken down to some extent in the gut. Soluble fibre is acted on by bacteria, forming by-products, some of which are thought to enter the bloodstream. These include certain fatty acids believed to play a role in lowering blood cholesterol.

The degree to which insoluble fibre is broken down varies, but as it passes through the digestive tract it absorbs large quantities of water – up to 15 times its own weight. The water adds bulk to waste matter and helps to move it through the system. There is also evidence that by helping to expel waste matter swiftly, insoluble fibre may play a role in preventing cancer of the colon.

MAKING THE ADJUSTMENT

I'm trying to include more fibre in my diet, but I've come up against an embarrassing problem – wind. Is there any way around this, or should I cut back on offending foods such as beans, broccoli and cabbage?

Increasing the fibre in your diet is a very positive step to take, so don't be put off because you are experiencing wind. It is only a sign that your system is adapting to your new, healthier way of eating. Flatulence – and sometimes bloating and diarrhoea – is a very common problem for people who suddenly start eating more fruit, vegetables, pulses and other gas-inducing high-fibre foods.

The amount of gas produced depends on the predominant species of bacteria in the gut. When you start to include more fibre in your diet, the populations of bacteria change and there appears to be a period of extra gas production. Once things settle down again, the problem should resolve itself, as less-gas-producing bacteria will thrive in the more acid environment created by fermentation of fibre in the colon. The time the adjustment takes varies from person to person, depending on the existing bacterial population.

In the meantime, experiment with a variety of high-fibre foods – you may find that some cause less trouble than others. Or try adding any potentially gas-inducing foods to your diet a little more gradually, giving your system time to adjust to them one by one. On no account avoid nutritious foods such as broccoli, beans and cabbage – if necessary, eat smaller portions to start with.

Ensuring a proper mix of fibre

To get a good combination of soluble and insoluble fibre in your diet, as well as a wide range of nutrients, eat a variety of fruit, vegetables, pulses and grains. Remember, the body does not like sudden changes, even if they are for the good – increase your intake gradually to guard against digestive upsets.

● Eat plenty of wholegrain, unrefined foods, such as wholemeal bread and pasta, and brown rice.

● Start the day with a wholegrain or bran cereal, porridge, or wholemeal bread or toast. Wholemeal bread has three times the fibre of white.

● Make your own breadcrumbs and croutons from wholemeal bread.

● Eat plenty of fruit and vegetables and, where possible, scrub and eat the skins instead of peeling them.

● Eat whole fruit instead of drinking juice. A whole orange contains about six times as much fibre as a glass of juice.

● Try eating more of the stems of vegetables such as broccoli and asparagus. Slice them finely if you find them tough in large pieces.

● Add cooked beans, peas and lentils to soups, stews and salads.

● Add grated or sliced vegetables to casseroles, sauces and salads.

● Eat wholemeal bread or fruit for snacks.

FIBRE SUPPLEMENTS

If fibre is such an important part of the diet, should I consider taking supplements?

It is probably not a good idea, for several reasons. Though fibre pills are sold widely as laxatives and slimming aids, not enough is known about the fibre components of food and how they work to be able to say with any certainty that you can get the same benefits from a concentrated supplement.

While fibre may be good for you, it is possible to have too much of a good thing. In addition to causing wind and other intestinal upsets, excessive amounts of fibre can reduce absorption of minerals such as iron, calcium, magnesium and zinc. Eaten in food form, fibre is not likely to be consumed in amounts that could cause mineral absorption problems – but the same cannot be said for supplements. The best way to get fibre, as with all dietary requirements, is from a good variety of natural foods – not from pills.

Fruit and vegetables

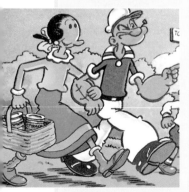

Reinforcing a fallacy
Generations of children were brought up to believe with Popeye that spinach could make them strong. It can't – but it is still a good food.

HOW MUCH TO EAT

You so often hear advice to eat more fruit and vegetables, but what does it actually mean? What's a good daily target?

Current nutritional advice is that everyone should try to eat at least five portions of different fruit and vegetables a day. One portion counts as a single fruit such as an apple or orange, a cup of small fruit such as grapes or raspberries, two or more heaped serving spoons of cooked vegetables, a wine glass of pure fruit juice, or a good bowl of salad.

The value of fruit and vegetables lies in their ability to prevent illness and maintain long-term good health. They are a valuable source of fibre, minerals and vitamins – in particular of the antioxidants beta-carotene (a form of vitamin A) and vitamin C which, according to current theories, may protect cells from ageing and disease (see page 404).

To get your five portions, try having one piece of fruit at breakfast, another as a mid-morning snack, a salad or portion of vegetables at lunchtime, and a couple of portions of vegetables or a large salad in the evening.

CANNED AND FROZEN

I find frozen and canned vegetables very convenient – but are they as nutritious as fresh ones?

Frozen vegetables are a good substitute for fresh produce – they are processed quickly after harvest (within two-and-half-hours in the case of peas) which means that vitamin losses are kept to a minimum. Provided they are correctly stored, frozen vegetables have a vitamin content comparable to that of fresh, or even superior. Canned varieties have been exposed to high temperatures which destroy a substantial proportion of many vitamins, although mineral content is relatively unaffected. Dried vegetables and pulses will also inevitably lose some vitamins.

Remember that the nutritional content of fresh vegetables is variable too. Always try to buy the freshest produce available and avoid anything tired, wrinkled or limp. Store and cook with care – see panel, opposite.

THE PROBLEM WITH PESTICIDES

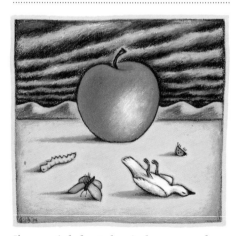

I'm worried about chemical sprays used on fruit and vegetables. How much of a risk to health might they actually pose?

More than 400 different chemicals are currently licensed for use as pesticides in Britain alone. Because there has been no research carried out into the potential effect of accumulated residues over a long period of time, it is impossible to predict how the widespread use of chemical pesticides will affect our long-term health, but most nutritionists agree that the benefits gained from eating plenty of fruits and vegetables outweigh by far any possible health risks posed by minute amounts of pesticides they could contain.

These days there is also a more responsible attitude towards pesticides. Many more controversial chemicals, such as the long-lasting cumulative poison DDT, have been banned throughout the European Union. Maximum Residue Levels (MRLs) have been set for all British and imported foods, and all the large supermarkets test their produce regularly to ensure that the levels remain within strict limits. Safety limits are expressed in terms of an Acceptable Daily Intake (ADI) based on average adult eating patterns.

Even so, it is still wise to do what you can to avoid consuming residues unnecessarily. Washing produce in clean running water, and peeling fruit and root vegetables, will remove a large proportion of any pesticides on or just below the skin, although you will also lose some of the nutrients in the outer flesh. If you still feel concerned, you could consider buying organic fruit and vegetables instead, which are grown without pesticides.

ORGANIC PRODUCE

My neighbour claims that organically grown fruit and vegetables are safer than others, and taste better too. Are they really worth the extra money?

People buy organic produce for many reasons and only you can decide which factors will or will not make it worth spending any extra money on them.

Organic fruit and vegetables are grown in ways intended to protect wildlife and the environment. Instead of chemical fertilisers, farmers use natural compost and farmyard manure. Pests control is achieved by using resistant plant strains, natural predators and techniques such as crop rotation.

Sales of organic produce are increasing in Britain, even though prices can be as much as three times as high as for conventionally produced food. There are several reasons for the extra cost. Firstly, although increasing, demand for organic food is still relatively low. Secondly, much organic food is imported, so transport costs are high. Organic farming is also more labour intensive, yields are generally lower, seed is more densely sown, and production costs are substantially higher.

There is relatively little difference in the nutritional value of organic and other produce. Some surveys have suggested that organic fruit and vegetables may have lower water content and so be more concentrated in terms of vitamins and minerals – and possibly also flavour. However, low water content could simply be a sign of dehydration owing to poor storage or transportation.

In the end you will need to make your own decision – whether on the grounds of health, taste or concern for the environment. Whatever you decide, store, prepare and cook vegetables carefully (see panel, right).

SYMBOLS OF ORGANIC FOOD

All food that is sold as organic has to be produced to recognised European Union organic standards. Wherever you buy your food and however it is packaged, there are two official symbols to look for that indicate food produced in line with official standards and inspected for quality.

....

The Soil Association

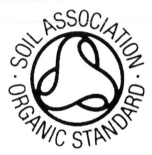

When it was established in 1946, the Soil Association was one of the world's first environmental organisations and it has stayed in the lead ever since. It has its own certification scheme and its standards have become widely respected by farmers, food retailers, consumers and the government. The Soil Association's standards are set with both environmentally sound farming and animal welfare in mind.

United Kingdom Register of Organic Food Standards (UKROFS)

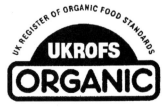

The Register was set up by the government in 1987 to impose standards for organic food and to provide official certification. Its standards are almost identical to those of the Soil Association.

DO'S AND DON'TS

for preserving vitamins

Do store leafy greens and salads in plastic bags or ventilated containers in the bottom drawer of the refrigerator. Tougher vegetables such as potatoes and carrots need only be kept in a cool, dark, airy place such as a larder.

Do cook vegetables until only just tender. Microwaving with a minimum of water, stir-frying and steaming are all excellent methods for preserving nutrients.

Do use vegetable cooking water for soups, stews and stock.

Do get into the habit of eating vegetables raw some of the time. Have them as snacks, with dips or in salads.

....

Don't chop up vegetables until you are ready to start cooking, and don't chop more finely than necessary.

Don't leave vegetables (especially chopped ones) standing in water – water-soluble vitamins will leach out.

Don't add vegetables to water before it is boiling. The higher the temperature and the shorter the cooking time, the fewer nutrients will be lost.

Eating the Mediterranean way

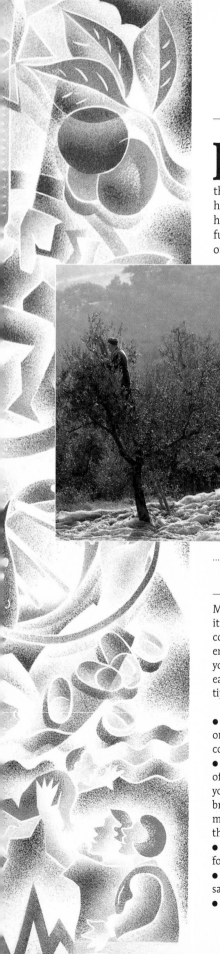

I N recent years, numerous studies have shown that Mediterranean areas such as southern Italy, Spain, Greece and the south of France have some of Europe's healthiest populations. Many explanations have been put forward, from a less stress-fuly way of life to genetic inheritance, but one above all stands out – diet.

Not that there is really such a thing as *the* Mediterranean diet, any more than there is *the* British diet. Mediterranean peoples eat in various ways, yet something pro-tects them all from heart disease, cancer and other killers in a way north European diets do not.

You don't have to make any dra-matic changes to start benefiting from Mediterranean eating styles. Everything you need is obtainable from any high-street supermarket and the basic principles of the diet are extremely simple to apply.

Harvesting olives The health-giving powers of this staple Mediterranean crop, especially the oil pressed from it, have been known for centuries.

MAKING THE CHANGE

Mediterranean cooking is not only healthy – it is also delicious. Dishes are neither time-consuming nor extravagant, and the ingredi-ents offer a vast range of choice. So whatever your culinary preferences, you should find it easy to accommodate them. Here are some tips to help you to make the change.

● Make the main part of each meal a cereal or starchy food such as rice, bread, potatoes, couscous or pasta.
● Serve a large mixed salad or a good variety of vegetables with each meal. Try to vary your range – if you have not already tried braised fennel, roasted red peppers, wild mushrooms or baked aubergine, now is the time to start.
● Eat less red meat and more fish and sea-food, beans and lentils, and chicken.
● Use olive oil (see page 37) for cooking, salad dressings, pasta sauces and dips.
● Have a wide variety of both fresh and dried fruit available for snacks and desserts.
● Use varied garnishes – sundried tomatoes, pine-nut kernels, anchovies, olives, nuts such as almonds and walnuts, and seeds such as sesame and sunflower.
● Use herbs, spices and garlic generously in your cooking. If possible, grow your own fresh herbs, such as parsley, sage and basil.

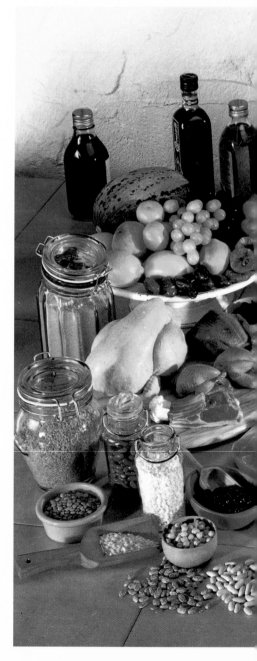

● Keep well stocked with basic supplies: canned tomatoes, tomato purée, pasta, rice, onions, canned or dried pulses, olive oil and red or balsamic vinegar. Canned fish, such as tuna is also a useful standby.

● Red wine is the main alcoholic drink in the Mediterranean, often diluted with water. If you drink, be sure to keep your intake within safe limits (see page 155).

Flavours of the sun The enormous variety of Mediterranean ingredients makes changing to this way of eating both easy and inviting.

Key to foods shown

1 Olive oils, wine vinegar and balsamic vinegars.
2a Fresh and dried fruit.
2b Raisins, dried figs and dried apricots.
3a Bulgur and couscous.
3b Rice.
3c Pulses.
4a Poultry, small game birds and lamb.
4b Ham and sausages.
5 Fish, calamari, prawns, mussels.
6a Fresh pasta.
6b Dried pasta.
7 Regional breads.
8 Red wine.

9 Vegetables, herbs, salads, edible flowers, fresh and dried mushrooms.
10 Cheeses – including mozzarella, ricotta, feta, Parmesan, goat's milk.
11 Savoury garnishes – sundried tomatoes, olives, capers, anchovies.
12 Nuts and seeds.

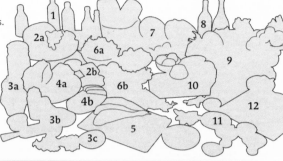

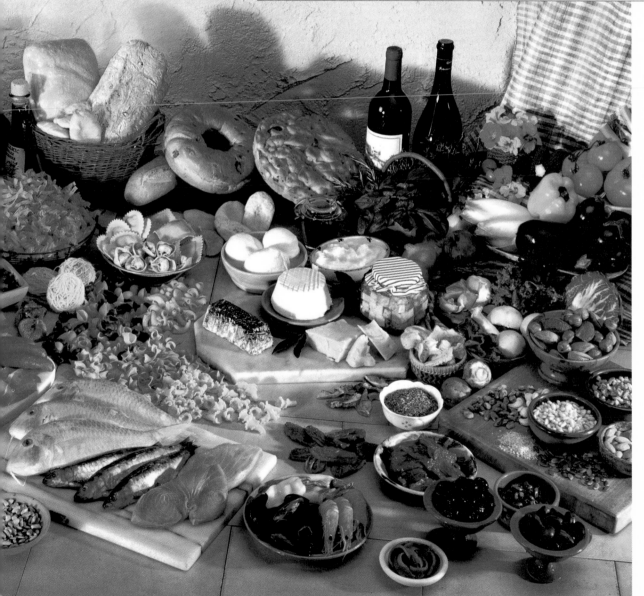

Meat, poultry and game

HOW MUCH MEAT?

I usually eat red meat four or five times a week. Is that too much?

If you are in good health, and if the rest of your diet is low in saturated fats (the type that can increase your cholesterol levels – found in meat fat, full-fat dairy products and hydrogenated or hardened vegetable oils and margarines), four or five *small* servings of lean red meat over the course of a week is probably not excessive.

The fat of red meat (beef, lamb, pork and game) is relatively highly saturated – about 50 per cent, compared with some vegetable oils which are almost entirely unsaturated – (see pages 36-37). But meat is also a valuable source of high-quality protein, vitamins and minerals, and can make a valuable contribution to a healthy diet.

You also have to take into account the fat content of the meat you are eating. Products such as pies, sausages, ordinary mince and burgers are generally very high in fat. It is better to serve smaller portions of lean meat than large portions of such products.

Nutritionists suggest we try serving small amounts of lean meat with lots of rice or pasta, accompanied by plenty of vegetables or salads, in the Mediterranean tradition.

Another way of cutting down without feeling too deprived, is to use meat just as a garnish, for example, chopped ham or beef sprinkled over a salad.

PIES AND PÂTÉS

I love sausages, pâtés and pies, but often wonder: are they healthy to eat?

The main aspect to consider when buying processed meat products is the amount of fat they contain. Sausages are especially high with around 1 oz (30 g) of fat per 3½ oz (100 g) of sausage. Pâtés can also contain a great deal of fat. As a general guide, if the label of a meat product indicates that there

FACT
— OR —
FALLACY?

'You will put on muscle rather than fat if you eat more meat.'

Fallacy Although both lean meat and muscle tissue are made of protein, eating more protein does not automatically create larger, stronger muscles. The only really effective way to increase muscle size and strength is through exercise and the best fuel foods for *that* are carbohydrates such as bread, potatoes, pasta and rice. Far from building bigger and better muscles, excess protein is simply converted into fat and stored in the body.

LOW-FAT COOKERY WITH MEAT

All the important nutrients in meat – the protein, vitamins and minerals including iron and zinc – are mainly in the lean while most of the calories are in the fat. If you trim or skim meat fat, nothing vital is lost, and the result is a healthier diet. So cut down on fatty meats such as sausages, bacon, lamb chops and standard minced beef, and buy lean meat such as game or lean cuts. Always trim any visible fat before cooking.

Roasting and grilling
When roasting or grilling, place the meat on a rack and allow the fat to drip clear.

Soups and stews
Skim surface fat from the tops of soups and stews before serving. Alternatively, prepare soups and stews a day early, refrigerate and simply lift off solid fat from the surface. Reheat thoroughly before serving.

Mince
Buy the leanest mince available or pick out a lean cut of beef yourself and ask the butcher to grind it for you. Substitute precooked or tinned beans or lentils for some of the mince in the recipe. Fry mince without added oil in a non-stick pan, then skim off any fat that separates out. If boiling mince, drain off any fat that rises to the surface of the water.

Burgers and sausages
If possible, make your own burgers from lean mince. Select thin sausages which lose more fat during cooking, or buy low-fat varieties. Cook by grilling or baking.

Tastier leaner cuts
Smear lean meat with olive oil before roasting or grilling, to protect the surface and seal in juices. A sprinkling of fresh or dried herbs, and crushed garlic rubbed over the surface of meat, adds extra flavour. Alternatively, marinate lean cuts in wine, oil herbs and spices.

Chicken and poultry
Remove skin before or after cooking. Cover with foil during cooking to keep in moisture. Brush the surface of skinless chicken with barbecue or chilli sauce before cooking to seal in the moisture.

is no more than 10 g of total fat per 3½ oz (100 g) of food, the product is fairly low in fat. It is also wise to watch out for the salt or sodium content (see page 39) – processed meats often have a great deal of added salt.

Products such as pâtés and pies do also have rather a bad reputation for food poisoning, but you can reduce any risks substantially with a few simple precautions. Buy your meat only from a clean, reputable supplier. Always check the 'sell by' and 'use by' dates and take care never to exceed them. Store all meat products exactly as instructed on the label. If you heat up a pie or cook sausages, always make sure that the food is piping hot all the way through before eating, and don't heat up any leftovers a second time. Avoid any takeaways that have been kept warm, or that are not fully heated up.

DRUGS IN MEAT

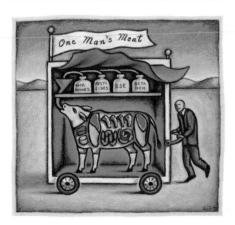

Am I consuming artificial hormones, antibiotics and other drugs when I eat red meat? Could they have any bad effects?

Some of the meat we buy in Britain may contain tiny amounts of drugs such as antibiotics and hormones given to farm animals. There is no evidence, however, of any ill effects on consumers. Growth-boosting hormones are banned in Britain and in the rest of the European Union but there are still some worries about illegal use, and about meat imported from other countries.

It is legal to feed antibiotic drugs to livestock both to minimise disease rates and to increase growth (a side effect of antibiotics). Fears have been expressed that by continually consuming small amounts of antibiotics we may be encouraging the development of drug-resistant strains of bacteria in the population. Others argue that any such effects would probably be experienced more by the animals involved than by humans. But so far the evidence is lacking to decide the issue conclusively one way or the other.

Where drug residues occur, they tend to accumulate in the liver, kidneys and fatty tissue. Low levels are not believed to pose any risk but if you are concerned you may wish to avoid products such as sausages and patés which contain a high proportion of fat and offal. Alternatively, you could consider buying organic meat from animals farmed without drugs and fed on pesticide-free feed.

THE RISKS OF BSE

Every so often the 'mad cow' disease scare resurfaces. What, if any, are the actual risks of eating beef?

It is not yet known whether humans can develop illness through eating the flesh of animals with so-called mad cow disease, or BSE (bovine spongiform encephalopathy). The disease is one of a group of disorders that affect the brain and nervous system of different species – scrapie causes similar effects in sheep and a related illness known as Creutzfeldt-Jacob disease affects humans. BSE was identified in Britain in 1986 and it is thought that it may have arisen from cattle being fed on meal containing carcases of sheep infected with scrapie.

In 1988, infected foodstuffs and all sheep-meal were banned as cattle fodder in an attempt to eliminate the source of the infection. In 1989, the Ministry of Agriculture, Fisheries and Food decreed that adult cattle brains and spinal cords (the parts thought most likely to harbour infection) should be removed and burned after slaughter.

Although they have not eradicated the disease, these measures appear to be showing some results and rates of infection for 1994 were lower than those for 1993. Nevertheless, the problem does remain and, although it is rare, calves can be born with the disease. Even so, it is still legal in Britain to use calf brains, spinal cords and spleens in products such as pies, pâtés, soups and stock cubes.

The BSE organism cannot be destroyed by cooking and its presence cannot be detected by either sight or taste. Although we have been eating scrapie-infected sheep for years without any signs of infection, BSE may behave differently. It has a long incubation period and it is thought that, were human cases to arise, they might take ten years or more to detect. At present, however, there is no evidence that infection can be transmitted to humans through eating beef.

Cooking meat and poultry safely

Meat that has been infected with bacteria – such as salmonella and listeria (see page 57) does not necessarily look or taste bad. The only way you can be sure it is safe to eat is to cook it to a high enough temperature to kill any bacteria, and to serve it piping hot, without keeping it warm or heating it a second time.

The best way to check whether cooked meat has reached the correct temperature is with a meat thermometer. Cooking time and appearance are not reliable measurements.

● **Poultry and game** are cooked properly when a thermometer inserted in the thick part of the thigh muscle – but not touching the bone – registers 80°C (176°F).
● **Pork** should always be heated to a central temperature of 85°C (185°F) for safety.
● **Lamb** should reach 80°C (176°F).
● **Beef** may be eaten in the traditional 'rare' manner, but it is still advisable to use a meat thermometer to establish that the central temperature has reached 70°C (158°F).

The lower temperature of 60°C (140°F) needed for very rare beef is not sufficient to kill bacteria. There is also a risk of food poisoning if you choose to eat uncooked beef in a dish such as steak tartare. Elderly people and pregnant women should never take this risk.

CHARRED MEAT

My family love summer barbecues, but I've recently become worried after reading that charred meat might be unhealthy. Just how dangerous is charring?

There is no need to deprive your family of the occasional summer barbecue – but it may be inadvisable to have them on a daily basis. It has yet to be definitively established whether charred meat poses any real health risks to humans. What is known is that as soon as meat shows any charring, whether through barbecuing, frying or grilling (and to a lesser extent through roasting), chemical compounds are produced which have been linked to cancer in laboratory animals.

There is a theory that while other animals are clearly not adapted to consuming cooked meat humans, who have cooked their prey since cave-dwelling days, may have developed some protective mechanism. However, no such mechanism has ever been identified and at present the theory is based on nothing more than speculation.

The potentially cancer-causing compounds that form in the dark, highly-flavoured areas of charred meat are known as HAAs (heterocyclic aromatic amines). Moist techniques of cooking meat, such as poaching, boiling and microwaving, do not cause charring and produce virtually no HAAs. Frying, grilling, roasting and barbecuing, however, can all expose meat to the higher temperatures that give rise to charring and HAAs.

If fat from meat on a barbecue drips onto the hot embers or heating element underneath, other potentially unhealthy chemical compounds called PAHs (polycyclic aromatic hydrocarbons) can also be created. They mix with the rising smoke and settle on the surface of the meat above. To reduce the formation of PAHs, choose lean meat without any visible fat, and precook it lightly – to ensure it cooks all the way through – before placing it on the barbecue.

Alternatively, cook your meat in a casserole, or braise or microwave it so that it does not char, and then add a barbecue seasoning to provide extra flavour. For regular use, this method is a lot less trouble than a barbecue and doesn't need a fine summer day. It is also safer for frequent consumption.

CAUTION Smoked fish, bacon, sausages, ham, cheese and other smoked foods can also contain PAHs. As a precaution it is wise not to eat them very often. Smoke-flavour seasonings and sauces are generally safe.

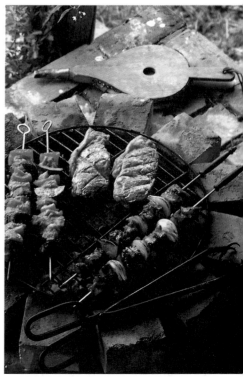

Outdoor eating Barbecues can be healthy. Use lean meat and part-cook it first so that it doesn't stay on the fire long enough to char. Always check that it is cooked to the centre.

ADVANTAGES OF GAME

My supermarket has recently started to keep a variety of game. Is it a healthy alternative to other types of meat?

Game is generally a healthy type of meat but if you choose with care other types can be just as good. Because wild animals such as pheasant, partridge, grouse, deer, rabbit and hare have endless exercise in their hunt for food, they become very lean and muscular, and consequently their meat contains little fat. What fat it has is also relatively low in saturates. Much game sold in supermarkets is farmed rather than wild, but even so it is still usually lean and healthy. By the same token, however, new breeds of farm animals have been developed which also yield very lean meat. As a result there no real reason to buy game unless you prefer it.

Pheasant, partridge and grouse contain between 4 and 6 per cent fat, about the same as chicken or turkey. Venison contains about 6 per cent fat, compared with an average of around 4 per cent for lean beef (brisket is 9 per cent and shin just 2.5) and as little as 1.7 per cent for lean ham.

If you don't eat meat

GIVING UP MEAT

My husband and I seldom eat meat and are thinking of becoming completely vegetarian. What, if any, would the health benefits be?

Vegetarian diets are gaining popularity and can be very nutritious. A study of 6000 vegetarians and 5000 meat-eaters, published in the *British Medical Journal* in 1994, found that the vegetarians lived longer and had less chance of developing cancer than the meat-eaters. The researchers noted, however, that the health benefits of a vegetarian diet may well be due to the high intake of vegetables, fruit, cereals, pulses (beans, peas and lentils) and nuts – rather than the absence of meat. The meat-eaters were also more likely to be overweight and to smoke. The findings were not considered to justify advising anyone to stop eating meat. Even so, they do appear to suggest a link between eating habits and the risk of cancer and heart disease. We could all improve our diets by following these guidelines, which possibly come more naturally to vegetarians than to others:

● Eat less saturated fat, thought to be a primary cause of high blood cholesterol and heart disease. Saturated fat is found in eggs, dairy products and hydrogenated vegetable oils as well as in meat products.
● Eat more fruit and vegetables. They are rich in vitamins and minerals, including the antioxidants beta-carotene and vitamin C, which may help to protect body tissues and cells against ageing and damage which can lead to heart disease and certain cancers.
● Eat more fibre in the form of unrefined grains and grain products, vegetables, fruits, salads, beans, peas and other pulses. Fibre helps to prevent constipation and possibly also cancer of the bowel.

CHEESE WITHOUT RENNET

I sometimes see 'vegetarian' Cheddar cheese for sale – what exactly is this?

Ordinary hard cheese and cottage cheese are made with an enzyme called rennet, which is extracted from the stomachs of cows and calves when they are slaughtered for meat. Rennet has been used for many centuries to convert liquid milk into solidified curds and watery whey, the first step in cheese production. Vegetarian cheese is still made with the same basic ingredient, milk, but the rennet is replaced by enzymes produced from fungi. Some other cheeses are also made without rennet, including Dolcelatte, cream cheese and low-fat or skimmed-milk soft cheese.

VEGETARIAN TEENAGERS

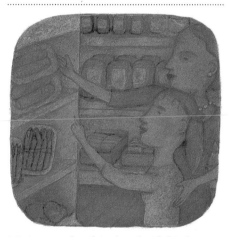

My teenage daughter has decided to become a vegetarian, but will she get enough protein without eating meat?

The first thing to do is to establish what your daughter *means* by vegetarian: she may still be happy to eat some fish, or even chicken, or she may intend to give up all forms of flesh. With very little effort, either of these options can make a perfectly nutritious diet, even for a growing youngster. On the other hand, if your daughter wants to follow the more extreme vegan diet – excluding animal-derived foods such as milk, butter and eggs – her diet will need more care and attention.

If your daughter is still eating fish, or even just eggs and dairy products, you really have no need to worry about protein. Even if she wants to be vegan, she can get plenty of protein from soya products, wholegrains, nuts and pulses. Most foods contain some protein, and deficiency is almost unheard of in the West. It is far more important to make sure that she gets enough iron, calcium and vitamin B_{12} – see panel, page 31.

Whether your daughter is vegetarian or vegan, encourage her to eat a good variety of vegetables, fruits, pulses, wholegrains, nuts

---

DO'S
—— AND ——
DON'TS

for becoming a vegetarian

Do learn how to cook a good variety of vegetarian dishes, including interesting foreign dishes such as Italian risottos, Indian curries and Chinese stir-fries made with grains, vegetables and pulses.
Do consider including fish in your diet. It is a good source of lean protein, vitamins and minerals, and oils that help to protect the heart and circulation.

Don't just switch from meat to large quantities of full-fat cheese, whole milk and nuts, or your diet will be just as high in fat. Eat more pulses and grains instead.
Don't assume that all vegetarian food is healthy. Fast foods such as pizzas, chips, oat flapjacks and vegetable samosas are high in fat, and so are many salad dressings and dips.

What does it mean to be a vegetarian?

There are several types of vegetarian diet.

Lacto-vegetarian
Milk and milk products are eaten, as well as plant foods.

Lacto-ovo-vegetarian
This includes milk, milk products and eggs.

Vegan
All foods in any way derived from the animal kingdom are excluded, even honey.

Pescatarian
Fish and other seafood are eaten, but no other flesh. Pescatarians may or may not include dairy products and eggs.

Semi- or demi-vegetarian
A half-way option that involves excluding red meat but not fish or poultry.

and seeds in her daily diet. Grains eaten in combination with pulses, nuts or seeds are excellent for protein – for example, rice with a bean casserole or lentil curry, or a peanut-butter sandwich or beans on toast.

A SAFE PREGNANCY

I have been a vegetarian for several years, but now that I am pregnant people keep suggesting that I ought to go back to eating meat. Is this really necessary?

There is no need to start eating meat again just because you are pregnant. Although certain nutrients are required in increased amounts during pregnancy, it is quite possible to obtain all of them from other sources. The most important areas to watch include:

PROTEIN Include milk, cheese, eggs, pulses, soya milk, tofu, wholegrains and nuts. No increase is needed from your normal diet.

IRON Eat wholegrains, pulses, green vegetables and dried fruit. Iron is better absorbed if taken with a good source of vitamin C, such as fresh fruit and vegetables.

CALCIUM AND VITAMIN D Be sure to include milk, cheese, yoghurt, tofu, green vegetables, wholegrains, pulses, dried figs, almonds and sesame seeds to increase calcium intake. Vitamin D is essential for calcium absorption and can be manufactured from sunlight or obtained from margarine and dairy foods.

FOLIC ACID Women who are or may become pregnant need to take 400µg of folic acid (also known as folate) daily until the twelfth week, to reduce the chances of spina bifida. Green vegetables, beans, eggs, wholegrains and fruit also contribute to intake.

VITAMIN B_{12} Eat dairy produce and eggs for a regular supply. Some brands of soya milk, margarine, yeast extract and vegetarian burger mixes are fortified with B_{12}.

CAUTION Vegan mothers-to-be, who eat no animal products at all, may need to take calcium and vitamin B_{12} supplements. Doctors can advise.

RAISING A VEGETARIAN BABY

We've just had our first baby and we'd like to raise her as a vegetarian. Is this safe? Are there any special rules to follow?

Well-planned vegetarian diets have been shown to be safe and healthy for children of all ages. In any case, all babies are vegetarian for the first four or five months – having only breast or formula milk before they are

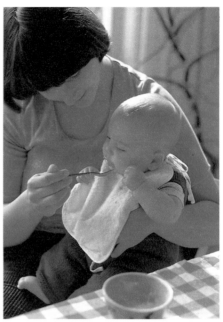

Early learning Babies and children can thrive on a vegetarian diet with plenty of iron.

gradually weaned onto solid foods.

Babies are born with enough iron to last about six months. After that it is important to include good sources of iron in the diet, including green vegetables, puréed apricots, cereals, mashed lentils and beans. Vitamin C helps the body to absorb vegetable iron, so include plenty of citrus fruit, broccoli, cabbage, potatoes and tomatoes. Baby juices also contain vitamin C but give them in small amounts (too much acid can harm teeth).

You will want to get your baby used to the vegetarian food groups: cereals, beans, nuts and seeds, dairy and soya products, and fruit and vegetables. Introduce new foods gradually, however, and remember that not all are suitable at all ages. This is a rough guide:

● Four to five months – give one teaspoon of baby rice or puréed apple, banana, pear, potato or carrot after or during a milk feed.
● Five to six months – try mashed lentils with some added vegetable oil. Gradually start introducing a wider variety of fruit and vegetables.
● Six to eight months – start giving wheat and oat-based cereals such as bread and porridge. Try tofu, smooth nut butters, cheese and hard-boiled eggs.
● Eight to twelve months – begin giving well-cooked mashed peas and beans. Pieces of peeled apple, raw carrot or bread crusts will help with teething. Introduce cow's milk and milk puddings only after the age of one.

VITAL NUTRIENTS FOR VEGETARIANS AND VEGANS

Human beings don't need to eat meat to stay fit and active and there is no reason at all for vegetarians and vegans not to be just as healthy as meat-eaters. Even so, there are three nutrients in particular that they do need to take a little extra care to obtain.

Iron

Everyone needs a good supply of iron to keep up the production of haemoglobin in red blood cells. Iron is especially important for teenage girls when menstruation starts, as some is lost each month once periods start. Shortage of iron can lead to tiredness and anaemia. Non-meat sources of iron include beans and lentils; wholemeal flour and other products; oatmeal, wheatbran, dried fruits (especially peaches, apricots and figs), dark green leafy vegetables (especially spinach, watercress and kale), nuts, parsley, egg yolk and cocoa. The body needs vitamin C to convert iron from non-meat sources into a usable form, so try to include some fruit, vegetables, salads or fruit juice in every meal.

Vitamin B$_{12}$

You cannot have a healthy nervous system and a strong red blood cell count without plenty of Vitamin B$_{12}$. Deficiencies are rare, but can lead to anaemia and nerve damage. B$_{12}$ occurs naturally only in foods of animal origin. While vegetarians can get this vitamin from milk and eggs, vegans need to take a supplement or to eat specially fortified-foods such as certain soya milks, breakfast cereals and yeast extracts.

Calcium

Healthy bones and teeth need a diet rich in calcium. The main vegetarian sources are milk and other dairy products. Vegans can get it from fortified soya products, nuts (especially almonds), broccoli, dark green leafy vegetables, sesame and sunflower seeds, dried fruit and white bread (white flour is fortified with calcium). Vitamin D is essential for the absorption of calcium – most people get enough from exposure to sunlight, but people who seldom go out need to make a special effort to include margarines and cereals with added vitamin D.

Feeding a vegetarian in the family

● Base everyone's meals on starchy foods such as potatoes, rice and bread, together with vegetables or salads, and serve meat as a side dish for those who want it.
● Get into the habit of making a vegetarian version alongside a meat dish such as a casserole. Make the two identical but substitute canned or cooked beans, soya mince or tofu for meat in one of them.
● It won't do any harm for everyone to have a meatless meal now and again. Easy favourites include vegetable risotto; vegetarian pasta dishes; omelettes; and baked potatoes with cheese or baked beans.

Food from the sea

FISH FOR HEALTH

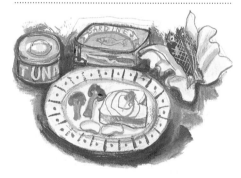

I keep hearing about the benefits of eating fish. Why is it supposed to be so healthy? And are some sorts better than others?

As long as you don't always eat it in the traditional British manner (fried in batter and served with greasy chips) fish is an excellent food, rich in protein, vitamins and minerals.

White fish such as cod, haddock and plaice are also exceptionally low in both fat and calories, making them ideal for slimmers. Oily fish such as sardines, pilchards, herrings, mackerel, trout and salmon contain more calories and fat than white fish, but the fat is mostly unsaturated. It also contains valuable oils known as omega-3 fatty acids that are believed to provide some protection against heart disease, when consumed regularly. Research has shown that eating oily fish twice a week can cut the risk of a heart attack by almost a third. Steaming, grilling, baking and poaching are all good cooking methods for preserving the oil. Oily fish are also rich in vitamin A (needed for good eyesight and healthy skin) and vitamin D (for bone growth and maintenance).

Don't forget about canned fish as an alternative, either. It has many of the same benefits as fresh types, and one extra – the bones of canned salmon, pilchards and sardines can be mashed and eaten to provide a rich source of calcium. If you are watching your calorie or fat intake, buy the sort canned in brine rather than oil.

FACT OR FALLACY ?

'Eating fish is good for the brain.'

Fact – possibly. There is some truth, albeit rather flimsy, in this old wives' tale. Recent research has shown that certain polyunsaturated fatty acids found in oily fish are important for brain and nerve tissue development while a foetus is still in the womb. Once the brain is fully developed, however, there is no evidence that eating fish will do it any special good.

Do buy seafood only from a reputable dealer.

Do buy only fish that is displayed on ice so that it does not spoil and go off quickly. Whole fish may lie directly on the ice, but cut fish and shellfish (in or out of the shell) should be kept on trays or on paper or plastic film.

Do examine fresh fish closely. They should smell clean and slightly sweet, not sour and 'fishy'. Look for the following signs of freshness: firm flesh, clear bulging eyes, moist and shiny skin without dry scales, and bright red or pink gills. There should be few or no traces of blood anywhere. Fillets and steaks should feel moist – but not slimy – and have a glistening shine.

Do rinse fish at home. Dry it with paper towels, put on a clean plate, cover and refrigerate.

Don't buy fish lying in its own juice.

Don't buy shellfish you are at all doubtful about. Fresh uncooked prawns should have undamaged shells and be pale and translucent. Select only live oysters and mussels – the shells will be tightly closed, or will close when tapped.

Don't keep unfrozen seafood longer than a day before eating.

Don't freeze fish unless you are certain it has not been frozen before.

HOW TO COOK FISH

There are many healthy ways to cook fish, and all of them are quick and easy. When the flesh comes away from bone – or flakes easily – the fish is properly cooked.

Baking

Owing to its high moisture content, fish can be cooked without any added liquid. Wrap it in foil or parchment and allow it to cook in its own juices. Never use lemon juice or wine if you are cooking fish in aluminium foil. The acid in the liquid will dissolve some of the aluminium and taint the flavour of the fish.

Poaching

White fish is particularly suited to gentle poaching in fish stock or milk. The cooking liquids are full of nutrients and make delicious sauces and soups.

Steaming

This is an excellent method for fish, as the hot vapour cooks the flesh quickly, while retaining nutrients and flavour.

Grilling

Use this method for whole fish like sole or thick cutlets, lightly brushed with oil. Oily fish such as mackerel work just as well, as their oil makes them virtually self-basting and keeps them moist.

Stir-frying

Cut the fish into strips and fry in a little oil for a few minutes. Then add chopped vegetables and sliced fresh garlic and root ginger to taste. Season with soya sauce.

SHELLFISH POISONING

Shellfish have such a healthy reputation – and yet they're notorious for causing food poisoning. Why is that?

Because they are high in protein and low in fat shellfish (especially molluscs such as oysters, mussels, scallops and cockles) would be among the healthiest of foods – if it were not for the risk of contamination by protozoa (microscopic sea animals), bacteria, viruses and even toxic algae.

Molluscs are filter feeders, and because gallons of water pass through them each day, they can easily accumulate harmful levels of viruses and bacteria if the water is in any way polluted by sewage. Crustaceans such as prawns and lobsters generally cause fewer problems because we do not eat the filtering organs where micro-organisms accumulate.

All shellfish that are sold commercially have to come from waters clean enough to meet strict European Union standards. Each country is responsible for monitoring its own waters and prohibiting the sale of shellfish from any areas that do not measure up. Despite these precautions, eating raw or lightly cooked molluscs does put you at slight risk of contracting a variety of bacterial and viral infections. For most people, the result is no worse than an occasional moderate stomach upset. But for the very young, the elderly and those with conditions such as liver problems, cancer or diabetes, there could be serious, or even fatal, consequences. Food safety experts therefore recommend steaming molluscs for at least six minutes.

Provided that you are in good health and accept that you may be taking a slight risk, the advantages of eating shellfish, which are particularly nutritious and low in fat, probably outweigh any risk of food poisoning.

CHEMICAL CONTAMINATION

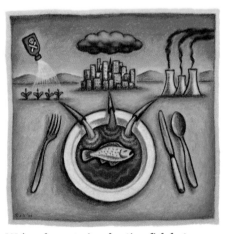

We've always enjoyed eating fish but recently we have been put off by hearing that some types can accumulate chemical pollutants in their flesh. How serious a risk is this, and which species of fish are most affected?

It is a sad fact of modern life that very few foods, however nutritious in themselves, are not affected to some extent by chemicals in the environment. Fish – even deep-sea ones – are no exception. Although the benefits of including fish in your diet still far outweigh any risks, some people do prefer to take precautions, just to be on the safe side.

● Buy fish from a reputable dealer. Look for fish with the Seafish Quality Award symbol, which ensures high standards.

● You may wish to vary the types of fish you eat (freshwater, deep-sea, local or imported) to limit possible risks.

● Choose younger, smaller fish, which will have accumulated fewer contaminants than larger, predatory long-lived fish such as shark, swordfish, halibut and tuna.

● Before cooking fish you may prefer to remove the skin and the layer of fat beneath it, as well as any dark-coloured fatty tissue. Pollutants tend to accumulate in fat.

● Some women who are pregnant or breastfeeding choose to avoid fish such as shark, swordfish and halibut which can build up higher levels of mercury – a potential risk to the foetal nervous system.

Don't let this advice put you off eating fish or giving it to children. It is still one of the safest and most nutritious foods available.

EATING FISH RAW

I enjoy eating raw fish dishes in Japanese restaurants – but someone told me that raw fish can carry parasites. Is this true? And, if so, are they dangerous?

Yes it is true. But the risk is very slight. If you eat raw fish in Japanese dishes such as sushi or sashimi, there is a possibility of swallowing parasites that would normally be killed by heat during cooking. The main culprit is a roundworm called anisakis which can live in the lining of the human stomach, where it forms a fibrous mass that eventually causes symptoms of pain and fever.

Even so, it is very rare indeed to consume live anisakis parasites in Britain. And if you take care to eat raw fish only in reputable Japanese restaurants, you can be certain that your food is prepared by an expert sushi chef who will have been well trained to spot and remove the anisakis worm.

Taking supplements

Fish oils contain fatty acids known as omega 3s that help to protect the heart and circulatory system (see pages 36-37). While the benefits of eating oily fish are not in question, taking highly concentrated supplements may not be a good idea. It is thought that large doses may slow down wound healing, and there is a danger of consuming toxic amounts of vitamins A and D (see page 44). Seek advice before dosing yourself.

Dairy products and eggs

LOW-FAT MILK

I know that skimmed milk is supposed to be better for you than the full-cream variety, but it tastes so watery to me. Is there really an important difference from the health point of view?

Yes, there is a significant difference. Milk fat is very high (62 per cent) in saturates, which are associated with raised blood cholesterol, blocked arteries and heart disease. While full-cream milk is 3.9 per cent fat, skimmed is only 0.1 per cent, so making the change will greatly reduce both the overall fat content of your diet and the content of saturates – especially if you drink a lot of milk. And if you are concerned about weight, a pint (570 ml) of skimmed milk has only 194 Calories, as compared with 387 in a pint of whole milk.

If you dislike the thinner texture, try stirring in a little skimmed milk powder to compensate – you will add a few calories but very little fat. Another compromise is to use semi-skimmed milk, which tastes creamy but is only 1.6 per cent fat (under half as much as whole milk) and has 270 Calories per pint.

Reduced-fat milks have the same amount of calcium and protein as whole milk, but – except for some enriched types – less of the fat-soluble vitamins A and D.

CAUTION Do not give skimmed milk to children under the age of five, or semi-skimmed milk to those under two. Children need the energy supplied by the extra calories in whole milk.

MILK INTOLERANCE

My six-year-old son has been diagnosed 'lactose intolerant'. Does this mean that he cannot eat any dairy products at all?

Lactose intolerance is a reduced ability to digest the sugar in milk (lactose), owing to a shortage of the enzyme lactase in the small intestine. When milk is drunk or foods containing milk are eaten, the patient develops symptoms such as abdominal pain, bloating, flatulence and diarrhoea. The condition usually develops in early childhood, and may get worse with age. It is also not uncommon to lose the ability to digest lactose during childhood, as may be the case with your son.

The simplest way to avoid problems is to give up milk and milk products, although many people who have a lactose intolerance do find that they can tolerate dairy products in which bacteria have already broken down most of the lactose. Bearing this in mind, your son could experiment cautiously with yoghurt; firm, ripened cheeses; and hard

Egg safety

Follow these simple guidelines to reduce the risk of salmonella food poisoning from contaminated eggs.

● Always wash your hands before and after handling eggs.
● Store eggs in their carton in a refrigerator, and eat within two weeks of purchase.
● Wipe shells clean if they are dirty. Discard eggs with cracks or other damage to the shell.
● Don't exceed use-by dates. If in doubt, test for freshness. A fresh egg should sink when submerged in cold water. If it floats or smells, discard it.
● Avoid using raw eggs in recipes where no cooking or only light cooking is involved.
● Eat egg dishes as soon as possible after preparation, or keep them refrigerated.
● Cook eggs until both white and yolk are firm. This means scrambling for 3-4 minutes, poaching for 5-7 minutes and boiling for 7-10 minutes.

cheeses such as Cheddar. He should not be tempted to try high-lactose cheeses such as cottage cheese, fromage frais and processed cheese spreads. If you have not already done so, you and your son should also see a dietician who will be able to draw up a list of safe foods and provide information about checking food labels – your doctor will be able to refer you. You will also need advice about ensuring your son receives a good supply of calcium, either by taking supplements or by including fortified soya products in his diet.

Some lactose-intolerant people find that they can eat dairy products if they also take lactase, in either liquid or pill form. Again, a dietician will be able to advise.

BUYING YOGHURT

There are so many yoghurts to choose from these days that I feel confused. Are they all the same nutritionally?

You may be surprised to learn that although yoghurt has a reputation for being one of the great health foods, some types are relatively high in fat and sugar. The amount of fat depends on the milk used. Virtually fat-free yoghurts have only traces of fat, low-fat types about 1 per cent fat, whole-milk yoghurt about 3.5 per cent fat, and Greek yoghurt as much as 10 per cent fat. Most flavoured yoghurts are also high in calories from added sugar, although some use artificial sweeteners instead – check the label. Alternatively, buy plain yoghurt and add fresh fruit.

One of the top health benefits of yoghurt comes from types that contain live *Lactobacillus acidophilus* bacteria in addition to the *Lactobacillus bulgaricus* and *Streptococcus thermophilus* used in making all yoghurts. While the latter two are completely harmless, *Lactobacillus acidophilus* is actually beneficial to the human body. It helps you to fight off infections by strengthening the population of 'good' bacteria in the gut, and by limiting the growth of harmful ones.

Beneficial bacteria are easily killed off by antibiotic drugs, so if you ever have to take a course of antibiotics, eating live *acidophilus*-containing yoghurt is a good way of replenishing your stock of beneficial intestinal bacteria. Heat-treated yoghurts (those marked pasteurised, sterilised, long-life or UHT), will not have the same effect, as the bacteria have been killed off by high temperatures.

Don't forget that as well as being a good breakfast, dessert and snack food (provided you choose well), yoghurt is also an excellent substitute for cream on puddings or

stirred into soups and sauces just before serving. Flavoured with chopped herbs, mustard, garlic or other seasonings it also makes a healthy dressing for a salad or jacket potato.

WHAT FREE-RANGE MEANS

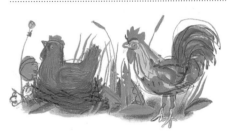

Are free-range eggs worth the extra money?

The answer depends upon your reasons for buying them. If you want a more nutritious or safer kind of egg then, no – nutritional differences are insignificant, and there is no guarantee that one type is less likely to carry salmonella (see below) than another. But if you want to support a better life for hens you may feel it is worth paying more.

If you do decide to buy free-range eggs, be aware that the labelling of egg boxes can be very misleading: 'country fresh' and 'farm' are legally acceptable descriptions for ordinary battery eggs. Only the three terms 'free-range', 'barn' and 'perchery' actually refer to less intensive methods of production.

Free-range eggs
Hens must have continual daytime access to open-air runs and the total amount of space must amount to 12 sq yd (10 m²) per hen.

Barn or perchery eggs
Hens are kept uncaged in an indoor enclosure and do not have any access to outdoor runs. They have the same amount of space as free-range hens do when indoors.

AVOIDING SALMONELLA

I've heard that runny eggs can cause food poisoning. How does this affect custard, mayonnaise and other soft-egg foods?

It has been estimated that about one egg in every 7000 harbours the salmonella bacteria that can cause food poisoning if eggs are not properly cooked. This may not sound much of a risk – until you consider that in Britain people consume more than 170 million eggs each week of the year. Cases of salmonella food poisoning (which contaminates both the yolk and white of affected eggs) are not uncommon. Eggs and products that contain eggs that have not been completely cooked are thought to be one of the main culprits.

Current government advice is therefore to avoid eating raw eggs in any form, including mayonnaise made by the traditional method of beating up raw egg yolk with oil and vinegar, and desserts featuring raw, whipped egg whites such as mousse, homemade cheesecakes, homemade sorbet and ice cream, and cold soufflés. Products manufactured commercially are generally considered to be safe, as they use pasteurised egg.

Runny fried, scrambled or poached eggs and soft-boiled eggs are not suitable for pregnant women, babies, the sick or the elderly – all of whom may be more at risk from food poisoning. They should eat eggs only when cooked until both white and yolk are solid.

As salmonella thrives in warm temperatures, eggs should always be refrigerated. A temperature of 5°C (41°F) or below will prevent salmonella bacteria from multiplying either inside the egg or on the shell.

LISTERIA FROM CHEESE

Some while ago there was a scare about listeria infection in cheese made from milk that had not been pasteurised. Are soft unpasteurised cheeses safe to eat?

They are just as safe as any other soft cheese – which in most cases means quite safe. Listeria is a food-borne infection that is generally not very serious (symptoms are flu-like), except in pregnancy, when it may precipitate miscarriage. However, there is no evidence that unpasteurised milk in any way increases the risk of infection. Rather, contamination occurs as a result of poor hygiene during processing. When present, the bacteria are usually found on the rind or near the surface, having been introduced by human handling.

Hard cheese such as Cheddar or Parmesan is seldom affected, but soft cheeses such as Brie, and blue-veined types are more easily contaminated owing to lower acidity. They should be avoided during pregnancy.

Fats and your health

WHY FAT MATTERS

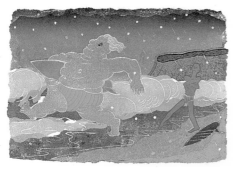

You are always hearing advice about how to cut down on the amount of fat that you eat. Just what is so bad about fat?

There are many reasons to control fat intake. Britain has one of the highest rates of heart disease in the world – a condition caused by clogged arteries and closely linked with fat consumption. If arteries in the brain rather than the heart are affected, the result can be a stroke. For reasons that are not well understood, high fat intake is also related to some killer cancers – breast, prostate and colon.

The type of fat we eat is wrong too. Butter, cream, hard cheese, sausages, pâtés, pastries, cakes and meat fats are all extremely high in saturates that increase cholesterol and block arteries. Vegetable oils, on the other hand, such as olive, corn and sunflower, and oils from fish such as salmon, mackerel and herring are safe – in some cases even beneficial.

Fat is also the most concentrated form of food energy, containing weight-for-weight more than twice the calories of either carbohydrate or protein. Dietary fat is easily converted into body fat and stored as excess weight – another health concern in Britain, where one in three adults is overweight.

But although most of us would probably benefit from cutting down on all fat, no one should try to avoid it completely (impossible, anyway, since some fat is present in virtually every food). Fats and oils are needed to make hormones, and for the absorption of the fat-soluble vitamins A, D, E and K. We also need to obtain certain essential fatty acids (the basic constituents of fats) from the diet, since they cannot be made in the body. Fat also enhances the flavour of food and creates a pleasant feeling of fullness.

All in all, the best advice for most people is to keep a watch on the overall amount of fat they eat (see panel, right), substitute lower-fat foods for higher-fat ones (see page 38), and increase the proportion of fish and vegetable oils to animal and dairy fats.

Calculating the fat in your diet

No more than 35 per cent of our calories are supposed to come from fat, yet few foods give the percentage on the label. Here's how to calculate it from two figures that *are* usually given, the Calories (kcal) and the grammes of fat per 3½ oz (100 g):

Multiply the fat figure by 9 (the number of Calories in 1 g of fat). Divide the result by the calorie figure, and multiply by 100. For example, if the label says there are 450 kcal and 10 g of fat per 3½ oz (100 g) of food:
10 x 9 = 90
90 ÷ 450 = 0.2
0.2 x 100 = 20
So 20 per cent of the calories come from fat – low enough to make it a healthy food.

HOW MUCH FAT IS IN THE FOOD YOU EAT ?

According to the Department of Health, fat should account for no more than 35 per cent of your total calorie intake. Based on average daily requirements for moderately active adults, this means women should eat no more than about 76 g of fat a day, and men no more than about 99 g a day.

When you do eat fatty foods, try to choose those with a relatively high proportion of unsaturated fatty acids to saturated fatty acids, which can harm the heart and circulatory system if eaten in excess. No more than about 10 per cent of your daily calories should come from saturates, which amounts to around 22 g of saturates a day for women and 28 g a day for men.

The chart below is designed to help you to keep track of the amount and kind of fat you are eating, and to compare different foods.

FOOD	TOTAL FATTY ACIDS (g)	SATURATED FATTY ACIDS (g)	UNSATURATED FATTY ACIDS (g)
Milk – ½ pint (285 ml)			
whole	11.1	6.8	4.3
semi-skimmed	4.6	2.8	1.8
skimmed	0.3	0.3	0.0
Cheese – 2 oz (60 g)			
Brie	16.2	10.1	6.1
Cheddar	20.6	13.1	7.5
reduced-fat hard	9.0	5.6	3.4
cottage	2.4	1.4	1.0
Egg – size 2	6.5	1.9	4.6
Spreads and oils – ⅓ oz (10 g)			
butter	8.2	5.4	2.8
soft margarine	8.2	2.6	5.6
low-fat spread	4.1	1.1	3.0
olive oil	10.0	1.4	8.6
Bacon – 1 oz (30 g)			
lean, grilled	5.6	2.3	3.3
lean and fat, grilled	10.2	4.0	6.2
Meat – 3½ oz (100 g)			
beef, lean, roast	4.4	1.4	3.0
beef, lean and fat, roast	12.0	4.1	7.9
chicken, roast, no skin	5.4	1.6	3.8
chicken, roast, with skin	14.0	4.2	9.8
lamb, lean leg, roast	8.1	3.9	4.2
lamb, kidney	2.7	0.9	1.8
pork, lean chop, grilled	10.7	3.8	6.9
ham	5.1	1.9	3.2
pork sausage, grilled	24.7	9.5	15.2
Fish – 3½ oz (100 g)			
cod, poached	1.1	0.5	0.6
cod, battered and fried in oil	10.3	0.9	9.4
herring, grilled	13.0	3.7	9.3
tuna, canned in brine	0.6	0.2	0.4
prawns	1.8	0.4	1.4
Sweets and cakes – 3½ oz (100 g)			
milk chocolate	30.3	17.7	12.6
iced cakes	14.9	9.3	5.6
chocolate digestives	24.1	12.2	11.9

SATURATES AND UNSATURATES

There is a lot of talk about different kinds of fats, such as saturates and unsaturates. What do these terms really mean and how much of each type should we be eating?

Most of the fats in your body, as well as in food, are made up of compounds called fatty acids. These are basically chains of carbon atoms, which may or may not be chemically bonded to hydrogen atoms. Fatty acids are said to be saturated if they contain as many hydrogen atoms as possible. If one or more pairs of carbon atoms is free, that is, not completely bonded to hydrogen atoms, the fatty acid is said to be unsaturated – if just one pair is free it is monounsaturated, if several pairs are free it is polyunsaturated.

Fats in food
The fats and oils that we eat all contain a mixture of fatty acids. In general, harder fats (butter, dripping, harder margarines) have more saturates and soft fats (vegetable oils and fish oils) more unsaturates. Foods relatively high in saturates include meat, most dairy products, animal fats, and palm and coconut oil. Olive oil, rapeseed oil, peanuts and avocados are rich in monounsaturates; while sunflower and corn oil, oily fish such as mackerel, and nuts in polyunsaturates.

Heart health
As far as your heart and circulation are concerned, saturates increase blood cholesterol while both monounsaturates and polyunsaturates can help to reduce it, particularly the harmful LDL type (see page 364-365) which is responsible for blocking arteries.

Poly or mono?
The only fatty acids you actually need in your diet are two polyunsaturates (called essential fatty acids, or EFAs). All others can be manufactured in the body even if you eat no fat or oil at all. Even so, there is no need to eat large quantities of polyunsaturates and there may be good reasons not to (a very high intake of polyunsaturates may be correlated with an increased risk of cancer, and polyunsaturates also reduce beneficial HDL cholesterol as well as harmful LDL cholesterol). Monounsaturates, by contrast, appear to have a purely protective effect and should make up most of the fat in your diet.

While the average total intake of polyunsaturates is considered about right, nutritionists advise increasing the proportion we obtain from oily fish such as mackerel and herring. Fish oils are the major source of two particular fatty acids (both belonging to the family known as omega 3s), which appear to counteract heart disease and may relieve certain inflammatory illnesses such as rheumatoid arthritis. Apart from this, you will get all the polyunsaturates you need from a varied diet including foods such as nuts, seeds, cereals, lean meat and even green vegetables.

IRON AND CALCIUM

I've been told to cut down on fat, but won't I lose other important nutrients as well if I avoid foods such as red meat and milk?

If you cut these foods out of your diet altogether, you will obviously be missing out on a number of important vitamins and minerals. Meat, for example, is a rich source of iron, B vitamins and protein; while milk and dairy products are rich in calcium, vitamins and protein.

A much better move would be to switch to reduced-fat alternatives which are still highly nutritious in other ways. Leaner cuts of red meat, for example, contain as much iron, B vitamins and protein as regular or fatty cuts. Lower-fat white meats are lower in iron so you need to make sure you include plenty of other iron-rich foods in your diet, such as leafy green vegetables, pulses and cereals.

Low-fat milks contains as much calcium, protein and B vitamins as ordinary full-fat milk but less of the fat-soluble vitamins A and D. Few people in Britain are at risk of deficiency in these vitamins but if you are concerned look for enriched brands of milk (some are also enriched with extra calcium). Reduced-fat hard cheese also contains less vitamin A and D but you can easily compensate by including more brightly coloured vegetables and fruit for beta-carotene (a form of vitamin A) and making sure you get some exposure to sunlight for vitamin D.

In other respects few reduced-fat foods are any less nutritious than their high-fat equivalents. For most people the benefits of cutting down on fat far outweigh any slight differences in the case of meat and milk.

BUTTER OR MARGARINE?

Is it true that margarine is no longer considered a healthy alternative to butter?

The long-running controversy over whether butter or polyunsaturated margarine is better for your health has caused a great deal of confusion. The two spreads have about the same number of calories (only reduced-fat spreads have significantly fewer), but butter is higher in saturated fatty acids that can contribute to the development of heart disease.

Until quite recently, margarine made from polyunsaturated vegetable oils was recommended as a healthy alternative – but now these products have come in for criticism. During margarine manufacture, liquid oils are turned into a solid spread by a process called hydrogenation, which involves bubbling hydrogen gas through them. The process has the effect of changing the chemical structure, creating saturated fatty acids and some unsaturated compounds known as trans-fatty acids, which affect the body in a similar way to saturated fats. It is thought that, like saturates, trans-fatty acids may increase the risk of heart disease. While there is as yet no conclusive proof of a link between trans-fatty acids and heart disease, the British Heart Foundation is taking the possibility seriously enough to have started its own research programme.

Tiny amounts of trans-fatty acids do occur naturally in butter, whole milk and the fat of beef and lamb. Butter and margarines that are labelled 'high in polyunsaturates' have about the same amount of trans-fatty acids (5-10 per cent of fat content), while ordinary margarines and hard margarines have about 15 per cent. Some margarine manufacturers are reformulating their products in order to reduce the trans-fatty acid content, and you can buy non-hydrogenated margarines from health shops, but they tend to be very soft. The best advice is to cut down on all yellow spreads on bread, and to substitute vegetable oils such as olive and rapeseed for butter and margarine in your cooking.

Trans-fatty acids will also be present in all processed foods that contain hydrogenated oils. If you want to avoid them, get into the habit of reading labels, and stay away from products that list hydrogenated vegetable oil.

CHOOSING OLIVE OIL

Why is olive oil supposed to be so good for you and how should I choose among all the different types on sale?

European heart disease rates are lowest in Mediterranean regions – where, unlike the milk and butter cultures of the north, olive oil is a staple. Olive oil is rich in monounsaturated fatty acids (see page 36) which lower blood cholesterol and protect the heart.

Olive oil is graded according to the means of extraction and the acidity level – the lower

How to choose the best vegetable oils

Cooking oils vary greatly in composition. Here are some hints to help you to choose among the main types.

Oils that are high in monounsaturates
These oils protect the heart and lower harmful LDL cholesterol levels. They are increasingly used in margarines and other blended products.
● **Olive** (70 per cent) – many types; good for all uses. See also below, left.
● **Rapeseed** (57 per cent) – neutral taste; suitable for all uses.
● **Blended oils** (typically 57 per cent) – suitable for most uses but quality varies. Look for types made mainly from rapeseed oil.
● **Peanut** (49 per cent) – suitable for all uses.

Oils that are high in polyunsaturates
Although these oils are a good source of vitamin E and can reduce cholesterol there are some health reasons not to eat them in very large amounts (see left).
● **Grapeseed** (73 per cent) – mild flavour, good for salads.
● **Safflower** (72 per cent) – light and delicate; good for fish and shellfish.
● **Sunflower** (63 per cent) – All uses; widely found in margarines.
● **Corn** (58 per cent) and soya (57 per cent) and – all uses; also quite high in monounsaturates (24 per cent). Corn oil can tolerate high temperatures well and is specially good for frying.

Should your children cut down on fat?

Probably not. Children are growing and need the concentrated energy that fat provides. Many high-fat foods such as cheese, whole milk and nuts also provide valuable vitamins and minerals and are much better for children than sugary snacks. (But avoid giving nuts to children under five, who could choke.)

Unlike sweets and cakes, nuts, cheese and milk are safe for teeth. Dentists recommend them as fillers between meals or instead of a pudding because they counteract mouth acids that lead to tooth decay.

Advice to cut down on fat is aimed mainly at adults, who have different nutritional needs and are more often overweight.

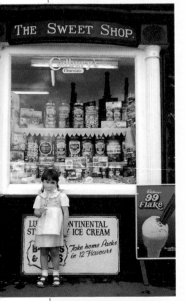

Sweet treat Ice cream is fine once in a while – children need more fat and calories than adults.

the acidity the better the taste. Extra virgin and virgin oil both come from the first pressing, but extra virgin has lower acidity and is considered finer in flavour. Both types are suitable for salad and pasta dressings, marinades and for sprinkling over grilled fish or vegetables, or for eating with bread in the Mediterranean style.

Olive oil labelled 'pure' is extracted chemically from the paste left after the pressing of virgin oil. The taste is mild and less favoured for table use, but it is perfectly acceptable for cooking. Those who find the taste of virgin oil too strong may even prefer it on salads.

Whichever you opt for, buy your olive oil in small bottles so it stays fresh. Stored in a cool dark place it should last for a year or so.

CAN FRYING BE HEALTHY?

I've heard that stir-frying is a healthy way to cook food, but also that heating oils to high temperatures can be dangerous. Is there any truth in this and, if so, should I avoid frying altogether?

The Chinese method of stir-frying has long been recognised as an extremely healthy way of cooking. Finely sliced vegetables sautéed quickly in a very small amount of oil stay crisp and keep almost all of their nutrients. Stir-frying is also an excellent way to cook small pieces of meat, fish and poultry, as the heat of the oil will kill any food poisoning organisms that may be present.

Other methods of frying can also be reasonably healthy provided you cook with care and don't rely on fried food excessively. Shallow frying enables meat, fish, chicken and other ingredients to retain moisture, flavour and vitamins; and deep fried chips actually keep more vitamin C than boiled potatoes.

Understanding the dangers

The main health risks of frying are to do with the amount of oil used, the temperature it is allowed to reach and the length of time for which it is kept very hot. When oils reach smoking point or are kept at very high temperatures for 15 minutes or more, chemical changes occur that lead to the formation of substances that are thought to be potentially cancer-causing.

The same applies to polyunsaturated oils such as sunflower if they are frequently reheated. Highly saturated fats such as lard, beef dripping and butter do not undergo damage of this sort, but should be eaten in moderation because of potentially harmful effects on the heart and circulation.

CUTTING DOWN ON FATS

Most people eat too much fat – in particular, too much saturated fat – but cutting down is not difficult. Some simple changes to a normal diet can reduce fat intake considerably without noticeably affecting eating habits. The tips below are designed to make the adjustment to a healthier diet as easy as possible. After the first few weeks, they will become automatic habits.

Meat and poultry
Cut down on high-fat meats and meat products such as sausages, burgers, bacon and minced beef. Buy lean meats and trim off any visible fat. As a substitute for red meat, eat more fish and poultry – and remove the skin from poultry. Skim the fat from soups, stews and curries before serving.

Dairy products
Eat full-fat dairy foods in moderation, especially cream, cream cheese and hard cheeses such as Cheddar. Replace whole milk with skimmed or semi-skimmed and use low-fat yoghurt or fromage frais instead of cream.

Spreads, dressings and oils
Try to use butter, margarine and even low-fat spreads sparingly. Use less mayonnaise and high-fat salad dressings, and less cooking fat and oil. When you do use oils, choose types such as olive, corn, sunflower, soya, rapeseed and peanut, which are low in saturates. Avoid coconut and palm. Never reuse cooking oil – reheating oxidises fats and creates potentially harmful substances.

Invisible fats
Beware of fats in processed foods such as biscuits, cakes, snacks, pastries and dips. Read food labels and look for lower-fat options.

Cooking methods
Wherever possible, try to use low-fat cooking methods such as grilling, poaching, steaming, roasting, baking, boiling and stir-frying. If you do fry chips or other foods occasionally, cut them into large pieces. Before serving, drain off as much fat as possible, and pat off excess oil with kitchen paper.

Better methods

To keep frying as healthy as possible, choose vegetable oil rather than animal fat, and use fresh oil each time. Never heat any oil to smoking point and don't fry at a very high temperature for more than a few minutes.

Choose oils according to taste: sunflower, rapeseed and peanut have a delicate flavour, while olive tastes stronger and can be heated to higher temperatures without smoking. Sesame and nut oils are highly distinctive – just a few drops are all you need in a stir-fry.

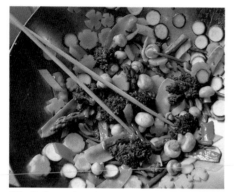

Stir frying The Chinese technique of frying finely sliced ingredients lightly in vegetable oil creates healthy and endlessly varied meals.

AVOIDING CHOLESTEROL

Is it important to keep a watch on how much cholesterol you eat?

When high blood cholesterol was first linked with the development of heart disease, many people became concerned about cholesterol in food. Now we know that the situation is rather more complex and that food cholesterol does not automatically turn into blood cholesterol. What does undoubtedly push up blood cholesterol levels is eating fats high in saturates (see pages 36-37) – and it is these that you need to watch, particularly if you have heart or circulation problems.

Only in rare cases of severely raised blood cholesterol do doctors advise limiting cholesterol consumption as well as saturates. This means avoiding squid, mussels, prawns and similar shellfish and crustacea; fish roe; egg yolk; liver and kidney. But for most people – even many of those with high blood cholesterol – there is no evidence that it helps to cut down on these (except possibly in the case of egg yolk, which is also high in saturates). Liver and kidney are lean and nutritious, and shellfish are a good source of protective omega-3 oils – see pages 36-37.

Salt and seasoning

SALT AND BLOOD PRESSURE

How much salt is needed in the diet? Do I have to watch my salt intake even if my blood pressure is normal?

Salt is made up of two components – sodium and chloride. Some sodium is necessary to regulate the fluid balance of the body and to help to transmit nerve impulses and enable muscles to function properly.

In Britain and in many parts of the world we eat far more salt than we need for these purposes. Under normal circumstances, the kidneys can get rid of any excess, but if large quantities of salt are consumed over years an excess can build up, causing fluid retention in blood vessels and exerting pressure on the vessel walls – and on other tissues. This can result in a rise in blood pressure.

The Department of Health estimates that we need 0.5 g-1.6 g of sodium a day, equivalent to about a quarter to one teaspoon of salt – a quantity we easily get from the natural salt in food alone, without adding any extra. In one study, researchers calculated that if we all cut our sodium intake by two-thirds it would result in 40 per cent fewer deaths from strokes overall and 30 per cent fewer deaths from heart disease – both conditions closely related to high blood pressure.

Watch what you buy

Most of our salt comes from processed foods and only about 25 per cent is added to home cooking or at table, so one of the most effective ways of cutting down is to get into the habit of checking labels.

High sodium foods do not always taste particularly salty, and include a huge range of products such as bread, cheese, breakfast cereals, biscuits, soups, stock cubes, prepared sauces, cured or smoked meat, canned foods, crisps, snacks, nuts and convenience foods.

● Food labels generally give sodium content rather than salt content. To calculate the salt equivalent, multiply the sodium figure by 2.5 if given in grammes (g). If it is given in milligrammes (mg) multiply by 2.5, then divide the result by 1000.

FACT — OR — FALLACY?

'Sea salt is better for you than common table salt.'

Fallacy Although sea salt has a fractionally higher content of certain minerals found in sea water, such as iodine, the actual amount is so minute that it will make absolutely no difference to the quality of your diet. Sea salt is sold in health shops more because it is *perceived* as natural and therefore assumed to be better than for any real benefit.

Do hot, spicy foods harm the stomach?

Not at all. There is no evidence that the digestive tract is harmed in any way by eating hot peppers, chillies or other pungent spices.

Such foods may make the mouth burn, the eyes water and the nose run, but research in Mexico, Thailand and India, where hot dishes are daily staples, shows no higher rate of ulcers or gastric problems than in countries with blander diets.

HEALTHY SEASONINGS

Unsalted food tastes bland to me. Is there a healthier way to pep up the flavour?

Yes, there are many healthier alternatives to salt – alternatives which will enhance the natural flavours of the food you prepare. Healthy seasonings include freshly ground black pepper, lemon juice, wine or balsamic vinegar, herbs (fresh or dried), spices, garlic, onions, wine and vegetable purées. Experiment in your cooking and at the table to see which ones you prefer. As a start, you might like to try some of the following suggestions:

● Cider or wine vinegar with salads.
● Lemon juice with steamed broccoli.
● Garlic with salads, dips and sauces, and in Mediterranean-style savoury dishes.
● Chopped parsley or salad onions sprinkled over boiled or mashed potatoes, fish, stir-fries or casseroles just before serving.

● Fresh root ginger, fennel seeds and Chinese five-spice with stir-fried foods.
● Tarragon with poultry or fish.
● Nutmeg with mashed potato.
● Rosemary with meat.
● Crushed coriander seeds.

Condiments such as soya sauce, ready-made mustard and Worcestershire sauce are poor salt substitutes as they also generally contain large amounts of sodium – if in doubt, check the label although it will not always state the amount. Low-sodium salt substitutes based on potassium chloride rather than sodium chloride are better, and are available in many health shops and supermarkets.

CAUTION While most people could do with an increase in potassium consumption, for a few people it could be dangerous. If you plan to use a potassium substitute regularly, check with your doctor first, particularly if you have had kidney or heart trouble.

Vitamins, minerals and supplements

Don't forget about these minerals

The body's need for minerals such as iron and calcium is well known but you also need small amounts of many other substances. Some of the most important ones include:

● **Magnesium** – from milk, leafy vegetables, nuts, seeds and grains.
● **Phosphorus** – from dairy products, eggs, meat, fish and grains.
● **Sulphur** – from meat, fish, eggs and pulses.
● **Copper** – from liver, kidney and seafood.
● **Fluoride** – from tea, canned fish (with bones), tap water.
● **Iodine** – from seafood, dairy products, vegetables, iodised salt.
● **Manganese** – from whole grains, fruit, tea, vegetables and pulses.
● **Molybdenum** – from liver, kidney, seafood, meat and whole grains.

DAILY REQUIREMENTS

What exactly is meant by the term RDA on food labels? And how should I use this information in my everyday diet?

The initials RDA stand for Recommended Daily Allowance and refer to the amount of a nutrient sufficient to meet the needs of practically all healthy people. (Some people with a particular illness have higher requirements than average, and these are not covered by the figure.) The figures are arrived at on the basis of ongoing long-term research and reflect an amount that is known to be adequate for 98 per cent of the population, including a substantial safety margin. They also take into account any known ill effects of high doses and the possibility that some vitamins and minerals can interfere with the absorption of others.

Among nutritionists in Britain RDAs have been partially phased out in favour of DRVs, or dietary reference values (thought to be a less misleading term), but as European legislation is based on RDAs they are likely to remain on food labels. By law, manufacturers can make claims such as 'a rich source of vitamin C' only if a food product provides at least 15 per cent of the RDA figure. The best way of using information about RDAs is not to worry too much about numbers and calculations, but just as a guide to help you to be more aware of which foods are particularly high in certain vitamins and minerals.

WHAT ARE ANTIOXIDANTS?

What are the 'antioxidants' and 'free radicals' that get so much attention in the Press these days?

Antioxidants are active compounds found mainly in fresh fruit, vegetables and wholegrain cereals, and thought to be important in maintaining long-term good health and protecting the body from some of the effects of ageing and disease. The principal antioxidants are the vitamins C and E, and beta-carotene, which is turned into vitamin A by the body. Other antioxidants obtained from food include substances known as flavonoids (found in fruit), and the minerals selenium, zinc, iron and copper.

According to an increasingly popular view, antioxidants may protect us from the damaging effects of free radicals – unstable molecules created as a by-product when oxygen is used in the course of countless reactions in the body. Free radicals are also thought to be created through exposure to environmental factors such as sunlight, cigarette smoke, radiation, traffic emissions and other atmospheric pollutants. Although free radicals are used by the immune system to kill invading bacteria and viruses, they may also, according to the theory, be responsible for some of the effects of ageing and disease on the body.

For good or ill, free radicals are chemically unstable. Stable molecules have pairs of electrons, which makes them relatively nonreactive. Unstable molecules such as free radicals have unpaired electrons. In order to reach a stable state, they 'steal' electrons from other molecules – sparking off a chain reaction.

Many scientists believe that free radicals play a part in the development of conditions such as heart disease, cataracts and possibly certain cancers, as well as aspects of ageing such as wrinkles and muscle deterioration.

Antioxidants are thought to help by neutralising free radicals without becoming unstable. Afterwards they are broken down into harmless substances. While little is known about how antioxidants actually work, it is clear that they have a protective effect. There is little proof that taking supplements is helpful, however – the best way to increase your antioxidant supply is to eat more fruit and vegetables (see panel, right).

TAKING VITAMIN PILLS

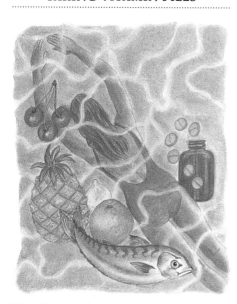

Vitamin and mineral supplements seem very popular. Are they really necessary if you are eating a good, varied diet anyway?

Doctors and nutritionists agree that a varied diet which covers your energy (calorie) needs should supply all the vitamins and minerals we need for good health. Supplements are just what their name implies – extras to be used when there is some special need. They cannot turn a poor diet into a good one, nor can they supply anything like the nutrient and energy content of food. Taken on their own, vitamins and minerals are not generally as well absorbed as those in food; taken with food, supplements are better absorbed. But supplements can also be expensive, especially if taken regularly. Most people would do better to spend their money on food.

Even so, there are arguments in favour of supplementation. Skipped meals and erratic eating habits can affect nutrition, particularly if they become a way of life. Poor soil quality in certain regions also means that fruit, vegetables and cereals can vary considerably in their vitamin and mineral content. In addition, significant vitamin losses can occur during food storage, preparation and cooking. Certain groups of people in particular may benefit from supplements.

● People who often miss meals, who regularly rely on fast food, or who do not eat much fresh fruit and vegetables, may benefit from a combined supplement.
● A multisupplement is a good idea for heavy drinkers or those getting over illness.
● Women who are pregnant or contemplating becoming pregnant are advised to take a daily 0.4 mg dose of folic acid (also known as folate), to reduce the risk of spina bifida in the baby. Supplementation should continue up to the 12th week of pregnancy.
● Teenage girls and adult women who have heavy periods may benefit from additional iron, but this should be prescribed by a doctor as there can be side effects.
● Smokers have an increased requirement for vitamin C because they process this vitamin at a higher rate than non-smokers.
● Housebound people with little opportunity to get out in the sun may need vitamin D supplements.
● People over 60 have a decreased ability to absorb nutrients, so a multivitamin and mineral supplement is a good idea.
● Anyone on a restricted diet, such as slimmers and vegans. Vegans need vitamin B_{12} supplements or fortified foods.

As a general rule, if you think your nutrition could be improved, take a close look at your diet before considering supplements. If you have any distinct symptoms, see a doctor – don't assume a nutritional cause.

CAUTION Pregnant women should seek medical advice before taking supplements.

Where to find antioxidants

Vitamins and minerals with antioxidant properties can protect the body. Here are the foods to eat to make sure of a good supply.

Beta-carotene
A form of vitamin A, this yellow-orange pigment gives carrots, apricots, mangoes, cantaloupe melons, pawpaws, sweet potatoes and red peppers their colour. It is also found in dark green leafy vegetables such as spinach, spring greens and broccoli.

Vitamin C
Good sources include citrus fruit and juice, strawberries, blackcurrants, Brussels sprouts, broccoli, cabbage, potatoes, tomatoes, peas, green peppers and leafy greens.

Vitamin E
Vegetable oils (especially sunflower, safflower and rapeseed), sunflower seeds, almonds, peanuts and peanut butter, avocados, wheatgerm, wholemeal bread and other wholegrain products such as pasta, and green leafy vegetables are all rich sources of vitamin E.

Iron, zinc, copper and selenium
To ensure a good supply of these four antioxidant minerals, include a variety of these foods in your daily diet: liver, kidney, shellfish, meat, eggs, poultry, fish, whole grains, nuts and seeds.

Foods that fight disease

SINCE at least the 14th century BC, when garlic was placed in the tomb of the Egyptian pharaoh Tutankhamun with other treasures for use in the afterlife, certain foods have been prized for their healing and health-promoting properties.

Scientists now believe that the way you eat can either contribute to or help to prevent a wide range of illnesses, from constipation and tooth decay to cancer, heart disease, osteoporosis (loss of bone mass) and high blood pressure. Although investigators are only just beginning to understand how the foods on these pages may help to prevent or to combat illness, all are highly regarded. Make sure to include a good variety of them in your diet.

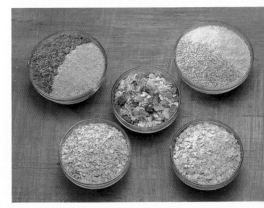

Oats   However you eat them, oats are good for your bowels and digestion. Oat bran contains soluble fibre that can reduce blood cholesterol.

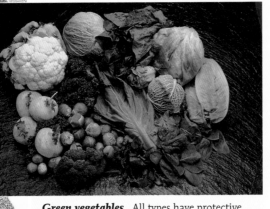

Green vegetables   All types have protective antioxidants. The cabbage family also contain sulphur compounds, thought to fight cancer.

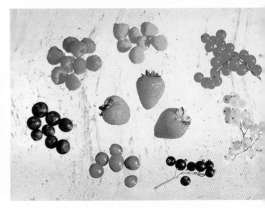

Berries   A high content of vitamin C and substances called flavonoids helps to ward off infections and to protect against some cancers.

CURES FROM YOUR KITCHEN

You don't have to turn to drugs when you feel under the weather. Common kitchen herbs and spices can sometimes be just as effective at relieving mild symptoms. Those on the right are some that have been tried and tested over centuries, and that appear to work well for many people. You can either eat them as foods or drink them as infusions (apart from chillis, turmeric and mustard, which are too hot or strong to be palatable to most people). To make an infusion, place about a tablespoon of chopped fresh herb, or a teaspoon of dried, in a cup of boiling water and leave to steep for two or three minutes. Drink in small sips.

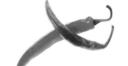

Chilli peppers   Fresh or dried, chillis are said to help the respiratory system and heart.

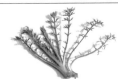

Camomile   An infusion of camomile is said to help against tension and insomnia.

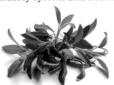

Sage   The herb is said to aid digestion, combat stress and be a nervous system tonic.

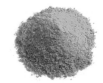

Turmeric   Try including turmeric in your cooking if you suffer from catarrh.

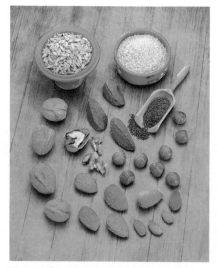

Nuts and seeds These are nature's food supplements – rich in protein, minerals and heart-protecting unsaturated fatty acids.

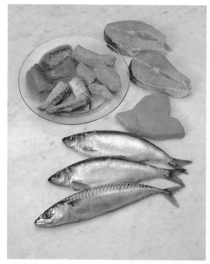

Oily fish Mackerel, tuna, sardines and other oily fish contain omega 3 fatty acids that protect the heart and circulation.

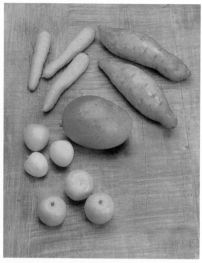

Orange fruit and vegetables The colour is due to beta-carotene, an antioxidant that can protect against many diseases.

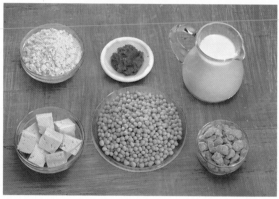

Soya Tofu, miso, soya burgers and other soya products are high in protein and low in fat. They also contain genistein, a chemical under investigation for anti-cancer properties.

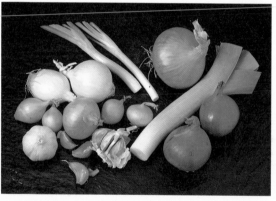

Onion family Leeks, shallots and other members of the onion family can reduce blood clotting, lower cholesterol and fight infections. Garlic may be anticarcinogenic.

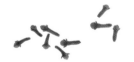

Cloves This antiseptic and anti-inflammatory spice is often used to ease toothache.

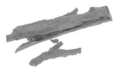

Cinnamon The antiseptic and stimulant properties are said to fight off colds and flu.

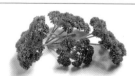

Parsley Infusions of parsely (a diuretic) can be helpful against fluid retention.

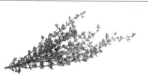

Thyme Use an infusion as an antiseptic and a stimulant to the body's natural resistance.

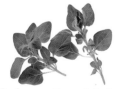

Marjoram Try an infusion to relieve a cold, indigestion or minor respiratory infection.

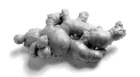

Ginger root An infusion of fresh or dry ginger is said to stave off colds and nausea.

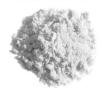

Mustard Eating foods with mustard may give relief from cold and flu symptoms.

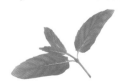

Mint Try a mint infusion after a rich meal or when you have a stomach upset.

What do amino acid supplements do?

Amino acid supplements are sold in many health shops and chemists, mainly as aids for athletes. They cost a lot, but there is little evidence that they can do much good.

Amino acids are the building blocks of proteins and since muscles are protein tissue there is a school of thought that more protein means more muscles, especially when the protein is highly concentrated, as in supplements.

It has been claimed that pure amino acids are absorbed faster than protein in food, since they don't need to be broken down any further. But since it takes hours to build muscle protein anyway, nutritionists believe this is unlikely to have any noticeable effect.

Supplements have also been claimed to deliver amino acids more efficiently, as well as faster. There is no evidence for this but even if it were true, food supplies such vastly greater quantities that it would still be a much better source. Most capsules contain about 0.5-1 g of amino acid. One small tin of tuna or a 4 oz (115 g) serving of cottage cheese gives 25 to 50 times as much.

Supplements can be harmful too, creating chemical imbalances in the body. Everyone, including athletes, is better off getting amino acids from food.

VITAMINS FOR STRESS

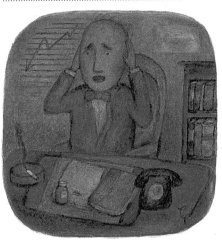

My husband believes that vitamin B capsules help him to get through stressful periods at work. Are they really beneficial?

Some B vitamins do play a role in the functioning of the nervous system, but there is no evidence that supplements help people to cope better with stress or give them more energy. The production of stress hormones such as adrenaline and corticol may slightly increase the need for some vitamins and minerals, but not the B group specifically.

In any case, the slightly increased requirement can easily be met from a well planned diet that includes plenty of fresh fruit, vegetables and wholegrains, and smaller quantities of protein foods such as lean meat, fish, chicken, eggs, cheese and other dairy products. A multivitamin and multimineral supplement can provide extra insurance, but it will not make up for a poor diet.

Encourage your husband not to skip meals or rely too much on fast food or fatty snacks bolted down in a free moment. If he eats regularly in restaurants, there are some simple ways of choosing healthy options (see page 52). Finding time for exercise and relaxation is also important, and not drinking or smoking more than usual. For further stress relief measures see pages 190-195.

HIGH DOSES

I've read that some supplements can be harmful if taken in high doses. Which are the ones that can cause problems?

You are quite right, some supplements can be harmful when taken in large amounts, because they build up to dangerous levels in body tissues. A toxic effect is rare with the water-soluble vitamins B and C because they cannot be stored in the body in significant amounts – any excess is simply excreted in the urine. Even so very high doses of vitamin C have been known to cause diarrhoea and increase the production of kidney stones in people who are already susceptible.

Similarly, when taken in very large quantities for months or years (as some women have done in attempting to combat premenstrual syndrome) vitamin B_6 can cause some severe nervous system disorders. The problems cease without leaving any lasting effects once dosage stops, however.

Fat-soluble vitamins (A, D, E and K) are potentially more of a risk since they are not excreted but stored in the liver and in fatty tissue. The most serious reported dangers arise with vitamin A. Excessively high doses can result in damage to the liver and bones, hair loss, double vision, vomiting and headaches. There is also a risk of birth defects in babies of women who overdose themselves during pregnancy. Government advice now directs that pregnant women avoid all vitamin A supplements, and also liver and liver pâté, as animal feed is often highly supplemented with vitamin A. For the rest of the population, the best advice is simply to avoid vitamin A supplements. Nearly everyone gets more than enough anyway, from foods such as oily fish, liver, butter, margarine and milk.

Vitamin D can also have ill effects in very large quantities. Most people obtain enough from exposure to sunlight, which causes it to be manufactured in the body, and from foods such as oily fish and egg yolk. Pregnant and nursing women, who need extra, and people who are confined at home are generally advised to increase their intake by diet.

Although also fat-soluble, vitamins E and K appear remarkably free of side effects.

DO 'WONDER FOODS' WORK?

I've heard startling claims about the benefits of supplements such as ginseng and evening primrose oil. What are these substances and can they really make a difference to your health?

Supplements of this sort are extremely popular but few of the claims made for them have ever been proved. Legislation now prohibits such claims except where supporting scientific evidence exists. These are some supplements you may come across.

● Blue-green algae – a tiny plant grown wild in lakes and cultivated in ponds. It contains some protein and beta-carotene but the protein is of relatively poor quality and there is little evidence for any of the miraculous effects that have been claimed.

● Coenzyme Q10 – a substance found naturally in every cell in the body and involved in energy production. Some believe it boosts energy and has other good effects but evidence is lacking. The chemical structure is similar to vitamins E and K.

● Evening primrose oil – an extract of evening primrose seeds. It is rich in valuable fatty acids, especially gamma-linolenic acid, which has been shown to help to treat eczema. Other claims remain unproven.

● Ginseng – herbal product obtained from the root of a plant grown in the Far East. Many claims have been made for tonic and therapeutic properties and there is some evidence to suggest that it may stimulate the production of hormones, increase stamina and help to combat some diseases.

● Guarana – an extract from the seeds of an Amazonian shrub. It has been claimed to increase energy, endurance, stamina, vitality and alertness – not surprising, since it contains a caffeine-like substitute.

● Royal jelly – the food of the queen bee, sold in capsules, liquids or with honey. Claims have been made for energy-giving and infection-fighting properties but although an excellent food for bees there is little evidence it can do much for humans.

GARLIC FOR THE HEART

Is it true that garlic is good for your heart, and if so are the capsules sold in health shops as effective as the fresh bulb?

Garlic has long been renowned as one of nature's most effective cure-alls and is among the oldest herbal folk remedies for ailments such as coughs, colds, stomach upsets and sore throats. Modern research also suggests that garlic could be good for your heart.

Garlic helps to keep blood flowing freely by discouraging blood platelets from clumping together. It appears to increase the level of beneficial HDL cholesterol in the blood and to reduce the level of more harmful LDL cholesterol, so helping to keep arteries clear and reducing the risk of heart disease. Garlic also appears to help to reduce high blood pressure and therefore to offer some protection against heart attacks and other circulatory problems such as strokes.

The benefical effects of garlic are largely due to a pungent substance called allicin, which is produced only when fresh garlic is cut, crushed or heated. As allicin loses its potency rapidly, it is better to get your garlic in the fresh form, whether cooked or raw, than to use products such as dried flakes, garlic powder or garlic salt.

Studies indicate that eating between one and three fresh garlic cloves a day provides enough allicin to reduce the risk of a heart attack significantly. These findings seem to be confirmed by the relatively low incidence of heart attacks among people who eat a Mediterranean-style diet (see pages 24-25) that is rich in garlic.

Garlic capsules, which do not release their allicin until they reach the stomach, are a good alternative to fresh garlic if you are worried about bad breath or do not like the flavour of the fresh herb.

CAUTION However good garlic may be for the heart, it cannot work miracles by itself. You still need to eat a healthy diet, take regular exercise and avoid smoking.

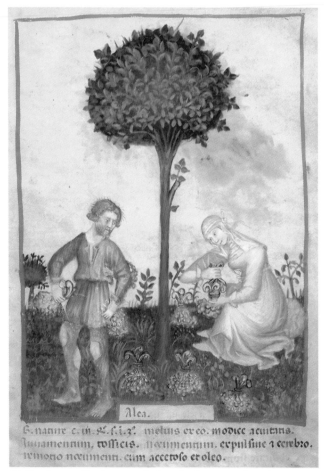

Gathering garlic Centuries before the discovery of antibiotics, or even the germ theory of disease, medieval herbals such as this 14th-century Latin manuscript extolled the virtues of garlic.

CHOOSING THE RIGHT FOODS FOR VITAMINS AND MINERALS

The vitamins and minerals listed here are all important for good health. If your diet is varied, balanced and has adequate calories, you probably do not need to worry about meeting your vitamin and mineral needs. If you are pregnant, have a chronic illness or other condition, or are following a special diet, however, you may need to take supplements. Consult your doctor.

Fat-soluble vitamins are found mainly in oil and fat-containing foods. Since the body stores these vitamins in its fatty tissues, you don't need to eat them every day. Overdosage with supplements can be toxic, so try to make sure you get a good supply from food.

NUTRIENT	GOOD SOURCES		MAIN ROLE
Vitamin A (retinol)	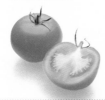	Full-fat dairy produce; liver; kidney; eggs; fish-liver oils. Also formed in the body from beta-carotene in brightly coloured and dark green fruit and vegetables.	Needed for healthy skin, mucous membranes, bones, teeth and hair; vision; and reproduction.
Vitamin D (calciferol)	Manufactured by body when exposed to sunlight. Also found in liver; fish-liver oils and oily fish such as kippers, mackerel, sardines, tuna, tinned salmon; margarine; egg yolk; evaporated milk; full-fat cheese, milk and other dairy products.	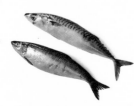	Helps absorption of calcium and phosphorous; needed for bone growth and maintenance.
Vitamin E (tocopherol)	Most foods, but especially vegetable oils, egg yolks, wholegrain cereals, wheat germ, green vegetables, nuts and seeds, margarine.	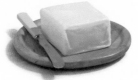	Helps to form red blood cells; acts as an antioxidant.

Water-soluble vitamins are found in a variety of plant and animal foods. Because the body stores them in small amounts and quickly excretes any excess, they need to be part of your diet nearly every day. Cook vegetables carefully (see page 23) – these vitamins are easily lost.

NUTRIENT	GOOD SOURCES		MAIN ROLE
Thiamin (B_1)		Wheat germ and wholegrain cereals, including brown rice; fortified white flour and products; brewer's yeast and yeast extracts; seafood; liver, meat, poultry; pulses; nuts; potatoes; milk.	Needed for nervous system function; helps release energy from carbohydrates.
Riboflavin (B_2)	Liver, kidney, meat, poultry; eggs, cheese, yoghurt; wholegrain cereals; fortified cereals; brewer's yeast and yeast extracts; fish; green vegetables; pulses such as beans and lentils.	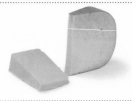	Helps the body to release energy from food.
Niacin (nicotinic acid, B_3)	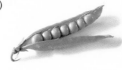	Rice; fortified white flour and products; meat, especially liver and kidney; poultry; yeast extract and brewer's yeast; eggs; fish; nuts; peanuts; cheese; peas, lentils and beans; dried fruit.	Needed for nervous and digestive system functions; helps to release energy from foods; controls blood cholesterol.

NUTRIENT	GOOD SOURCES		MAIN ROLE
Folic acid (folate)	Liver, kidney and other meat; and vegetables; fresh fruit; brewer's yeast/yeast extract; wheat germ; beans and lentils.	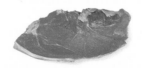	Helps to form red blood cells and genetic material.
B$_{12}$ (cyanocobalamin)	Many foods of animal origin, especially liver, kidney and other meats; fish; egg yolk; dairy products, especially cheese; fortified breakfast cereals.		Helps to form red blood cells, metabolise nutrients and keep nervous system healthy.
C (ascorbic acid)	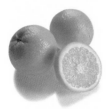 Best raw; fruits and fruit juices, especially citrus fruits and blackcurrants; rose hips and syrup; vegetables, including potatoes; green vegetables and peppers.		Promotes growth, formation and maintenance of bones and teeth, repair of tissues, resistance to infection.

The body needs dozens of minerals and elements for good health, some in relatively large amounts and others in minute quantities. These four are some of the most important to include in your diet. See page 40 for information about some others.

NUTRIENT	GOOD SOURCES		MAIN ROLE
Calcium	Dairy products; hard tap water; fish, and especially sardines, pilchards and other fish whose bones are eaten; leafy greens; fortified cereals, white flour and flour products.		Needed for bone and teeth formation and bone maintenance; plays a role in muscle contraction and clotting of the blood.
Iron	Red meat, especially liver and kidney; beans, peas and lentils; dried apricots and figs; cocoa; bread and cereal products; fortified breakfast cereals; nuts, especially almonds.		Helps to form red blood cells and to transport oxygen in blood and muscles.
Potassium	Most foods, especially fresh fruit; vegetables, including potatoes; meat; wholemeal flour, cereals and products; milk; coffee; tea. Salt substitutes and preservatives.	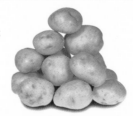	Helps to transmit nerve impulses, control muscle contraction, and maintain proper blood pressure.
Zinc	Most foods, but especially liver and red meat; egg yolk; milk and other dairy produce; wholegrain flour, cereals and products; seafood, particularly oysters.	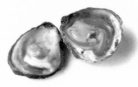	Needed for metabolism and digestion; aids in wound healing, growth, tissue repair and sexual development.

Buying vitamin and mineral supplements

Buying vitamin pills and food supplements is not always easy. Consider these points before you part with your money:

Single or multi supplements?

Unless otherwise advised by your doctor, a multivitamin and mineral supplement is better as some nutrients are absorbed only in the presence of others.

A good supplement should include vitamin A; the B-vitamins thiamin, riboflavin, niacin, pantothenic acid, pyridoxine, vitamin B_{12}, folic acid and biotin; vitamins C, D and E; and the minerals calcium, iron and zinc.

Natural or synthetic?

In most cases, there is no chemical or nutritional difference between natural and synthetic vitamins. The exception is vitamin E, where natural is more potent than synthetic.

Is 'time release' better?

Some supplements are designed to release nutrients over a longer period of time. They are more expensive but there is no proof that slow release makes them any better for you.

Should you buy chelated or 'food state' minerals?

These are combined with amino acids to make them more like minerals in food. They cost more and are supposed to be better absorbed but there is no evidence for this.

FIGHTING ANAEMIA

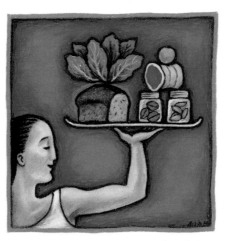

I think I may be anaemic, as I often feel tired and I suffer from heavy periods. Would iron pills help?

Iron pills could help you, but it is essential to talk to your doctor first to have a proper diagnosis. Your GP may give you a blood test to establish why you feel so tired. As you are having heavy periods, it is possible that you are losing more iron each month than you are able to absorb from your normal diet. However, there are a number of different types of anaemia and only one caused by iron deficiency. Even if this is what you have, it is advisable to get a doctor's recommendation before taking iron supplements as high doses can sometimes cause side effects.

Even if your doctor recommends you take supplements, it is still important to eat foods that are rich in iron. The body absorbs iron from red meat much more easily than from non-meat sources such as pulses, wholemeal bread, wholegrain breakfast cereals, dried fruit, nuts and dark green leafy vegetables. Absorption is improved, however, if you eat these foods with a source of vitamin C, such as tomatoes, potatoes, sweet peppers and citrus fruit or juice. It might also be worth cutting down on tea and coffee, which can reduce the absorption of non-meat iron if drunk with a meal, or just before or after.

WHEN TO TAKE A SUPPLEMENT

Is it better to take supplements with food or on their own – or doesn't it matter?

Supplements are generally better absorbed when they are taken with food. Many people also find it easier to remember to take them with a meal – usually breakfast. Ideally the fat-soluble vitamins A, D, E and K should be taken with fat – which, in practice, means at almost any meal. Otherwise there is no need for any special measures, except perhaps to avoid taking supplements with bran and other concentrated forms of fibre, which can hinder absorption – see page 22.

PROTECTING YOUR BONES

Although I'm only 25, I worry about developing osteoporosis, as both my mother and aunt suffer from the disease. Could taking calcium supplements help to prevent trouble in later life?

There is no guarantee that any special diet or supplements will stop you developing osteoporosis – but ensuring an adequate intake of calcium throughout your life will help to reduce the risk.

A calcium-rich diet is particularly important during childhood, adolesence and early adulthood in order to establish an optimal peak bone mass (PBM). A low intake of dietary calcium may result in a lower PBM and increase the risk of developing osteoporosis later on in life. After PMB has been reached (between the ages of 30 to 40 years), it is still important to consume enough calcium to keep the bones strong and to slow down the inevitable losses that age brings. The best food sources of calcium are milk, cheese and yoghurt but useful amounts are also found in green leafy vegetables such as spinach and broccoli, canned fish with soft edible bones (such as salmon and sardines), beans and lentils, enriched white bread and flour, dried figs, and many types of nuts and seeds.

It is also important to make sure you get enough vitamin D, which helps the body to absorb and make use of calcium efficiently. Sources of vitamin D include fortified margarines and cereals, oily fish and eggs.

Being physically active, however, can have a far greater effect on bone strength than changing your diet is likely to. During adolescence and early adulthood, regular exercise can actually increase peak bone mass. After PBM has been achieved, exercise can protect against loss of bone mass. Weight bearing exercises such as brisk walking, running, aerobics classes, dancing, weight training and racquet sports are best. Studies have shown that even a daily half-hour walk will have a measurable effect.

CAUTION Smoking increases the risk of osteoporosis. If you smoke, take steps to stop now (see page 157).

The drinks in your diet

WATER FOR HEALTH

How much water should you drink each day? Does the water contained in tea and coffee count?

There are currently no official guidelines for the amount of water we should drink, but most people would probably benefit from drinking a little more. Individual needs vary, but as a rough indication, moderately active adults will need at least 3½ pints (2 litres) of water every day. Drink more water in hot weather and when you exercise to replace liquids lost through sweat. The rule of thumb is an extra 1¾ pints (1 litre) of water for every hour of exercise.

British tea-drinking habits provide many people with their main fluid intake. However, it is healthier to drink tap or bottled water rather than downing endless cups of tea or coffee, because the caffeine in these drinks makes you urinate more frequently, counteracting the beneficial effects of drinking extra fluids.

The simplest way to judge whether or not you are drinking enough water, is to check your urine: it should be a pale lemon yellow. If it is dark gold, you probably need to drink more. Note, however, that vitamin supplements with riboflavin will turn your urine bright yellow – this is completely normal.

CAUTION As people grow older their response to thirst diminishes and the danger of dehydration increases. Signs to watch for include dry lips and skin, thirst, infrequent urination, confusion and high temperature. To prevent dehydration, have at least one cup of fluid every two hours.

A raging thirst, frequent urination and continual fatigue are symptoms of diabetes. Consult a doctor if they occur.

CHOOSING FRUIT JUICE

I'm confused by all the different types of fruit juice on sale. What is the difference between more expensive freshly squeezed juices and others?

Any product labelled 'fruit juice' must, by law, contain 100 per cent fruit juice. Freshly squeezed juice must come straight from the pressed fruit. It has the highest vitamin content compared with other types of fruit juice and has to be kept at 5°C (41°F) or less to preserve the vitamins. Since it has not been concentrated or heat-treated, it has the best taste. It will usually keep for five days (two once opened), but check the 'use by' date.

Reconstituted chilled juice
Other types of chilled fruit juice sold in cartons or plastic bottles are usually made from reconstituted concentrated fruit juice. The concentrate is produced by evaporating some of the water from fresh juice, reducing the bulk and making transport easier and cheaper. Once the concentrate arrives at its destination, manufacturers dilute it to original strength and package it. The process is less costly than producing freshly squeezed juice but there is a slight deterioration in both vitamin content and flavour. Reconstituted juice keeps refrigerated and unopened for seven to ten days (check the datemark) and for three to four days once opened.

Long life or UHT juice
These non-refrigerated juices are also made from reconstituted concentrate. The juice is heated above boiling point for a few seconds, and packed in cartons. It will keep at room temperature for several months – check the 'best before' date. Keep refrigerated after opening and use within five days. Long-life juice is cheaper than chilled reconstituted juice and has similar vitamin C content.

Fruit drinks
So called fruit 'drinks' may contain many ingredients and are usually only 5 to 10 per cent juice. The rest is water, sugar, flavouring and colourings. The label does not have to specify the actual fruit juice content. The sugar and calorie content is usually about the same as that of the juice from which the drink is made.

Points to remember
All fruit juices have the potential to cause tooth decay, but you can reduce the danger by choosing juices with lower sugar content and drinking them with meals. Avoid giving sweetened or acidic drinks to children.

Also bear in mind that eating whole fruit is better than drinking juice. It is safer for your teeth, provides more fibre and contains bioflavonoids that aid vitamin C absorption.

**DO'S
—— AND ——
DON'TS**

for mineral water

Do drink mineral water only if you prefer the taste – it is no healthier than tap water.

Do treat mineral water as a perishable food. Check the use-by date, store it in the fridge and drink it within three or four days of opening. Bacteria levels build up once it is opened.

Do ask your doctor's advice about bottled water if you are on a low-salt diet. Some types are high in sodium.

Don't leave bottles of mineral water in direct sunlight. Light and heat can encourage bacteria and algae to grow.

Don't regularly give water with more than 1.0 mg of fluoride per litre to children, as it may harm their teeth.

THE TRUTH ABOUT TEA

Is there any reason to limit the number of cups of tea that I drink during the day?

The main reason to restrict your intake of tea is the same as for coffee: the caffeine content of these drinks is high, and large doses of caffeine can adversely affect health (see below). Up to six cups of tea or coffee per day is considered a safe intake and is unlikely to have any harmful consequences.

Note that tea contains less caffeine than coffee – approximately 40 mg in a cup compared with 60-80 mg in coffee; even a strong cup of tea will seldom contain more than 60-80 mg of caffeine.

Tea also contains tannin, which in high doses (for example from two or more cups in one go) can reduce absorption of iron from non-meat sources. If you need to get more iron from vegetable sources such as pulses and cereals, wait a while before drinking tea. Tannin does have its good side, however. It is

an antioxidant (see pages 40-41), so it seems that tea might reduce the risk of various diseases, and could even, as some studies have suggested, help to prevent heart attacks.

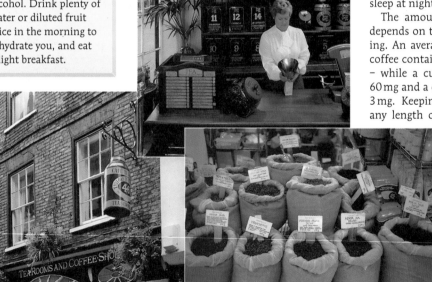

Social drinking Tea and coffee are an integral part of our culture and social life, and specialist dealers (above) and teashops (left) do a thriving trade. Provided your intake is reasonable, neither drink is a risk to your health.

CONCERN ABOUT COFFEE

I enjoy two or three cups of coffee a day, but wonder if this is unhealthy for me. Should I try to give it up?

You'll be glad to know that two or three cups of coffee in a day will not do you any harm. Around four cups per day is considered by nutritionists to be a moderate amount, and research suggests that even as many as six cups is probably quite safe. That said, larger amounts may have some health effects.

Caffeine
Coffee contains caffeine, which is a mild stimulant. The amount in a couple of cups of coffee has been shown to improve mental alertness, concentration, reasoning, reaction time and memory. Caffeine is also found in tea, cola drinks, cocoa and chocolate. Some people are more sensitive to the effects than others, and find that too much caffeine can make them feel anxious, restless or unable to sleep at night.

The amount of caffeine you are getting depends on the type of coffee you are drinking. An average cup of freshly ground filter coffee contains most caffeine – about 80 mg – while a cup of instant coffee has about 60 mg and a cup of decaffeinated coffee only 3 mg. Keeping percolated coffee warm for any length of time will not affect the caffeine content or strength of the beverage as is sometimes supposed, but the flavour is likely to deteriorate significantly and become bitter.

Other health concerns
A considerable amount of research has been carried out into the effects of coffee on health. According to one unproven theory coffee can raise the blood cholesterol level and increase the risk of heart disease. The main focus of concern is on Scandinavian-style coffee-making methods that involve long periods of boiling without filtering afterwards.

Claims that coffee may contribute to causing cancer of the pancreas, breast or colon have not been proved either. In several studies, the subjects were also heavy smokers, so any increased risk of cancer was more likely due to smoking than to coffee drinking.

Pregnant women are sometimes advised to avoid coffee, to reduce any risk of miscarriage or retarded foetal growth. But cutting out caffeine altogether is not essential, says the Royal College of Midwives; they advise a mother-to-be simply to cut down.

Some people who suffer from heart palpitations also choose to avoid coffee although there is little real evidence that it can cause or exacerbate the problem.

Coffee is not addictive, as often claimed. But giving it up abruptly can cause symptoms such as irritability and headaches. If you want to cut down, do it gradually.

COFFEE WITHOUT CAFFEINE

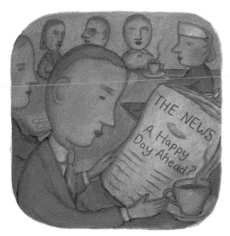

Is it true that some decaffeinated coffees contain harmful chemical residues?

This is not really a problem any longer. The chemical that caused all the concern in the early 1980s was the solvent methylene chloride, which was used during the process of removing the caffeine from coffee. Methylene chloride has been linked with cancer in some research studies, but although European leglisation still permits its use at what is considered to be a safe level, it is in fact rarely used nowadays for decaffeination.

In Britain most coffee manufacturers now use either liquid carbon dioxide or steam to remove caffeine from beans. Neither process involves harmful chemicals.

The European Union imposes strict limits on the level of permitted residues in decaffeinated coffee, so products offered for sale will contain only very small amounts – often none at all. The label will not tell you which method of decaffeination was used, but you can take it that all are now perfectly safe.

HERBAL AND FRUIT TEAS

Are herbal and fruit teas safe to drink, or can there be any side effects?

The herbal and fruit teabags sold in supermarkets and health shops are generally considered to be safe, and a good alternative to caffeine-containing tea and coffee. Always treat herbal preparations with respect, and don't forget that herbs have powerful medicinal properties. Apart from mild infusions of well-tried herbs such as those on pages 42-43, don't try to dose yourself medicinally.

Most people who buy herbal and fruit teas do so for the taste and for the beneficial properties traditionally ascribed to plants such as mint and camomile. Herbs owe their health properties and flavour to the essential oils they contain. Most of the herbs used in teas are of medicinal grade and have had to pass rigorous quality and safety tests. However, the essential oil content can vary considerably from brand to brand, and there is no legal minimum requirement. Always buy herbal teas from a reputable supplier.

Pregnant women are usually advised to avoid herbal teas, with the exception of peppermint, lime and camomile – said by some actually to relieve morning sickness.

WINE ADDITIVES

I know that winemakers use different additives in the fermenting process. How can I tell exactly what I'm drinking?

You can't. Current European legislation permits 27 different additives in wine without requiring any to be listed on the label. The additives include preservatives, and processing aids such as gelatine and isinglass which are used to clarify wines, but not colourings. Cheaper wines generally contain more additives than expensive and traditional wines.

Preservatives and antioxidants are often used to prolong the shelf life of a wine. The most common chemicals added are sulphur dioxide (E220) and potassium metabisulphite (E224), which helps to prevent the wine from browning, stops bacterial growth, stabilises the colour and prevents the wine from going bad (oxidising).

In some asthma sufferers, sulphites can provoke attacks of wheezing. It is possible to exceed the acceptable daily amount of sulphur dioxide after just a few glasses of wine. These additives have to be declared on the label in the United States and some other countries, but not in Britain and Europe.

Coffee substitutes

As well as decaffeinated tea and coffee, and herbal and fruit teas, there are several beverages available that don't contain caffeine. They come in the form of granules, powders and extracts and are all low in calories and fat, with only very small amounts of other nutrients. It may take you a little while to get used to the taste of some.

● Dandelion – this coffee-like compound is made from dried and roasted dandelion roots. Some brands have lactose (milk sugar) and flavouring added to improve the taste and texture.

● Chicory – the chicory root is split, cut, dried and roasted for coffee-style drinks. Brands such as Bamba also add dried figs, wheat, barley or acorns to the mixture.

● Cereals – a variety of roasted cereal grains can be used to make drinks such as Barley cup (barley, rye and chicory), Postum (bran, wheat molasses and maltodextrins) and Caro Extra (barley, malted barley and chicory).

● Vegetable extract and yeast extract drinks – these are fortified with B vitamins and are useful for vegans because they contain vitamin B_{12} (not available from any plant food). Some are high in salt.

● Meat extracts – some brands are fortified with folic acid, which is recommended in pregnancy.

ALCOHOL AS A FOOD

I've heard that alcoholic drinks used to be given as food supplements. Does this mean that they are a good food source?

No, though alcoholic drinks *were* once used by doctors to supplement the diet of certain patients unable to eat a normal healthy diet. Modern dietary supplements are far more suitable. Alcoholic drinks are rich in calories, but they are 'empty' calories – all that they provide is an easily accessible energy source for a short period of time.

Some alcoholic drinks contain traces of vitamins and minerals: wine contains the B vitamins niacin and riboflavin, and the minerals iron, calcium and potassium; beers and stout contain some B vitamins, iron and potassium. But they hardly count as foods.

Eating out and prepared meals

Terms to watch out for if you wish to avoid fatty foods

Á la crème – served with a cream sauce.
Alfredo – with a cheese, cream and egg sauce.
Au gratin – sprinkled with a mixture of cheese and breadcrumbs.
Béarnaise – served in a creamy sauce.
Béchamel – in white sauce made with butter, flour and milk.
En croute – cooked in a pastry case.
Florentine – with spinach in a white sauce with cheese.
Hollandaise – in a rich buttery sauce.
Sautéed – pan-fried.

HEALTHY DINING CHOICES

My wife and I love eating out, but we're trying to cut down on fats. Which dishes should we choose?

There is certainly no need to deprive yourselves of the pleasures of eating out. Most restaurants offer dishes that are low in fat, even if they are not labelled as such.

For a starter, choose a fruit or vegetable dish (for example, grapefruit, melon or crudités), smoked salmon, parma ham, or clear plain soups such as vegetable, minestrone or chicken and sweetcorn consommé. Avoid any very creamy soups and dishes with rich, oily dressings. With your main course, include some jacket, boiled or new potatoes; boiled or steamed rice; boiled noodles; or pasta. Order lots of vegetables (without butter) or salads (without high-fat dressings). Choose grilled or roasted lean meats, or grilled or poached fish. Avoid battered foods, anything cooked in breadcrumbs and thick or buttery sauces. If you are having pasta, choose a tomato sauce rather than creamy or cheese–based one. Here are some additional tips for particular types of restaurants:

● In a Chinese restaurant, order several vegetable dishes and a little meat, chicken, tofu or seafood to go with some rice or noodles. Stir-fried dishes are low-fat. Avoid duck and spare ribs, which are usually fatty, and any battered or deep-fried dishes – the word 'crispy' on the menu is a warning sign.
● In an Indian restaurant choose dishes based on vegetables, rice and pulses such as lentils and chickpeas. Other good choices include chapattis, tandoori chicken or chicken tikka. Avoid dishes made with a lot of ghee (clarified butter), or with coconut, cream or oil – ask your waiter's advice.
● In an Italian restaurant, pasta with lightly cooked vegetables, chicken or fish makes a good choice. Ask the waiter if low-fat pasta dishes are available. Avoid sauces with cheese, cream and fatty mince – all high in saturated fat. Pizza can be high in fat and very salty, especially if topped with anchovies and olives. Tuna, prawns and vegetables are the best choices for toppings.

SELECTING A SANDWICH BAR

I've heard that some sandwich bars are not as hygienic as they should be. How can I tell if the food is safe?

Unfortunately, it is impossible to tell if food is safe just by looking at it. The reliability of sandwiches and other ready-to-eat takeaway foods depends largely on good standards of hygiene during preparation, and on a safe storage temperature – aspects that consumers cannot monitor. Here are some tips and

Eat out in good health If you embark on a new healthy diet there is no need to give up eating out. Apart from special health-food establishments, many ordinary restaurants have healthier options on their menus, such as salads and pasta.

guidelines to help you to judge the level of hygiene when you next visit a sandwich bar:

● Ready-made sandwiches should be wrapped and labelled with a 'use-by' date. They should be kept refrigerated.
● Fillings for made-to-order sandwiches should be moist and fresh and kept in a refrigerated cabinet or display counter.
● Staff should avoid touching food by hand as far as possible. Many hygiene-minded caterers wear thin protective gloves and use spoons or tongs.
● Food handlers should have their hair tied back and preferably covered completely.
● Crumbs and spilled sandwich fillings should be cleared up quickly.
● When new fillings are needed, a fresh container should be brought in. New food should not be tipped on top of what is left.

QUICK NUTRITIOUS MEALS

I don't have the time to cook after work in the evenings, and I often rely on ready-made meals. Will these give me all of the nutrients that I need?

Fortunately, it is possible to base a healthy diet on convenience meals – provided that you also eat fresh or frozen vegetables and salads, and plenty of fruit as snacks. Many supermarkets sell bags of ready-washed salad leaves and chopped vegetables all year round – all you have to do is toss them in a little olive oil or a low-fat dressing for a quick, light meal.

Bear in mind that although ready-made meals may be convenient, many are high in salt, low in fibre and low in energy-giving carbohydrates. Many varieties are also high in fat, including harmful saturates, so check the label. They also tend to be much more expensive than similar homemade meals. 'Slimmer' meals are often meagre and unsatisfying – the lower calorie count is often simply the result of a small portion size.

Try not to depend on ready meals. Instead, cook abundant dishes and freeze them in handy portions. Jacket potatoes can also be frozen if you wrap them in foil. Consider investing in a microwave oven – it will cook potatoes and other vegetables in minutes.

There are also many meals you can make for yourself in less time than it would take to heat up a ready-made dish:

● Baked beans on toast.
● Jacket potato with cottage cheese, baked beans, tuna, reheated chicken or salad.

● Pasta with ready-made sauce, or with your own sauce, made by mixing together tomato purée, red wine and seasoning, with tinned tuna or frozen vegetables added to make it more substantial.
● Scrambled or poached eggs, or an omelette, with salad or vegetables.
● Pilchards or sardines on toast.
● Low-fat or tofu burgers with salad and potatoes or low-fat oven chips.

FAST FOODS FOR CHILDREN

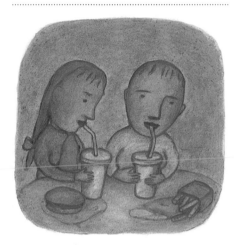

My children love fast-food restaurants. Is there really any harm in letting them have burgers and pizzas if that is what they would like to eat?

There is no harm in indulging your children from time to time, as long as you set healthy eating standards at home. Fast foods such as burgers, pizzas and sausages are generally high in fat, and high-fat foods need to be balanced by starchy foods such as potatoes, rice, pasta and bread.

When at home, try to make sure that your children have the opportunity to sample and enjoy main meals that are relatively low in fat, such as roast chicken served without skin, lean ham and lean roast pork. Mashed potatoes, pasta, toast soldiers and bread fingers add valuable starch and no extra fat. Serve with plenty of vegetables and salads. Children particularly like crunchy sticks of carrots, cucumber and other vegetables.

If your children demand burgers at home, consider using lean mince mixed with beans, lentils, or bread crumbs. In this way, you can make a burger that provides an excellent basis for a healthy meal. A really simple way to cut down on fat is to oven-bake or grill foods that you normally fry, such as burgers, sausages and fish fingers.

Some points to look for in a healthy and hygienic salad bar

● Fresh salads should look moist and crisp. Limp lettuce leaves or slightly dry slices of tomato are unlikely to give you food poisoning, but they do suggest that a restaurant is not taking as much care of its food as it should.
● The salads should be kept on a refrigerated counter, or the food bowls surrounded by broken ice.
● Every bowl should have its own serving spoon or tongs with long handles, to prevent customers' hands or sleeves from contaminating the food.
● All salad bars should have a glass panel (called a 'sneeze screen') in front of them to protect the food from customers' breath as they serve themselves.

Processing and packaging

IRRADIATED FOOD

I read a while ago about plans to introduce irradiated fruits and vegetables to Britain. Are they now on the shelves?

Irradiated foods were introduced in Britain in 1990. Irradiation is permitted by law on a wide variety of foods, including vegetables, fish, shellfish, cereals, and herbs and spices. However, these are not yet widely available, since most food companies and retailers do not wish to use irradiation.

Even though irradiated foods have been exposed to a radioactive source (in a process similar to having a medical X-ray), they are not at all radioactive themselves. Research has shown that irradiated foods are safe for consumption: in spite of the view of some scientists, who argue that high irradiation doses cause chemical changes in the food and could form cancer-causing substances, there is so far no convincing evidence that irradiation will affect long-term health.

The effect that mild irradiation has on the flavour or appearance of the food itself is somewhat more controversial. Slight chemical changes risk producing a pulpy texture in cucumbers, for example, or an off taste in high-fat foods. Irradiation can also cause a small loss of nutrients – though no greater than in many other processes.

In its favour, however, irradiation is an effective way of killing any bacteria, insects and moulds, so reducing the risk of food poisoning and the need for chemicals in food production. It can also prolong shelf life by delaying the ripening of fruit and vegetables and the sprouting of onions and potatoes. By enabling produce to stay fresh for so much longer, irradiation reduces the need for preservatives and other additives.

All foods and ingredients that have been irradiated are obliged by law to be labelled 'irradiated' or 'treated by ionisation'.

BUYING DENTED CANS

My local supermarket reduces the price of dented cans. Are the contents safe to eat?

The only completely safe policy is to avoid all damaged cans. Although moderate denting will not necessarily create a health risk, all cans have a lacquered inside surface which can be damaged by denting. As a result food may come into contact with metal, causing tainting (especially if the food is acidic). In addition, if seals on the top, bottom or sides are damaged they can provide an entry route for air and bacteria. Never eat the contents – take the can back and exchange it. The seller needs to improve checking procedures.

CAUTION Never try to open a 'blown' or bulging can, and be careful not to drop it. The contents are under pressure and the can could burst. Dispose of it immediately.

GENETIC ENGINEERING

What exactly is meant by genetically engineered food? Is it widely available and is it harmful to eat?

Genetic engineering is the manipulation of animal or plant genes to produce new characteristics in food products. There are two types of genetic engineering.

The first involves within-species breeding of animals or plants. For example, by identifying the relevant genes, scientists can help farmers to breed leaner livestock or are able to devise ways to develop crops that need less fertiliser, survive better in droughts or are more resistant to disease.

The second type of genetic engineering is the transferal of genes from one species to another. Sweeter-tasting tomatoes have been created by introducing the genes from a sweet berry grown on the Ivory Coast. It is also possible to transplant genes from animals to plants. Frost-resistant tomatoes have been developed by inserting an 'antifreeze' gene from the Arctic flounder fish!

Two genetically engineered 'foods' are at present available in UK shops – an enzyme used in the production of vegetarian cheese in place of animal-derived rennet, and a modified baker's yeast for bread-making.

Genetic engineering is still a fairly new process and is carefully controlled, although how safe the foods developed by this process are is still not certain. The Ministry of Agriculture, Fisheries and Food (MAFF) assures consumers that such products are safe and believes it would be unrealistic to label every food produced with genetic modification. As yet, no British or European directive exists requiring this type of labelling.

DO YOU KNOW WHAT A FOOD LABEL IS TELLING YOU?

To protect consumers – from both allergic reactions and false claims – regulations are now strictly enforced to ensure accurate and helpful information on packaged foods. In most cases ingredients have to be listed (dairy products and alcoholic drinks are notable exceptions), as well as additives. Labelling must also include a datemark and the weight. A nutritional breakdown need only be given if the manufacturer makes a special claim (such as 'low calorie') about the product.

MUESLI

INGREDIENTS
Wheatflakes, raisins, oatflakes, dates, sultanas, barley kernels, almonds, brazil nuts, roast hazelnuts, toasted coconut, pumpkin seeds, malt extract

NUTRITION INFORMATION
TYPICAL VALUES AS SOLD

	PER 100g	PER 60g SERVING
Energy	1499 kJ	900 kJ
	355kcal	213kcal
Protein	8.0g	4.8g
Carbohydrate	64.7g	38.8g
of which sugars	28.2g	16.9g
Fat	7.1g	4.3g
of which saturates	2.0g	1.2g
Fibre	6.1g	3.7g
Sodium	trace	trace

High in Fibre

500g ℮

Best before end
DEC 95 14615

Product name or description
The terms used must clearly identify what the product is, be accurate and mention any processing it has been subjected to, such as smoking, pickling, drying or ultra-heat treatment.

Ingredients
The ingredients are listed in descending order of weight. In this muesli, there is most wheat and least malt. Apart from food ingredients, labels must identify additives – substances not normally counted as food. Most additives fall into these categories:

ANTIOXIDANTS These prevent fats and oils from going rancid, and fruit juice turning brown.

COLOURINGS Artificial colours are added to thousands of food products including yoghurts, jams, drinks and processed foods such as tinned peas.

EMULSIFIERS The use of emulsifiers allows fats to blended smoothly with water to make products such as margarine, ice cream and chocolate.

FLAVOURINGS Flavourings can be added to improve the taste of bland food or to restore flavour lost in processing. Thousands of flavourings are permitted and do not have to be individually identified on the label.

PRESERVATIVES These are added to prevent bacteria and moulds from growing on food. They are used particularly in bacon, dried fruit, dairy desserts and soft drinks.

STABILISERS Pectin and similar substances prevent runny foods such as yoghurt from separating.

THICKENERS A wide variety of ingredients is used to improve the consistency of foods such as soups, sauces and pies. Modified starch and guar gum are two of the commonest.

Nutritional information
If the product makes a claim such as 'low in fat' or 'high-fibre', the manufacturer must declare the energy, protein, sugar, carbohydrate, fat, fibre, saturated fat, and sodium content as well as that of any other nutrient for which a claim is made. This is to protect consumers from being misled – a product that advertises that it is 'rich in vitamin C' may also have a high sugar content, for example. The figures are given per 3½oz (100g), and also often per serving (in which case the serving size must be identified).

If no claim is made, the manufacturer need not give any nutritional information. But if it is voluntarily given, the label must list energy, protein, carbohydrate and fat content.

Weight
All packages must show the weight of their contents. The 'e' indicates that the weight is an average per pack, so it may not be the exact weight of that particular pack.

Datemarks
The 'best before' date is for foods that do not actually go bad but that might lose flavour or texture over time. The 'use by' date is placed on foods that could become harmful with time. It is illegal to sell food after the 'use by' date. Both dates are calculated on the assumption that the food has been correctly stored. Any special storage requirements, such as refrigeration, should also appear.

FOOD ADDITIVES THAT CAN CAUSE TROUBLE

Legally permitted food additives have all undergone stringent safety testing and are generally considered very safe although, of course, it is impossible to test a food for 20 or 30 years of daily intake so long-term effects are less well known. People with allergies or conditions such as asthma may be advised to stay away from some additives. Use the chart below as a guide.

▲ – May increase hyperactivity in affected children.

■ – Asthmatics sometimes react badly.

● – Take care if you are sensitive to aspirin.

▼ – Be cautious if you suffer from allergies or intolerances.

★ – May not be suitable for babies.

ADDITIVE	FUNCTION AND USES
E102 Tartrazine ▲ ■ ●	Yellow/orange colour very widely used in drinks, cakes, biscuits, puddings, meat products, smoked cod and haddock, sauces, confectionery, snacks.
E104 Quinoline yellow ▲	Greenish-yellow colour used especially in smoked fish and Scotch eggs.
E110 Sunset yellow ▲ ●	Yellow colour used in chocolate and orange drinks, packet soups and desserts, biscuits, breadcrumbs and preserves.
E120 Cochineal ▲	Natural red colour from dried insects and egg yolk. There is a synthetic form used in confectionery and cakes.
E122 Carmoisine ▲ ■ ●	Reddish-purple colour used in raspberry drinks, jam, desserts and sauces, and in brown sauces and packet soups.
E123 Amaranth ▲ ●	Red colour used in drinks, fruit-pie fillings, jellies, cakes, puddings, packet soups, gravy mixes and beefburgers.
E124 Poncea ▲ ■ ●	Red colour used in meat pastes, tomato soup, strawberry products such as pie filling, jellies and puddings, and in cake mixes.
E127 Erythrosine ▲	Red colour used in glacé cherries, tinned fruits, packet desserts, biscuits, ham and pork products and some potato snacks. It is also used in tablets to reveal plaque on teeth.
128 Red 2G ▲	Red colour used in pork pies, sausages and other meat products.
E131 Patent blue V ▲ ■ ● ▼	Violet-blue colour used especially in Scotch eggs and canned vegetables.

ADDITIVE	FUNCTION AND USES
E132 Indigo carmine ▲ ■ ● ▼	Blue colour used in meat products and gravy mixes.
133 Brilliant blue ▲	Blue colour used mainly in bacon-flavoured snacks and tinned peas.
E151 Black PN ▲	Black colour used in fruit sauces and in cheesecake mixes.
E153 Carbon black or vegetable carbon ▲ ▼	Black colour from burnt vegetable matter used in juices, jams, jellies and brown sauce.
E154 Brown FK ▲ ▼	Brown colour used in kippers and other smoked fish.
155 Chocolate brown HT ▲ ■ ● ▼	Brown colour used in a wide range of processed foods.
E210-E219 Benzoic acid and its derivatives ▲ ■ ▼	Benzoic acid occurs naturally in teas and raspberries, but is made synthetically for use in the food industry. Together with various derivatives it is used in a wide range of foods including fruit products, pickles, marinated fish, salad dressings, beer and coffee essence. Also used as an antioxidant.
E320 Butylated hydroxyanisole (BHA) ▲ ■ ▼ ★	Antioxidant used in raisins, potato snacks, margarines, biscuits, breakfast cereals, pastry, sweets, bottled sauces, ice creams, soft drinks and prepared fried foods.
E321 Butylated hydroxytoluene (BHT) ▲ ■ ● ▼ ★	Antioxidant similar in use to E320.
E413 Tragacanth ▼	Emulsifier, thickener and stabiliser extracted from the gum in the trunks of certain *Astralagus* trees. Used in processed cheeses, cake decorations, sherbet and salad dressings.

Food hygiene and safety

PROBLEM IN PERSPECTIVE

Is 'food poisoning' rather a grand name for an ordinary stomach upset, or is it really more serious?

Food poisoning takes many forms. It can be a mild digestive upset that makes you feel a little 'off colour', or it can be a very unpleasant illness that could land you in hospital. In some instances, food poisoning can even be fatal. It is caused by consuming food or drink that has been contaminated by germs (harmful bacteria or viruses), or by toxins (poisons) produced by bacteria or the foods themselves, or by chemicals.

The symptoms vary from case to case but usually include abdominal pain, nausea, vomiting and diarrhoea. Other symptoms include headache, fever and aching joints. You can start to feel ill just a few hours after eating contaminated food or many days later – and the illness can last from one day to a week, or sometimes even longer.

RECOVERING FROM SICKNESS

What should you do if you think you may have contracted food poisoning?

If you are only slightly ill, drink plenty of fluids and avoid eating until you feel better. See your doctor if the illness continues more than a day or you feel worse. If you are violently sick or have serious diarrhoea, see a doctor as soon as possible.

In most cases, it is a sensible precaution to stay away from work until you are fully recovered. To prevent spreading the infection, avoid preparing food for other people. Until you are better, don't dry yourself on towels used by other members of your household. If your job involves working with food in any way, it is illegal to go to work until a doctor has given you the all clear.

Your doctor will automatically report any cases of food poisoning to the local council's environmental health department. You can report your illness to the department yourself if you prefer. Environmental health officers (EHOs) have wide powers to investigate any infection that seems to be linked to a particular food, shop or restaurant, to insist on changes that affect hygiene, and to take unhygienic companies to court.

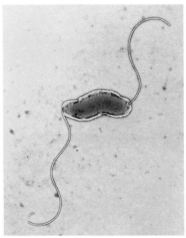

Campylobacter jejuni These germs are the commonest cause of diarrhoea and other gastric symptoms in Britain.

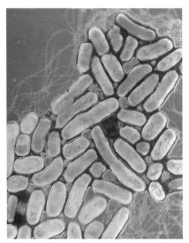

Salmonella Poultry contaminated by salmonella causes many cases of food poisoning. Eggs can also be affected.

DATE MARKS FOR FRESHNESS

My brother is convinced that 'use by' dates are a sales ploy to make consumers buy more food. Is he right, or is it dangerous to eat food after it has passed it 'use by' date?

Far from being a sales trick, 'use by' dates are a legal requirement for many foods, to protect the public from food poisoning. Most foods that deteriorate quickly must by law be marked with a 'use by' date. They include packed fresh poultry, meat and fish; cooked meat, fish and poultry; prepared meals and salads; pâté and soft cheeses. You would run a high risk of food poisoning if you decided to eat or drink food that has gone past its 'use by' date, even if it looked, smelled and tasted all right. Do remember too that date marks are reliable only if you also follow any storage instructions on the packaging.

Foods that have a longer shelf life, such as butter, cake, bread, dried fruit and canned foods, are labelled with a 'best before' date indicating the period when the food will be in ideal condition. Some foods may remain safe to eat, even if they have become rather stale or soggy, when they are older than their 'best before' date. The Food Safety Advisory Centre recommends you check that a date-expired food looks and smells wholesome: if you have any doubt, throw it out.

In addition, a 'display until' mark is used voluntarily by some food retailers to help to

The danger zone

The bacteria that cause food poisoning grow easily at temperatures between 5°C and 63°C (41°F and 145°F), so a golden rule of food hygiene is to keep highly perishable food out of this temperature danger zone as far as possible. A refrigerator should run at between 1°C and 4°C (34°F and 39°F) to slow down bacterial growth. However, even in freezers at about -18°C (-1°F) not all bacteria die and they rapidly multiply as soon as the food begins to thaw – so food should be thawed quickly to keep it out of the danger zone. Bacteria start to die at temperatures warmer than 63°C (145°F): few bacteria survive when food is cooked thoroughly at 75°C (167°F) or hotter.

ensure that only the freshest food is offered for sale. If a product has a 'display until' date as well as a 'use by' date, you can safely keep and eat it until the expiry of the 'use by' date.

NATURAL TOXINS IN FOOD

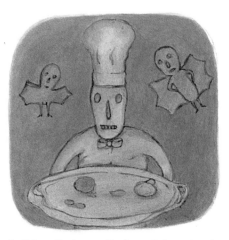

Is it true that some foods contain natural poisons? If so, which ones should I avoid?

Some plants and foods from other sources do naturally contain traces of poisons, called toxins, that can make us ill, or even cause death, if eaten in excess. However, it is usually easy to avoid the risk.

When potatoes sprout, they produce a bitter tasting natural chemical, called solanine, that can cause abdominal pains, diarrhoea and in some rare cases even death. The Food Advisory Safety Centre advises against eating green or sprouting potatoes.

Although rhubarb and spinach are both excellent foods and can safely be eaten once or twice a week by most people, those with kidney stones would be wise to avoid them because of high levels of oxalic acid, which can aggravate the problem. Rhubarb is also a mild laxative – you will probably know if you are eating too much of it.

Red kidney beans are safe only if soaked for five hours, then boiled vigorously for 10 minutes in clean (unsalted) water and simmered until soft (a further 1-1½ hours). If not cooked properly, they can damage red blood cells. Canned beans are ready-cooked.

If you enjoy picking mushrooms, learn to recognise the types that could make you ill. The death cap fungus kills more than half the people who unwittingly eat it. Don't eat any nuts sold as bird feed. They could be contaminated by poisonous mould called aflatoxin. Seafood can also be risky – follow the safety precautions on pages 32-33.

Keeping food covered

All food should be covered to prevent contamination and to loss of natural food moisture.

● Glass, ceramic and plastic are good for storing most foods: ensure that the container is scrupulously clean.
● Greaseproof paper and waxed paper make useful coverings, especially for wrapping fatty foods, such as cheese.
● Paper is good for storing mushrooms.
● Aluminium foil is safe for all but extremely acidic foods.

TO DRY UP OR NOT

When washing up, I always dry the dishes and put them away, but my daughters say I should rinse the dishes and leave them to drain. Is their suggestion more hygienic?

Yes, their suggestions are best for hygiene - even though you have probably come to no harm by following your own method.

After washing up, rinse all utensils, crockery and cutlery in clean hot water to get rid of invisible traces of food that could nourish germs. Hygiene specialists say it is preferable to leave dishes to drain on a clean draining board or draining rack because tea towels quickly collect microscopic particles of food which are transferred to other plates and utensils, and can evenutally cause food poisoning. If you rinse everything in hot water, your washing up could be dry in less than one minute – saving you time and effort as well as improving hygiene in your kitchen.

However, if you still prefer to dry your dishes by hand, do rinse them in very hot water first, and use a clean tea towel for every new batch of washing up. Replace the tea towel as soon as it starts to feel damp or greasy, and at the end of each day.

CHOPPING BOARD PERILS

I've read that wooden chopping boards are unhygienic. Are they safe to use?

Most hygiene specialists advise against using wooden chopping boards and other wooden kitchen utensils because wood is absorbent and can rapidly develop the tiny cracks and crevices that often harbour food poisoning bacteria. Instead, they recommend chopping boards made from polypropylene – a tough type of plastic. However, even polypropylene can become contaminated and will need to be replaced if the surface gets badly scored.

To be on the safe side, use wooden boards only for slicing bread. Consider buying at least two other, polypropylene boards – one solely for meat and poultry and the other for general use. Colour-coded boards – red for meat, green for vegetables, white for general purpose - are available at most department stores and specialist kitchen shops.

Always scrub and rinse synthetic boards in very hot water and consider regularly disinfecting boards used for meat and poultry in a taint-free kitchen disinfectant. Whenever it is possible, leave boards to dry in the open air. Do not leave wooden boards immersed in water: they will develop tiny cracks.

USING CLING FILM

I'm confused whether it is safe to wrap and store food in cling film and whether cling film can be used in a microwave oven?

It is a little confusing because there are three types of cling film, each with a safe and an inadvisable use.

Furthermore, both food safety experts and the government are cautious about cling film because some of the components it is made with, called plasticisers, are known to migrate into food. There is still little knowledge or conclusive evidence to show whether or not this could cause health problems. With this in mind, the best general advice is:

● Check the manufacturer's instructions about using each type of cling film.
● Never wrap any kind of cling film around fatty foods such as cheese, butter or meat with visible surface fat.

As a general rule, the thinnest and stickiest cling film is safe for covering food bowls and containers because it creates a tight seal. It should not touch the food. A heavier cling film, sometimes called 'food wrap', is more suitable for wrapping around non-fatty food. Take care – if you are wrapping sandwiches with a cheese filling, for example, don't let the film touch the filling. The third type of cling film is made for use in a microwave oven – but it should not touch the food.

LOOKING AFTER FOOD AT HOME

Food hygiene is not just an issue when eating out – you also need to take some precautions at home. By following these simple guidelines for storing, preparing and cooking food you should be able to avoid most problems and keep your kitchen as germ-free as possible.

Selecting food

● Check the date marks to ensure that the food is fresh: don't buy more fresh food than you can eat within the 'use by' period.
● Avoid buying food in dirty or damaged packaging – the food could have been contaminated.
● Avoid buying frozen food that has a lot of ice around the packaging: at some stage it has been allowed to become too warm, encouraging harmful bacteria to grow.
● Take the food home and store it as quickly as possible: use insulated bags for refrigerated and frozen foods.

Safe storage

● Keep your refrigerator clean and use a thermometer to ensure it is operating at between 1°C and 4°C (34°F and 39°F). This will slow down the development of any harmful bacteria.
● Check that your freezer is running at between -18°C and -22°C (-1°F and -8°F) and that it is not packed above the load line (if there is one), because the temperature could be too warm for safe storage.
● Clean cupboards regularly and check that food has not gone past its safe storage date.
● Don't allow food to spill or drip on to other food or work surfaces.
● Keep food covered.
● Keep cold food at a cool temperature – at below 4°C (39°F). Leave food in the fridge until just before you need it.

Kitchen hygiene

● Clean the kitchen regularly. Disinfect surfaces that come in contact with raw food, such as chopping boards, and that you touch frequently by hand, such as fridge handles. When preparing and cooking food, clear up any mess as you go.
● If you cannot eat cooked food immediately, keep it hot – at 63°C (145°F) or warmer to prevent the growth of food poisoning bacteria.
● Reheat food once only. Ensure that it is piping hot right through to the centre. Avoid giving reheated food to anyone who is recovering from illness.
● Keep pets out of the kitchen.
● Empty rubbish bins regularly.
● Disinfect dish cloths and mops regularly to avoid spreading harmful bacteria.

Personal hygiene

● Wash your hands before and after handling food, after going to the toilet and coughing, sneezing or wiping your nose. Wash your hands between jobs involving different raw foods.
● Avoid wearing outdoor shoes and coats in the kitchen – you could bring soil or bacteria into the kitchen.
● Use spoons, forks and tongs to move food: avoid using your bare hands.
● Don't smoke in the kitchen.
● If you can, try to avoid preparing food when you have a stomach upset.

Storage times for tinned food

Canned foods without a 'best before' date can be safely stored for several years, although the quality may gradually deteriorate.

● **Use within 2 years**
Baked beans.
Potatoes.
Citrus fruit.
Soft fruit, such as strawberries.
Apples.
Tomatoes.
● **Use within 3 years**
Sweetcorn.
Carrots.
Spinach.
Potatoes, unpeeled.
Pineapples.
Peaches.
Meats.
Fish in brine or tomato sauce.
● **Use within 4 years**
Pulses.
Peas, beans.
● **Use within 5 years**
Salmon.
Corned beef.
Fish in oil.

CAUTION Once a tin has been opened, place any leftover food in a covered container in a refrigerator.

EXERCISE AND PHYSICAL FITNESS

For a strong heart and a healthy body, you need regular physical activity. Exercise improves your mood, enhances muscle tone, keeps joints supple and helps to prevent illness.

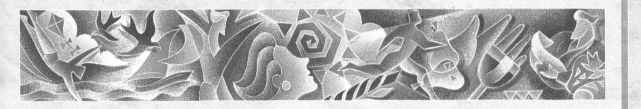

Are you as fit as you could be?

You don't have to work out in a gym or go to aerobics classes to keep fit, but you do have to make exercise and activity of some sort part of your daily life. Here is a simple quiz to help you to rate your everyday habits for fitness value. In each case, tick the box that most applies to you and check your score as shown below.

1 How often do you use a car for short journeys when you could walk?

a) Always. ☐
b) Sometimes. ☐
c) Never. ☐

2 How often do you take part in sports or other activities such as golf, tennis, squash, bowls, swimming or dancing?

a) Never or very rarely. ☐
b) A few times a month. ☐
c) Once a week or more. ☐

3 When you have to go up a few floors in a building how often do you take the stairs?

a) Never, or only if the lift is broken. ☐
b) When feeling specially energetic. ☐
c) Always. ☐

4 How often do you exert yourself enough to make you slightly breathless for at least 20 minutes (for example, by cycling or fast walking)?

a) Never or rarely. ☐
b) Once a month to once a week. ☐
c) More than once a week. ☐

5 If you have to run 100 yd (100 m) for a bus how long does it take you to get your breath back?

a) 3 minutes or more. ☐
b) Under 3 minutes. ☐
c) Unlikely to be out of breath. ☐

6 How often do you walk 2 miles (3 km) or more at a time?

a) Never or infrequently. ☐
b) Once or twice a month. ☐
c) Once a week or more. ☐

7 How would you describe your normal daily routine?

a) Mostly sedentary. ☐
b) Variable, but generally fairly active. ☐
c) Always on the move. ☐

8 On average, how many hours a week do you spend watching television?

a) 24 hours or more. ☐
b) 10 to 24 hours. ☐
c) Fewer than 10 hours. ☐

9 How often do you engage in vigorous tasks such as floor-scrubbing, digging the garden or washing windows?

a) Never or rarely. ☐
b) A few times a month. ☐
c) Once a week or more. ☐

10 Which of these ways of spending a Sunday afternoon is most usual for you?

a) Sleeping or watching television. ☐
b) Pottering around the house or garden. ☐
c) Walking or playing sport. ☐

SCORING

Award yourself 0 for all (a) answers; 1 for all (b) answers; 2 for all (c) answers. Add up your score.

14 to 20: Your way of life is almost certainly active enough to keep you fit.

7 to 13: You are probably fairly fit, but there is plenty of scope for improvement. Try to make time for some physical activity every day.

6 or less: You don't seem to be very active, but any sort of activity is better than nothing. Try increasing the amount of walking that you do, and spend more time on the move rather than sitting down.

The value of fitness

WHAT FITNESS MEANS

Everyone seems to have different ideas about exercise and fitness. What does being fit really mean?

At its simplest, fitness means the ability to get on with your life without becoming exhausted by normal daily activities. For most people 'being fit' also means feeling well and looking good.

Physical activity helps to protect against those chronic illnesses such as heart disease and osteoporosis (loss of bone density) that can result from leading a sedentary existence. So it is also fair to say that being fit helps to maintain your general health and wellbeing, while at the same time improving the quality and length of your life.

BENEFITING FROM EXERCISE

Does exercise really do you any good?

Yes – medical research and personal experience confirm it. Millions of ordinary people have discovered that exercise gives them benefits ranging from greater physical strength to a sense of inner peace and confidence.

Studies by doctors and fitness specialists throughout the world show that regular exercise can not only improve how you feel and look, but can also protect you against all kinds of ailments and chronic diseases. It can, for example:

- Protect against heart disease, stroke, hypertension, blood pressure, blocked arteries, obesity, gall stones, diabetes and osteoporosis.
- Prolong life expectancy.
- Decrease pain associated with menstruation, childbirth and a range of complaints, such as backache.
- Increase stamina and reserves of energy.
- Improve physical strength.
- Provide the suppleness that allows a wide range of comfortable movements.
- Assist in lifting depression.
- Help you to relax, improving sleep patterns and reducing tiredness.
- Enable you to deal more easily with stress.
- Improve concentration, mental agility and physical coordination.
- Help to enhance your sex life.
- Help to improve your confidence and self-esteem, often enabling you to socialise with greater ease.
- Help you to look good and feel well.

LEVELS OF FITNESS

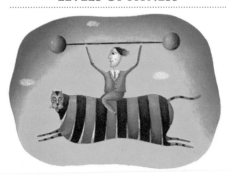

Is there one fixed level of fitness that applies to everyone, or does it vary from person to person?

Just as people's lives are varied, so the level of fitness needed to cope with that way of life varies. Being fit for an elderly person may involve simply staying strong enough to do the daily shopping, cooking and cleaning, and staying supple enough to play the occasional game of bowls. But a world-class athlete may need a daily programme of structured exercise to cope with the strenuous physical demands of competitive events.

Personal fitness also changes throughout your life. It will be dependent upon your age, weight, body type, stress levels, state of general health, degree of any injury or disability, and the amount of physical activity you are involved in generally.

But whatever your circumstances, you can usually improve your level of fitness simply by taking more exercise.

EXERCISE AND LONGER LIFE

Is it true that people who take regular exercise live longer and visit the doctor less frequently than those who don't?

Many studies show that people who exercise regularly live longer than those who lead an inactive life. Exercise seems to reduce the risk and severity of some potentially life-threatening conditions, while helping people to stay active well into their later years. Of

Finding out about the nation's sports

There are nearly 400 governing bodies for sports in Britain, which can provide information about all aspects of participation. For information contact the Sports Council, 16 Upper Woburn Place, London WC1H 0PQ, or:

- Local libraries.
- Sports and leisure centres, gyms, and sports and health clubs.
- Local adult education colleges.
- GPs, physiotherapists and other practitioners.
- Specialist magazines.

course, a long and healthy life is also determined by genetics, nutrition, stress and environment, but your efforts can make a difference. Even a little exercise is better than none, and you do not have to spend all your leisure hours in a gym.

Studies show that gentle walking, climbing stairs, cycling at a moderate pace and other active recreational pursuits help people to stay healthier and more alert, and to outlive their sedentary counterparts.

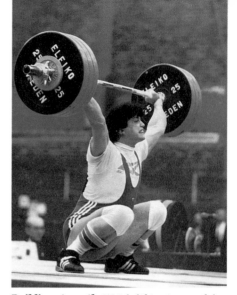

Building strength Weightlifting is one of the purest anaerobic, or strength, exercises. To be truly fit, you need aerobic exercise too.

FIVE KINDS OF FITNESS

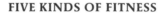

What does fitness consist of?

True fitness involves a combination of activities that enable you to perform physical tasks well. It has several components.

STAMINA A healthy heart provides stamina, or endurance. The best exercise for the heart is aerobic – meaning that it burns oxygen. To be effective, aerobic exercise has to be energetic enough to make you slightly breathless. Walking, running, cycling, swimming and aerobics increase stamina.

SKILL Being fit also means being able to control and coordinate our movements, and being able to balance and react quickly. We use these skills whenever we move, but many sports and physical activities also develop mental and social skills.

MUSCULAR STRENGTH Powerful muscles can improve posture and protect against injuries and back pain, as well as helping with everyday activities such as carrying the shopping. Muscle-strengthening exercise is called anaerobic – it does not require extra oxygen. Activities such as swimming and cycling combine anaerobic and aerobic exercise.

MUSCULAR ENDURANCE Repeated movements, such as pedalling a bike, inflating a tyre with a foot pump or beating up a cake mixture, improve your muscles' ability to keep on working hard without tiring.

SUPPLENESS Flexible muscles are strong and healthy, and help to preserve mobility and independence in later life.

Developing endurance

The big muscles of the body, such as the quadriceps in the thigh and the biceps in the arm, need slow, rhythmic exercise to build their ability to keep going. Cycling, swimming and walking all serve the purpose.

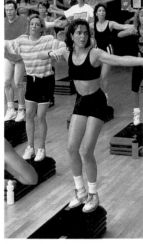

Increasing stamina Step classes and other aerobic activities strengthen the heart and increase lung efficiency.

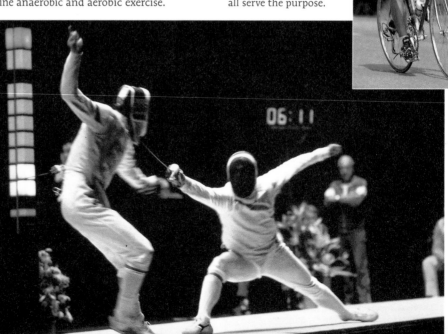

Honing skills Fencing demands lightning-quick perception and muscle response. Participants also develop poise and agility – and get an excellent workout too.

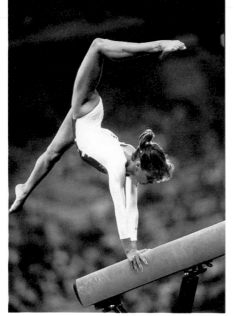

Staying supple You don't have to be a gymnast to develop flexibility and balance. Simple stretches will help, as will activities such as golf, badminton, dancing and skiing.

GETTING ENOUGH EXERCISE

How much exercise does an ordinary person need to become fit and stay fit?

As a rough guide, adults need at least one hour's moderate or energetic exercise every week. This does not have to be taken all at once. Fitness experts say that 20 minutes of physical activity carried out at least three times a week would make an excellent fitness routine.

This way you are likely to get just enough exercise during each session to gain aerobic benefit – strengthening your heart and improving your blood circulation.

AM I FIT ENOUGH?

I have never played a sport or taken any exercise classes, but I feel perfectly fit. Is it really necessary to make more effort?

Energetic housework, gardening, polishing the car, climbing stairs and walking can all play an important part in your overall fitness. However, you need to ensure that you have activities that make you:

● Breathe harder.
● Lift, push and carry fairly heavy objects.
● Stretch and bend.
● Keep exercising or moving continuously, for at least 20 minutes if possible.

Even if you can be certain that your daily activities provide you with all the exercise you need, you could still be missing out on the fun and feeling of achievement that goes with taking part in an active recreational pursuit. It is also worth considering that if you are not currently involved in any fitness activities outside your home or working life, you run the risk of becoming sedentary in later life, with all the linked risks of immobility, ill-health and disease. You don't need to become a slave to exercise, but you do need to do about 20 minutes of fairly vigorous activity three times a week – and the best forms of energetic activity are sports and fitness programmes.

CHANGING SEDENTARY HABITS

I have a sedentary existence and I am short of free time. Can I get fit without changing my whole way of life?

Yes – but the hardest 'exercise' will probably be the act of breaking your old sedentary habits. If you really cannot make any immediate changes, try to make your existing activities a little more active:

● Use the stairs instead of the lift.
● Walk up stairs two at a time.
● Cycle or walk at least part of a journey.
● Meet friends and colleagues for a regular walk instead of meeting for a meal.
● Wash and polish your car or the windows of your home with extra vigour.
● Do some discreet stretches or warm-up exercises while you wait for a meeting to start or a kettle to boil.

A little exercise is better than no exercise at all, and if you are unfit it is best to begin gently. In the long term, however, try to make time for an hour of energetic activity at least once a week; there are many health benefits from being fit, while inactivity can quite literally be fatal.

EASING STIFF JOINTS

Since I retired, my joints have become stiffer. Is this a feature of getting older?

No. Many older people are just as fit and flexible as younger ones. Unless it is caused by a medical condition, such as arthritis, the stiffness in your joints can be reversed by exercising – check with your doctor, who can advise about safe forms of exercise. Gentle, loosening exercises are a good start, and then you may want to consider walking, dancing, swimming, Keep Fit, or T'ai Chi – all good for suppleness. The chart on page 72 can help you to choose.

The chart on page 72 can help you to choose.

It's no excuse

Even though exercise provides a wide range of health and fitness benefits, people find all kinds of excuses to avoid physical activity. Few are ever valid.

● **I haven't got time.** Just 20 minutes of activity three times a week will make a measurable difference to your fitness.

● **I feel too tired.** Exercise can help you to relax and sleep better. It also releases brain chemicals called endorphins that make you feel less tired.

● **I've left it too late** or **I'm too old to start now.** It is never too late to start exercising, and if you have been sedentary for years, you will make very rapid gains.

● **I am too fat.** Combine good aerobic exercise with a healthy diet low in fat and sugar, and you will almost certainly lose weight. And you'll keep it off – more than can be said for most diets.

● **I don't look good in lycra and leotards.** Don't worry – sensible exercisers dress for comfort, not for fashion. In most gyms and classes you'll have plenty of company if you wear a baggy tee shirt and old leggings or shorts.

RELIEVING STRESS

My wife is going through a difficult phase at work, and comes home feeling tired and stressed. Would exercise help her?

Even though the long-term solution is probably to tackle the cause of the stress, some gentle daily exercises and a nutritious diet could help to make her life a great deal more tolerable. It seems that exercise triggers the release of endorphins – chemicals in the brain that reduce pain, improve mood and interrupt the cycle of anxiety that leads to stress. The chemicals may also help you to relax by decreasing some needless muscle activity. Many people find that exercising reduces tension, helps them to sleep better, and temporarily distracts them from the problems causing the tension. Any physical activity that is repetitive and rhythmic and lasts for about 20 minutes would probably give your wife more energy. Try encouraging her to fit a little walking or stair-climbing into her day, with relaxation exercises (see pages 190-192) in the evening.

Exercise for life

INACTIVE CHILDREN

My grandchildren seem to play so many computer games and so few outdoor games that I'm concerned they may not be getting enough exercise. Is there anything I can do?

Your grandchildren could well be among the many youngsters in Britain and the United States who are not as active as they could be. Studies show that inactive children usually become unfit adults – at high risk from serious diseases, such as coronary heart disease, osteoporosis (loss of bone density) and diabetes, and all the problems of immobility. Even if inactivity does not hamper youngsters during their school years, they need to develop good exercise habits that will help to protect them in later life. Perhaps this is where you come in.

Even encouraging your grandchildren and their parents to walk, instead of going by car, would improve the exercise habit. Alternatively, ask your grandchildren to join you on a regular ramble, swim or cycle ride. If someone in the family plays a sport, why not try

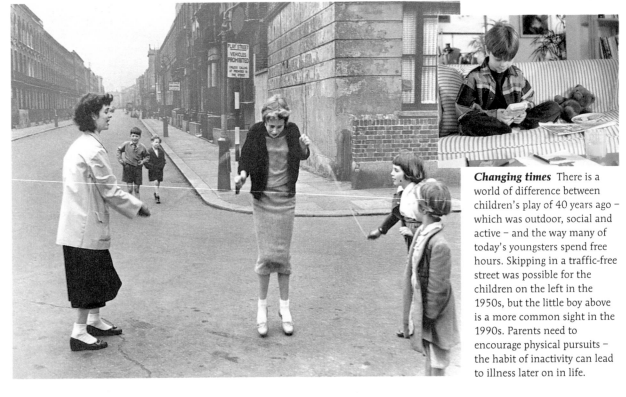

Changing times There is a world of difference between children's play of 40 years ago – which was outdoor, social and active – and the way many of today's youngsters spend free hours. Skipping in a traffic-free street was possible for the children on the left in the 1950s, but the little boy above is a more common sight in the 1990s. Parents need to encourage physical pursuits – the habit of inactivity can lead to illness later on in life.

to involve the children? But avoid putting pressure on them. When children are forced into an activity, they tend to give up quite quickly. Of course, exercise does not have to be highly structured, excessively vigorous or expensive, so try to interest young children in simple ball games, tag, hop-scotch or hide-and-seek. (If you are unfit, these games will give you some exercise too.)

Most older children enjoy skipping games and leap-frog, as well as team games, such as cricket, football, netball, hockey and rounders. In the end, it does not matter which activities your grandchildren do, as long as they take some form of exercise regularly.

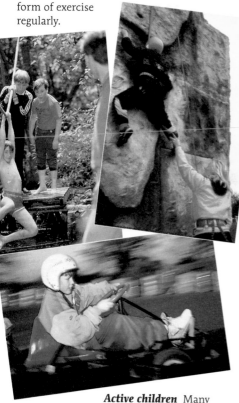

Active children Many schools and clubs organise exciting activities for children. An adventure weekend (top left) teaches cooperation; rock climbing (top right) demands stamina, skill and confidence; and kart racing (bottom) is invigorating fun.

EXERCISE BENEFITS FOR WOMEN

Are there any particular advantages of exercise for women?

Women now participate and compete in more and more sports and physical activities, giving them the chance to discover a sense of wellbeing and achievement that was often denied to older generations. Although everyone needs exercise, many women stand to gain even more health benefits than men. Women – particularly Caucasian and Asian women – are prone to osteoporosis (thinning of the bones, due to calcium loss) and exercise helps to prevent the condition by strengthening the bones. Some women find that exercise relieves the symptoms of premenstrual tension (PMT) and period pains, although others find that exercise is ineffective at these times.

Women who get and stay fit before and during pregnancy often experience less back and labour pain than women who are unfit. Fit mothers-to-be usually avoid becoming overweight, and regain their shape quickly after giving birth (see page 276).

Many women say that exercise helps them to boost their self-confidence, to improve their appearance and to meet people outside their immediate family circle. Some women-only exercise classes also teach self-defence skills.

MENSTRUATION AND EXERCISE

My 14-year-old daughter does two dance classes a week and swims and roller skates at the weekend. I've heard that too much exercise can delay the onset of a girl's menstrual cycle. Is this true?

Vigorous exercise can delay the start of menstrual periods or upset their regularity. Girls and mature women involved in gymnastics, running, ballet and similar activities in which low body weight is traditionally encouraged seem to be most affected by amenorrhoea – lack of periods.

However, it tends to affect only those in regular, vigorous training or with eating disorders (see page 205). A low body weight and the physical and psychological pressures of training block the production of the hormone oestrogen that is needed for menstruation to occur each month.

Usually, the menstrual periods start or return to normal once training intensity is eased or the participant gains weight. In the long run, the disruption seems to have little effect upon fertility.

Girls' periods usually start at some time between 10 and 15 years, and your daughter's activities do not seem excessive for her age. Children and young people need plenty of exercise – for their own enjoyment and to help them to stay fit and healthy throughout their lives. Your daughter's chosen activities also develop her concentration, memory, analysis, coordination and balance. But if

The booming business of exercise

About two-thirds of the population (almost 36 million adults and children) take part in some kind of sport or physical recreation. This proportion has increased in recent years, mainly because more women now take part. Women are more likely to take up indoor activities, such as Keep Fit and aerobics, and they are largely responsible for the rapid growth in these activities.

People aged between 16 and 29 take part in most sports, showing a particular liking for energetic and team sports. Swimming, jogging, cycling, fishing, ten-pin bowling and fitness exercise – such as Keep Fit and aerobics – are favoured by people in the 30-44 age group, while walking, swimming, bowls, golf and snooker appeal particularly to those aged between 45 and 59. For the over-60s, walking and bowls are the main fitness activities.

Students and professional job-holders tend to play more sport than unskilled and semiskilled job-holders.

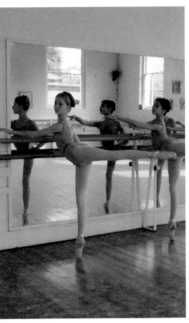

In danger? Normal ballet classes are perfectly safe for young girls, but extreme training programmes can sometimes affect health. The risks are increased if the diet is strictly controlled to prevent weight gain. Similar risks are also associated with intensive gymnastics and athletics training, or even obsessive attendance at aerobics classes.

you believe that she is seriously underweight for her build and age group, or that her periods should have started by now, have a talk with the doctor.

A FIT PREGNANCY

I would like to maintain my fitness during pregnancy. Can you tell me if all exercise is safe and beneficial for mothers-to-be, or are there some activities that should be avoided?

Women who are fit before their baby's conception and remain so during pregnancy often have an easier labour and regain their shape more rapidly after giving birth than women who are unfit. But that won't necessarily apply in every birth: what is safe for one woman may be unwise for another.

Every mother-to-be should regularly check with her midwife or doctor throughout her pregnancy, but the following advice is well worth considering:

Health benefits
Moderate exercise during pregnancy helps you to:
● Avoid putting on unnecessary weight.
● Improve blood circulation – reducing the risk of varicose veins, thrombosis and swollen ankles.
● Strengthen muscles – supporting the back in its new posture (with the extra weight of the foetus and change of balance).
● Improve cardiovascular efficiency – giving more oxygen to the baby and improving your stamina.
● Relax and deal with any stress.

Recommended
The best antenatal exercises are those that strengthen and keep flexible the muscles that will take extra strain – muscles in the back, abdomen, shoulders and pelvis – and activities that improve the circulation. Doctors and midwives usually recommend swimming and water exercises (in warm water), walking, movement to music and toning exercises. Most hospitals run antenatal sessions that include breathing, posture, and strengthening and relaxation exercises.

Risky
Avoid vigorous exercise, such as squash, even if you were very active before pregnancy. Don't do any activities where you risk falling, knocking yourself or frequently jarring your body. Horse riding, hockey, high-impact aerobics, skiing, hang-gliding and motorcycling are risky. Decrease the intensity of your exercise: switch from running or jogging to low-impact aerobics or brisk walking. If your balance is upset, change from bicycling to using a stationary exercise bike.

Don't do any exercise where you have to lie on the floor and lift your legs: such an exercise can deprive the foetus of blood. Take care when stretching: hormonal changes may make it easier to stretch, but you run the risk of overdoing it.

Precautions
Talk to your midwife or doctor about your exercise plans. Drink plenty of water before, during and after exercise. Keep your pulse below 140 beats a minute during exercise. Stop immediately if you have pain or any loss of blood – then seek advice from your doctor.

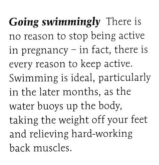

Going swimmingly There is no reason to stop being active in pregnancy – in fact, there is every reason to keep active. Swimming is ideal, particularly in the later months, as the water buoys up the body, taking the weight off your feet and relieving hard-working back muscles.

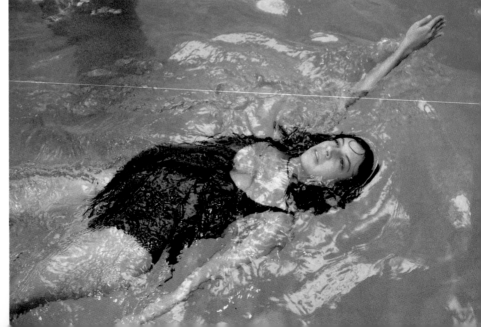

DARTS AND BILLIARDS

My parents have both retired recently. They say that playing darts, bar billiards, snooker and pool will keep them fit into their nineties and beyond. I don't want to spoil their enjoyment but wonder whether these games will really keep anyone fit?

Although these games do not make major demands on the body, don't dismiss the small contribution that they can make towards general fitness and wellbeing.

The games require concentration and co-ordination, helping your parents to remain alert and in control of their movements, and probably helping them to sleep soundly at night. Darts gently exercise the shoulders and wrists while pool, snooker and billiards give the back a little exercise, helping your parents to stay flexible. Even standing watching a game will help a little towards keeping their leg bones strong.

It is important that retired people should organise plenty of absorbing activities to avoid becoming lethargic and immobile. Your parents' favourite games are sociable, competitive activities that provide fun and a chance to excel. So don't put them off, but do encourage them to avoid heavy drinking and smoking while they play, and to take some additional exercise regularly several times a week – walking to the games venue would be a healthy, inexpensive option.

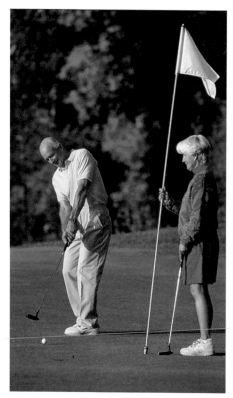

The fun way to get fit You don't have to lift weights or leap on a bicycle to keep yourself in good health. A round of golf can provide excellent exercise – and whatever activity you choose, you are much more likely to keep at it if it is something that you enjoy.

Choosing the right exercise

TOTAL FITNESS TRAINING

Is there any one particular sport or physical activity that could give me complete all-round fitness?

No single sport or physical activity can give you total fitness, although some forms of exercise do give better all-round results than others. Swimming, rowing, aerobic exercises, cross-country skiing, and certain kinds of dance – contemporary, jazz and ballet, in particular – use nearly all the major muscle groups, improve circulation and strengthen the heart and skeleton.

An ideal fitness routine includes exercises that improve cardiovascular efficiency (the heart and circulation system), create muscular strength and endurance, and improve suppleness. For most people, this means doing a number of different physical activities each week. This is called 'cross-training' – but you do not have to spend all your leisure hours in a gym, at an exercise class, or on a sports field. Walking to work, carrying the grocery shopping, washing the car, gardening and other similar physical activities will all help you towards total fitness. If you find it hard to combine activities to give yourself an all-round workout, you might benefit from circuit training (see below).

CIRCUIT TRAINING EXPLAINED

What is circuit training, and who is it for?

Circuit training, sometimes called 'circuits' for short, is a sequence of fitness activities providing aerobic and anaerobic exercise (see page 64) by working every part of the body.

Footballers, tennis players, golfers, canoeists, dancers, cyclists, track athletes and many others do circuit training to maintain general fitness, work particular muscle groups, and provide variety in their training. Most gyms and leisure centres provide an indoor circuit of between four and twenty 'stations', including mats for warming up, cooling down and stretching; steps, treadmills and fixed cycle machines to raise the heart rate; and a variety of machines to increase muscular strength and endurance.

Circuit training usually lasts between 40 minutes and an hour. Outdoor circuits, often found in parks, usually include bars for balance, steps to work your leg muscles, and a horizontal ladder or parallel bars to work your arm and shoulder muscles.

TONING MUSCLES

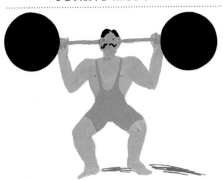

More and more people at my health club are using weights. What are the benefits?

You do not have to aspire to look like Arnold Schwarzenegger to try exercising with weights. As well as improving muscular strength, weight training is a good way to change the body's appearance – by toning your muscles, you make your body firmer, and so tend to look slimmer.

Lifting the weights creates a resistance for the muscles to work against – a type of exercise that is largely missing from many sports and physical activities. Some people do intensive weight training for body building, but many others use light weights in a programme for general fitness. However, if weight training is your main form of exercise, you will also need to do some activities that provide aerobic exercise (working your heart and lungs) and improve your flexibility (see chart, page 72).

Many women now use weights for body building and muscle toning. The lower levels of the hormone testosterone in women's bodies prevent their muscles from bulking up, so unless women do about four hours'

intensive weight training every day, they will not end up with bulging muscles.

CAUTION When lifting free weights, such as dumbbells and barbells, have a partner standing by to prevent accidents.

HELP WITH WEIGHT CONTROL

Which exercises would be the best to help me to lose weight?

Exercise increases the speed at which your body breaks down food, so that less of it is stored as fat. Combined with a healthy diet, all exercise can eventually help you to reduce and control weight.

It was once thought that energetic activities were the only effective fat-burners. But it is now known that sustained, gentle, rhythmic exercises, such as slow walking, cycling and swimming, are equally good. However, the less vigorous the exercise the longer it will take to gain the full benefit.

CHOOSING AN ACTIVITY

I want to do something to get fit, but I am not drawn to any one activity. What should I consider when choosing between all the options on offer?

The most important thing is to find an activity that you enjoy and that makes you feel good – the benefits of health and fitness then become a by-product of your enjoyment. Until you develop a strong preference, why not find a taster course covering one or more sports or physical activities? These are often run by sports centres, gyms and adult education colleges, and sometimes include sessions for women only, the over-50s or parents with children of primary school age.

Look for activities that particularly suit your way of life:

● Choose something that you can do regularly – at least once a week.
● Match the activity to your particular fitness needs – for example, choose yoga, Keep Fit or jazz dance for flexibility; weight training for strength; or cross-country running for endurance. (The chart on page 72 outlines fitness values of various sports.)
● Find physical activities that also fulfil some of your social, mental and spiritual aims – try team games or join a class or club to meet people; consider dance to stimulate your concentration, coordination, balance and memory; try long-distance walking,

cycling or swimming to let your mind roam freely; try T'ai Chi for inner peace; consider hang-gliding, climbing or whitewater canoeing for excitement.

BENEFITS OF TEAM GAMES

What are the advantages of taking part in a team game rather than an individual activity, and do you need to have a particularly hearty personality to get on well in team sports?

You do not have to be the back-slapping type to enjoy team sports and do well at them – even though some sports, such as rugby, do have a reputation for lively off-pitch behaviour. Of course, it helps if you feel comfortable as part of a group, cooperating with others to achieve a shared ambition.

Some people produce their best performances when part of a team, but others find the team spirit overwhelming rather than a spur to excellence. If you also enjoy achieving things on your own, you might get on well in sports that have both team and individual competitions, such as tennis, golf, running, rowing, swimming and canoeing. Most popular team sports, including soccer, rugby, cricket, hockey and netball, provide an excellent combination of aerobic and anaerobic exercise, so they are good for your heart, circulation and stamina while strengthening bones. But few of the most popular team sports are good for flexibility.

CHOOSING A RACQUET SPORT

I'd like to get back to playing tennis, badminton or squash at weekends. Which one of these racquet sports would give me the best all-round exercise?

All racquet sports will help you to stay fit, but they do not rate as highly as swimming, rowing and cross-country skiing for all-round exercise. Tennis, squash and badminton are stop-start activities that provide a good mix of aerobic and anaerobic exercise (see page 64), build muscular strength and endurance, and improve balance and coordination.

Squash is the best aerobic exercise. Because it makes heavy demands on your heart and the major muscles in your arms, legs and back, you should be fairly fit before you start to play. Tennis and badminton create bursts of intense aerobic exercise but rarely keep your heart rate within your training zone (see page 75) – the rate that helps most to improve heart strength and circulation.

DRY-SLOPE SKIING

I'm planning to take lessons on a dry slope before I go on my first skiing holiday. Are there any differences in the techniques I'll need on real snow, and can I learn snowboarding and cross-country skiing on a dry slope?

The techniques taught on a dry slope are the same ones you will use on snow – but you will probably find snow a great deal more slippery. You can learn about downhill skiing, snowboarding and mono-skiing on a dry slope and, although you cannot practise cross-country skiing on a dry slope, you can learn the basic techniques. You can prepare for cross-country skiing by using a cross-country skiing machine. Don't be put off if you feel insecure at first: even experienced cross-country skiers initially find it hard to balance. It is a good idea to take lessons on a dry slope well ahead of your holiday – to condition your body and to gain confidence.

ROLLER SKATING

My children enjoy roller skating, and I wonder whether it is doing them any good?

Both roller skating and ice skating help to build strong ankle and leg muscles and develop balance and coordination. More specialised activities such as ice dance and roller dance are also good for flexibility.

Other fitness benefits, such as strengthening the heart and lungs and improving the circulation of the blood, are seldom abundant except for those who skate very vigorously. So if skating is to be your children's primary form of exercise you should also try to encourage them to take up some aerobic activities, such as brisk walking, jogging, skipping, dancing or energetic cycling.

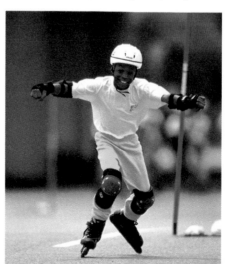

On a roll Youngsters who roller blade are getting some valuable exercise, though it may need supplementing. There is some element of risk, but provided that skaters stay well away from traffic and wear the right protective clothing, spills are not likely to do much harm.

GETTING THE MOST FROM SPORTS AND EXERCISES

Different activities develop the body in different ways, and to different levels. This chart shows how much benefit various sports and physical activities will give in five vital fitness categories – from stamina, through muscle endurance and strength, to suppleness and coordination. For example, circuit training comes out top in all categories, but jogging and running, though good for aerobic stamina and muscle endurance, will not do much for your flexibility or coordination.

●	POOR
●●	FAIR
●●●	GOOD
●●●●	VERY GOOD
●●●●●	EXCELLENT

ACTIVITY	AEROBIC FITNESS	MUSCULAR ENDURANCE	MUSCULAR STRENGTH	FLEXIBILITY	COORDINATION
Aerobic exercises	●●●●	●●●●	●●●	●●●	●●●●
Badminton	●●●●	●●●	●●	●●●	●●●●●
Bowls	●	●●	●●	●●	●●●
Circuit training	●●●●●	●●●●●	●●●●●	●●●●●	●●●●●
Cricket (batting)	●●	●	●●●	●●●	●●●●
Cycling:					
5 mph (8 km/h)	●●●	●●●	●●●	●●●	●●●●
12 mph (19 km/h)	●●●●	●●●●●	●●●	●●●	●●●●
Dancing (jazz)	●●●●	●●●	●●●	●●●●●	●●●●●
Football (soccer)	●●●●	●●●●	●●●	●●●	●●●●
Golf (carrying clubs)	●●	●●●	●●●	●●●	●●●●
Hockey	●●●●	●●●●	●●●	●●●	●●●●
Horse riding	●●	●●●	●●●	●	●●●●
Jogging and running:					
5 mph (8 km/h)	●●●●	●●●	●●●	●	●●
9 mph (14.5 km/h)	●●●●●	●●●●	●●●	●	●●
Judo/karate	●●	●●●	●●●●	●●●●●	●●●●●
Rowing	●●●●	●●●●●	●●●●●	●●	●●●
Rugby	●●●	●●●●	●●●●	●●●	●●●
Sailing	●●	●●●	●●●	●●	●●●●
Skiing:					
Downhill	●●●	●●●●	●●●●	●●●●	●●●●●
Cross-country	●●●●●	●●●●	●●●●	●●●●	●●●●
Skipping	●●●●	●●●●	●●●●	●●	●●●
Snooker/billiards	●	●	●	●●	●●●
Squash	●●●●	●●●●●	●●●	●●●●	●●●●●
Swimming (fast crawl)	●●●●	●●●	●●●●	●●●●	●●●●●
Tennis	●●●	●●●	●●●●	●●●●	●●●●●
Walking (brisk)	●●●	●●●	●●●●	●●	●●
Weight training	●	●●●●	●●●●●	●	●●●●
Yoga	●	●●●	●●	●●●●●	●●●●

Getting started

MEDICAL TESTS FIRST?

I am 46 and healthy, but I have not taken much exercise since I left school. Should I take any medical tests before I start fitness training?

Even though you are in good health, it is worth having a chat with your doctor before you start any new vigorous physical activity – if only to gain reassurance. Your doctor will probably measure your blood pressure and weight, check if you smoke and consider whether anything in your medical history could affect your safety while exercising.

Of course, medical tests cannot always identify potential illnesses, such as heart disease. It is therefore up to you to exercise sensibly: start with gentle activities, and slow down or stop if you feel any discomfort.

If you have any fears about your health once you have started training, don't hesitate to get more advice from your doctor or a qualified fitness specialist.

AGE, FITNESS AND CHECK-UPS

Should everyone have a medical check-up before starting a programme of exercise?

There is no harm in getting your doctor's advice, whatever your age and current level of fitness. But generally speaking, people who are under 40, who do not smoke, who are not overweight, and have no personal or family history of heart problems can usually take up exercise safely without having to consult a doctor first.

For most other people, it would be wise to see the doctor before starting any new kind of physical activity, particularly if they are affected by any of the following problems. Consult your doctor before taking up fitness training if:

● You are under 40 and in good health but have been inactive for some time.
● You are over 40, regardless of your general health – a check-up is a sensible precaution, because the risk of heart disease increases as you get older.
● You are overweight.
● You have high blood pressure, or high cholesterol levels.
● You are taking regular medication.

● You are pregnant.
● You have a history of heart disease or cardiac problems, such as a heart murmur.
● You have any long-term or chronic illness, such as asthma, arthritis or diabetes.
● You have experienced dizziness or chest pains during exercise or at any other time.
● You smoke.
● You are unaccustomed to exercise.
● You have muscle, ligament or tendon strains or sprains.
● You have an injury or are recovering from a recent illness.

ALLERGIC TO EXERCISE

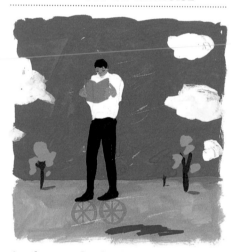

Are there people who should not exercise?

No. Activity is crucial to our physical and mental wellbeing. Our bodies are designed to be active, and most people benefit from some kind of exercise (see page 65). However, in some people exercise can trigger off an asthma attack with coughing, breathlessness or wheezing. Even so, with modern prescribed drugs, many sufferers can continue to exercise safely.

WHEN TO AVOID EXERCISE

Are there any circumstances when it is unsafe or ill-advised to exercise?

The answer depends to some extent upon your personal medical history and your current level of fitness, but as a rule it is best to avoid exercising whenever you have a high temperature or a fever. It is also wise not to

---

Exercises to avoid

You might have tried these exercises without ill effects, but fitness experts now say they could be dangerous.

Danger to the neck
● The plough – never lie on your back and lift your legs over your head so that they rest on the floor behind you.
● Neck extension – avoid dropping your head back as far as it will go.
● Sit-ups with hands behind the neck – to be safe, position your hands at the side of your head close to your ears.

Danger to the knees
● Hurdler's stretch – avoid sitting on the floor with one leg bent behind you and the other extended in front while you stretch your arms and body out over the straight leg. The danger is to the bent knee.
● Deep knee bends, or squats – don't bend your knees past 90° (so that your buttocks are lower than your knees).

Danger to the back and knees
● Flat back stretch, sometimes called windmills – avoid positions where you keep your legs straight with feet apart while stretching a hand across to the opposite foot.

Danger to the back
● Sit-up with straight legs – make sure you bend your legs for safety.
● Double leg lift – never lie on your back and lift both legs up while keeping them straight.

take exercise when you have a heavy cold (see page 100), have just eaten a heavy meal (see page 91), or drunk alcohol. You should also need to take some precautions when exercising in extremely hot or cold weather (see pages 84 and 85). If you are pregnant, or recovering from an illness or injury, or taking certain prescribed drugs, or affected by certain complaints, such as high blood pressure, you should get your doctor's advice about the type and intensity of exercise that is safe to undertake.

CHOOSING A GYM

There are dozens of local gymnasiums, fitness centres and clubs in my area. How should I choose between them?

You are far more likely to exercise regularly if you join a gym, club or class that is easy to get to. Make an initial choice of between three and five that are nearby and try to visit them at a time when you would be most likely to use the facilities. This will allow you to talk to those who use the gym regularly and to see how crowded it gets. Take advantage of the chance offered by many gyms to sample the facilities free of charge. This will help you to find out whether the staff are genuinely interested in you, your aims and any problems you have, and to see how carefully they supervise the use of exercise machines, the swimming pool and fitness classes (see page 115).

Ask lots of questions, find out whether the changing facilities are clean and warm with secure storage space for your clothes. Check the membership fees, any additional charges, and arrangements for spreading costs. At the end of the day, however, you may well find that the best gym is the one with the right feel or atmosphere.

FREE FITNESS TESTING

My local gym is offering free fitness testing. What would this involve and how useful would it be?

Although this is a promotional lure, the test could, in fact, give valuable clues about what you need to do to maintain or improve your level of fitness. Use the opportunity to get as much free information as possible about the kind of activity that would give you the greatest benefit.

The trainer will probably ask about your general health and any history of injury, the type of exercise you do, how you spend your leisure time, and what sort of diet you have. The trainer will probably test your blood pressure, measure your body fat with calipers and ask you to carry out some simple tests and activities, such as cycling on an exercise bike, running briefly on a treadmill, stretching, gripping and lifting.

You may receive a computer print-out that shows your aerobic fitness, and your strength, flexibility, blood pressure, resting heart rate and percentage of body fat.

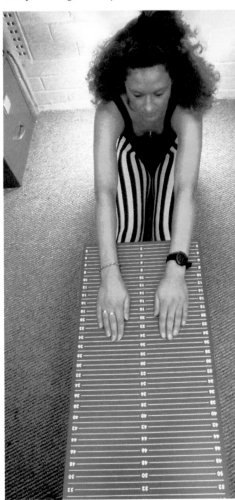

Reaching for fitness 'Sit and reach' tests monitor overall flexibility, including movement in your shoulders, arms, back, pelvis and legs.

EXERCISING ALONE

I am worried. Is it safe to exercise on my own or could it lead to me injuring myself?

You are quite right to be concerned, but provided you are sensible with the exercises you are undertaking then you won't have much to worry about. However, if you are starting any new kind of exercise, or if you have been inactive for some time, it would be wise to first join a class or club where a qualified teacher can help you to get the best out of the exercise and to avoid injury.

Once you are familiar with the possible risks of your chosen activity, you will be in a far better position to make your own decisions about safety when you are working out on your own. Of course, some sports, such as long-distance running, are traditionally solo activities, and with these there is an additional hazard. Apart from the danger of twisting an ankle and lying injured and unaided, there is the possibility of your being attacked by a mugger. As remote as this may be, it is still worth being prepared. Make a mental note of where any telephone boxes are positioned along your proposed route and, whenever possible, ask friends to help by accompanying you on different stages. If you are involved in a solo sport or activity, such as windsurfing, tell someone where you are going and the time you aim to return.

HOW FIT ARE YOU? – TESTING YOUR RESTING PULSE RATE

Use your resting pulse rate as a measure of fitness. The fitter you are the slower and stronger the beat will be. Take your pulse before getting up in the morning (see the panel, right). If your resting pulse rate is higher than the top 'unfit' figure in the chart, below, consult a doctor.

MEN	AGE	UNFIT	FIT	VERY FIT
	20s	86 or more	60 - 85	59 or less
	30s	86 or more	64 - 85	63 or less
	40s	90 or more	66 - 89	65 or less
	50s and older	90 or more	68 - 89	67 or less
WOMEN	AGE	UNFIT	FIT	VERY FIT
	20s	96 or more	72 - 95	71 or less
	30s	98 or more	72 - 97	71 or less
	40s	99 or more	74 - 98	73 or less
	50s and older	103 or more	76 - 102	75 or less

ARE YOU WORKING HARD ENOUGH? – THE TRAINING ZONE

To get aerobic benefit from exercise you need to raise your heart rate to within the 'training zone' – 60-90 per cent of its maximum capacity. If you are over 60, very unfit or have a heart condition, consult a doctor before taking up any new activity or attempting strenuous exercise.

BOTH MEN AND WOMEN	AGE	MILD WORKOUT (60-70%)	MODERATE WORKOUT (70-80%)	STRENUOUS WORKOUT (80-90%)
	20 - 24	118 - 140	140 - 157	157 - 180
	25 - 30	114 - 137	137 - 152	152 - 171
	31 - 35	111 - 132	132 - 148	148 - 170
	36 - 40	108 - 129	129 - 144	144 - 166
	41 - 45	105 - 125	125 - 140	140 - 161
	46 - 50	102 - 122	122 - 136	136 - 157
	51 - 55	99 - 118	118 - 132	132 - 152
	56 - 60	96 - 115	115 - 128	128 - 148
	61 and older	up to 111	up to 127	up to 143

Testing your pulse

You can find your pulse by placing your first or second finger on the thumb side of your wrist (the radial artery) or on your neck behind your Adam's apple about half way between your chin and ear (the carotid artery). Look at a watch that shows seconds, and count the throbs in your artery for 15 seconds. You may have to do this a few times to feel confident you have counted correctly. Multiply by four to obtain your pulse rate.

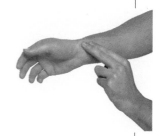

Fingertip touch The easiest place to find your pulse is on the radial artery on the inside of your wrist. Press lightly with your first and second fingers on the artery to feel your pulse.

What your heart rate says about fitness

Your heart rate is an important guide to your level of fitness. When adults are inactive, their hearts beat at an average 72 beats every minute, while children's hearts beat faster and old people have a slower heart rate. Exercise increases your heart rate temporarily but helps your heart to work more efficiently in the long term, improving your performance when you are active and helping to protect you from illness.

HOW FAST DO YOU GET BACK TO NORMAL? – THE RECOVERY RATE

The rate at which your heart returns to normal after exertion is a good measure of fitness. To rate yourself, step on and off a step about 8 in (20cm) from the ground once every 2-3 seconds, for 3 minutes. Then rest for 30 seconds and take your pulse. Stop if you feel dizzy or sick.

MEN	AGE	UNFIT	FAIRLY FIT	VERY FIT
	20s	102 or more	76 – 101	75 or less
	30s	104 or more	80 – 103	79 or less
	40s	106 or more	82 – 105	81 or less
	50s and older	108 or more	84 – 107	83 or less
WOMEN	AGE	UNFIT	FAIRLY FIT	VERY FIT
	20s	112 or more	88 – 111	87 or less
	30s	114 or more	89 – 113	88 or less
	40s	116 or more	90 – 115	89 or less
	50s and older	118 or more	92 – 98	91 or less

Good ways to warm up

THE NEED TO WARM UP

Why do I need warm-up exercises ?

For two important reasons – to allow you to move easily (so that you can perform to your full capabilities) and to protect your body from injuries, aches and stiffness. A warm-up routine simply involves gentle movements that prepare your body for more strenuous activities later. It is rather like putting a car into first gear to get started.

Most muscles in the body work in pairs and, as one contracts, the other relaxes. This can be seen in such muscles as the biceps and triceps of the upper arm, or in the muscles at the back and front of the thigh.

If you go straight into vigorous exercise without warming up, the contracting muscle obeys the signals it is sent, but the relaxing muscle may be a little slower and it, or its ligament, risks being pulled. That is why sprinters, with their powerful thigh muscles, will sometimes damage a hamstring at the back of the thigh.

A warm-up allows your body to make complex adjustments in readiness for exercise. When you are inactive, your blood flows fairly evenly around your body. As you become more energetic, the blood circulation increasingly favours the working mus-cles, providing them with the oxygen and fuel (glucose) that they need to work properly. The temperature of your muscles also increases, helping you to stretch and move your joints easily and safely.

HOW TO WARM UP

What warm-up exercises should I do?

Your warm-up does not have to be complicated, but it does need to include two main parts – *general* exercise and *specific* movements or stretches for your sport or activity.

An ideal warm-up for sport, dance and fitness exercises would start with gentle movements to work all the major muscle groups – neck, shoulders and upper back, arms, lower back, legs and feet – followed by more energetic movements to raise the pulse rate (see pages 86-87). Only then should you start on specific exercises for your chosen activity.

The principle for this second stage is to do movements that imitate those of your sport or activity. A golfer or tennis player would choose movements that stretch and mobilise the upper body, such as deltoid and triceps stretches (see page 81), elbow circles (page 78) and hip swings (page 79). The golfer could then practise imaginary shots, while the tennis player could practise serving or hitting the ball back and forth to another player or against a wall. A footballer could follow a general warm-up with a leg exercise, such as hamstring stretches (see page 81) and gentle jogging (page 79).

Even though it may seem extreme, physiotherapists recommend that we warm up before *every* new moderately energetic physical activity – whether it is gardening, spring cleaning, joining in a charity fun race or going out dancing. The reason is that however fit you may be, the body is not instantly ready to cope with the demands of exercise, and you would be vulnerable to strains, sprains, fractures, aches and stiffness if you were to rush into any sudden exertion. The only exceptions are gentle walking, which can provide a warm-up in its own right, and warm-up exercises themselves.

Before gentle activities such as mowing the lawn, cleaning the windows or washing the car, there is no need for an elaborate fitness routine, even so, the warm-up exercises on pages 78-79 could help you to benefit from the mild exercise you will be getting.

TIMING A WARM-UP

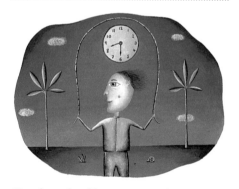

How long should my warm-up last?

Carry on with warm-up exercises for as long as it takes for you to feel warmer and looser. If you are planning to do any vigorous exercise, then your warm-up should also leave you slightly breathless.

There are no fixed rules for the length of a warm-up: different activities require different amounts of preparation, and people warm up at different rates – for instance, youngsters usually warm up faster than older people. But as a rough guide, energetic sports and fitness activities (such as tennis, rowing, squash, rugby and aerobics) and demanding forms of dance (such as jazz, contemporary, tap or ballet) require a warm-up of about half an hour – longer than most people expect. Less energetic sports (such as bowls

and golf) require about ten minutes' worth. Activities such as gardening and window cleaning need at least five minutes.

Always warm up immediately before you start your chosen activity. And even when the activity is under way, try to build the intensity of your movements gradually to avoid pulling muscles or losing your balance.

ALREADY WARM ENOUGH

I get hot and sticky enough when I exercise, so do I really need to bother with a warm-up before I start?

You certainly do. The 'warming up' done for exercising is not the same as feeling warm – even though the two types of warmth are linked. When you take exercise, your muscle movements create heat. Although your muscles need to be warm to move to their full extent, your body tries to keep its temperature at about 37°C (98.6°F). As your body cools, you get sticky with sweat.

If you exercise energetically without doing a warm-up, your body will not have prepared itself properly. You will quickly become hot and sticky as your body tries to cope with sudden energy demands, and you risk injuring muscles that are not yet flexible enough for the activity you are forcing upon them.

SAUNA OR WARM-UP?

If I have a hot bath or sauna before I exercise, does that mean I can do without warm-up exercises?

No – the only way to do a warm-up is through physical activity. Nothing else has been proved to have any beneficial effect, though dancers and sports people have tried massage, aromatic baths, whirlpool baths, saunas and steam baths.

It could in fact be dangerous to take a bath or sauna before energetic activity. Although the heat will make you feel warm and increase your heart rate, it will also lower your blood pressure, restricting oxygen to your muscles and possibly causing you to faint if you exert yourself.

However, some people find that a warm shower before they start their warm-up routine helps them to relax and clear away any distracting thoughts so that they perform better. A shower is considered safe before starting exercise because you stand and move about under the water, but its value is largely therapeutic and it is not a substitute for a proper exercise warm-up.

SIMPLE EXERCISES FOR A SAFE WARM-UP

Warming up is an essential part of preparing your body for vigorous activity. It increases muscle flexibility and protects against injury. Any good exercise class should include a warm-up session, but if you are playing a sport or working out on your own – or just getting ready for some energetic gardening – you will need to devise your own programme. This sequence of exercises provides a gentle warm-up suitable for most sports and physical activities. Move smoothly and rhythmically, avoiding any sharp twists or jolts. Try to relax – smiling occasionally might help – and breathe easily. Follow this warm-up with appropriate stretching exercises (see pages 81-82).

HEAD TURN

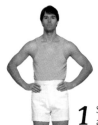

1 Stand with your feet about hip-width apart and your knees slightly bent. Rest your hands on your hips and look straight ahead of you.

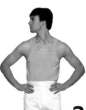

2 Without dropping your head, straining, or moving your shoulders, gently turn your head to the right as far as possible. Hold for a count of 2, then turn back to the centre.

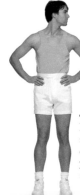

3 Count to 2, then make a similar turn to the left, moving slowly and smoothly. Repeat 4 times to each side, always keeping your chin level and your shoulders square.

ELBOW CIRCLE

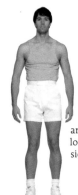

1 Stand with your feet about hip-width apart, your knees slightly bent and your arms hanging loosely by your sides.

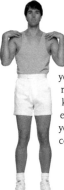

2 Bring your hands to your shoulders and rest them there, keeping your elbows as close to your body as is comfortable.

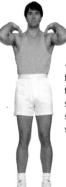

3 Now bring your elbows forward, raising them as you do so. Try not to shrug your shoulders.

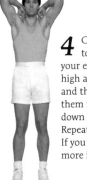

4 Continue to raise your elbows as high as possible, and then sweep them round and down again. Repeat 6 times. If you can, do 6 more in reverse.

HEEL DIG

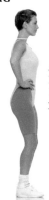

1 Stand with your feet a little apart and your knees slightly bent. Rest your hands on your hips.

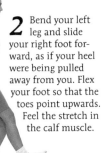

2 Bend your left leg and slide your right foot forward, as if your heel were being pulled away from you. Flex your foot so that the toes point upwards. Feel the stretch in the calf muscle.

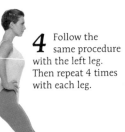

3 After a count of 2, slide your right foot back to the starting position.

4 Follow the same procedure with the left leg. Then repeat 4 times with each leg.

MARCHING ON THE SPOT

1 Stand upright, with your feet very slightly apart. Starting with your left leg, raise the heel, as if you were peeling your foot off a sticky surface.

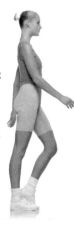

2 Lift your foot off the floor, but no more than a few inches, and swing your arms loosely as if marching. Return to the starting position, toe first, as if sticking your foot to the floor.

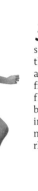

3 Lift your right foot, starting with the heel, again as if peeling from the floor, and begin getting into a marching rhythm.

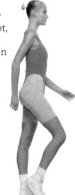

4 Keep marching for between 30 seconds and a minute, moving your feet and arms smoothly. Don't be tempted to jog at this stage – it is too early in your warm-up.

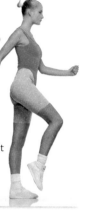

HIP SWING

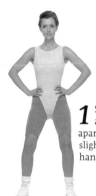

1 Stand with your feet about shoulder-width apart and your knees slightly bent. Rest your hands on your hips.

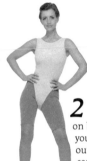

2 Swing your hips to the right, with weight even on both feet. Don't stick your stomach or buttocks out – imagine you are sandwiched between two large sheets of glass.

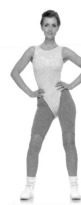

3 Smoothly swing your hips back through the starting position to the left. Keep your stomach muscles pulled in and your shoulders relaxed. Repeat 8 times each side.

LEG AND ARM CURL

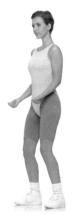
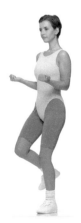
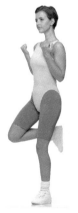
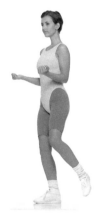
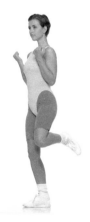

1 Stand with your feet slightly apart, your knees slightly bent, your arms slightly raised in front of you and your fists gently clenched.

2 Keeping your elbows by your sides, raise your hands towards your shoulders. At the same time, begin to swing your right foot.

3 Continue raising arms, bringing fists up to shoulder level. Raise your right knee as if trying to tap your buttocks, but don't strain.

4 Slowly and smoothly return your leg and arms to the starting position. Then follow the same routine with the left leg.

5 Continue at a comfortable speed, stepping gently from side to side on alternate legs, for at least 8 lifts with each leg.

STRETCHING TO WARM UP

My sister says that 'warming up' is just another term for stretching. Is she right?

No. Stretching is an essential part of the warming up process, but it is not the whole story. You also need to do pulse-quickening exercises such as the marching on the spot exercise and leg and arm curls on page 79. These will indirectly help you to stretch your muscles by increasing their supply of oxygen and fuel. It is easy to overstretch and injure yourself when you begin to warm up, so you must stretch gently at this stage.

Later on, when you have exercised more fully, you can stretch farther – it is especially important to do so during your cool-down (see page 89) to ease away any muscle tension that has built up during exercise and to increase your flexibility. (See below and pages 81-82 for more on stretching.)

Why you need to stretch

A VALUABLE STRETCH

Is stretching good for you?

Yes, although it is all too often a neglected part of exercise. It is well known that stretching increases flexibility, but less well known that it helps to make muscles strong. We need strong muscles to balance and stand upright, move from the spot, bend and lift. The strongest muscles are the ones that have been stretched.

Of course, stretching is only one part of fitness. You also need aerobic and anaerobic exercise (see page 64) to build muscle strength and endurance, but stretching makes many contributions to fitness:

● Increased flexibility, which allows a wider range of comfortable movements and helps to maintain mobility into old age.
● Prevention of injury, because muscles and joints can move easily without straining.
● Reduced soreness and stiffness, because muscle tension is eased after exercise.
● Increased power for jumping, lifting and bending, because well-stretched muscles have greater power when contracted.
● A sense of wellbeing after the release of muscle tension.

WHEN TO DO DEEP STRETCHES

I've heard other people refer to deep stretching. What is this and when should I do deep stretches?

There aren't any precise measurements, but a small (or shallow) stretch is an undemanding movement – as gentle as dropping your head towards one shoulder – while a deep stretch requires more effort to elongate a group of your muscles to their full extent. A muscle is like a bundle of elastic bands. If you stretch it too hard or too far, it could tear and weaken or even snap. So the general principle for stretching is to start with small stretches and to progress slowly and gently, without straining, towards deeper, longer ones, where you either bend more or position your arms or legs farther apart.

Before you exercise, your muscles are tight and cold and unprepared for exertion. As you start to warm up, they loosen and become more flexible – rather like a warm elastic band, they start to 'give' more easily. Ideally, your warm-up will be followed by stretches (see examples on pages 78 and 79 and opposite) for your chosen activity, which will further elongate the muscles. By the end of your exercise session, the constant contractions and extensions will have left your muscles tight, although not as tight as they started. So you should stretch again during your cool-down, to ease the tightness and avoid discomfort and cramp later.

With experience you will soon feel the difference between shallow and deep stretching and learn the limits of what is safe and comfortable for your body .

STRETCHING SAFETY

Is it true that some kinds of stretching can be dangerous? If so, what should I do to avoid hurting myself?

Although stretching is a natural activity for both humans and animals, specialists now know that certain positions and techniques can cause injuries.

Generally speaking, fitness experts recommend a stretching technique called static stretching, or the stretch-and-hold method.

Continued on page 82

A STRETCHING ROUTINE FOR BEFORE AND AFTER EXERCISE

To be fully fit, your muscles must be flexible as well as strong – and only stretching can do this. Whichever activity you choose, make stretching exercises a regular part of your routine, both after warming up and before cooling down. The techniques below will give a good stretch to most muscle groups. Hold each position at maximum stretch for a count of 4, relax and repeat 8 times each side.

GLUTEAL STRETCH

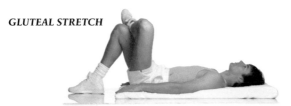

1 Lie on your back on a mat or soft floor with knees bent and feet flat on the floor. Raise your left leg and rest it against your right knee.

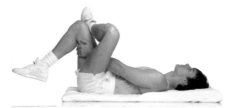

2 Grasp your right thigh with both hands and ease the leg gently in towards you, lifting the foot off the floor. Go only as far as comfortable.

HAMSTRING STRETCH

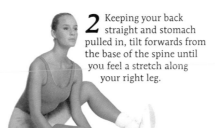

1 Sit upright with your right leg straight. Bend your left leg, letting the knee drop a bit to the side but keeping the foot flat. Rest your arms on either side of your right leg.

2 Keeping your back straight and stomach pulled in, tilt forwards from the base of the spine until you feel a stretch along your right leg.

DELTOID STRETCH

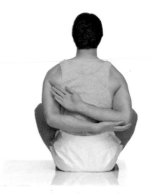

1 Sit straight with your right arm bent behind you and your hand flat against your back. With your left hand, draw the right elbow across your back.

LOWER CALF STRETCH

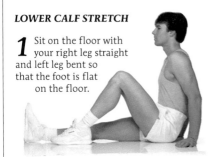

1 Sit on the floor with your right leg straight and left leg bent so that the foot is flat on the floor.

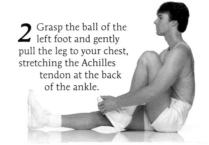

2 Grasp the ball of the left foot and gently pull the leg to your chest, stretching the Achilles tendon at the back of the ankle.

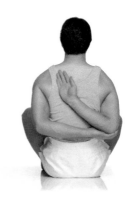

2 As you pull the elbow across, try to reach up between the shoulder blades until you feel a good stretch on the outside of the right shoulder.

TRICEPS STRETCH

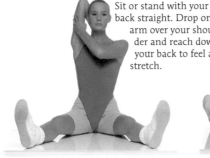

Sit or stand with your back straight. Drop one arm over your shoulder and reach down your back to feel a stretch.

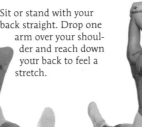

Alternatively, hold the elbow with the other hand and gently pull it behind your head until you feel a stretch.

Continued on page 82

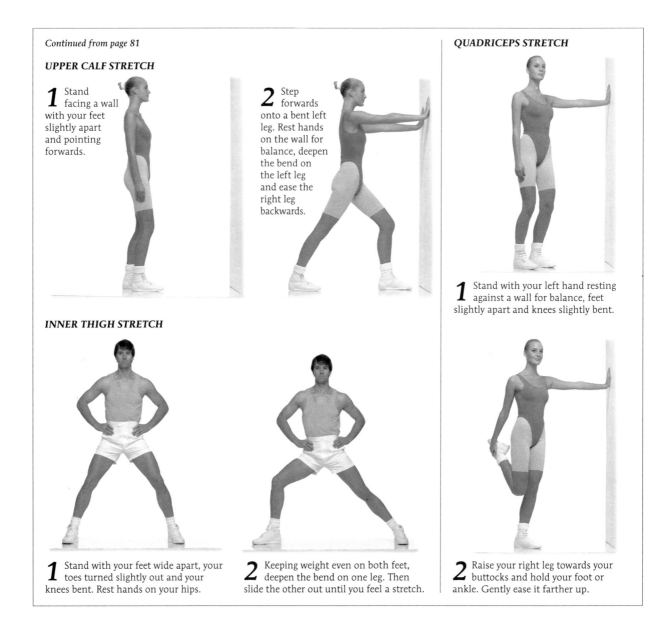

Continued from page 81

UPPER CALF STRETCH

1 Stand facing a wall with your feet slightly apart and pointing forwards.

2 Step forwards onto a bent left leg. Rest hands on the wall for balance, deepen the bend on the left leg and ease the right leg backwards.

INNER THIGH STRETCH

1 Stand with your feet wide apart, your toes turned slightly out and your knees bent. Rest hands on your hips.

2 Keeping weight even on both feet, deepen the bend on one leg. Then slide the other out until you feel a stretch.

QUADRICEPS STRETCH

1 Stand with your left hand resting against a wall for balance, feet slightly apart and knees slightly bent.

2 Raise your right leg towards your buttocks and hold your foot or ankle. Gently ease it farther up.

Continued from page 80

This involves moving smoothly into positions where it is possible to stretch without pain, and hold the various stretches without straining – for between six and fifteen seconds each initially.

You should feel a gentle pull but not a tug or wrenching sensation, and you should be able to breathe normally. Relax after each stretch, then repeat, holding the position for up to 30 seconds.

Exercise specialists now warn against the stretching technique that uses a sequence of small bouncing movements – called ballistic stretching. The technique was once very popular among fitness enthusiasts, but is now known to encourage overstretching, tearing of the muscle fibres, and sometimes even long-term injury.

It has also been discovered that certain other stretches and postures, which you may have tried in the past without suffering any ill effects, can also sometimes cause damage to the neck, back and knees.

Some of the commonest are described in the box on page 73, and – unless you are particularly fit and involved in frequent, regular training, undertaken with expert supervision – it is safest to avoid all such stretches and exercise routines. Fortunately, there are plenty of safe alternatives, as you will note from the various exercise suggestions given throughout this chapter.

How to get the best from exercise

STEP BY STEP

I am about to start exercising at a gym. Should I take it easy at first?

Having made the decision to improve your fitness, you naturally want to get on with it. But take care: you cannot get fit instantly – and it would be risky to try. You will gain little but discomfort and possible injury if you start by exercising flat out. However, by warming up (see pages 78-79), exercising for short periods at the beginning, and cooling down methodically (see pages 89-90), you will gradually be able to increase the intensity, frequency and duration of exercise.

You don't need to exercise vigorously every day: your body needs time to recover, and this could take as long as a week when you start. By practising a little patience now – and ideally with some help from a fitness specialist at the gym – you will soon learn how far you can safely push yourself.

AGREE TO PERSEVERE

Despite good intentions, I always give up exercising after a month or so. I want to get fit, so what can I do to encourage myself to carry on?

You are not alone. In fact, many people give up classes even earlier than you. The most sensible way to prevent those discouraging lapses is to have a plan – a plan in which you AGREE with yourself to get fit. This is the way it works:

Aim at clear and realistic goals.
Graduate your programme of exercise.
Reward yourself for effort and progress.
Encourage yourself and others.
Enjoy yourself.

Aims
Although it is legitimate to say 'I just want to feel fitter', you will find it easier to carry on exercising if you have a clear reason and some concrete goals to achieve: to do a sponsored swim for charity, to get into smaller clothes, or to avoid being left at the bottom of the stairs by a young colleague. Of course, you must be realistic. If you have been sedentary for years, don't expect to win a race with a fit teenager. But if you feel like giving up, remind yourself of your target.

Graduated stages
Many people abandon exercise, even when they enjoy it, because they feel they are not progressing. Devise a programme – with the help of a specialist if possible – to suit your way of life and current level of fitness. Build up the intensity and frequency gradually.

Rewards
Eventually, the benefits of fitness will be their own reward, but when the going gets tough, give yourself an incentive – a reward or a bribe. It could be an extra half-hour in bed on a Sunday, buying special training shoes – anything that you value, provided that it is not fat-laden or sugary snacks, or alcohol. When you feel discouraged, reward yourself for effort – for simply going to the gym, pool or class, or for walking instead of driving. When things are going well, reward yourself for your progress.

Encouragement
Other people can sometimes encourage you when you cannot persuade yourself to keep going. Why not join a class with a friend? Perhaps you could arrange to have a healthy snack and drink after exercising – it might give you more to look forward to. Alternatively, get involved in a sponsored event. You won't want to let others down and when you succeed once exercise becomes a habit.

Enjoyment
Find an activity that you enjoy for its own sake. If the first form of exercise you try does not give you pleasure, keep looking for one that does. If you find it difficult, remind yourself that being fit will enhance your sense of wellbeing and help you to get more enjoyment from life in general.

WHEN BEST TO EXERCISE

My son tries to discourage my wife from jogging in the afternoon. He says that it is better to exercise in the morning. Is he right?

Our bodies have 24-hour biological rhythms that are largely unaffected by what we do on any one day. Body temperature is generally warmest – which is best for muscles – in the late afternoon or early evening. Blood circulation, metabolism – the rate at which our bodies convert food into energy – and muscle

---

FACT
— OR —
FALLACY?

'No pain, no gain.'

Fallacy It is quite common to believe that exercise will do you good only if it hurts, but this is a risky attitude to take. Good exercise does involve exertion: if vigorous enough, it will make you breathless and cause sweating, and afterwards you might ache slightly. But if exercise hurts (or 'burns'), or you feel exhausted for days afterwards, you are pushing yourself too far, and you could cause long-term injury. Ease off if you begin to feel pain. And, if the pain persists, see a doctor.

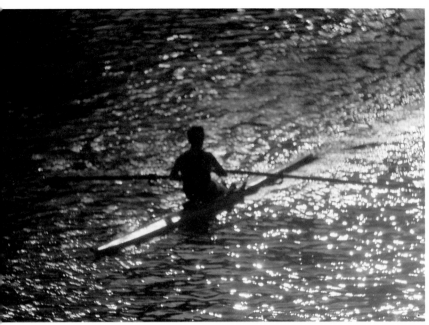

Night train to fitness To get
the most from training, all
really serious sportspeople
synchronise sessions with
times when their body
rhythms are at a peak. For
this particular sculler, that
means late evening.

of people do exercise safely when it is hot. It
is largely a matter of making sure you take
the following sensible precautions.

● Before you start any sort of exercise
programme, drink plenty of water. Sip water
whenever you feel dry during the exercise,
and afterwards, drink more water or diluted
fruit juice. Avoid alcohol, coffee, tea and
soft drinks, such as cola, that contain
caffeine – all of these dehydrate you. The
amount of liquid you should consume
during exercise – whether it is playing
tennis or golf or doing aerobic exercises –
will depend on the heat and how long the
session lasts. Normally, a person requires
around 3½ pints (2 litres) of fluid a day,
but add an extra 1¾ pints (1 litre) for every
hour of exercise.

● Avoid the hottest times of day. Try to
exercise when it is coolest – usually early
morning or evening.

● Always wear a hat or scarf of some kind
when exercising beneath a blazing sun.
Wear loose-fitting clothes that allow air
to circulate, and protect exposed areas of
skin with a sunscreen.

● Do not over-exert yourself, and stop at
once if you feel faint, sick, disorientated,
or extremely hot or thirsty. If you do feel
ill, move into the shade and drink water.
If the symptoms persist, see a doctor.

strength are also at their peak in the afternoon or the early evening. However, mental
powers have a more complex pattern: some
mental skills are at their greatest at about
midday, while others reach their peak in the
afternoon or evening.

The precise relationship between all these
body rhythms and performance in physical
activities is not fully understood, although
research suggests that the best time for physical performance is from midday to about
9 pm, but it is doubtful whether biorhythms
make any difference to someone who exercises just for fitness and pleasure. However,
serious or competitive sportspeople might
benefit from adjusting their training times.

Your wife should jog whenever she feels at
her best – her body will respond better and
recover faster. Failing that, she should simply
jog whenever she can find the time, so long
as she is not putting herself in danger.

HEAT PRECAUTIONS

*My wife and I usually enjoy taking part in
the tennis classes which are run at our
summer holiday hotel in southern Spain.
But now I've started to wonder whether it
is wise to play or exercise in intense heat?*

Dehydration is the greatest danger you face
from exercising in hot weather. If you exert
yourself without drinking enough water, you
could drive your body temperature so high
that you begin to suffer heat exhaustion or
heat stroke (see page 464). However, plenty

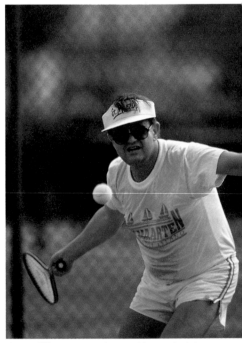

A sensible return A hat and loose clothing,
along with plenty of fluids, are essential when
playing tennis or exercising in the blazing sun.

SAFETY IN THE COLD

How safe is it for my family to go hiking when the weather is very cold?

Outdoor exercise in winter can be extremely invigorating. Provided you assess the conditions carefully and take sensible precautions against becoming wet and cold, it should be quite safe to take exercise in cold weather.

● Assess the conditions. Check the weather forecast before setting out. If it is icy or foggy, go for a short walk along local roads, and hike on another day. Turn back if the weather deteriorates while you are hiking.
● Dress warmly. Wear a hat: up to 40 per cent of the heat lost from the body can escape from an uncovered head. Keep your neck, hands and feet well covered. Wear layers: a thermal sports vest will provide warmth and draw perspiration away from your body. A fleece over a jumper is also a good option: it will provide more warmth and keep moisture away from your skin. You also need an outer windproof, waterproof jacket. Waterproof leggings may be necessary too. If you do not own these specialist clothes, build up layers of tee-shirts under a jumper and waterproofs. Asthma sufferers could tie a scarf across the nose and mouth to help to prevent an asthma attack triggered by cold air.
● Protect your skin. Rub moisturising cream into your face before setting out. Petroleum jelly on lips provides a useful barrier against wind and rain. Apply sunscreen if necessary.
● Make sure that you drink plenty of water before you go out: you can become dehydrated even in very cold weather. Take warm drinks with you.
● Prepare for your hike by doing warm-up exercises (see pages 78-79).
● Keep a careful watch on any young or old members of the family or anyone who has recently been ill. If anyone shows signs of disorientation, drowsiness, or loss of coordination or concentration, or becomes pale with numb fingers or toes, turn back immediately and treat the person for hypothermia (see page 464).
● Cool down. Continue moving around for about five minutes when you return indoors so that your circulation can return fully to your fingers, toes and nose. Alternatively, try the cool-down exercises on pages 89-90.
● Carry emergency items. Take a flask of warm drink, an extra jumper, a snack, a whistle and a torch. (See the advice on page 106.) If anyone in your family is asthmatic,

take tablets and inhalers with you, since cold weather can sometimes prompt an asthma attack.

CAUTION For safety's sake, let someone know if you are going for a long walk, and tell them what time you plan to return.

FEELING WORSE

Since I started exercising I feel more unfit than ever. Is something wrong with me?

It is not unusual to feel tired and experience a few aches when you start exercising, especially if you have been inactive for a long time. The exercise should make you feel temporarily tired but elated – not exhausted and discouraged. If you still haven't recovered fully after resting for two or three days, then you have done too much.

However vague your symptoms are, it is a good idea to see your doctor, who will probably check your pulse rate and blood pressure, and will advise you on the suitability of what you are doing. Of course, exercise is not the only thing that affects how fit you feel. Do you sit awkwardly, placing a strain on your back so that you feel tired? Do you eat enough food at the right time (see page 91) and drink enough water to ensure that you have enough fuel and fluid for exercise? Do you give enough time to leisure pursuits?

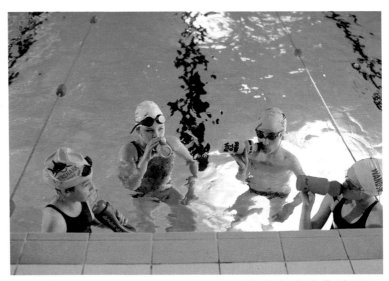

Whatever your answers, don't be put off the idea of exercise. With patience – and perhaps a little help from a fitness expert at a local gym – you should be able to find an enjoyable exercise routine that will improve your fitness without draining your energy.

Restoring body fluid With any sort of exercise, the body loses fluid. Swimming is no exception. To replenish the fluid they have lost, these children take regular drinks during breaks in training.

AN AEROBIC WORKOUT TO TRY AT HOME

Once you have warmed up you can then start working out. You don't have to buy a fitness video or go to classes, the exercises shown on these pages can be done at home, but must be performed for at least 20 minutes to give you the maximum aerobic benefit. The exercises are not in any particular sequence, but it is advisable first to carry out all the exercises done on the floor, or in a sitting position, before tackling the standing or moving-on-the-spot exercises. Apart from that, simply follow the routine that suits you best.

BOX PRESS-UP

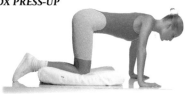

1 Kneel on a mat or soft surface with your weight evenly balanced over your knees and arms. Don't arch your back or move your hips.

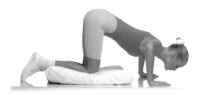

2 Bend your arms and try to touch the floor with your nose before returning to the starting position. Repeat at least 5 times.

LATERAL RISE

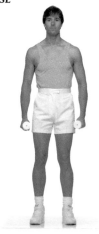

1 Hold a dumbbell or medium-sized baked bean can in each hand by your sides.

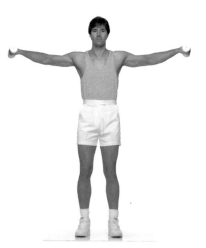

2 Slowly lift the weights to shoulder height and lower gradually. Repeat at least 10 times.

KNEE LIFT

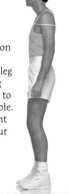

1 Aim to march on the spot by stepping from one leg to the other, lifting your knees as close to your chest as possible. Keep your arms bent to the side with your hands near your shoulders.

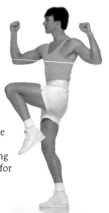

2 As you lift one leg, twist your upper body and try to raise your knee to the opposite elbow. Get your knee as close as possible to your elbow without bending your back. Continue for 16 lifts.

BICEPS CURL

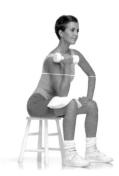

1 Sit on a stool with feet flat on the floor. Hold a dumbbell or a medium-sized baked bean can in your right hand with your elbow supported on your right knee.

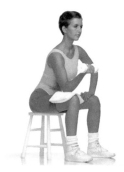

2 Lean forward slightly from the base of your spine, but don't round your back. Lift the weight slowly towards your chin, without leaning backwards.

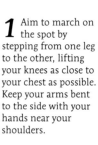

3 Slowly lower the weight back to the starting position. Repeat about 10 times, then switch to the left hand.

LEG LIFT

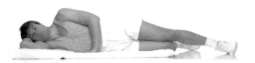

1 Lie on your side on a mat or soft surface with your right leg bent at a comfortable angle to your body. Rest your head on your right arm and place the left hand on the floor in front of you.

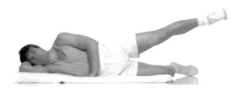

2 Slowly lift your left leg, keeping it straight. Hold for a count of 2 then lower your leg to about 2 in (5 cm) off the floor. Repeat 7 times, then turn onto your other side and repeat with the right leg.

TWIST AND JUMP

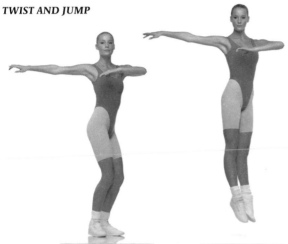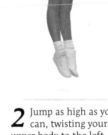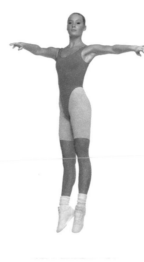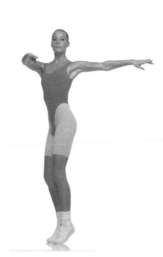

1 Hold your right arm straight out to the side and your left arm bent in front of your chest. Bend your knees before you jump.

2 Jump as high as you can, twisting your upper body to the left. Bend your knees to help you land and take off again.

3 As you jump, swing your arms across and twist to the right. Bend your knees as you land and always twist towards the straight arm.

4 Repeat the exercise to the right and left at least 8 times.

CRUNCH

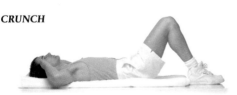

1 Lie on a mat or soft surface with your knees bent and feet flat on the floor. Rest your fingers lightly on the side of your head, around your ears.

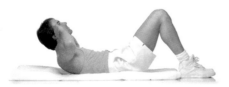

2 Lift your shoulders and head so that you can see your knees for a moment. Return to the starting position gradually. Repeat about 8 times.

STAR JUMP

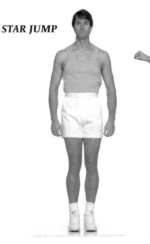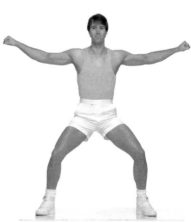

1 Stand with your feet slightly apart, knees slightly bent and arms by your side. Bend your knees to help you to jump and land.

2 Jump your feet wide apart as you raise your arms to the side and land in a star shape. Jump back to the starting position. Repeat 8 times.

ACHING TO SKI

Every time I go on a skiing holiday, I ache like mad after the first day, and return home with stiff legs and arms. Is this an inevitable part of skiing?

The excitement and brevity of a ski trip combine to encourage people to exert themselves to the full on the slopes. If you have been inactive before the holiday, the result is that

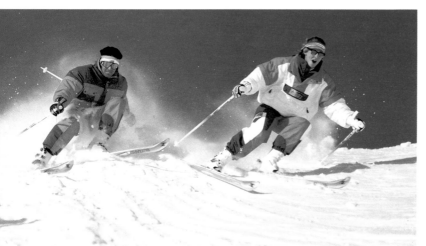

you place excessive demands upon your body. Good sense and preparatory fitness will help you to avoid the aches and pains.

● Stay generally fit throughout the year with weekly sessions of fairly vigorous exercise.
● Ideally, before the holiday practise on a dry slope or use a cross-country skiing machine. Whichever sort of exercise you choose, make sure to work your leg and arm muscles, and do flexibility exercises for your lower back: a combination of water exercises (see pages 110-111) and jogging, dancing or cycling.
● Before you ski, warm up thoroughly and do arm and leg stretches (see pages 78-82).
● After skiing, cool down and do stretches.
● During the holiday, don't try to do everything on the first day: pace yourself and gradually increase the intensity of the skiing. If there is a pool nearby, swim once or twice a week to ease any muscle pains.
● After the holiday, don't revert to a sedentary life: do at least one session of moderate exercise each week.

Fit for the slopes? For true exhilaration, there's nothing quite like a long ski run. To enjoy it to the full, and to avoid aches and injuries, be sure to reach adequate fitness before your trip begins.

Cooling down

PROTECTIVE MOVEMENTS

Is cooling down after exercise just a fad, or does it have some real value?

It is not just a fashion trend. The reason that you might have heard more about it in recent years is that fitness specialists have now conclusively established its protective value. Cooling down – or 'warming down' as it is also called – involves simple movements that return your body gently to its resting state after activity. In the first stage of cooling down, your movements should gradually restore your breathing to its normal (inactive) rate and return your circulation to an even flow throughout your body. This also helps to clear lactic acid, a waste product created when your muscles are exercised without getting enough oxygen.

Ideally, you should then do a series of cool-down stretches to ease any tension in your muscles and protect you from soreness and long-term injury. It is in fact dangerous to stop vigorous exercise suddenly, as you

will know if you have ever dashed for a train and then slumped with relief into your seat, only to feel faint or have a tingling sensation in your face, feet or hands. When you suddenly stop moving, your heart is still pumping rapidly – faster than you need it to – and blood is concentrated in the parts of your body you have been using most, such as your legs or arms. As a result, you may feel sick or giddy, or get pins and needles or cramp. The key to avoiding this is to slow down gradually, to allow your body to readjust gently to the changes in your energy demands.

LENGTH OF A COOL-DOWN

Do I need to cool down after every type of exercise and, if so, for how long?

The important point to bear in mind is that you should not suddenly stop moving. If you do, you might faint, feel sick or get cramp. You also increase the risk of aching muscles

Continued on page 90

EXERCISES FOR A GENTLE COOL-DOWN

After exercising it is important to gradually bring your breathing and heart rate back to normal. Don't stop suddenly – cool down gently with simple exercises such as these. If you have played a sport as energetic as squash, start with vigorous arm circles, gradually slowing down the speed. Stretches, arm rises and curl hugs are ideal for winding down after less active exercises.

ARM CIRCLE

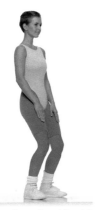 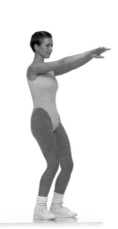 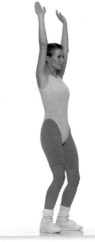 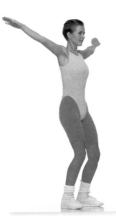

1 Stand comfortably with your feet about hip-width apart and your knees slightly bent.

2 In a continuous movement, raise your arms towards your head and breathe in.

3 Continue to raise your arms above your head, as high as possible, still breathing in.

4 Complete the circle by bringing your arms back down to your sides as you breathe out. Repeat 10 times.

SIDE STRETCH

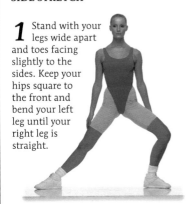 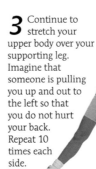 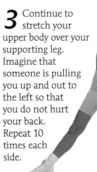

1 Stand with your legs wide apart and toes facing slightly to the sides. Keep your hips square to the front and bend your left leg until your right leg is straight.

2 Raise your right arm above your head and reach up, then start to reach over towards your supporting leg.

3 Continue to stretch your upper body over your supporting leg. Imagine that someone is pulling you up and out to the left so that you do not hurt your back. Repeat 10 times each side.

ARM RISE

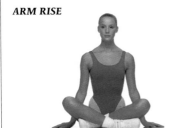 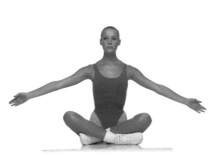 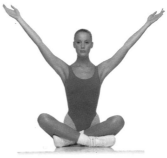

1 Sit with your legs crossed on the floor keeping your back straight. Concentrate on sitting upright, but relax.

2 As you breathe in, slowly raise your arms to the side and above your head. Keep your shoulders relaxed.

3 Breathe out as you lower your arms. Adjust the speed of the arm rises to suit your breathing. Repeat 20 times.

Continued on page 90

Continued from page 89

INNER THIGH STRETCH

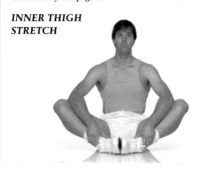

1 Sit with your back straight and feet together. Rest your hands on your ankles. Use your inner thigh muscles to ease your knees down. Hold for a count of 4, relax and repeat 7 times.

CURL HUG

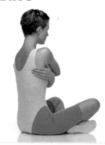 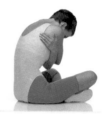

1 Sit on the floor or in a firm chair with your back straight and your legs crossed. Fold your arms across your body, as if hugging yourself, and breathe in.

2 Drop your head forward, breathing out and allowing the weight of your head to curl your body forward. Relax and let your breath become slow and rhythmic.

THIGH HUG

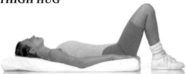 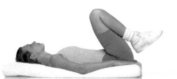 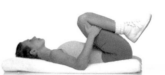

1 Lie on your back on a mat or soft surface with your knees bent and your feet flat on the floor. Try to press the hollow of the back against the floor.

2 Keeping your back as flat against the floor as you can, gradually lift your knees towards your chest. Breathe slowly and rhythmically.

3 Alternatively, clasp your hands behind your knees and gently squeeze your thighs to your chest. Stay in this position until you feel relaxed.

Continued from page 88

the following day. But the length of time and the amount of energy you need to put into your cool-down depend upon the intensity of the exercise you have just done. If you have just played a vigorous game of tennis or football, for instance, or done an aerobics or dance class, you will probably need to cool down for between five and ten minutes to get your pulse back to its normal resting rate and to give your muscles an adequate post-exercise stretching.

If you have been playing bowls or golf or taking a leisurely walk, by contrast, you might need to do only two to five minutes of cooling down. But whatever the activity you have been doing, you should continue to move around immediately after exercise and resist the temptation to flop into a chair or your car, or to lounge in a bath.

A warm shower is fine after cooling down, but if you prefer a bath, you should wait a further 20 minutes. Relaxing in a warm bath tends to lower the blood pressure, and if you settle down to a good wallow too soon after exercising, there may be a slightly increased risk of fainting when you stand up again.

AN IDEAL COOL-DOWN

Which are the best exercises for cooling down after you have been playing sport?

Any rhythmic movements that help to reduce your pulse rate will make an excellent start to your cool-down. If you have been involved in an energetic activity, such as squash, hockey or aerobics, you should start with more vigorous movements than you would if simply cooling down after a gentle bike ride, walk or swim. If you are unsure what is best, choose movements that mimic what you have been doing. For instance, if you have been running, start your cool-down by slow jogging on the spot. If you have been playing golf or a racquet sport or been canoeing, try movements in which you swing your arms and work your upper body. Gradually reduce the intensity of the movements until breathing returns to normal. Afterwards go on to do some stretches, to ease any remaining tension from your muscles and to maintain your flexibility.

Many people also like to finish their cool-down with simple breathing and relaxation exercises (see pages 190-192).

Eating for fitness

FOOD SUPPLEMENTS FOR SPORT

Should I take food supplements, such as vitamins, now that I exercise regularly?

The promotion of sports foods, drinks and pills in Britain might persuade you that you do need supplements. Some products claim to give extra energy or allow you to train for longer, while others say that you will build muscles or absorb your food more easily.

Most sports nutrition experts are sceptical about the claims, saying that an ordinary, nutritious diet should provide most people with everything the body needs, whether or not they lead an active life.

Until conclusive evidence is recognised by medical, sports and nutrition specialists, it is probably best to treat product claims with caution and to concentrate more on improving your everyday diet.

CAUTION If you believe that you need supplements, consult your doctor before taking any. Some have unpleasant side effects, such as constipation.

WHICH FOOD FOR SPORT ?

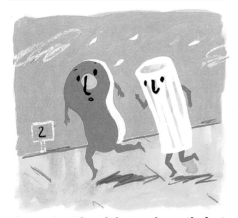

At one time I heard that steak was the best food for athletes and other people in sport. Now everyone talks about pasta. Is one really better than the other when it comes to sport for fitness and leisure?

To remain healthy, everyone needs a mixture of carbohydrate (from foods such as pasta, potatoes and rice) and protein (from foods such as eggs, meat, cheese, nuts and seeds), as well as some fat, vitamins and minerals, and plenty of water. Protein's main function is to form, grow and repair the body's cells and tissues, while carbohydrates provide the main source of energy for physical activity, whether vigorous or not. The body's own fat reserves provide a second fuel larder, with protein supplying emergency energy if necessary – when glycogen (a muscle fuel that comes from carbohydrates) is exhausted by long or intense exercise, or when there are insufficient carbohydrates in the diet.

Most people in Britain have enough protein in their diets to more than satisfy their body's requirements, but sports nutritionists now believe that top weightlifters, marathon runners and others involved in strength or endurance sports might need more protein than sedentary people.

However, to compare your requirements with those of a highly trained sportsperson could be equivalent to comparing the fuel requirements of a Formula One racing car with those of a family saloon. Increasing the protein in your diet is unlikely to improve your performance in sports or other physical activities, and it might merely increase your body fat. It is, therefore, far better to increase your carbohydrate intake to improve your energy levels before, during and after exercise (see page 92).

WHEN TO EAT FOR EXERCISE

I have two children, work every afternoon and do not have time for a meal before my aerobics class. Although I often feel hungry before class, the exercise kills my appetite. How will this affect my fitness?

Good food and regular exercise are inextricable parts of being fit, so you will need to juggle your mealtimes and what you eat to suit your way of life.

Even if you could find the time to eat a meal just before your class, it would not be sensible to do so. Your body cannot digest large amounts of food while you are exercising because it diverts blood from the digestive system to your muscles. With food left in your stomach, you can feel lethargic, sick or dizzy when you become physically active.

However, you should not miss out food altogether: in fact, that could be dangerous. When you have been very active, but have not eaten for about five hours, your glucose

Measuring energy from food

The energy value of food is measured in calories, but because one calorie is very small, figures are usually given in terms of 1000 calories – a quantity called a kilocalorie (kcal) or Calorie (Cal). You may also see the unit kilojoule (kJ) used – equal to about 4.2 kcal. Moderately active women need about 1940 kcal a day, and men about 2550 kcal.

Give yourself a 'top up' before exercise

In mild weather, a moderately active adult loses nearly a pint (570 ml) of liquid a day, mainly through perspiration. During exercise, this loss increases, to around 1¾ pints (1 litre) an hour. The body could lose as much as 4 pints (2.3 litres) every hour during vigorous activity in hot weather. You cannot prevent this happening, even when swimming, but you can prepare yourself by topping up with liquids in advance.

Food before exercise

Your body needs plenty of fuel for exercise. Carbohydrates provide the best energy store, so include them in a main meal about three hours before exercise or as small, snack-like meals up to one hour before exercise. The following foods are rich in carbohydrates:

● Banana sandwich – on wholemeal bread.
● Bowl of porridge or breakfast cereal with skimmed milk.
● Raisins.
● Baked or boiled potato, with a low-fat filling, such as cottage cheese.
● Crispbreads, crackers, toast, bread or rice-cakes with jam, honey or fruit spread.

Food after exercise

Try to eat within two hours after exercising. If exercise suppresses your appetite, have a carbohydrate-rich snack as soon as you can, then eat more later if you feel hungry. Some ideal after-exercise foods are:

● Banana sandwich using wholemeal bread.
● Oatmeal biscuits.
● Fruit cake, fruit loaf.
● Pasta with vegetables, fish or chicken.
● Baked potato with a low-fat filling, such as cottage cheese or beans.
● Tofu and vegetable stir-fry with noodles.
● Cold salad of boiled rice and sweetcorn.
● Fruit crumble with topping made from oats.
● Vegetable stew.
● Wholemeal toast.

(or blood sugar) level can drop so low that energetic activities could be too demanding and might make you dizzy. Even if you escape such obvious ill effects, your concentration and stamina could suffer during the class and afterwards. If you continually do energetic exercise without eating enough food, you will tire quickly, whatever you are doing, and will feel generally run-down.

Nutrition experts recommend that we eat regularly, although this does not necessarily mean three large or formal meals a day.

On your exercise day the most important thing is to make sure you have a nutritious breakfast and lunch. If possible have lunch earlier than usual. Eat several small, carbohydrate-rich snacks (see panel, left) at about two-hour intervals during the afternoon to boost your energy levels before exercising.

Many top-ranking sportspeople like to eat a small carbohydrate snack of about 1½ oz (50 g) between five and twenty minutes before competing to give fast energy. Try this about an hour before your class, but no later, or you may feel sick while exercising.

Drink plenty of water throughout the day, including one or two glasses within an hour of starting the class.

Try to eat a snack or light meal that contains plenty of carbohydrate within about two hours of finishing the class. The body is geared to refuelling at this time, so glycogen and glucose, which fuel the muscles, can be replenished quickly (see panel, left). However, try to avoid eating a large meal after about 9.30 pm. You are unlikely to need all the energy that a large dinner would supply before bedtime and the excess will be stored by your body as fat.

CARBOHYDRATE POWER

Which sort of carbohydrates will give me the most energy before and after sport?

Carbohydrates are digested at different rates, so the body's blood-sugar level – an indicator of energy – may rise slowly or rapidly.

In general, starches (or complex carbohydrates), from foods such as potatoes, bread and rice, release their energy slowly, while simple carbohydrates (sugars), such as those from jam, honey, fruit, juice and other sweet foods, give a quick energy boost. But the full picture is much more complicated.

For one thing, some types of complex carbohydrate – such as those in potatoes and bread – produce a more rapid rise in blood-sugar levels than some simple carbohydrates do, such as the sugars in apples and dates.

For another, the mixture of carbohydrates, protein, fat, water and soluble fibre that we consume affects the rate at which carbohydrates are broken down. What is more, many dishes contain a combination of simple and complex carbohydrates – think of rice pudding, for example.

You can follow a simple guide – the glycaemic index – that identifies which foods create a slow, moderate or fast rise in blood-sugar levels. Generally speaking foods with a high rating are best before exercise, foods with a moderate or high rating straight after, and foods with moderate or low rating later.

High glycaemic rating

Most sugary foods fall into this category, including raisins, bananas, honey, jam, glucose, sweets and chocolate bars, and sweet biscuits. Both white and brown rice have a high rating, as do bread, most breakfast cereals, sweetcorn, potatoes and broad beans.

Moderate glycaemic rating

These foods include pasta, oats, sweet potatoes, crisps, porridge, bran cereals, grapes, oranges and oatmeal biscuits.

Low glycaemic rating

Foods that rate low include milk, yoghurt, ice cream, apples, plums, grapefruit, dates, figs, dried apricots and pulses such as kidney and butter beans, lentils and chick peas.

HOW MUCH WATER?

I've been told to drink water whenever I get thirsty during an exercise session, but doing so makes me feel sick. Is there a way around this, and how much should I drink?

If you drink enough water well before exercising, you are unlikely either to get thirsty or to feel sick during your exercise session. It is important never to become dehydrated. If you do, you could damage your ability to perform well or even safely.

As your body's fluid level drops, you could be sick or feel faint, or suffer from diarrhoea, breathing difficulties, mental confusion or heat exhaustion – which in extreme cases could lead to a heart attack and even death.

How much you need to drink when you take exercise depends upon the type, intensity and duration of the activity, the weather, your fitness and how much you sweat.

As a rough guide, adults need between 1¾ pints (1 litre) and 2½ pints (1.4 litres) a day if sedentary and between 3½ pints (2 litres) and 5½ pints (3.1 litres) if active. Drink an extra litre for each hour of exercise you take. If you are drinking enough your urine will be pale yellow, as if diluted. If it is darker, you probably need to drink more.

If you exercise for more than an hour, take water with you, and take a few sips when you get the chance or when your throat gets dry. In time, you may be able to tolerate bigger mouthfuls during your chosen activity.

Try to get into the habit of drinking several glasses of a carbohydrate and electrolyte solution (see right) or of diluted fruit juice after exercising, even if you do not feel very thirsty. Your body needs to replace all the fluids and minerals that it has lost. Studies suggest that you recover fastest if you drink immediately after exercise rather than waiting until you get home.

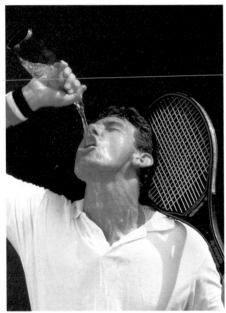

Don't get dehydrated You need to drink as much as possible during and after exercise to replenish the fluid you lose by sweating.

THE VALUE OF SPORTS DRINKS

My son spends a big chunk of his pocket money on sports drinks for use after football training and matches. What's in them and will they do him any good?

Commercial sports drinks typically consist of water with varying quantities of carbohydrates (glucose polymers or sugars) that provide energy, and/or electrolytes (mineral salts such as sodium, potassium, magnesium and chloride) that help to restore the balance of body fluids. Various flavourings and some vitamins are also often included. These drinks will not do your son any harm. They will help to replace the fluids and minerals he has lost during exercise, and some of them may help to sustain his energy level.

He is right to drink plenty of liquids after exercise, because so much body fluid is lost by perspiring and breathing hard. But why not encourage him to drink plenty of water instead, or diluted unsweetened fruit juice, or a home-made isotonic drink (see panel, right) before, during and especially in the two hours after taking part in sport? These are cheaper and just as effective.

Eating a high-carbohydrate snack, such as a banana sandwich, could also help to boost depleted energy reserves and replace some of the electrolytes lost in sweat.

But don't worry if your son prefers drinking a commercial sports drink. It is probably better than drinking sugary soft drinks and caffeinated drinks – such as cola, tea and coffee – which will temporarily dehydrate him and prolong the time needed to rehydrate after exercise. The main thing is that he is drinking the right kind of fluids.

SPORTS DRINK GUIDE

Special sports drinks often have scientific-sounding descriptions. What, if any, are the differences between these drinks, and where do 'energy' drinks fit in?

The terms used of commercial sports drinks – hypotonic, isotonic and hypertonic – refer to how concentrated the drink is by comparison with the body's fluids. This determines how quickly the body absorbs the liquid.

Hypotonic
These liquids are less concentrated than the body's fluids so they are absorbed faster than water or any other fluid. They are ideal for rapidly rehydrating during long exercise sessions and immediately afterwards. Diluted fruit squash is hypotonic (see panel, right).

Isotonic
These liquids are absorbed fairly quickly, as they are in balance with the body's fluids. They are ideal for rapid rehydration after exercise. Water sweetened in the right proportions is isotonic (see panel, right).

Hypertonic
These liquids are more concentrated than body fluids, and are absorbed slowly. Commercial hypertonic beverages are sometimes marketed as 'energy' drinks, because their high carbohydrate content can increase your

---

Making your own sports drinks

You don't have to spend money on commercial sports drinks. Some homemade versions are just as good.

Hypotonic drink (for before, during or after exercise)
- 4 fl oz (120 ml) orange squash.
- 1¾ pints (1 litre) drinking water.
- Small pinch of salt.

Shake all the ingredients together in a container with a lid. Refrigerate until required.

Isotonic drink (for before, during or after exercise)
- 2 oz (50 g) granulated sugar or glucose.
- 1¾ pints (1 litre) drinking water.
- Small pinch of salt.

Warm 4 tablespoons of the water and mix it with the salt and glucose or sucrose. Add the rest of the water and chill.

Hypertonic drink (for restoring energy after exercise)
- 1 pint (570 ml) unsweetened orange or apple juice.
- Small pinch of salt.

Shake ingredients in a container with a lid. Chill until needed.

blood sugar. They are suitable for replenishing energy stores after exercise, so that you recover faster. Hypertonic drinks such as fruit juice are not good for rehydration, so if you take them after exercise, you should also have water or isotonic or hypotonic drinks.

ALCOHOL – SAFE FOR EXERCISE?

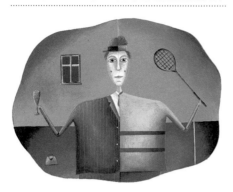

I really look forward to having one or two beers with a friend after a workout, but now I hear that I could be undoing all the good I've achieved. Is this true?

Experts advise against drinking after playing any contact sport such as boxing or rugby where there is a risk that you may have sustained a head injury. But generally speaking, a moderate amount of alcohol after exercise is unlikely to damage your fitness or health. Drink plenty of water or isotonic or hypotonic drinks (see page 93) *before* going to the bar, to replace the fluids that you have lost while exercising and to protect against the dehydrating effects of alcohol. It is not always appreciated that alcohol is a diuretic – it flushes liquids from your body.

Since it is very important to rehydrate and not dehydrate after exercise, choose long drinks such as beer rather than spirits such as gin. Stretch alcoholic drinks with non-alcoholic ones: try mixing wine with soda, or lager with lemonade, or alternate a glass of water with every pint of beer. Sports nutritionists also suggest that you eat something with your drink – ideally a carbohydrate-rich snack such as a banana – to slow down your liver's metabolising of the alcohol.

Drinking before exercise probably presents greater dangers than the occasional social pint afterwards. Alcohol can impair your balance, coordination and judgment, and is responsible for many accidents. It can also dehydrate the body for many hours. So, if you intend exercising in the morning, keep to sensible limits (about 2-3 units) in the evening and make sure you rehydrate with water before you go to sleep. (See page 155 for sensible drinking limits.)

Weight control through exercise

MUSCLES AND WEIGHT GAIN

Is it true that people who exercise regularly put on weight, and when they stop regular exercise their muscles turn to fat?

It is true that people who take regular exercise may initially gain a little weight, partly because muscles weigh more than fat. Also, the volume of blood in circulation increases (fat people and fit people have more blood). But in the longer term, exercise helps you to lose weight, by burning calories that would otherwise be stored as fat. Well-toned muscles usually make you look slimmer too.

Physical activity increases your metabolic rate – the rate at which your body turns stored food into energy. Fit bodies can therefore draw upon reserves of fat far sooner than unfit bodies. When you exercise regularly, the increase in metabolic rate lasts longer than the period you spend exercising, so you use more body fat, even at rest.

If you stop taking regular exercise, your metabolic rate will decrease and you will not draw so quickly upon your fat stores. As a result you may gain weight if your diet stays the same. As muscles lose tone, they become softer and start to look flabbier. However, muscle is always muscle and fat is always fat. Although they work together to provide you with energy, one cannot turn into the other.

SHEDDING THE POUNDS

Are some sports and physical activities particularly good for slimmers?

All forms of exercise can help you to lose weight by using up energy (calories) stored in the form of fat. Aerobic exercise – the sort that makes you feel slightly breathless – is the best way to increase your metabolism, and so burn up more body fat for energy.

Walking, jogging, swimming, cycling, aerobics, rowing and many kinds of dancing are all good choices. To burn fat, you need to do the exercise for at least 20 minutes at a time and vigorously enough to increase your heart and lung rate, making you a little out of breath. Long periods of activity such as a day of hillwalking or a long, slow jog are best for losing fat. Short, intense bursts are unlikely to help much with slimming. For people who are overweight, cycling and swimming are two good choices – excellent for burning calories and also providing support for the body.

WEIGHT IN THE FAMILY

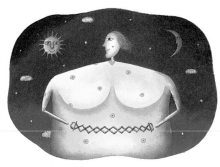

My grandmother says everyone in our family is so heavily built that there is no point in trying to lose a little weight by exercising. Is she right?

We inherit our body types, so a heavy-boned, broad-shouldered, wide-hipped person will not become a slender lightweight through exercise. However, you will certainly not be wasting your time. Exercise can help virtually anyone to improve general health and fitness, burn off fat, and feel and look better. While you will still have the same number of fat cells, they will not be so well stocked.

Don't expect an overnight miracle, and try to be realistic about what you can achieve. Remember that to lose weight you will also need to control what you eat. Joining a slimming group or a fitness club will help you to set a realistic goal and decide on the best way to achieve it. (See also pages 152-153.)

SWEATING WEIGHT AWAY

I have heard of people going into sweat-baths to lose weight. Does it really work?

You can lose weight temporarily by sweating. But it is not a good method of weight control, because the reduction is due solely to the loss of water, which the body will replenish within a few days. To lose weight and keep it off you must lose fat – ideally by combining exercise and a slimming diet.

SLIMMING GRADUALLY

I've been dieting and exercising for three weeks now, but have lost only two pounds. Does this mean that I'll never get slimmer?

No – but losing weight makes complicated demands upon the body, so you will need to have a little faith and patience.

Most nutritionists recommend that you lose only one or two pounds a week. If you lose weight any faster, it rarely stays off, and you may suffer from feelings of dizziness and nausea, nutritional depletion and various other problems.

At the start of a slimming diet, you could shed several pounds through water loss, only to be disappointed to find the weight back again several days later, once the body has re-balanced its fluid levels.

If you continue a slimming diet without taking some form of regular exercise, some more body weight may be lost, but your body will soon reduce its metabolic rate – the rate at which it converts food stored as fat into energy. It is as if the body does not know when it will next get fed, so it stocks up a store cupboard of fat as a precaution against possible future starvation. Exercise breaks through this defensive process by increasing the metabolic rate, so that more calories are used up even when at rest.

CRAVING FOR FOOD

My best friend refuses to take any exercise while she is on a slimming diet because she is convinced that it will increase her appetite. Is she right?

Exercise affects people in different ways. For some, activity temporarily suppresses hunger before their appetite rises, while others crave food immediately.

Your friend may feel more hungry after she exercises, but in the long term, she must take exercise if she is to retain any benefits from dieting.

Until she stops craving food, your friend could try 'browsing' or 'grazing', particularly on days when she exercises. Instead of eating full meals, she could take several mini-meals or snacks, ideally of foods with a high carbohydrate content, such as fruit, low-fat oat flapjacks, rice and sweetcorn salad, plain or fruit yoghurt, or a wholemeal sandwich. She should also drink plenty of water.

Note too that if she avoids eating just before bedtime, she will reduce the build-up of calories stored in her body as fat.

Burning calories

Your body needs energy every minute of the day, so it is constantly using up calories, even when you are sitting reading or fast asleep in bed. However, the number of calories that you use up in a day depends upon your fitness level – fit people burn fat faster than unfit people – and also upon the intensity and duration of any physical activity that you take part in.

The following examples are therefore only a rough guide:

How many Calories per hour will everyday activities burn up?
- Sleeping – 70
- Eating – 96
- Standing – 108
- Driving a car – 168
- Vacuuming – 250
- Cleaning the windows – 300
- Walking at 3 mph (5 km/h) – 300
- Walking at 5 mph (8 km/h) – 480

How many Calories do gentler sports burn off in an hour?
- Golf (if you are walking and carrying golf clubs) – 300-360
- Ballroom dance – 360
- Swimming (doing either front crawl or backstroke) – 360-750

How many Calories per hour do the more strenuous sports use?
- Aerobics – 360-480
- Tennis – 480
- Rowing – 480-840
- Cycling at 12 mph (19 km/h) – 600
- Jogging – 600
- Circuit training – 600
- Squash – 600-900

DO'S
— AND —
DON'TS

for weight control

Do consult your doctor before starting a new type of exercise if you are overweight, obese or underweight.

Do consider swimming and cycling: they are excellent for overweight people because the body is supported.

Do start with moderate types of exercise that do not stress the joints.

Don't attempt vigorous activities, such as squash, until you are fitter and slimmer.

Don't forget that ordinary household activities can also burn calories, particularly if done vigorously.

DEALING WITH EMBARRASSMENT

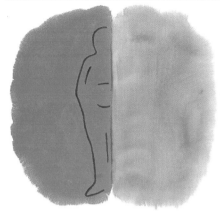

My father has put on a lot of weight and his doctor says that he needs more exercise. He wants to get fitter but cannot bear to go to a gym. What other options are there?

Overweight people such as your father are often reluctant to reveal their bodies, and need a lot of encouragement to start or continue any kind of exercise. A starting activity should be gentle, allow him to keep his body covered and provide an interest other than just getting fitter. If you, another member of the family, or a friend could join in as well, it would give your father the moral support and encouragement that he probably needs.

Walking or cycling would be good choices until your father feels less self-conscious. Both activities improve the efficiency of the heart, lungs and circulation, and are good for fat-burning. You could suggest joining a short guided walk to combine exercise with learning about an area of interest. Later on, you could encourage your father to try a ramble or cycle along country lanes. Try to get him more interested in exploring the area than thinking about his own body.

He could try exercising at home with a beginner's video tape (see page 103). Or if he can afford it, he could consider buying equipment such as an exercise bike, rowing machine, or multigym (see page 102).

You could encourage your father to watch an aerobics or swimming class that has been specially designed for elderly, unfit or overweight people. (Contact your local council and leisure centres for details.) He will see that the world is not full of perfect bodies, and most people are too busy exercising to take much notice of others. If he is still too daunted to try out any such activities, urge him to do more at home: gardening and decorating can provide a good workout, provided that he does not overdo it.

The role of rest in a fitness programme

Try to take at least one full day off from exercise per week. Rest days are a vital part of a balanced fitness plan. Time off allows your muscles to recuperate and replenish their energy stores, so resting will enhance your fitness. Also, the time that you take off from your chosen activity will probably mean an increase in your enjoyment when you are exercising. Overtraining is counterproductive: it will reduce both your performance and your enjoyment, and it can make you more vulnerable to injury.

Healthy attitudes to exercise

MENTAL EXERCISE

Is physical exercise good for the mind?

It is still unclear whether exercise can bring about any specific changes in the brain. But it is very well known that exercise can make people feel better, more alert and more confident, as well as fitter. People who exercise regularly are less likely to experience anxiety or depression, and fitness training has been used to relieve symptoms in those diagnosed as clinically depressed. Research also shows that exercise may help older people to stay mentally astute and to reduce memory loss.

EXERCISE ADDICTION

Is it possible to become addicted to exercise?

Yes – some people can become dependent on exercise, just as on gambling, or dieting, to the point of obsessiveness. What starts out as a way to improve daily life begins to take over, and may lead to the neglecting of work, personal relationships, studies and important events.

Rest days are an important part of a fitness routine because they allow the body to recover and the muscles to refuel. Someone who cannot go a day without some form of strenuous exercise, or who insists on exercising despite injury or illness, could be developing an addiction. Other signs can include inability to talk about anything else, sleeplessness, loss of weight, digestive problems, menstrual irregularities, and anxiety.

People obsessed with exercise usually need professional help to break the habit without losing their fitness and wellbeing. A qualified trainer can help by developing a routine that includes rest days and a variety of types of exercise – most obsessive exercisers concentrate on just one form of activity, such as weightlifting, and neglect all-round fitness. In severe cases, counselling may be needed to deal with deeper emotional issues unconnected with fitness training.

VISUALISING SUCCESS

Are there any mental techniques or exercises that would help to improve my performance in various active leisure pursuits?

Many experts suggest that mental preparation is as important as physical training for competitive events. Techniques used by top competitors may help you or anyone else who exercises for fitness and pleasure.

Concentration and determination to succeed are just two mental qualities that have an obvious effect on physical prowess and sports performance. Research has also shown that people who can learn to relax before a stressful competitive event end up focusing more clearly on it when it begins, and therefore performing better.

Before you start your exercise session, why not try some simple breathing and mental relaxation exercises (see pages 190-192). Aim to put the day's events out of your mind as you gradually ease tension from your body.

The technique known as 'visualisation' (see page 192) is particularly effective – just imagine the moves that you will be making in your chosen sport or physical activity.

For example, if you are about to play golf, conjure up a mental image of swinging the club and hitting the ball with just the right amount of force. Imagine too how you feel, or could feel, when you achieve what you set out to do. Treasure these feelings of relaxed control, confidence and success while you exercise: with a little practice, you will find they can help you to get even more satisfaction out of your chosen physical activity.

Preventing pain and injury

FIRST AID FOR INJURIES

What can I do to help myself recover if I hurt myself during exercise?

The first rule is that if you are in great pain, or believe you could have a serious injury, you must get medical advice straight away.

If you believe that the injury is a minor one, follow some simple steps to recovery. They are easily remembered by the acronym RICE – Rest, Ice, Compression, Elevation.

● Rest the injured area. Do not continue exercising, even if you can tolerate the discomfort: you will delay your recovery, and could cause more serious damage. Keep your weight off injured areas until any pain or swelling reduces.
● Use ice cubes in a plastic bag or a bag of frozen vegetables as an ice pack. Spread petroleum jelly over the injured area or cover it with a cloth to protect the skin and apply the pack for up to 12 minutes every two to three hours for the first day, then several times a day for the next 48 hours.
● After applying the ice pack wrap the injured area in an elastic bandage. Use the bandage for up to 72 hours, after which the pain and swelling should have gone down.
● When you apply an ice pack to your injury, keep the injured part of your body raised, to prevent it from swelling with fluids and blood. If you have a leg injury, for example, support the leg on a cushion.

After the first 48 hours you should try gentle exercise in order to rehabilitate the injured area and keep it mobile. Gradually increase the amount you attempt to do. If movement remains painful, seek medical advice.

RISKS OF INJURY

I've heard that thousands of people are hurt every year while exercising. Just how dangerous are Britain's most popular fitness activities, and is injury inevitable?

Millions of people in Britain enjoy sports and fitness activities without coming to any harm. But exercise injuries do occur often enough to cost more than £600 million each year in health care and days lost from work.

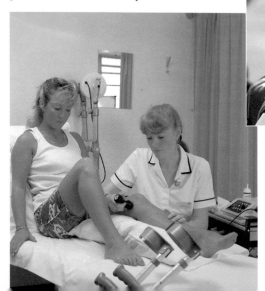

Treating injury An ice pack is a simple form of first aid to relieve pain, but for more serious or recurring problems, sports injuries may require expert attention from a physiotherapist.

High-risk activities

This list is based upon the number of injuries for every 1000 times someone engages in each activity, the highest-risk sports are:

1 Rugby
2 Soccer
3 Hockey
4 Cricket
5 Martial arts
6 Badminton
7 Squash
8 Tennis
9 Jogging, running (road or cross-country), orienteering
10 Weight training
11 Horse riding
12 Fitness exercise (such as aerobics, Keep Fit, yoga, circuit training or using exercise machines)

Of all sports, rugby produces the greatest number of injuries which need treatment or which prevent the player from working or taking part in normal daily activities. It is three times more risky than soccer, the activity with the next highest injury record for adults (see panel, below left).

About half of all new injuries result from colliding with another person or an object or by falling. Over three-quarters of recurring injuries, and about half of all new injuries, are due to the way people exercise – such as over-exerting themselves or over-stretching: so many injuries could be avoided by exercising more safely (see panel, left).

CAUSES OF CRAMP

Every time I exercise I get terrible cramp in my legs. What am I doing wrong?

The cause in your case is probably that you are not doing a thorough warm-up before your session and a proper cool-down afterwards. Cramp is the sharp pain of a sudden contraction, or spasm, of a muscle. If you follow this simple advice, you should be able to avoid cramp, whatever its cause may be:

● Warm up thoroughly (see pages 78-79). Cold muscles are particularly vulnerable to cramp and injury.
● Do some stretches to lengthen and loosen your muscles before you begin a workout (see pages 81-82).
● Build the intensity of your exercise gradually to allow your body to adjust to the more strenuous physical demands.
● Don't overdo it. Ease off if you experience any discomfort. Get plenty of rest between sessions of activity.
● Do some cool-down exercises at the end of a workout (see pages 89-90) to balance the body's fluids and rid the muscles of the lactic acid produced by exertion.
● Try some deep stretches (see pages 80-82) after exercising, to ease muscle tension that has built up during vigorous activity.
● Ask an expert to check that you are moving safely: awkward technique may be responsible for cramp.
● Vary the exercise you do. If you cannot fit in more than one type of fitness activity each week, avoid working one set of muscles (such as your leg muscles) to the exclusion of others.
● Drink plenty of liquid before and after exercising or you risk dehydration, which can contribute to cramp.
● Refuel with a carbohydrate-rich snack and

an isotonic drink (see page 93) shortly after exercising to replenish the mineral salts which are lost in sweat, and glycogen, a form of energy stored in the muscles.
● Wrap up after exercising: a sudden drop in temperature can make muscles contract.
● If cramp continues or if you experience prolonged muscle spasms, ask your doctor's advice – you might have a trapped nerve.

VULNERABLE FEET

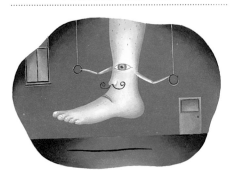

I've seen several people hobbling around my gym after fitness classes. Is there anything in particular I should do to avoid injuring my knees, ankles and feet?

Feet take the brunt of most fitness activities, yet are often overlooked during a warm-up routine. This neglect puts extra strain on the knees, ankles and feet during exercise.

To warm up your feet and legs before exercise do some heel digs and marching on the spot (see pages 78-79). If possible, wear shoes designed specifically for your activity. If this is not possible, wear well-cushioned general-purpose training shoes. Avoid fashion shops when shopping for sports shoes, and change running shoes regularly. Ask your instructor to check that your shoes are suitable for the exercise that you are doing.

You need to use your feet properly. Ask your instructor to check your moves: one common fault is to slap your feet down flat, putting excessive force on the knees, ankles and feet. Instead, try to move through the whole length of the foot as you put it down.

A FRESH START

I have been unable to do any exercise for months because of a minor injury. Is there anything I should avoid when I restart?

Yes – you cannot expect to be as fit as when you were taking regular exercise. Whenever you have had to stop exercising because of illness or injury, you should start back at a more modest level than the one at which you left off, so you will need to scale down the intensity of your exercise at first. Also be prepared for the possibility that you may need to exercise less frequently and for a shorter time until you regain your fitness.

Build up your strength slowly, over several weeks, and try not to be despondent if you are not quickly back on peak form.

It is sensible at first to avoid highly aerobic exercise and activities that pound the joints, so do not play squash or tennis, go running or take part in high-impact aerobics until you are back in condition. Swimming, walking and cycling are often the safest forms of exercise for people who have not fully recovered. Always make sure that you do a proper warm-up and cool-down, and don't push yourself too far, too hard or too fast.

If you are injured and unable to continue with a favourite sport, it is best to try to prevent a serious decline from occurring by keeping your fitness up in other ways while you recover. If you have ankle strain from running, for example, you could still keep fit by swimming and weight training for a few weeks until you are fully recovered.

PREVENTING A STITCH

I often get a stitch in my side when I am running. Is it dangerous, and how should I prevent it?

A stitch is a form of cramp. It is not dangerous, but the pain is the body's warning to slow down or stop for a moment, so do not ignore it. Try bending over slightly to relax the muscles, then walk until you can breathe slowly and rhythmically. Do not start jogging again until the pain has gone.

A stitch is unlikely to last long, and it can be avoided. Common causes include:

- Running or jogging too energetically before your muscles are properly warm. To avoid the problem warm up and stretch properly before you exercise (see pages 78-82).
- Incorrect breathing techniques – often caused by an inadequate warm-up.
- Weak abdominal muscles, or undigested food in the stomach and intestine. Avoid exercising immediately after a meal, and do some abdomen-strengthening exercises.
- Dehydration - drink enough water.

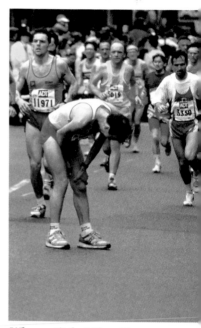

When a stitch strikes Slow down or stop. Try bending over to relax the muscles which are causing the pain.

Illness and exercise

AVOIDING HEART DISEASE

How safe is it for people who have heart disease or a high cholesterol level to take part in exercise?

People with a high cholesterol level or who are suffering from heart disease must ask their doctor's advice about safety before they start any new type of exercise.

The main cause of heart disease and heart attacks is a build-up of fatty deposits, called plaque, in the arteries. This accumulation of plaque is partly caused by high levels of cholesterol in the blood (see page 363).

The relationship between exercise, cholesterol and heart disease is a complex one. It seems that exercise and a low-fat diet can help to control cholesterol levels and so protect against heart disease. Aerobic exercise helps to raise blood levels of high-density lipoproteins (HDL cholesterol), the sort of cholesterol believed to protect against the build-up of plaque in the arteries. Exercise is also thought to reduce blood levels of low-density lipoproteins (LDL cholesterol), the sort that produces plaque.

More sustained endurance exercises such as hill walking, swimming or jogging are particularly useful, as they encourage the body to use up its fat stores.

BLOOD PRESSURE CONTROL

Does exercise reduce or increase blood pressure, and how does this affect someone with high blood pressure, or someone at risk from a stroke?

Regular exercise will generally lower blood pressure in the long term but increase it in the short term while you are exercising. Aerobic activities (which burn oxygen), such as walking, will raise your blood pressure less than muscle-strengthening anaerobic exercise (which does not require extra oxygen), such as weightlifting.

People who have high blood pressure or are very overweight are generally warned to avoid vigorous anaerobic exercises such as press-ups. Instead they are usually advised to take aerobic exercise to strengthen the heart, reduce resting blood pressure and improve the efficiency of the blood circulation.

FIGHTING COLDS

If I did more exercise, would it prevent me from catching colds and flu?

It could do, although there is no conclusive scientific evidence that it will. It is thought that regular, moderate aerobic exercise helps to build up the body's immune system, so that it can resist infection. Many people who take regular exercise report catching fewer colds and similar conditions.

However, people who do a great deal of exercise may find that they are actually more susceptible to infection. One possible reason is that doing too much physical exercise may use up the body's stores of energy, proteins and vitamins at the expense of the immune system, making illness more likely.

It is debatable whether you should exercise once you have caught a cold: it largely depends upon how ill you feel, and how you respond to physical activity at such times. Exercise can help to drain and clear your nose and respiratory system. It can also help you to relax by altering your breathing patterns and releasing natural painkilling substances known as endorphins. However, for most people, exercising with a cold leaves them feeling listless.

CAUTION Most doctors advise against exercising when you have flu or a fever because you could increase your temperature, make yourself feel worse, and even possibly delay your recovery.

STRENGTHENING BONES

I have heard that exercise can help to build up stronger bones and counteract the development of osteoporosis. Is this true? Is any particular sort of exercise best?

Taking regular exercise throughout life helps to protect the skeleton against osteoporosis (diminishing bone mass). But even if you have been inactive in earlier years, starting exercise in later life will help to maintain your bone mass. Swimming is a good exercise for those who already have osteoporosis because it is a non-contact, low-impact form of activity. Before starting any form of exercise, sufferers must check with their GPs.

If you currently lead a sedentary life, it is well worth taking up some form of physical activity, such as walking, dancing, aerobics or even cycling, that will help to strengthen and maintain your bones. Remember, however, that bones will weaken very quickly whenever people are inactive, this is particularly noticeable in those who are confined to bed or to a wheelchair for more than a few weeks at a time.

Women are much more susceptible to osteoporosis than men. At particular risk are Caucasian and Asian women, women with a low body weight, women whose periods have stopped (for example, some ballet dancers and gymnasts) and women who have passed menopause (see also pages 48 and 390-391).

EXERCISING NEAR TRAFFIC

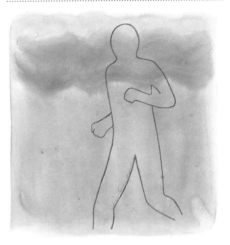

My morning jog takes me through areas with a lot of traffic. What are the risks in jogging in polluted air?

Even healthy people find that traffic pollution can cause breathlessness, coughs, stinging eyes, sore nose or throat, or a feeling of tightness across the chest. Anyone who suffers from a heart or respiratory ailment risks developing some rather more serious problems from exercising when the air quality is poor. They must be extremely careful.

People who are particularly sensitive to air quality for any reason should take precautions such as reducing or avoiding physical activity on hot, humid, windless days when pollution levels tend to rise (see pages 302 and 351). If you have to wait to cross a busy road, step back from the kerb to avoid inhaling exhaust fumes directly.

Also consider altering your jogging times to avoid the morning rush hour and middle-to-late afternoon when sunlight will have reacted with morning pollution to increase ozone levels. The early evening could be the safest time for you to go jogging. If this is not convenient, and you are worried about air pollution in the area, consider doing some of your jogging on a treadmill indoors.

SAFE EXERCISE FOR ASTHMATICS

How safe is exercise for young children who suffer from asthma?

In all but a very few asthma cases the benefits of taking exercise are thought to be much greater than the risks. Although activity may sometimes trigger an attack of breathlessness many people, including children, find they can deal with the problem by exercising less energetically for a while, and by taking medication. So if a child uses an inhaler it should always be close to hand.

Adults should also encourage asthmatic children to slow down and rest for short periods, especially if they show signs of becoming breathless. Most children's games and activities, such as hide-and-seek, hopscotch, cricket, football, climbing and swimming do provide natural rest periods.

Asthma sufferers should also avoid triggering factors such as running in very cold air or cycling along busy roads where the air quality is bad. On the whole, unless a doctor has banned vigorous exercise, it is definitely beneficial for asthmatics to stay active.

KEEPING FIT WITH BACK PAIN

Will exercise help to ease back pain, and are there any exercises that people with weak backs should avoid?

Exercises can help to relieve back pain, but do check with your doctor before beginning an exercise programme. Generally speaking, the exercises for backs on pages 143-144, and the warm-up and cool-down exercises (see pages 78–79 and 89-90) are safe for people who have back trouble.

Warming up thoroughly before any exercise is particularly important for people with vulnerable areas such as a weak back. What you are able to tackle safely depends on your health, fitness and susceptibility to injury. In most cases, physiotherapists will warn you to avoid these exercises:

● Head rolls.
● Dorsal rises, where you lie face down and lift your head and shoulders or your chest.
● Any exercise where you lie face down and lift your legs and/or arms.
● Full and partial press-ups.

REAL LIVES

GETTING FIT AT 60 – HOW EXERCISE CHANGED A LIFE

After 20 years of illness Inge Killick could barely walk round the block – even when holding a walking stick in one hand and her husband's supporting arm in the other. Three hip operations to tackle the consequences of chronic osteoarthritis, as well as the problems of angina (a form of heart disease) and chronic bronchiectasis (a bad chest complaint), had made Inge into what she describes as 'a frail and truly old woman of 60'. After trying all kinds of conventional and 'alternative' treatments without obtaining any lasting relief, the once-lively mother of two and former teacher could only look ahead to more pain, tiredness and a severely restricted social life.

At her daughter's suggestion, but without much hope, Inge went for an assessment at a health and fitness club. The results confirmed what she already knew – she was terribly weak and unfit. The trainer was, however, encouraging.

He said that a programme of carefully supervised, very gentle, regular exercise might improve her mobility, but he warned her not to expect a miracle.

Inge started going to an aqua-aerobics class. It was fun, and she found that she could do more than she expected because the water partially supported her weight. She progressed to two sessions a week, gradually gaining confidence as well as strength. Some of her pain seemed to ease, and Inge's trainer suggested that she start using exercise machines, such as a fitness bike. At first she could manage only a few feeble movements, but after 18 months she had improved enough to begin using machines with weights.

'I used to be just half a person,' says Inge. 'By two or three o'clock in the afternoon, I used to be absolutely finished. I had to do everything in the morning. Going out was a drag – I just didn't have any energy.'

Now Inge can once again enjoy looking after her large Hertfordshire house and garden and her family's animals: indoor and outdoor fish, a cat, a dog and two invalid owls.

She says: 'I am a new person, full of energy, free from any pain; and to crown it all, my fourth hip operation became unnecessary. The muscles in my legs have become really strong, and it seems that the hip joint has repaired itself. I have forgotten what became of my walking stick, and I can walk without pain – something that was denied me for 20 years. I used to need as many as ten angina tablets on a bad day. Now I have not needed a tablet for a year or so. It is an understatement to say that exercise is good for you and reverses the process of ageing. I wish that more people would take my story of success to heart and help themselves to a better, happier and fuller life by taking up some form of regular exercise.'

Home and office exercise

THE HIDDEN HOME GYM

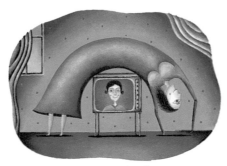

I am too busy with my family to get to a gym regularly. How can I keep fit at home without buying an exercise machine?

Consider turning your home or garden into a minigym. All you need is enough space to move about in without hitting or slipping on anything, and good ventilation if your gym is indoors. Wear loose, comfortable clothes.

Ideally you should try to exercise for at least 20 minutes a time. Include the warm-up exercises on pages 78-79, some of the workout exercises on pages 86-87, some deep stretches (see pages 81-82) and some cooling down movements (see pages 88-89).

With a little imagination, you can turn a variety of household objects into exercise aids. Why not use food cans as dumbbells, or make a length of old washing line into a skipping rope? You can use a wall, cupboard or chair to help you to balance during various exercises.

If you cannot put aside 20 minutes at one go, try a few simple movements while you wait for a kettle to boil, or even when you are on the telephone.

HOME EXERCISE EQUIPMENT

How should I go about buying a home exercise machine?

Shop around and try as many machines as possible to find one that feels comfortable and gives the kind of exercise you want. It should also be easy to store and use.

Type

If you want to lose weight, select a machine that encourages aerobic exercise. If you want to build muscles, look for equipment that provides anaerobic exercise. For general fitness, select a machine that provides a combination of the two. Some machines, such as climbers, treadmills or cycles, give you aerobic exercise while working muscles in one particular part of the body. Others, such as rowing and cross-country skiing machines, give you a good all-round workout, as well as aerobic exercise. Multigyms, work benches and free weights allow you to do a variety of anaerobic exercises.

Design

Machines that use a flywheel instead of a hydraulic system tend to be fairly expensive. But they are less strenuous to operate, so your muscles tire less quickly and it is easier to exercise long enough (about 20 minutes at a time) to get aerobic benefit. Check that the relevant features – handlebars, pedals, saddles, weights, height, resistance and gradients – can be altered to suit you.

Safety features

If a machine has moving parts, such as cogs, chains and flywheels, and safety rails (on treadmills and climbers), try to find a model in which they are safely enclosed.

Monitors

It can be helpful to monitor your heart rate, recovery rate, and energy consumption, and also aspects of your performance, such as your speed, distance, or time. These features can help you to set and achieve targets, but don't be tempted to buy more gadgetry than you are really going to need.

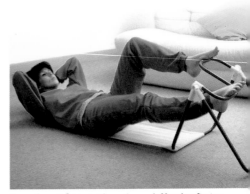

Exercise at home If you have difficulty fitting exercise into a busy schedule, the answer may be to buy an exercise machine to use at home.

CHOOSING A FITNESS VIDEO

I'd like to do some exercise to music at home, but I'm bewildered by the number of fitness videos in the shops. What should I look for?

From aerobics to 'boxercise' to 'cardiofunk', 'dancercise' and so on – with so many exercise tapes available, it is no wonder you feel confused. But all you need to do is to check four aspects of any tape that appeals to you:

TYPE OF EXERCISE Ideally, you should choose a style of exercise that you have already tried under the supervision of a proper teacher.

LEVEL Look for a programme that suits your ability. Don't be tempted to try advanced routines unless you are already fit and experienced, or you could end up hurting yourself. If you decide to try something entirely new to you, be sure to check the box first for any special health or fitness warnings.

DESIGN Don't be diverted by an attractive, famous face on the cover. It is more important to check up on the qualifications and experience of the person who *designed* the exercises. Make sure that both warm-up and cool-down exercises are included in any programme before you buy it.

DATE Avoid programmes that were designed before 1990, because they will be more likely to include any exercises that specialists now say are risky.

SURVIVING A SEDENTARY JOB

I drive to work, then sit at a desk all day. Although I get plenty of exercise at the weekend, should I do anything during my working day to keep more active?

Yes, you should try either a radical or a more gentle strategy. The radical approach involves walking or cycling at least part of the way to work every day and spending one lunchtime a week in a gym.

If this seems too daunting or you are short of time, think of trying a gentler approach: some office exercises to keep your muscles and joints moving easily. You don't have to make an exhibition of yourself. Whenever you are tense or you feel stiff, try the exercises on page 193. You could also try some of the flexibility exercises for older people (see page 412). Neither set of exercises requires a warm-up or cool-down because they are so gentle. All can be done in working clothes, and require a minimum amount of space.

Whichever approach you choose, ensure that your office chair supports your back properly, and that you stand up and move about once every hour or so. If you get stuck in a traffic jam on the way to or from work, put the handbrake on, keep an eye on the road, and – if it is safe to do so – try a few shoulder shrugs or stretching exercises at your desk, such as those on page 193.

SKIPPING INTO FITNESS

I've heard that skipping is good for you. As I haven't done any skipping since I was at school, how should I get started?

Skipping is an excellent way to get aerobic exercise – the sort that leaves you slightly breathless and strengthens your heart and improves your blood circulation. Skipping also builds the strength of the muscles in your legs and upper body, assisting balance and coordination. As with any new kind of exercise, you should check with your doctor that it is suitable for you. Start slowly and increase the intensity gradually, even if you were a champion skipper at school.

Warm up by doing the exercises on pages 78-79, then try skipping for 20 turns of the rope. Rest for half a minute. If you feel fine, try 20 more skips, then cool down by doing some of the exercises on pages 89-90. From now on, try skipping every other day. Try to reduce your rest period by roughly five seconds each session until you can skip comfortably for five minutes without stopping.

At this stage, aim to turn the rope 60 to 70 times a minute. Later on, you could try 100 turns a minute, but don't worry if you cannot achieve this: you should always exercise at your own pace, slowing down or stopping altogether if you feel any pain, dizziness or sickness.

Skip on a soft surface, such as grass, to avoid jarring your joints. Bend your knees as you jump and as you land. Don't try to jump any higher than a couple of inches off the ground. Relax your neck and shoulders, use your wrists to help you to turn the rope, and remember not to hold your breath.

What you need for skipping

Most importantly, you must wear well-cushioned shoes, such as those designed for aerobics or tennis, or cross-trainers (see page 108), to protect feet, ankles and knees. Use a rope that reaches to your armpits when you stand with both feet on the middle. Some commercial skipping ropes have handles, sometimes with a swivel action that makes skipping smoother, but a length of old washing line would be fine to get you started.

Fitness in the home

Home exercise machines of various sorts offer privacy and convenience – at a price:

- A treadmill lets you run or walk as far and as fast as you want to.
- A multigym offers a range of exercises to strengthen muscles.
- Ski machines mimic cross-country skiing actions for an aerobic workout and muscle building and toning.
- Rowing machines work the upper and lower body at the same time.
- Exercise bikes give a good aerobic workout.
- Steppers and climbers will work your thighs and buttocks.

Walking for fun and fitness

A CHANGE OF PACE

Do I need to walk fast to gain any benefit from walking?

No – all walking is beneficial. It keeps your muscles and joints in working order and fit for most everyday activities. Whether it is a gentle stroll along a country lane, window-shopping in town, or a walk to work, it can do wonders for your wellbeing.

Studies suggest that even very gentle walking may add years to your life by keeping you mobile and burning calories you might otherwise store as fat. In fact, when it comes to using up unwanted fat or calories continuous walking for 30 to 45 minutes at a time seems to be as good as or better than brief bouts of vigorous exercise.

You should remember that you need to do some kind of aerobic sport or activity during the week to maintain the efficiency and strength of heart, lungs and circulation. As a rough guide, a moderately fit adult will gain aerobic benefit from walking at between three and four miles an hour for at least 20 minutes continuously, a minimum of three times a week. If this is too strenuous for you, do what you can at first. It is far better – for your fitness, your enjoyment of life and your mobility, especially as you get older – to do a little leisurely walking than to do none at all.

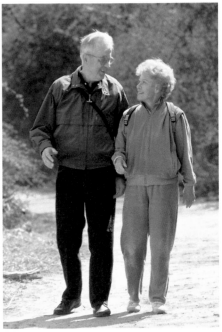

Leisure walking Even ambling along at a comfortable pace – usually at less than three miles an hour – and over fairly flat surfaces can provide good exercise if done regularly.

DIFFERENT STYLES

What is the difference between walking, rambling and strolling, and which one is the best way to start?

The number of descriptions for walking (hiking, strolling, power walking, race walking and so on) can make it seem that it is not just a matter of putting one foot in front of the other. But making a start is the main thing, whichever style you opt for.

If you have not done much walking of any sort before, you might like to consider taking a short guided walk (see panel, page 106) before tackling a strenuous uphill route or a long-distance hike. The challenge of completing a demanding walk can be exhilarating, but do remember the general principle of all exercise – to do things gradually. Start with shorter walks on familiar terrain, and build up from there.

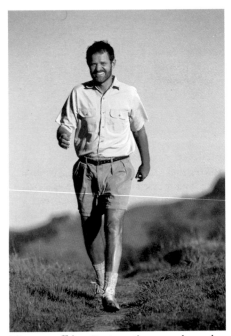

Fitness walking To strengthen muscles and burn calories you need to walk fast enough to make you pant slightly for 15-20 minutes.

Safety precautions

The Ramblers' Association notes that walking in Britain presents very few problems. However, they also suggest some precautions that you should take:

- Don't overdo it by attempting walks that will exhaust you. Build up slowly at first.
- Know where you are going and what to expect of the conditions.
- Use good maps, such as Ordnance Survey.
- Wear, or take with you, adequate clothing for all the likely weather conditions.
- Carry basic emergency and survival items with you (see page 106).
- Tell someone where you are walking and when you expect to be back.

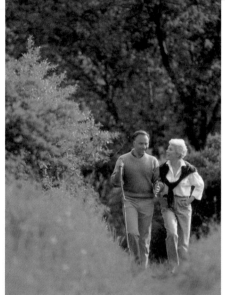

Rambling The fitness benefits of rambling depend on the terrain and distance that you cover. Ramblers' groups organise walks of different levels to accommodate all abilities.

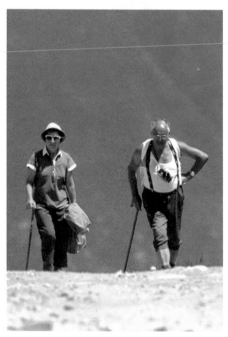

Hiking and hill walking For long, strenuous walks taking several days you need to be in good physical shape. Make sure you have adequate equipment and supplies.

CONTROLLING COST

I'm keen to take up walking. What do I really need to buy when I start, and what may be useful at a later stage?

Walking is a relatively economical form of exercise. It does not involve buying complicated equipment or expensive clothing. You need a comfortable, well-cushioned pair of shoes and a jacket to protect you from the weather. When you can afford it, invest in a pair of specialist walking shoes or boots. For leisure or fitness walking you may want to consider a pair of purpose-designed walking shoes or 'cross-trainers' (see page 108) – look for plenty of padding and some toe protection across the front.

If you are going to ramble, hike or hill-walk, buy walking boots, which will protect your ankles and knees when you are walking across uneven ground such as country tracks or hill paths. It doesn't matter if the boots are leather, synthetic or a combination of the two, but they should be water-resistant, and have a sturdy sole to provide a good grip. People new to walking often find lightweight boots more comfortable than heavy ones.

There is a wide choice of walking socks available, and it is best to experiment a bit with socks of different fabrics. Most experienced walkers wear two pairs of socks – and a larger-size boot – for extra cushioning and warmth. They usually wear a thin cotton pair next to the skin for comfort and a thick pair on top to give extra cushioning for the feet. Even though some of the special walking socks may seem expensive in comparison to everyday socks, they will repay their cost in the comfort they provide.

It is advisable to wear a hat of some kind in cold or windy weather since about 40 per cent of the heat lost from the body escapes through the head. Also, in sunny weather, a hat will help to protect you from sunburn and heat exhaustion.

It is important to protect yourself against wind and rain. Some jackets include thermal linings to ensure warmth, but these can feel quite heavy. You can also buy separate synthetic fleeces, many of which can be zipped into other jackets as a warm lining.

Many more expensive lightweight walking jackets are made from materials that prevent water getting in but allow perspiration to get out. Waxed jackets and some heavy-duty types will protect you against thorns. If you take up rambling or any other form of cross-country walking, you may also want to invest in a knee-length jacket or cagoule, or in waterproof trousers or gaiters.

Many walkers find a waterproof map case, a compass and a small rucksack useful (see page 106). Ask for advice about other useful pieces of equipment from those with experience, and look round some of the specialist outdoor shops. If you don't wish to spend much concentrate on the essentials – looking after your feet and protecting yourself against cold, heat and wet weather.

DO'S AND DON'TS
of walking

Do work through some warm-up exercises before taking a long or strenuous walk. Pay special attention to feet.
Do include some walking-on-the-spot exercises in your warm-up routine.
Do start slowly, to help you to warm up, and increase your pace gradually.
Do slow down or stop if you develop a stitch (see page 99).

Don't walk too fast: as a rough guide you should be able to hold a conversation comfortably with someone as you walk.
Don't flop into a chair the minute you finish a long or energetic walk: instead, do some cool-down movements.
Don't try to walk too far, too soon: it is best to increase gradually the duration and frequency of your walks.

GETTING EQUIPPED FOR A GOOD DAY'S WALKING

Various accessories can make walking more comfortable. Some of them, such as a torch, you will need only occasionally. But others, such as a flask, can come in handy at any time.
Summer: (s); Winter: (w); Summer and Winter: (s/w).

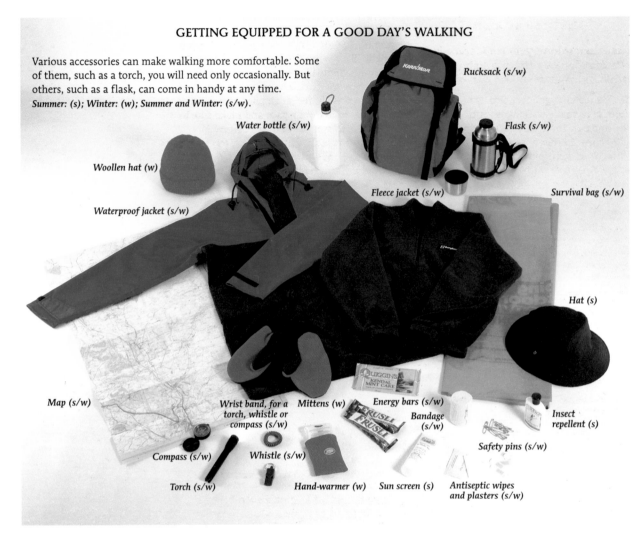

Rucksack (s/w)

Flask (s/w)

Water bottle (s/w)

Woollen hat (w)

Waterproof jacket (s/w)

Fleece jacket (s/w)

Survival bag (s/w)

Hat (s)

Map (s/w)

Wrist band, for a torch, whistle or compass (s/w)

Mittens (w)

Energy bars (s/w)

Bandage (s/w)

Insect repellent (s)

Safety pins (s/w)

Compass (s/w)

Whistle (s/w)

Torch (s/w)

Hand-warmer (w)

Sun screen (s)

Antiseptic wipes and plasters (s/w)

Turn walking into sociable fun

If you would like to walk with others, consider:

● **Guided walks** – get information from local tourist offices, newspapers, and listings magazines.
● **Rambles** – contact The Ramblers' Association (see page 190).
● **Orienteering** – get in touch with the British Orienteering Federation (see page 109).
● **Sponsored walks** – get fit and raise money for a good cause.

THE BEST WAY TO WALK

I enjoy walking, but I've read that to get the most out of it you need special techniques. Is this true?

There are both good and bad ways of everyday walking. A bad style can affect your posture, breathing, comfort and vulnerability to injury. You can improve, but it will take time and patience to correct any bad habits that you learned in childhood.

Your starting point should be the way you stand (see pages 142-143). It will also help your walking style if you remain relaxed and breathe normally. Whenever you walk, look up and ahead as much as possible; looking down could make your back and neck ache.

Avoid rolling your feet, either inwards or outwards, which puts stress on the ankles and knees and can lead to back pain. Try to use the entire foot by placing it down on the back of the heel and then moving through the length of the sole to the toes. It may help to imagine that you are peeling your foot forward off a sticky surface. If your feet still roll badly, take advice from your doctor or podiatrist. Orthotics (arch supports moulded to fit your own feet exactly) may be prescribed by a foot specialist to help solve any problems.

Keep your hands relaxed, not clenched, as you walk, and swing your arms up from the shoulders to give extra propulsion. Try shortening your stride when you go uphill to gain more power with less effort.

Power walkers and race walkers can sometimes achieve speeds of up to nine miles per hour (14 km/h), which is faster than most people can run. They adopt a pronounced hip-swinging style that uses the muscles of the abdomen, buttocks, arms and shoulders to give them extra power. This type of walking is highly specialised and should be practised only after special training.

ONE STEP AT A TIME

I have been sedentary for many years, but now I want to get fitter by walking for recreation. What is my best plan of action?

You've made a good choice for your new exercise regime – walking is gentle, inexpensive and easy to fit into your way of life.

Perhaps the most important point is not to let your new-found enthusiasm get the better of you. As with all forms of exercise, you should start gently and avoid overdoing it. This might mean walking for just ten minutes at a time every two or three days. If this does not seem much, do remember that it is better to do regular short walks than to wear yourself out on one long arduous walk and give up your new resolution.

There are no set rules about what you should achieve. It will depend upon your overall level of fitness and health. But you might like to aim for a walk of at least 20 minutes about three times a week. Don't try to do this immediately, and if you start to sweat heavily, or feel at all faint or sick while walking, reduce your pace and make sure to give yourself time to recover between trips.

If you can walk sufficiently briskly to feel just slightly breathless – though you should always be able to talk to a companion – you will be getting aerobic exercise, which will strengthen your heart and circulation and indirectly help every aspect of your fitness.

Why not try meeting a friend for a walk rather than for a drink or a meal? You could find that walking adds pleasure and purpose to social life as well as improving fitness.

Jogging and running

THE RIGHT TRACK

Would I do better to run or jog outdoors – or is a treadmill just as good for fitness?

While you can run or jog almost anywhere, smooth, even surfaces are the best and safest. Grass, asphalt, cinder, concrete paving, all-weather tracks, Tarmacadam, treadmills and even small-size trampolines are all suitable. However, softer surfaces, such as grass, jar your leg joints less severely than a hard surface such as a concrete pavement. Indoor and outdoor activity give equal aerobic benefit.

Exercising on a treadmill
● Provides you with an even surface to run on so that you are less likely to trip.
● Allows you to avoid extreme weather.
● Safe from traffic, pollution and crime.
● Gives you information about your speed, distance covered and (in some cases) your pulse rate, which should help you to regulate your fitness training programme.
● Allows you (in some cases) to set precisely the distance and speed that you run and the gradient that you run it over.

Running or jogging outside
● Allows you to exercise at no cost.
● Gives you a variety of terrain to run on.
● Can provide interesting surroundings to look at as you run.
● Allows you to exercise when it suits you.
● Gives fresh air if you run in the country.

Best of both
To benefit from the advantages of both types of running, and to introduce some variety, why not consider combining or alternating the two? You will probably get more exercise if you are not dependent on either one.

RUNNER'S HIGH

Friends say that jogging makes them feel wonderful in every way. Which benefits, other than fitness, can be gained from running and jogging?

When jogging and running popularity was at a peak in the mid 1970s, many people talked about a feeling of euphoria they experienced while exercising.

This feeling, which became known as runner's high, could be fleeting or it could last as long as several days. Joggers and runners also reported a sense of achievement in the distance covered, the short time taken and better sleep patterns.

These feelings of wellbeing are not just associated with running and jogging. Many people involved in other regular and fairly vigorous exercise report similar experiences, including feeling generally happier, calmer, more clear-headed and better able to cope with difficulties in other areas of life.

Scientists believe that bouts of energetic exercise triggers the release of endorphins – chemicals in the brain that elevate your mood and reduce pain and anxiety.

**FACT
—— OR ——
FALLACY?**

'Overweight people should not jog.'

Fact Without a doctor's express approval it is unwise for overweight or obese people to jog or run. The exertion is believed to put too great a strain on the heart. Instead, doctors tend to encourage overweight people first to lose some weight by changing their diet and taking gentler exercise, such as walking or swimming, before they give the all-clear to start jogging.

CHOOSING THE RIGHT SHOES FOR EXERCISE

Different sports make different demands on your feet. Racquet sports, for example, involve twists and turns, so they demand flexibility and strength, but walking on rough ground needs a stiff sole and firm ankle support.

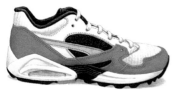

Running shoes These are built for lightness, speed and shock absorption.

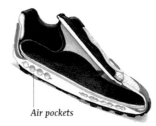

Air pockets

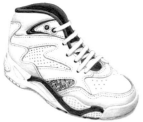

Step aerobic shoes The sole must absorb impact and the shoe light and flexible.

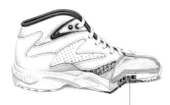

Honeycomb cushioning

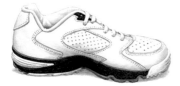

Cross trainers Good makes provide heel and toe cushioning, and firm support.

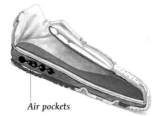

Air pockets

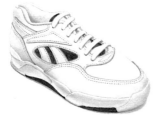

Tennis shoes There must be all-round foot support for twisting and turning.

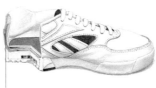

Firm heel support

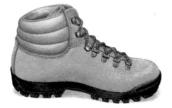

Walking boots Look for cushioning and a stiff sole to hold the foot steady.

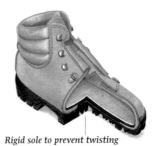

Rigid sole to prevent twisting

RUNNING RISKS

I have read newspaper stories about people dying of heart attacks while they are out running or jogging. Just how dangerous are these activities?

Some press reports can make jogging and running seem unsafe, and yet many studies in Britain and the United States show that most energetic activities, including jogging and running, help to *prevent* heart disease, high cholesterol levels, high blood pressure and a wide variety of other health problems. What's more, joggers and runners in Britain are far less likely to be injured than people taking part in rugby, soccer, cricket, hockey and the martial arts.

Some of the people whose deaths were most publicised were at risk from *any* vigorous exercise. Some had not taken enough notice of their poor personal health. Some were unaware of a health problem, such as a heart weakness, while others simply did too much for their level of fitness.

Jogging and running can give you many fitness benefits, so do not be put off by these stories. However, if you wish to take up jogging, running, or any energetic type of exercise, you should consult your GP if you have:

- a family history of heart disease.
- a personal history of being overweight or obese, or of having had high blood pressure, high levels of cholesterol or stress.
- any back or knee complaints.
- previously smoked or eaten a high-fat diet.
- been inactive and are 35 years or older – people over the age of 35, especially men, are at greatest risk of heart attack.

Don't do too much too soon. Start with brisk walking and some jogging. Make sure to warm up and cool down (see pages 78-79 and 89-90). Stop if you feel any pain.

If these precautions are observed, then running and jogging are not especially dangerous forms of exercise. The greatest risks are to knees, ankles and feet. This is because jogging and running are high-impact activities in which the feet constantly strike the ground with a force that is three or four times greater than when you are walking. Your knees bear most of the brunt of this pounding, though well-cushioned shoes can help to protect them.

If you run on roads, make sure you are highly visible by wearing reflective clothing. Also, if the road has a pronounced camber, alternate the direction in which you run to avoid straining one side of your body.

ORIENTEERING

What is orienteering, and is it a suitable form of exercise for people who jog?

Many orienteers would describe their sport as a way of making walking or jogging more interesting, because it involves a mental as well as a physical challenge.

Orienteering is a race across country. You choose your own route and pace, but you must visit a number of fixed control points in the correct order and endorse a special card at each. The location of the control points is shown on a map, and a description of each point is usually given too. You must choose the quickest and most suitable route between the control points, and cover the distance as fast as possible.

Orienteering events take place in town parks, the countryside, forests and moors, and permanent orienteering courses can be found throughout the country. Courses vary from just over half a mile (about 0.8 km) to more than 10 miles (16 km), and they can have between 10 and 30 control points. The courses are set with the age and ability of competitors in mind. Technically taxing but physically easy courses, for example, may be set for elderly competitors, longer taxing ones for experienced adults and short easy ones for children.

Be sure to wear comfortable walking or training shoes, and trousers to protect your legs from branches and undergrowth.

You might also need a ball-point pen for marking your course on the map, as well as a polythene bag to use as a map case. On some courses you may need a compass to help you to plan the route. The British Orienteering Federation is located at Riversdale, Dale Road North, Darley Dale, Matlock, Derbyshire DE4 2HX.

OVERDOING RUNNING

Last week I started running four miles a day. After three days I had to stop because I ached all over. What went wrong?

You did too much too quickly. But don't lose heart: running and other types of exercise need not be painful – build up more gradually, and try again. It is quite common to ache when you take up exercise, but the discomfort is usually mild and normally goes within a week. Just follow these golden rules:

● Warm up before you begin and cool down afterwards (see pages 78-79 and 89-90).
● Start slowly and gently, gradually building up your speed, distance and the number of times a week that you run.

A typical programme, supposing you were an unfit beginner, would start with brisk walking – about twice a week for two weeks. Then, as you get accustomed to exertion, you could progress to short periods of jogging and gradually build up to longer runs. You need to adjust the exercise intensity to your own level of fitness, but you might like to aim to run two miles in 20 minutes by about your seventh week.

Joining a running club can be a good idea. Members can give you advice, and you may be able to run with experienced runners.

Swimming and water sports

VALUABLE EXERCISE IN WATER

What does water exercise involve, and is it better for fitness than swimming?

Virtually any kind of sport or fitness activity in water counts as water exercise. However, the term is usually used to describe specialist fitness programmes that are carried out in water such as aqua-aerobics, hydro-aerobics, swimmercise or water keep fit.

You do not have to sign up for any of these, or even have to be able to swim, to have fun and get fit through water exercises. You'll see on pages 110-111 that you can adapt most land-based exercises to the water.

Although no single exercise can give you total fitness, swimming comes close to it by working most of the major muscle groups and giving an excellent aerobic workout.

Some water exercises are designed to help you to work particular parts of your body such as legs or arms, while others such as water jogging (see page 110), also give you aerobic exercise.

Which one is best for you depends upon your general level of health and fitness, what you enjoy and are aiming to achieve. It is best to think of swimming and water exercise as complementary activities. Together they offer variety, plenty of fun for all the family and an enjoyable way to stay fit.

GETTING FIT IN THE WATER – EXERCISES TO TRY IN A SWIMMING POOL

If you like being in the water but get bored swimming up and down lanes, or just want to vary your routine, consider trying some pool exercises. As well as bouying you up, water provides resistance to work against, so exercises are more effective than on dry land. Water exercise can also be safer and more comfortable for pregnant women and for people who are overweight or suffer from arthritis, back pain or other muscle or joint problems. Since your weight is partially supported and your movements slowed down, you are much less likely to injure yourself. Try the exercises here as a starter – if you enjoy them, consider joining a class.

UPPER BODY TONE-UP

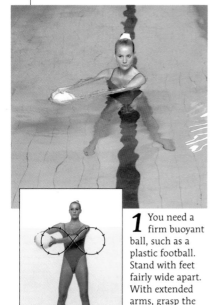

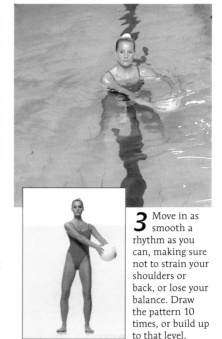

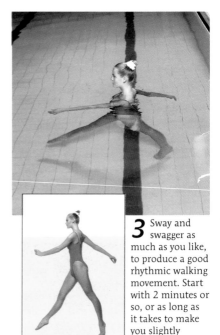

1 You need a firm buoyant ball, such as a plastic football. Stand with feet fairly wide apart. With extended arms, grasp the ball between your hands. Push it under the water.

2 Swing the ball in a figure-of-eight pattern through the water, keeping your arms straight. Breathe evenly. Feel the varying resistance on your arms and upper body.

3 Move in as smooth a rhythm as you can, making sure not to strain your shoulders or back, or lose your balance. Draw the pattern 10 times, or build up to that level.

WATER MARCHING

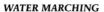

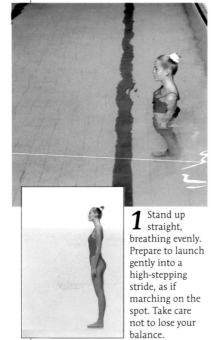

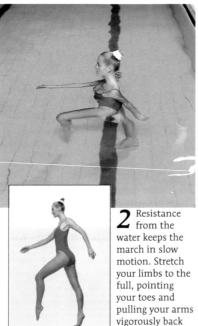

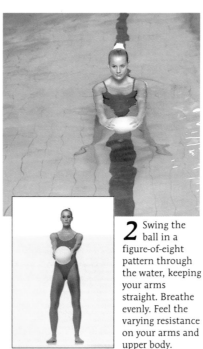

1 Stand up straight, breathing evenly. Prepare to launch gently into a high-stepping stride, as if marching on the spot. Take care not to lose your balance.

2 Resistance from the water keeps the march in slow motion. Stretch your limbs to the full, pointing your toes and pulling your arms vigorously back and forth.

3 Sway and swagger as much as you like, to produce a good rhythmic walking movement. Start with 2 minutes or so, or as long as it takes to make you slightly breathless

WATER STAR JUMPS

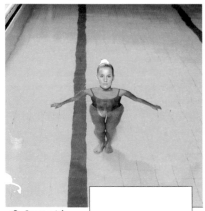

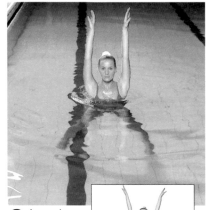

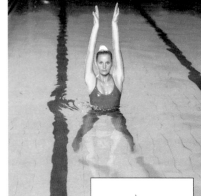

1 Start with your feet flat on the bottom of the pool and your arms relaxed by your sides. Bend your knees and spring up off the bottom of the pool as high as you can.

2 As you jump, kick your legs out to the side, pointing your toes down, and swinging your arms out to the side and up above your head, so that your limbs form a star shape.

3 Land with knees bent and feet apart. Then jump up again as high as you can and bring your feet back together and your arms back to your sides. Repeat the exercise 15 times.

POOLSIDE STRETCH

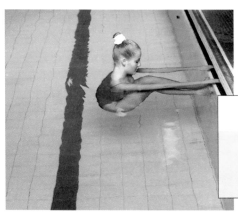

1 Face the side of the pool and grip the edge. Place your feet against the pool wall with your knees bent.

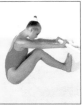

2 Straighten your legs, but take care not to lock your knees or elbows, or strain your back. Repeat 10 times.

WAIST TRIMMER

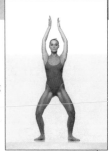

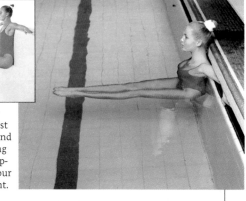

1 With your back against the pool wall and your arms along the edge for support, stretch your legs out in front.

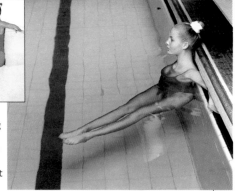

2 Breathing evenly, swing your legs to the right, then to the left, then back to the centre. Repeat about 15 times.

DO'S AND DON'TS
for water safety

Do supervise children and inexperienced swimmers.

Do wear a buoyancy jacket for water sports such as rowing and canoeing.

Do shower thoroughly and disinfect any cuts after swimming.

Do find out about tides and currents before going out on any kind of water.

Don't stay in the water if you feel cold.

Don't swim near locks or weirs: you could be pulled under.

Don't swim in gravel pits or any other places with steep sides.

Don't swim until at least an hour after eating.

Don't ignore beach warning flags – red means do not swim.

THE CUSHIONED EXERCISE

Is it true that many people who are unfit, overweight or elderly can exercise more safely in water than on land?

Yes – many people who would find it difficult, painful or even dangerous to exercise on land are able to exercise safely and in relative comfort in water.

Doctors often suggest water exercise for unfit, overweight, obese, elderly and physically disabled people. This is because water supports a person's body weight, cushioning vulnerable joints against the impact of the exercise and reducing the strain on them, that weight-bearing exercise would cause.

Even if someone has only limited mobility on land, they can usually stay afloat, with a little help, and move about in water.

The cushioning effect of water also makes this form of exercise a comfortable option for people suffering from arthritis and for many pregnant women. If you are recovering from illness or an injury, your doctor may recommend some stretching and strengthening exercises in water in order to help you to get back into good physical condition.

CAUTION Exercising in water is not safe for all. If you are unfit and aged over 35, overweight, recovering from illness, or suffering from a condition such as heart disease, check with your GP whether it is safe for you to swim or do water exercise.

ROWING OR SAILING?

I love sailing, and my sister is a keen rower. Is one a more 'complete' form of exercise than the other?

While no single sport can give you total fitness, some, such as swimming, rowing and cross-country skiing, do work all the major muscle groups and also give aerobic exercise.

Rowing is excellent for aerobic fitness and muscular strength and endurance – much better than sailing. Even so, sailing will help to improve your strength and flexibility, and it is good for coordination. Of course, any benefits depend upon how energetically you do either sport. An occasional leisurely row in a dinghy will not give you the aerobic exercise you would get from a regular 90-minute training session.

But in the end, as with all sports, the best water sport for you is the one that you enjoy most and take part in most regularly.

LEARNING LIFESAVING

I've always thought it would be useful to know how to help someone out of trouble in the water. Would lifesaving classes help me to get fit, and could even a weak swimmer benefit?

Lifesaving classes are a good way to get fit by swimming – but they are not suitable for beginners or weak swimmers. After all, you cannot hope to rescue other people from danger if you are unable to look after yourself. For that reason, The Royal Life Saving Society recommends that weak swimmers improve their swimming techniques and stamina before learning how to rescue others.

However, even if you are a weak swimmer, don't abandon your idea. You could learn about land-based lifesaving skills, such as how to look after somebody who has been rescued, or even resuscitation techniques, until you have improved your endurance and swimming ability. Your local pool should be able to advise you about swimming classes, clubs and lifesaving courses.

If you are already a strong swimmer, then lifesaving classes should give you the confidence and ability to rescue another person from trouble. You will probably also find the classes a wonderful incentive to become and stay really fit.

If you would like to find out more information about lifesaving, contact The Royal Life Saving Society UK, Mountbatten House, Studley, Warwickshire B80 7NN.

Water sports for fitness Windsurfing builds muscle strength and endurance, and kayaking gives excellent aerobic exercise for the heart as well.

POOL-BASED ACTIVITIES

I love swimming, but I sometimes get fed up with just going up and down the pool lanes. Are there any other kinds of exercise that I could do in a swimming pool?

Swimming with friends can be more enjoyable than just swimming up and down lanes alone. Try to find a nearby swimming club that runs a variety of events and swimming sessions, aqua-aerobics (see page 110-111), or lifesaving (page 112).

Many clubs meet and train at local pools. You could try water polo or canoe polo and there is also sub-aqua for underwater explorers. Octopush, a form of underwater hockey, is also played at some local pools. Contact these societies for further information:

● The Amateur Swimming Association, Harold Fern House, Derby Square, Loughborough, Leicestershire LE11 0AL.
● The British Octopush Association, Culver Farm, Old Compton Lane, Farnham, Surrey GU9 8EJ.
● The British Canoe Association, Adbolton Lane, West Bridgford, Nottingham NG2 5AS.
● The British Sub-Aqua Club Telford's Quay, Ellesmere Port, South Wirral, Cheshire L65 4FY.

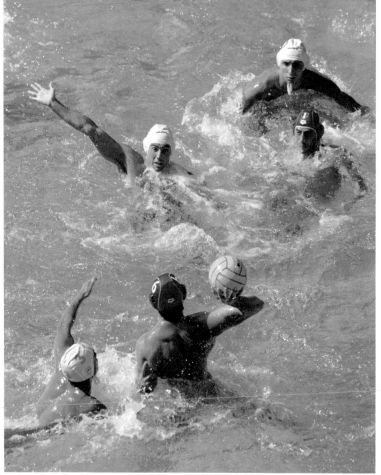

Competing for fitness Water polo is good fun and outstanding exercise. As you play, vigorous blocking, throwing and jumping moves raise your heart rate, and your muscles work hard to move you through the water in pursuit of the ball.

Cycling

CHOOSING A BICYCLE

Cycling seems a practical way to get around and stay fit, but what should I look for when I buy my first bike?

For safety and comfort, choose a bicycle that suits the kind of cycling you will be doing and is right for your body size. If you know any keen cyclists, ask their advice before you buy. Also, some helpful leaflets are produced by the British Cycling Federation, National Cycling Centre, 1 Stuart Street, Manchester M11 4DQ and the Bicycle Association, Starley House, Eaton Road, Coventry CV1 2FH.

Type
Decide where you will do the most cycling – city roads, country lanes or a mixture of terrain – and what you want to do with your bicycle – get to work, carry shopping, travel on a train. Then try out a number of models

designed for those purposes. The British Cycling Federation suggests beginners start with a lightweight bike that responds easily and can be lifted and carried without effort.

Frame size
The frame of your bicycle – measured from the bottom bracket spindle, where the pedal is fixed to the junction with the seat tube – should be about 10 in (25 cm) shorter than your inside leg measurement. You should be able to touch the ground with one foot when you are sitting on the saddle but not necessarily to place your foot flat. Make sure that you are able to place your heel on a pedal and straighten your leg without stretching.

Handlebars
Choose carefully – you need to be able to control your bike without shoulder ache. The British Cycling Federation advises dropped handlebars for beginners, so that they can

Cycling in safety

Safety is an essential part of cycling:

Get yourself seen
On the road, make sure that you are dressed to attract attention – fluorescent, light-coloured or reflective clothing is best.

Light up
By law you must have *at least* a white front light and a red rear light if you are cycling at night.

Protect your head
Wearing an approved helmet (see page 339) will significantly reduce the risk of sustaining a serious head injury.

hold on and steer from a number of positions. To estimate the handlebars' ideal position, place your elbow on the front edge of the saddle. You should be able to touch the handlebars or be within about 1 in (2.5 cm) of it. If the distance is much greater, ask the bicycle shop to adjust the position for you. If the gap is still too great but the cycle is the one you want, buy a handlebar extension.

Saddle

You don't have to suffer a narrow or uncomfortable saddle. Try out a variety of designs and makes, and consider buying one with gel that eventually moulds to fit your shape.

CAUTION It is dangerous for children to ride bicycles that are too large for them. They will be unable to steer safely and may lose control.

FITNESS RATING OF CYCLING

All my family look forward to leisurely weekend cycle rides. I'd love to know whether this kind of fun activity counts as real exercise?

It certainly does. Exercise does not have to be fast or furious to give you fitness and health benefits. Even gentle exercise, such as your weekend outings, will help. In fact medical experts maintain that cycling is one of the best types of exercise. Not only that: it is also simple to do, easy to squeeze into a busy weekly schedule and suitable for people of most ages and levels of fitness.

When you pedal your bicycle, you continually contract and relax the large muscles in your legs. This builds muscular endurance, tones your leg muscles, and even if you are moving only fairly slowly, usually gives you aerobic exercise, which helps to strengthen your heart, lungs and blood circulation.

With cycling, there is less risk of straining muscles or jolting joints than in running or jogging. Even so, your legs and arms do take some of your body weight while you ride, so you gain some protection too from osteoporosis – loss of bone mass.

INDOORS OR OUTDOORS

Which is better for fitness – an exercise bike or a real one?

There is little difference in terms of fitness. As long as you can adjust an exercise bike's resistance to simulate hills as well as flat surfaces, it can provide exactly the same fitness benefits as a real bicycle.

For many regular cyclists, the fitness value of their trip often takes second place to the pleasure they gain from the scenery or the places they can reach by bicycle. In contrast, most people using static exercise bikes are aiming to get fit and often have little time to spare. To counter the boredom of pedalling on the spot, they turn to watching television, listening to music or even looking at simulated scenery.

Exercise bikes are among the top-selling home fitness machines in Britain, possibly because you can cycle in any weather, night or day. There is no traffic to contend with and it does not matter if your eyesight is poor. Machines also often monitor the distance you have 'travelled', and some can even measure your heart rate as you pedal.

POLLUTION ON THE ROADS

I cycle to work every day to keep fit, but now I hear that traffic pollution could be damaging my health. Am I doing myself more harm than good?

The British Medical Association (BMA) recommends cycling as one of the best ways to become and stay fit. But it warns against riding on heavily congested roads, particularly if you have a heart or lung disorder.

Cycling makes you breathe more deeply, but the exhaust gases from cars reduce the amount of oxygen in each breath, and you take pollutants into your lungs. This can cause damage to the air passages in the nose, throat and lungs, and can also result in breathing difficulties, respiratory infections or a disrupted heart rate. However, it would be a great shame to give up an established routine that gives you such good exercise.

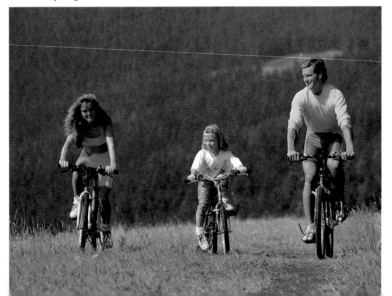

Travelling together Cycling makes a good group activity. Cyclists of different ages can keep up with each other quite easily, and there is plenty to look at as you go.

So if your journey takes you through busy streets, try to avoid the rush hour or find a less congested route. If you cannot avoid heavy traffic, keep as far away as possible from vehicle exhaust pipes. There are various masks available which are designed to filter out pollutants from the air before they reach your lungs, although there is some debate as to their effectiveness. Discuss the options with a knowledgeable bicycle dealer.

Exercise to music

AEROBICS DEFINED

My daughter-in-law is always talking about the benefits of her aerobics classes. What exactly is aerobics, and would classes be good for me?

Aerobics is an energetic type of exercise performed to music with a clear, simple beat. There are a number of varieties, including high and low-impact versions; step aerobics, in which you move on and off a small platform; 'cardio-funk' a dance-like version; aerobics with wrist and ankle weights and even 'aqua-aerobics' in water. New styles are constantly being developed.

The term 'aerobics' comes from ancient Greek roots meaning 'air-life', and suggests 'containing oxygen', but it is not the only form of aerobic exercise. Any continuous activity is aerobic if it makes you breathe harder and quickens your heart rate to pump oxygen-rich blood to the working muscles. The result is a long-term benefit of improving the efficiency of the heart, lungs and bloodstream, and helping to reduce heart disease and circulation problems.

An aerobics class would be good for you so long as you do not suffer any complaint that could make exercise dangerous (see page 73). Why not watch one of your daughter-in-law's classes and talk with the teacher afterwards? You will probably find a sociable atmosphere, and notice that you do not have to look like a Hollywood film star to enjoy and gain fitness benefits from classes. If you decide that aerobics is not for you, there are alternatives: why not consider Keep Fit or dance classes instead?

LOW AND HIGH IMPACT

Are high-impact and low-impact aerobics equally suitable for beginners?

These terms describe the force with which the feet hit the ground during any activity. In high-impact activities, such as vigorous aerobics, running, squash, and some forms of dance, the feet pound about five times more violently than when you walk.

Most exercise specialists recommend that beginners, and anyone who is unfit, should start with either a no-impact activity – such as swimming and cycling, where there is little risk of ankle, knee or hip injury – or a low-impact activity such as walking or gentle aerobics, in which one foot stays on the ground and you are unlikely to damage your joints. If you plan to exercise alone at home, it might be safer to stick to low-impact aerobics: any new, unsupervised form of exercise can be risky. If you do decide to join a class, have no serious medical problems, are fairly fit, and warm up thoroughly (see pages 78-79), there is no reason why you should not progress fairly quickly from low to high-impact aerobics.

CAUTION Doctors usually advise people who have heart disease, who are overweight or who have problems with their lower back, knees, ankles or hips to avoid any kind of high-impact exercise.

SELECTING THE BEST CLASS

What should I bear in mind when choosing a class for exercise to music?

Your choice will obviously depend partly on how wide a selection is available locally, and also on the relative costs. Do remember to check the safety and teaching standards too. Here are some features to check:

Your right level
The classes offered should each be graded for beginner, intermediate, advanced or professional levels, taking into account fitness and experience. Watch or take part in at least one sample class before signing up. Don't be afraid to move up or down a level.

The teacher's qualifications
There is no legal requirement for a qualification, but good teachers usually have at least three years' full-time training in the dance

or exercise style they teach and/or a nationally recognised teaching certificate. Training ideally includes anatomy and first aid. Lists of examining organisations for fitness exercise and dance are available from The Central Council of Physical Recreation, Francis House, Francis Street, London SW1P 1DE.

Good teaching

The best instructors:
- welcome newcomers and check whether they have any health or fitness difficulties.
- set modified exercises for anyone with problems, such as a weak back.
- include a warm-up and cool-down.
- build the difficulty and intensity of movements gradually.
- demonstrate moves and sequences, especially to beginners.
- invite and answer questions during or after the class.
- check how well participants move, and correct any potentially dangerous movements, warning everyone of the dangers.
- encourage class members to work hard, without prompting competition or tempting participants to ignore pain.

Physical conditions

You should have enough space to move and to see the teacher's demonstration. (If floor space is limited, the teacher should split the class for some activities, so that everyone has the chance to move to their full extent.) The floor should be semi-sprung, not concrete or carpeted. The room should have a comfortable temperature with adequate ventilation. Music should be clear but not so loud that you have difficulty hearing the teacher. Ideally, there should be facilities for changing and showering.

STEPPING OUT SAFELY

I have a friend who twisted her ankle badly while out running. Are there dangers of my doing the same with step aerobics?

It's unlikely – provided you exercise sensibly. When you step onto something, always put your heel down first and continue moving your foot until your weight is spread evenly throughout its full length.

When you step down from a height, place your toes down first, then the ball of your foot and then your heel until your weight is supported evenly. In particular, be sensible when jumping. Be sure always to bend your knees before you leave the ground and again as you land to make use of these natural

shock absorbers. Land on the ball of your foot, quickly lowering your weight through to your heels so that the whole foot supports you. Avoid sticking your buttocks out or rolling your knees together.

CHOOSING A DANCE STYLE

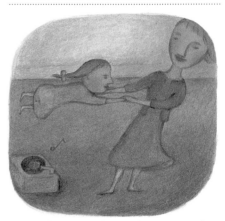

Although I am no longer that young, I love dancing around at home to all kinds of music. I would like to join a class but how can I tell what would be suitable for me?

Forget about your age, fitness or lack of formal dance experience, and indulge in a little day-dreaming to help you decide. As you swirl around the living room, imagine yourself as the star of a high-class cabaret, the dance partner of Patrick Swayze or Fred Astaire perhaps, the hostess of a Highland ball or a belly dancer at an exotic feast. In many parts of Britain, especially in or near large towns, you will find classes that allow you to begin or improve your dancing in any of these styles.

Why not look out for 'taster courses' in your area? You could sample dance classes in styles such as jazz (for the cabaret spot and Patrick Swayze), ballroom and tap (for Fred Astaire), or a variety of national and regional styles including Scottish (for the Highland ball), Egyptian (for belly dancing), Latin American (for salsa, lambada or jive) or Indian (for a range of traditional and contemporary styles).

Talk to the teacher and to the members of any classes you watch or sample, until you find a dance style that appeals to you. No one should worry about being younger, older, fatter, thinner, stiffer or less knowledgeable than other members of the class – everyone has to be a beginner at some time, and people involved in dance are seldom competitive or concerned with what other class members are wearing.

DO'S
—— AND ——
DON'TS

for exercise with music

Do warm up before strenuous exercise.
Do stop exercising if you feel pain.
Do ask a qualified teacher about regulating your breathing.

Don't try to stretch by using bouncing movements (see pages 80-82).
Don't continue using one set of muscles for long periods.
Don't force your body into positions that are uncomfortable.

THE PROS AND CONS OF DIFFERENT STYLES OF EXERCISING TO MUSIC

EXERCISE	ADVANTAGES	DISADVANTAGES
Aerobics	Improves general fitness. Especially good for aerobic fitness, muscular strength and endurance. Usually sociable.	Not suitable for people with back or joint complaints. Flexibility exercises tend to get low priority. Needs special shoes. Sometimes of limited variety in music styles.
Ballet	Excellent for flexibility, strength, endurance, coordination and concentration. Encourages self-discipline and musicality.	Physically demanding. Often not suitable for people with joint problems. Needs special shoes.
Ballroom, Old-Time	Good for general mobility. Sociable. No regular partner needed for some classes and functions. Suitable for most people.	Social dancing not always good for aerobic exercise. Limited muscular benefits.
Barn/square dance	Good for aerobic exercise. Relaxing, sociable fun. Suitable for most people.	Risk of pulled muscles if you do not warm up first.
Belly dancing	Good for flexibility and muscular strength, especially abdominal and lower back muscles. Fun. Suitable for most people.	Traditionally danced by women only.
Contemporary/jazz dance	Excellent general exercise. Wide variety of styles, techniques and music. Encourages rhythm and self-expression. Can be attempted by most people. Usually sociable.	Physically demanding. Might not be suitable for people with joint trouble.
Keep Fit	Improves general fitness. Encourages rhythm, interpretation, self-confidence and a positive attitude towards health. Sociable.	Does not always give a great deal of aerobic exercise. Benefit depends on intensity of session.
Latin American dance (including salsa, lambada and jive)	Good for aerobic exercise. Improves general fitness, strength, endurance, flexibility and rhythm.	Might not be suitable for people with lower back problems.
Rock, disco, rave, bhangra	Usually good for aerobic fitness. Sociable.	Risk of pulled muscles if you do not warm up first. Each type of dance uses mainly one style of music.
Tap/Irish step-dance	Good for lower body strength, aerobic exercise and coordination. Encourages rhythm.	High impact: not suitable for people with back or joint problems. Needs special shoes.

My grandson does ballet and contemporary dance classes. Wouldn't he get more out of playing football, cricket or another sport?

Dancing sometimes requires great physical strength, especially if the dancers have to lift each other. Both ballet and contemporary dance demand greater agility, flexibility, balance and coordination than either football or cricket. They also provide good aerobic and anaerobic exercise, and are good for physical endurance. In fact, these forms of dance are such good exercise that footballers, hockey players, ice skaters and martial arts participants are among those who regularly take dance classes to improve their overall fitness, flexibility and concentration.

Your grandson obviously enjoys dancing. And while he is learning about rhythm and interpretation, he is probably getting more fitness benefits than he would from playing football or cricket. Men have danced in most societies throughout history and these days are joining dance classes in increasing numbers, for both fitness and pleasure.

Fitness with rhythm Whether letting loose in a club (above) or performing in a Latin dance competition (left), young men will find that dancing can make them more agile, and probably fitter, than football or cricket.

Exercise from the East

Do ask your doctor's advice before starting yoga if you have a back problem or high blood pressure or are pregnant.
Do wear loose, comfortable clothes.
Do ease yourself into positions gently.
Do relax and breathe evenly.
Do practise regularly, ideally for at least ten minutes a day.

Don't force yourself into awkward, uncomfortable positions.
Don't try to compete with others in a class.
Don't hold your breath when you move into a yoga position.

STARTING YOGA

I want to join a beginners' yoga class. Is it better to make a start at home with a book, or should I wait until the class begins?

Books will give you a good idea of what to expect from a class and what you might be able to achieve. Even so, it is probably too soon to attempt yoga without expert supervision. As with other types of exercise, yoga involves positions that can cause injury. Trained and experienced participants can avoid hurting themselves, but newcomers could put themselves at risk. There is something to do in the meantime, however: you can prepare yourself by doing simple daily relaxation exercises. Some of these are described on pages 190-193. The basic exercise, used to begin most yoga classes, is one that you should master right away.

Simply lie on your back on the floor, with your legs either straight or bent at the knees, and arms resting a little way from your sides. Concentrate on breathing slowly and evenly for about ten minutes. The more relaxed you become, the easier you will find it to achieve the yoga positions when you eventually start to practise them, and the more refreshed you are likely to feel at the end of class. A word of caution: get up slowly off the floor once you have finished the exercise, in order to avoid an attack of dizziness.

THE VALUE OF YOGA

Is yoga useful as physical exercise, or is it mainly a technique for relaxation?

It is both – and for some people it offers mental and spiritual benefits as well. Yoga is excellent for coordination, balance, muscular strength and flexibility. It is especially good for strengthening the spine and back muscles and keeping them flexible, and it can help you to expand your lungs to their full capacity, and so allow you to breathe more efficiently.

However, yoga does not provide the sustained aerobic activity that is so beneficial for strengthening the heart and blood circulation. If you are aiming at overall fitness, you will need to supplement the benefits you get from yoga with a more vigorous form of exercise – such as aerobics, swimming or even brisk walking – that increases the heart rate.

Most yoga exercise in Britain is a form called hatha yoga, which uses breathing and relaxation techniques to help you to achieve yoga positions without strain.

Some people value yoga for its philosophical or spiritual aspects. Developed in India about 1500 years ago, yoga aims to help people to control and balance all that they feel and experience in life – the word yoga comes from the Sanskrit word for 'union'. Positions are designed to make you aware of your body's rhythms and, through this awareness, to reach a sense of peace or stillness and a more positive, yet relaxed, outlook on daily life.

T'AI CHI FOR FITNESS

I've seen television clips of Chinese people doing graceful exercises in a park. Are these exercises suitable for people of all ages who would like to stay fit?

The slow, controlled, dance-like exercise you have seen is T'ai Chi Ch'uan, usually shortened to T'ai Chi. Although not a martial art in the way most Westerners think of it, a few highly skilled practitioners can use it for self-defence. Because it is so gentle, T'ai Chi is usually a safe form of exercise for people of all ages. It is excellent for strength, coordination, flexibility, balance, posture and breathing, and is often used to relieve stress. You can use T'ai Chi for its fitness benefits alone, but many people find that it gives them an even greater sense of wellbeing – a spiritual harmony. Closely linked to the ancient Chinese philosophy of Taoism, T'ai Chi is based upon the belief that in order to remain fit and healthy we must balance the flows of mental (or emotional) energy and physical energy within our bodies.

The T'ai Chi movements are based upon observations of animals and linked into a sequence called 'the form', in either a short or a long version. Practising the form is said to lead to self-mastery through the balancing of internal and external energy.

You will need an experienced teacher to learn T'ai Chi. Classes are run in and around most main towns in Britain. If you have difficulty in finding a class, send an s.a.e. to The British Council of Chinese Martial Arts, 46 Oaston Road, Nuneaton, Warwickshire CV11 6J2, for details of the class nearest you. Before joining, watch some sessions and talk things over with the teacher.

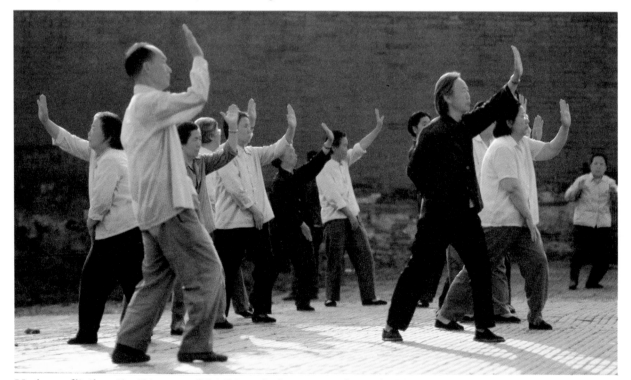

Moving meditation The Chinese art of T'ai Chi goes back centuries and trains both body and mind in balance, control and coordination. The movements are supposed to imitate animals and are performed slowly and deliberately, with a gentleness that makes T'ai Chi an ideal form of exercise for people of any age. It is also an excellent form of relaxation and stress relief.

LOOKING AFTER YOURSELF

Whether it's brushing your teeth or reaching for an aspirin, everyday habits can either prevent illness or contribute to it. So take good care of yourself, treat minor complaints properly and have symptoms attended to before they become serious.

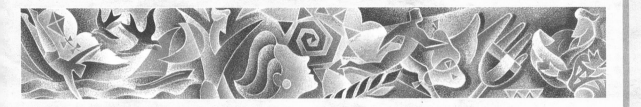

Are you living healthily?

Health is more than just a matter of not being ill – it's about feeling positively well and energetic every day. It's also about building up your immune system, and recognising problems before they become serious. Try this test to see if you know how to look after yourself. Tick the right box in each case, and check your score.

1 Which symptom does not usually merit a visit to the doctor?

a) Unusual fatigue. ☐
b) A winter cold. ☐
c) Chronic indigestion. ☐

2 How can you protect your ears when listening to a personal stereo?

a) Never listen at full volume. ☐
b) You don't need to – personal stereos do not play loudly enough to harm you. ☐
c) Never listen at a volume that makes it impossible to hear an outside conversation. ☐

3 How frequently do you normally change your toothbrush?

a) Once or twice a year. ☐
b) Every two or three months. ☐
c) When it starts to look worn. ☐

4 Which is least likely to protect you from colds and flu?

a) Washing your hands frequently. ☐
b) Having an anti-flu injection. ☐
c) Staying indoors in cold weather. ☐

5 Which is the best time to arrive at your destination if you want to avoid jet lag?

a) Early evening. ☐
b) Sunrise. ☐
c) Midday. ☐

6 How often should you rest your eyes when using a computer, reading or doing close work?

a) Every hour. ☐
b) Every 30 minutes. ☐
c) Every 10 minutes. ☐

7 Which statement is true?

a) You can get sunburned even on a cloudy day. ☐
b) You should use a sunscreen lower than factor ten if you want to tan. ☐
c) People with darker skins don't need to use a sunscreen. ☐

8 Which is most likely to help if you want to lose weight?

a) Skipping meals. ☐
b) Cutting down on alcohol. ☐
c) Avoiding starchy food. ☐

9 Which is the better way to breathe?

a) Through your mouth. ☐
b) Through your nose. ☐
c) Neither is better than the other. ☐

10 Which treatment is least likely to damage your hair?

a) Perming. ☐
b) Blow-drying. ☐
c) Bleaching. ☐

SCORING

Award yourself 1 point for each of these answers: 1(b), 2(c), 3(b), 4(c), 5(a), 6(b), 7(a), 8(b), 9(b) and 10(b). Add up your score.

8-10: You are obviously well aware of what makes for a healthy way of life – now make sure you are putting it all into practice.

5-7: You probably have a good basic knowledge about most aspects of healthy living, but there might be a few subjects you could brush up on.

4 or less: Don't despair, all is not lost – this chapter can help you to make safer and healthier habits a part of your daily life.

A long and healthy life

STAYING WELL

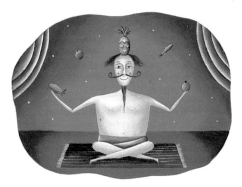

What steps can I take to help me to live a longer, healthier life?

There are many factors that influence health and lifespan. Some, such as environment and genetic inheritance, are difficult or impossible to control, but there are still many things you can do to increase the chances of a longer, healthier life.

● Eat a healthy, varied diet, including plenty of fresh fruit and vegetables. The more varied your diet, the more likely it is to contain all the necessary nutrients.
● Exercise regularly. Frequent, vigorous exercise helps to keep bones, joints and muscles in good working order, reduces the risk of heart disease, helps control weight, relieves stress and promotes a positive mental outlook.
● Try to keep your weight within the recommended range (see page 154). People who are overweight are more likely to contract disorders such as diabetes, hypertension, arthritis and heart disease. Those who are significantly underweight may have lowered resistance to infection.
● Find ways of dealing with the stresses of everyday life. Exercise, meditation, yoga and massage are just a few relaxation techniques that can help (see pages 190-191).
● If you drink alcohol, drink in moderation (see page 154). Heavy drinking over a long period of time can harm your mental, physical, professional, domestic and social wellbeing.
● If you smoke, stop. Smokers are substantially more likely to die from lung cancer, bronchitis and heart disease than non-smokers or ex-smokers.

● Visit your doctor regularly for any necessary health checks and screening tests.
● Avoid any unnecessary risks: use the correct safety equipment for potentially dangerous work or leisure activities; take medicines only when necessary; practise 'safe' sex (see page 258); don't drink and drive; have any recommended immunisations before travelling to developing countries (see page 171).

PREVENTIVE MEDICINE

I've heard a lot of talk about 'preventive medicine'. What exactly does it mean?

The focus of preventive medicine is on promoting good health rather than on treating problems once they develop. It is considered to be a part of community health and includes a variety of services.

● The provision of clean water.
● Health education to discourage smoking and excess alcohol consumption.
● The promotion of exercise.
● Advice on a healthy diet.
● Immunisation programmes against infectious diseases.
● Screening programmes to detect diseases such as cancer of the cervix and breast, high blood pressure, glaucoma and tuberculosis, before they cause symptoms.

A generation ago people were taught very little about the influence of nutrition, exercise and stress relief on health. Today, the impact of scientific studies on the causes of disease has changed that and governments across the world have started to realise the importance of health promotion as part of public policy. An irrefutable connection between smoking and lung cancer has inspired antismoking campaigns; the role of saturated fat in heart disease has been publicised; and the benefit of aerobic exercise is well documented.

In Britain, such policies are set out in the Health of the Nation document, which outlines goals such as reducing deaths from heart disease and strokes in people under 65 by at least 40 per cent by the year 2000. Screening for cervical and breast cancer already has a proven record of success, and family doctors offer practical advice on diet, exercise and health promotion to all patients.

Your body's warning signals

See your doctor if any of these symptoms develop. They do not necessarily indicate a serious complaint, but rather a condition that may call for professional diagnosis.

● Unusual bleeding or discharge, particularly rectal bleeding or blood in the faeces, urine, vomit or sputum. In women: vaginal bleeding between periods, during pregnancy or after the menopause; or bleeding or discharge from the nipples at any stage.
● Any marked change in bowel or bladder habits.
● Any change in a mole, or a sore on the skin that fails to heal within about three weeks.
● Any lump, swelling or thickening.
● Unusual fatigue.
● Persistent hoarseness or coughing that lasts more than a couple of weeks.
● Chronic indigestion or difficulty in swallowing, or recurrent vomiting.
● Sudden, unexplained drop in weight.
● Sudden or severe pain.
● Fever or sweating that lasts for more than a few days.
● Unexplained lightheadedness or fainting.
● Blurred vision; seeing halos around lights.
● Severe, unexplained shortness of breath.
● Bluish lips, eyelids or nail beds.
● Chronic ankle swelling.
● Yellowing of the skin or whites of the eyes.
● In men, frequent or painful urination.

BOOSTING THE IMMUNE SYSTEM

How does the immune system work and are there any ways of making it more effective?

The immune system is a system of specialised cells and proteins that work together to protect your body from potentially harmful microorganisms such as bacteria, viruses and fungi, and from certain poisons. The immune system also plays a role in the control of cancer, by recognising and destroying cells that grow out of control.

Not all immune reactions are beneficial, however – allergies and hypersensitivities are the result of an excessive or abnormal immune response, and it is the immune system that provokes rejection after an organ transplant. Nevertheless, immunity is essential to protect the body from hostile agents in the environment.

Some immunity is present from birth. The skin provides a general barrier to infection, while acids in the stomach and enzymes in the mucous linings of the mouth, throat, eyes, intestines, vagina and urinary tract destroy invaders on contact. Some antibodies are also acquired from the mother while the baby is still in the womb.

After birth, the body develops further resistance as it is exposed over time to potentially dangerous agents and organisms in the environment. When it recognises a foreign invader, the immune system produces antibodies to attack and destroy the threat. After the first exposure, a 'memory' remains that enables the body to recognise and fight off the invader more quickly the next time it is encountered. The natural process of acquiring immunity clearly carries a risk, since the body has to be exposed to a dangerous organism or substance before it can produce antibodies. Artificial immunisation, however, generally uses a weakened form or a very small dose of the germ or toxin to create immunity without the same dangers.

The efficiency of your immune system depends to some extent on heredity, but a good diet and a generally healthy way of life can go a long way to boosting its performance. Finding ways to defuse and deal with stress are equally important.

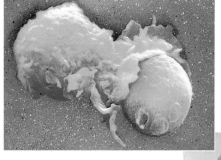

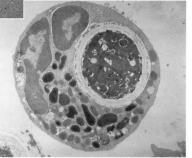

Natural defenders White blood cells are the warriors of the immune system. They collect at sites of infection to fight off foreign invaders such as the yeast spore being latched onto on the left. Eventually, the spore is completely engulfed and digested, as below.

Taking care of your eyes

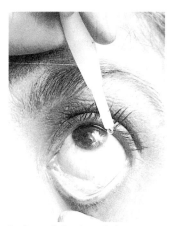

Seeing red Eyedrops help to relieve irritation, but prolonged use can actually increase redness.

TREATING IRRITATED EYES

I occasionally suffer from red and irritated eyes. Are eyedrops the answer?

If you have a mild eye irritation, eyedrops will cure the redness, but the relief is only temporary and not entirely without risk. Eye irritation has many causes, from dust and smoke to colds and allergies. Severe cases, especially when accompanied by a discharge, may be a sign of conjunctivitis, an infection that needs treatment with antibiotics. In any case, if the problem persists or recurs frequently, it is important to have a proper diagnosis.

Many over-the-counter eyedrops contain decongestants which reduce inflammation by shrinking blood vessels in the eye. These drops may trigger allergic reactions in some people, particularly contact lens wearers and people with glaucoma, who should consult a doctor or ophthalmologist before deciding to use them.

Try to use eyedrops only occasionally – excessive use can eventually exacerbate the problem, causing eyes to become more red more quickly as the effects wear off, and increasing the need for more drops.

Always use eyedrops carefully, to prevent any risk of infection. Remember that as soon as you break the seal of the sterilised container, you open the way to contamination from germs. Squeeze bottles are the safest dispensers, as long as you don't touch the nozzle; eye baths are the worst. Eyedroppers are acceptable provided you don't set the applicator end-down on a surface, or touch it. Wash your hands before and after applying drops, and don't touch your eye with the applicator. Never share eyedroppers.

TREATING STYES

My daughter seems to be susceptible to styes. How are they best treated?

Styes are intensely irritating, but extremely common. They are caused by a bacterial infection in an eyelash follicle. A small abscess forms on the edge of the eyelid and as it develops the spot becomes red and painful. Eventually a visible pimple appears and shortly after the stye comes to a head and discharges the pus that has built up. Afterwards the pain and irritation diminish and the abscess rapidly clears up.

There is no simple way of preventing styes, but the condition is reasonably easy to treat. The best time to start is as soon as the patient notices symptoms. To encourage the stye to come to a head, get your daughter to hold a warm compress to the area for about 15 minutes, three or four times a day. It is important that she is careful not to rub the eye, as this may cause the infection to spread.

Styes are painful while growing, but seldom need treatment with antibiotic drugs. If your daughter continues to experience problems, however, or if the styes cause her excessive pain, she should see her doctor.

BUYING SUNGLASSES

I need to buy a new pair of sunglasses. Are there any special features I should look for?

A good starting point is to look for a pair of glasses labelled British Standard 2724:1987. The label will also supply other useful information – such as how much light the lenses let through, whether there is any image distortion, and how tough the lenses are. For most ordinary uses any pair that conforms to the Standard should be quite adequate.

Department stores and larger chemists keep a good range of glasses and you should not need to pay more than about £15 unless you have special requirements. One feature that may be worth considering is polarised lenses to cut down glare from water, snow and other highly reflective surfaces.

Before you buy your glasses, examine the lenses carefully and avoid any with bubbles or scratches. Glass lenses are less susceptible to scratching than plastic ones, but they are heavier and more likely to break. Also check for colour distortion by looking at red and green objects in the shop – poor differentiation could make driving hazardous.

CAUTION Unlike glass, plastic is permeable to ultraviolet light. If you buy plastic lenses, make sure they are marked UV400. Other types may let through ultraviolet radiation which can contribute to cataracts and cause painful – though temporary – snow blindness.

WHEN YOU CAN'T SEE COLOURS PROPERLY

Complete colour blindness, in which the world is seen only in shades of grey, black and white, is extremely rare. Much more common is difficulty in distinguishing between colours, particularly red and green, although the degree of difficulty varies considerably. Colour blindness is largely an inherited defect and while it cannot be cured it is important for those affected to be aware of it.

Colour blindness is usually discovered accidentally but it is important to have a proper diagnosis if you suspect your colour vision, or that of a child, may be defective. Children whose close relatives are colour blind should always have a test. Although it is not a sign of disease or associated with any other eye problem, poor colour differentiation can cause difficulties in people who are unaware of having the condition.

Testing for colour blindness can be done by a doctor or ophthalmic optician using a method known as the Ishihara test, which was developed in Japan. The subject is shown a series of plates made up of coloured dots, in which numbers or patterns can be discerned, depending on colour perception.

Being colour blind has little effect on everyday life, except that motorists must learn to distinguish traffic lights by position. Careers such as being an airline pilot or train driver may also be problematic. Coloured spectacles and contact lenses may help to enhance contrast, but cannot correct actual colour vision.

Colour code In this Ishihara image, people with normal sight see a '6'. Those with red-green colour blindness see a jumble of dots.

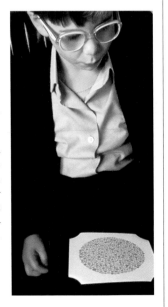

CHANGING TO CONTACT LENSES

I've worn glasses all my life, but am now considering getting contact lenses. How difficult is it to get used to them, and are there any health risks involved?

Recent advances in the design and cleaning of contact lenses mean that more people are now able to wear them. But even the most up-to-date contact lenses still cannot correct all vision problems, and remain unsuitable for some people, such as those with particularly sensitive eyes or those with unusual optical requirements.

Many eye doctors also advise against contact lenses for people who are clumsy with their hands – most children, for example – because of the risk of eye injury when putting them in or taking them out.

Dry climates, and even the dry air in aeroplanes, can make contact lenses feel gritty. They may also be unpleasant to wear when you have a cold, either because your eyes are watery or, conversely, because they are dry thanks to a decongestant you may have taken. For some women, contact lenses may become temporarily intolerable when the chemical composition of their tears changes slightly as a result of menstruation, the contraceptive pill, or pregnancy.

People who work in an environment where there are high levels of dust, chemical pollutants and other airborne irritants may find

---

THE BASICS OF CONTACT LENSES

The type of contact lens that is most suitable for you depends on several factors: your particular vision problem; whether you want to wear your lenses every day or only occasionally; and how easy you want them to be to look after. There are five main types of contact lens:

Hard lenses
These are the original contact lenses, and still offer the best vision correction for people with astigmatism and irregular corneas. They are durable (possibly giving more than five years of use) and inexpensive. There are drawbacks: it may be several weeks before they are comfortable to wear all day. They are not very porous to oxygen, and so should not be worn for longer than 20 hours at a time. And they fall out more easily than other lenses.

Gas-permeable lenses
These are rigid like hard lenses, but allow oxygen to pass through more easily and reach the surface of the eye, thereby reducing the risk of infection. They offer the sharp vision of hard lenses (though less durability – up to five years), with some of the comfort of soft lenses.

Soft lenses
Soft lenses allow oxygen to pass through them, and because of their high water content, most people find them comfortable almost immediately. Soft lenses can correct short and long-sightedness, but are not suitable for astigmatism. They are also very fragile, giving about two to three years of wear, and are more expensive than hard lenses.

Extended-wear soft lenses
These soft lenses have a very high water content, and can be worn for up to a month without removal. But they may increase the risk of infection, because they allow a contaminated lens to stay in contact with the eye for a long period of time.

Disposable soft lenses
These special soft lenses are replaced every two to four weeks. This disposability lowers the risk of eye infection and reduces the build-up of protein on lenses, which elsewhere can lead to blurred vision and eye irritation. Such lenses are increasingly popular. Disposable lenses must be cleaned in the same way as conventional soft lenses.

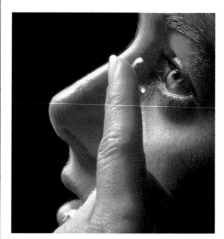

Eye contact Soft contact lenses are small and delicate – to protect them, keep your fingernails short and avoid folding the lens.

HOW DO VISUAL DEFECTS AFFECT YOUR SIGHT?

For most people, vision is never again as sharp as it is at the age of one. Problems often become apparent at about the time of puberty as the eyeball grows too long or not long enough, or becomes misshapen – the three commonest reasons for needing to wear glasses. The pictures below attempt to recreate photographically an image as it would be seen in each case.

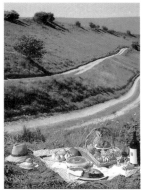

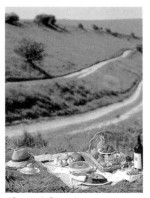

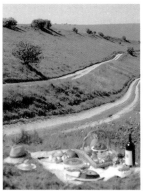

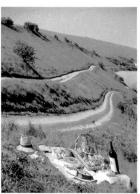

Normal sight The eyeball is perfectly shaped for light rays to converge exactly on the retina. The eye also reacts rapidly to changes in light.

Short sight Distance vision is blurred as the eyeball is too long and light rays converge short of the retina. Concave lenses correct the problem.

Long sight Close-up vision is blurred as the eyeball is short and light rays do not converge. Convex lenses can overcome the problem.

Astigmatism Vision is blurred both horizontally and vertically as the eyeball is irregular in shape. Cylindrical lenses correct the defect.

that tiny particles become trapped under contact lenses, causing discomfort and sometimes even scratches on the cornea. In such cases, protective goggles should be worn.

BIFOCAL GLASSES

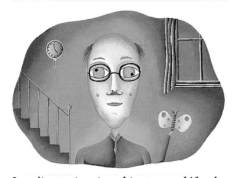

I can't seem to get used to my new bifocal glasses. Is it just a matter of time, or will I have to give them up?

Don't worry. Adjusting to bifocals just takes a little practice. The key to wearing them successfully is to get accustomed to looking through the appropriate section of the glasses for each task. Conventional bifocals have two distinct sections for each eye, the upper part of the lens being ground to correct for distance vision, the lower and usually smaller one for close-up vision.

Mid-range vision – the kind one relies on when descending stairs or stepping off a kerb – is sometimes blurry because it literally 'falls between the cracks' of the lenses.

The best way to adjust to bifocals is to wear them indoors at first, in safe and familiar surroundings. Practise going up and down stairs at home until you feel confident enough to move with ease in public places.

In seamless bifocals (also known as progressive lenses), one section of the lens blends into the other without a line in between. Some people find these glasses more attractive, but they sometimes prove difficult to get used to, and are also more expensive than the standard version.

LASER EYE SURGERY

I've grown tired of wearing glasses, and can't be bothered with the fuss of contact lenses. Is laser surgery the answer?

First of all, any type of surgery involves some degree of risk, and laser eye surgery is no exception. Secondly, it is only short-sighted people that can be helped by laser surgery, and not even all of them – you will have to be assessed by an eye surgeon.

The degree of short-sightedness is a key factor in assessing your suitability. A person with normal vision is said to have 6/6 or

20/20 vision. Deviation from the norm is measured in dioptres. The best candidates for laser surgery are those with up to –4 dioptres and no astigmatism or lens distortion, but surgeons will consider people with up to –6 dioptres and moderate astigmatism.

The procedure takes between 15 and 30 seconds for each eye. It is painless at the time, though the eyes may hurt in the following 24-48 hours. If so, painkillers will probably be prescribed. It takes approximately three months for the eyes to heal completely and for vision to stabilise.

After laser surgery there is a 50-60 per cent chance of perfect 6/6 vision, and an 80-90 per cent chance of 6/12 vision – enough to allow you to play most sports and to drive by day without glasses.

Laser eye surgery is not available on the NHS, so you are likely to run up considerable expenses – varying somewhat according to your particular vision problem.

There is a 1 to 2 per cent chance that people who have undergone surgery may experience distortions in night vision, such as radiating lines from street lamps, or even experience double vision. In such cases, patients may have to wear contact lenses until a follow-up operation takes place.

Even when treatment is successful and long-distance vision is improved, glasses still may be needed for reading.

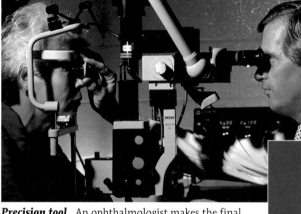

Precision tool An ophthalmologist makes the final adjustments to a focusing laser. It ensures correct alignment before the main beam is used for surgery.

Beaming into the eye
Once the focusing laser has been positioned correctly, as below, anaesthetic drops are placed in the eye in preparation for surgery. A surgical laser will reshape the cornea by shaving away fine saucer-shaped layers from its outer surface.

Nasal problems, ears and hearing

The right way to blow your nose

According to ear, nose and throat specialists, the safest way to blow your nose is to clear one nostril at a time – pressing gently on one side while blowing out through the other. Applying pressure when blowing your nose is dangerous: it may rupture an eardrum or send bacteria into the ears or sinus cavities.

If your nose is congested, clear it regularly, before mucus has a chance to build up.

NOSEBLEEDS

My nose bleeds frequently – and for no apparent reason. Why does this happen, and what is the best way to treat it?

An injury to the nose, a spell of vigorous nose blowing, a cold or other viral infection, or sometimes just being at a higher altitude than usual – any of these can rupture the capillaries inside the nose and cause it to bleed. If you live in a dry climate, or produce less mucus than average, the inside of your nose may also be more prone to cracking and bleeding.

Nosebleeds are fairly common in childhood, but are seldom serious. They then tail off, but become more common again and more serious during old age. If they really do represent a recurring problem, and are not clearly associated with any of the circumstances listed above, see your doctor. He or she may recommend 'cauterisation', in which prominent blood vessels in your lower nose are chemically sealed or destroyed.

To stop a nosebleed lean forward while pinching the tip your nose. If necessary, apply a cold flannel or ice-pack to the forehead or bridge of the nose. Keep the nose pinched for five to ten minutes, then release slowly to see if the bleeding has stopped. Resume if necessary. Keep your head still throughout this procedure, as a blood clot that has just formed is easily disturbed by movement.

CAUTION If the bleeding does not stop after 20 minutes, or if it is associated with a blow to some other part of the head, seek medical attention immediately.

CLEANING YOUR EARS

I was always told never to stick anything in my ears. What can I do then about all the wax that my ears seem to generate? Must I go to a doctor to get them cleaned?

Not necessarily. Ear wax is a natural protective substance produced in the ear canal, and need not be removed unless it starts to affect your hearing. It usually occurs in small amounts, and is regularly cleared away by the self-cleansing processes of the ear.

If an excessive amount of ear wax does build up, however, try softening it with a few drops of warm olive oil, or perhaps with sodium bicarbonate eardrops, available from chemists. After a few days, the wax should disperse by itself.

If your own efforts fail to reduce wax build-up, or if your ears remain blocked, see your doctor. He or she may use an instrument to remove the wax manually, or flush out your ears with a syringe containing warm water.

CAUTION Don't poke anything into your ears – not even cotton buds. You may drive wax deeper into the ear canal and just make the problem worse.

RINGING IN THE EARS

My husband has been tortured by an incessant ringing in his ears for some time. Can it be cured?

What he is suffering from is most probably tinnitus, a condition in which a ringing, buzzing or other noise is heard in one or both ears. Since it is clearly disturbing your husband, he should see his doctor immediately. No matter what the cause, tinnitus is usually treatable if not curable.

In some cases, the noise is just a symptom of an ear blocked with wax, something that is easily remedied. Occasionally there is a more serious cause, such as developing deafness, high blood pressure, the inner ear disorder Ménière's disease, or otosclerosis, a type of deafness that runs in families.

In other cases, tinnitus is brought on by old age or by drugs such as aspirin or quinine. Sometimes, even when there is no obvious cause, the condition seems to be aggravated by anxiety or depression.

The doctor will examine your husband's ears, conduct simple hearing tests and, if necessary, refer him to a specialist. Drug treatment may be offered, especially for Ménière's disease. If the problem is severe, the doctor may recommend a 'masker', an instrument that looks like a hearing aid and produces a low background noise to block out the ringing.

If you require further advice on or information about tinnitus, contact The British Tinnitus Association, 14-18 West Bar Green, Sheffield S1 2DA.

TREATING EARACHE

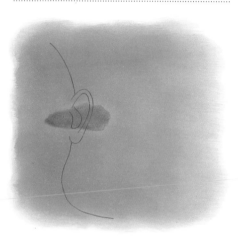

My son suffers from earache from time to time. What could be causing the problem and how should it be treated?

The most common cause of earache, particularly in children, is an infection of the middle ear. Symptoms include severe stabbing pain, dulled hearing and sometimes a discharge from the ear. Although many infections do clear up on their own, and require only pain relief, it is always advisable to consult a doctor. In some cases antibiotics may be prescribed. If the problem occurs frequently, your doctor will want to investigate the infection in turn. The most common causes are a cold, allergic nasal inflammation or enlarged adenoids. Consult your doctor immediately if:

● An earache persists after 4-8 hours' rest.
● There is any discharge.
● Pain develops after a discharge, or in association with a respiratory problem.
● Pain occurs after flying or diving.

Among the other possible causes of earache are dental problems such as an impacted wisdom tooth, a foreign object that has become lodged in the outer ear or a perforated eardrum. The eardrum can perforate after a blow to the ear, but the usual culprit is the discharge resulting from a middle ear infection that has failed to heal.

Using a personal stereo safely

Personal stereo headphones can damage your hearing if you keep the volume up too high and wear them all day. Noises that measure louder than 85-90 decibels (db) risk producing irreversibly impaired hearing. The general rule for safe use of headphones is this: make sure you can hear normal conversation through the music. The volume of normal speech is 40-60db, whereas personal stereos can generate a volume of 110-120db. Most listeners would tend to set them at around 80-85db, but a fairly large number insist on playing their personal stereos at up to 102db. Some manufacturers have devised 'danger level' indicators for the volume controls, which may go some way to reducing the risk.

Did you know…?

It is better to breathe through your nose than your mouth. The mouth is primarily an entry for food and water; it has few defences against germs and is not very good at warming the air you breathe. The nose, by contrast, acts as an air conditioner for the respiratory system. It filters out dust, traps incoming bacteria, adds moisture and warms the air up towards blood temperature.

Oral hygiene

FIGHTING TOOTH DECAY

Does sugar actually cause tooth decay, or is that just a myth? Is it a good idea to brush your teeth after eating something sweet?

Certainly sugar causes tooth decay, though not directly. The main culprit is plaque, a microscopic film of bacteria, food particles and saliva that forms on the surface of the teeth. Plaque does most damage when combined with sugar, and is especially harmful if left undisturbed for a long time. So whether or not you eat sugary foods, do brush and floss thoroughly at least once a day.

Sugar and plaque combine to increase dramatically the level of acid in your mouth. The acid eats into tooth enamel and decay begins. The crucial factor in the formation of acid is not how *much* sugar is consumed, but how *often*. Avoid consuming sugary foods and drinks throughout the day, or else mouth acid will remain at a high level and expose teeth continuously to attack. For the same reason, avoid giving babies fruit juice or other sugar-containing drinks to comfort them when they go to bed.

The only natural defence is saliva. It washes over the teeth, diluting and neutralising the acid in plaque that eats through tooth enamel. Salivation virtually stops when you are sleeping, so eating bedtime snacks and not brushing afterwards is an invitation to decay.

CHOOSING A TOOTHBRUSH

There is a bewildering array of toothbrushes on supermarket and chemist's shelves now. Are some better than others and, if so, which one should I be using?

When buying a toothbrush, you should take the following points into consideration:

- The brush head should be small, narrow and densely packed with bristles. For adults' brushes, the head should measure 22-28 mm x 10-13 mm, and for children's 20 mm x 10 mm.
- Choose synthetic bristles rather than natural ones if possible, since natural bristles do not dry out as quickly, and run the risk of collecting bacteria.
- Look for thin, flexible bristles that are rounded at the tip.
- Choose a soft or medium brush – hard bristles can scratch tooth enamel and cut your gums.
- The toothbrush handle should be long and slender, and if possible slightly flexible in order to moderate the pressure to your teeth and gums during brushing.

BLEEDING GUMS

Why do my gums bleed when I brush my teeth or use dental floss?

You most probably have gingivitis – inflammation to the gums, caused by infection.

Healthy gums are pink or brown and firm; with gingivitis they become red, soft and swollen, and often bleed on brushing. The condition is usually caused by a hazardous build-up of plaque around the base of the teeth. Bleeding can also be caused by rough brushing or flossing, or by a cut or other injury to the gums.

To solve the problem, make sure to brush your teeth regularly using the method on page 132, and floss using the technique explained in the panel, left. If your gums continue to bleed, see your dentist: untreated gum disease is one of the main causes of tooth loss. In any case, visit your dentist at least once a year to have your teeth checked and cleaned thoroughly.

AMALGAM FILLINGS

I have a mouth full of old amalgam fillings and am worried that the mercury they contain could be dangerous. Should I have them replaced?

According to the British Dental Association, there is no conclusive evidence to prove that amalgam fillings pose any risk to health. So the official view is that there is no justification for having amalgam fillings replaced with more expensive and less durable white composite fillings (made of porcelain or acrylic) – unless you are one of the very few people with an allergy to mercury.

Amalgam is a hardwearing mixture of silver, mercury and other metals, and is generally used to fill the back teeth where it will not show. For many years dentists and scientists have argued that because the mercury is 'locked' into the amalgam with silver, it is

---

Flossing technique

Flossing is an important part of dental hygiene: it removes the plaque that a toothbrush cannot reach. Use the following technique:

1 Break off about 12 in (30 cm) of floss. Wind it round the second finger of each hand, leaving about 4 in (10 cm) of floss in between.
2 Pull the floss taut and carefully insert it between two teeth. Draw the floss firmly between the sides of the teeth with a sawing action. Stop when the floss reaches the gum tip.
3 Curve the floss into a C-shape against one tooth. Gently slide it into the space between the gum and the tooth until you feel resistance. Do not jerk or snap the floss into the gums.
4 Hold the floss against the tooth. Gently scrape the side of the tooth, moving the floss away from the gum. Repeat for the rest of your teeth, using a fresh section of floss each time.

DENTAL CARE EQUIPMENT

The typical Western diet has so much sugar in it that it is almost impossible to prevent tooth decay completely. The main aids to limiting the damage are: good dental care, eating fewer sugary foods and having regular check-ups by a dentist.

As for your dental care equipment, a toothbrush and fluoride toothpaste are the bare minimum. Dental floss, tape or sticks are highly recommended – mouthwashes less so. All of the products below, and more, are available from a good chemist.

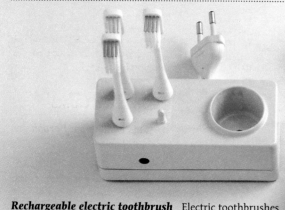

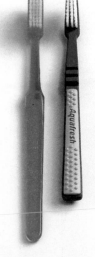

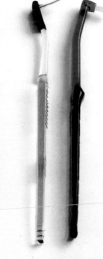

Rechargeable electric toothbrush Electric toothbrushes are particularly useful for disabled people. To get the best results, make sure to keep the batteries fully charged.

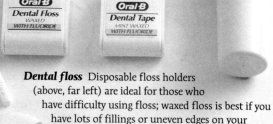

Dental floss Disposable floss holders (above, far left) are ideal for those who have difficulty using floss; waxed floss is best if you have lots of fillings or uneven edges on your teeth; dental tape is similar to floss, but wider.

Toothbrush Adults' and children's toothbrushes should have soft, rounded bristles and a long flexible handle. The smaller head is designed to suit a child's mouth.

Interdental brushes These clean the hard-to-reach areas, such as under a bridge. Incorrect use can damage gums, so consult your dentist beforehand.

Wooden dental sticks These toothpick-like sticks are helpful if you have large gaps between your teeth or if you don't like using floss.

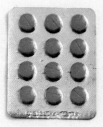

Disclosing tablets Chewing a disclosing tablet releases a dye that stains plaque red, indicating the areas where you need to improve your brushing.

not dangerous. In recent years, however, scientific studies have shown that some mercury does leach out of fillings, and may accumulate in certain organs, including the brain, and in foetuses, thereby increasing the risk of a miscarriage.

Whether or not the quantities of mercury leaching from amalgam are large enough to cause long-term mercury poisoning is unknown. At all events, in some European countries amalgam is being phased out, and in the United States and Britain some dentists have stopped using it altogether.

The evidence remains inconclusive, so it is difficult to decide. Two further considerations may give you pause. First, having your fillings replaced will be a fairly expensive procedure. Secondly, the removal of amalgam fillings tends anyway to release mercury vapour, and your exposure to it cannot be eliminated entirely. All in all, current medical opinion is against mass replacement.

CARING FOR YOUR TEETH

For the removal of plaque – an almost invisible film of bacteria that forms on the surface of the teeth, and a major cause of gum disease – you should brush your teeth for five minutes at least once a day. Use a medium-soft nylon toothbrush and a fluoride toothpaste, and pay particular attention to the gaps between teeth and just below the gumline.

Even regular brushing, however, will not remove all of the plaque that builds up between teeth and gums. As a supplement, use dental floss daily, following the technique on page 130.

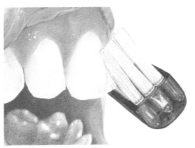

1 Place the head of the brush at a 45-degree angle against your gumline. Clean the front teeth by moving the brush in small circles for about 30 seconds.

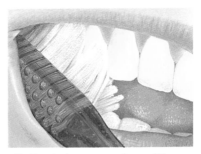

2 Brush the outer surfaces of the upper and lower back teeth, keeping the bristles of your toothbrush angled against the gumline.

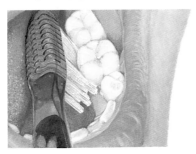

3 Clean the inside surfaces of the lower teeth, using small circular brushing movements. Spend about 30 seconds on each tooth.

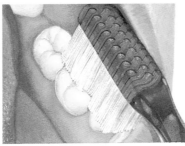

4 Brush the biting surfaces of the upper teeth, using firm to-and-fro strokes. Repeat the technique to clean the biting surfaces of the lower teeth.

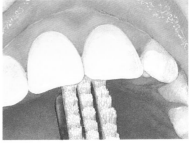

5 Use an up-and-down stroke to clean the inner surfaces of the front teeth, only this time tilt the brush vertically to make access easier.

FACT
— OR —
FALLACY?

'Cloves relieve toothache.'

Fact Cloves have been used to treat toothache since ancient times. Clove oil acts as a local anaesthetic and antiseptic.

Most toothaches are caused by a cavity or an infection, conditions to be treated by a dentist. For immediate relief, saturate a wad of cotton wool with oil of clove (available from chemists) and hold it on the tooth for a few minutes until the pain subsides.

MOUTH ULCERS

My teenage daughter suffers fairly regularly from an outbreak of mouth ulcers. Is there any reason for this, and how should they be treated?

There are many possible reasons why your daughter has recurring mouth ulcers:

● She may be feeling run down or suffering from stress.
● Mouth ulcers may run in your family.
● Hormones also play some part – ulcers often appear at puberty or during menstruation.
● Her diet may be lacking in vitamins B or C, or she may be anaemic.
● She may be brushing her teeth over-vigorously. Such brushing causes abrasions on the gums that can turn ulcerous.
● Her mouth may be suffering irritation from particular chemicals, spices, tobacco or even alcohol.
● Rather more serious, the culprit may be the herpes simplex virus, which also causes cold sores (see page 135). The first attack can be severe, with sore throat and ulcers inside the mouth. Subsequent attacks are less severe, with fewer and smaller ulcers.

For immediate relief, when ulcers appear, your daughter should avoid hot or spicy food and drink, and alcohol and tobacco, and use an analgesic mouthwash or mouth gel to ease the pain. If the ulcers coincide with feeling run down, your daughter should check that her diet is well-balanced (see pages 14-15) and possibly take more rest.

Mouth ulcers usually heal by themselves, but see a doctor if they persist for more than two weeks or are accompanied by a skin condition or by other symptoms such as white patches in the mouth or throat.

Ulcers that appear in the wake of medication also need immediate medical advice, as do any that bleed or become infected, or that are associated with lumps or growths in the mouth. A doctor or dentist may prescribe a stronger mouthwash or ointment to accelerate the healing process, or conduct blood tests to check for other disorders.

BEATING BAD BREATH

No matter how often I use a mouthwash, I still suffer from bad breath. What causes it and how can it be prevented?

Poor dental hygiene may well be the cause of your bad breath. Without proper brushing food particles become lodged between teeth and along the gum lines and decay, thereby forming plaque and emitting a foul odour.

A better toothbrushing and flossing technique will probably take care of your immediate problem, though a thorough clean by a dentist may be needed if plaque is extensive and if gum disease is advanced. Smoking is the second major offender. The residues of tobacco tars in the mouth combine with the tainted air being expelled from the smoker's lungs, and produce a stale smell. Bad breath can also be an early sign of a mouth infection or ulcer, or the side effect of a sore throat. In either case, use an antiseptic mouthwash until the condition heals.

Eating raw onions or garlic is another common cause of bad breath. Although toothbrushing may help, some of the pungency will remain in the blood, and thus in the lungs and breath, for up to 24 hours.

If bad breath is new to you and not due to any of the causes listed here, consult your doctor. In very rare instances, it may be a symptom of stomach and lung infections or perhaps serious internal ailments.

Colds, coughs and flu

AVOIDING INFECTIONS

Every winter without fail I'm laid up with one cold after another or, even worse, with bouts of flu. Is this something I have to live with or can it be prevented?

Colds and flu are infectious viral illnesses. Flu is the more severe – and the rarer – of the two. Both infections are more common in winter, when people spend a greater amount of time close together indoors. Although you cannot avoid exposure completely, there are several steps you can take that will reduce the chances of infection:

● Keep away from other sufferers.
● Wash your hands often. Turning a door knob or picking up a telephone recently touched by someone with a cold may be enough to infect your system, particularly if you rub your eyes or nose afterwards. The eyes and nose, rather than the mouth, are the most frequent routes of cold and flu infection. In fact, you are more likely to catch a cold by shaking hands than by kissing.
● Strengthen your immune system and keep your general level of health high (see pages 123-124). Cold weather, stress, lack of sleep and poor nutrition can all damage immunity and increase susceptibility to passing viruses.

WHEN TO SEE A DOCTOR

When, if ever, does a cold become serious enough to see a doctor?

Complications arising from a common cold are rare, but when they do occur you should see your doctor promptly. Such complications are usually caused by bacteria that multiply in the sinuses, ears or lungs, and lead to a 'secondary' infection that is sometimes more serious than the original problem.

A persistent fever above 38.5°C (101°F) in adults or 39°C (102°F) in children is usually the first sign of a secondary infection. Consider calling a doctor if any of the following symptoms develop: swollen glands, difficulty in breathing or swallowing, chest pains, skin rashes, a cough that produces coloured mucus, neck stiffness, earache, and thick white or yellow spots at the back of the throat. Even in the absence of such symptoms, consult your doctor if a cold lasts more than two weeks.

TREATING SNEEZES, COUGHS AND COLD SYMPTOMS

There is no cure – except time – for the common cold, yet there are an overwhelming number of remedies to be found on the shelves of chemists and supermarkets. Most can make the symptoms at least easier to bear. This chart lists the most common medications and a few home remedies.

CAUTION Over-the-counter cold cures are generally safe to use, but some may be inadvisable during pregnancy and for people with diabetes, high blood pressure, heart or thyroid disease and stomach ulcers. If in doubt, or if you are taking any other medication, consult your doctor.

SYMPTOMS	DRUG TYPE	ADVICE AND SIDE EFFECTS	ALTERNATIVES TO TRY
Stuffy nose.	Decongestant (tablets, capsules, nasal sprays and drops).	Decongestant sprays and drops are the most effective. However, long-term use may actually increase congestion. Decongestants taken orally can cause an increase in blood pressure.	Steam inhalation using a few drops of menthol or eucalyptus oil in a bowl of hot water.
Stuffy or runny nose, sneezing, watery and itchy eyes caused by an allergy.	Antihistamine (tablets, capsules, nasal sprays and drops).	Effective in relieving symptoms caused by allergy, but of little value in the treatment of the common cold; may cause drowsiness or dizziness, though non-sedative preparations are available.	Avoid known allergens; try cutting out dairy products; take vitamin B and C supplements.
Productive (producing phlegm) cough.	Expectorant (liquids, lozenges, tablets).	Effectiveness unproven. Increasing your fluid intake is more helpful.	Hot compress, using 3 parts hot water to 1 part cider vinegar, applied to the throat and chest to get rid of phlegm.
Dry cough.	Cough suppressant (liquids, lozenges).	Effective. Do not take for productive phlegm-producing cough. It will prevent you getting rid of phlegm and may delay recovery.	Steam inhalation, using a few drops of eucalyptus, thyme or cypress oil in a bowl of hot water. To soothe a sore throat, try gargling with a few drops of the same oils in a glass of water.
Pain, muscle aches and fever.	Painkillers such as aspirin, paracetamol and ibuprofen (tablets, capsules). (See also pages 165-166.)	Effective. Do not give aspirin to children under 12.	Rest in a warm room and drink plenty of fluids. Tea made from lavender flowers is said to ease a fever.

ANTI-FLU INJECTIONS

I have been offered an anti-flu vaccine at work, and am in two minds about whether to accept. How effective is the vaccine and are there any possible risks that I should be aware of?

Flu inoculations are very effective against the strains of the flu virus included in the vaccine. Studies have shown that the risk of contracting flu is reduced by about 75 per cent if you are vaccinated. Even when they do not completely protect you, the illness is generally less severe than usual, so it is hardly surprising that more and more employers are funding the vaccination for their staff. Since the serum does not contain live viruses, there is no danger of infection. Those who have an allergy to eggs, however, should avoid being inoculated, because the virus is cultured in eggs.

Flu inoculations are available on the NHS, but doctors tend to reserve their supplies for people who are particularly at risk. This group includes the elderly and those with chronic illnesses such as diabetes, asthma or heart disease. People who live or work in nursing homes, schools or other institutions where infections spread rapidly may also be offered a vaccination.

The flu vaccine provides only short-lived immunity against the strains expected to be prevalent each winter. It does not protect against unexpected strains of flu – those would not be included in the vaccine. To have an effect, the inoculation needs to be repeated every year during autumn, just before the beginning of the flu season.

PERSISTENT COUGH

I recovered from flu several weeks ago, but I am still coughing. Is it really necessary to see my doctor?

Yes, particularly if you have symptoms such as fever, earache, shortness of breath or chest pains. These are all signs that you may have a continuing chest or sinus infection, which needs investigating and possibly treatment with antibiotics.

Most robust people make a full recovery from flu within about two to three weeks. But occasionally – particularly among elderly people and those with underlying heart or respiratory problems – other infections take advantage of the system's temporary weakness. It is possible that this is what has happened in your case. And even if not, and your throat or bronchial tubes are just slightly irritated still, a visit to your doctor will at least help to put your mind at rest.

COLD SORES

Whenever I get a cold, I also suffer from an outbreak of cold sores. How are the two related, and can I do anything to prevent cold sores?

These small, itchy, sometimes painful skin eruptions that appear around the edges of the lips are not actually caused by colds at all, though they can be triggered by any form of stress, including a minor infection. Cold sores are, in fact, symptoms of infection by the herpes simplex type 1 virus – a virus related to, but different from, that causing genital herpes.

The type 1 virus infects most people early in life, but usually remains dormant for years at a time until it is reactivated by some type of minor physical or psychological stress, such as a bad case of sunburn, the onset of menstruation or anxiety.

An attack of cold sores usually begins with tingling and itching around the mouth, followed by the appearance of one or more blisters. Several days later, fluid in the blisters is secreted and a crusted scab forms. As the fluid contains live viruses, it is easy to spread the infection to other sites on the body or to someone else, so scrupulous hygiene at this stage is essential. Wash your hands often and avoid kissing. You should not share towels or face cloths, and on no account should you touch your eyes after touching a cold sore blister – the virus can harm the cornea and do permanent damage to eyesight. Cold sore outbreaks usually last about a week to ten days.

When you feel an attack coming on, get plenty of rest and avoid alcoholic drinks. An antiviral drug called Zovirax is now available without prescription at chemists. It can sometimes prevent a full outbreak if used as soon as the first tingling is felt.

If you experience a painful red eye or an extensive outbreak of blistering spots anywhere near your eyes, or elsewhere on your body besides your lips, be sure to see your doctor within 24 hours.

STAYING IN BED

How important is it to rest in bed when you have a bad cold or flu?

Bed rest does nothing to alter the course of the common cold, which usually takes about a week to clear up, whatever you do. But a day at home may make you feel better and perhaps prevent a more serious secondary bacterial infection such as bronchitis. If you are feeling miserable, you won't accomplish very much at work anyway.

Influenza, or flu, is a more severe viral infection, with symptoms that can include chills, fever, headache, muscle ache, severe fatigue, coughing and chest pains, as well as the usual sore throat and runny nose. Two or three days of bed rest are often necessary to get your strength back.

For the elderly and those with lung or heart trouble, a bout of flu cannot be treated lightly, and it is important to call a doctor as soon as symptoms develop. Complications such as bronchitis or pneumonia could be very serious.

Occasionally, flu can damage heart muscle. People who suffer from heart disease should make sure that they get plenty of rest until they have completely recovered.

Vitamin C

The idea that vitamin C, or ascorbic acid, can ward off colds and reduce their severity has been popular since the early 1970s. The theory's chief advocate, Dr Linus Pauling, a Nobel prize-winning chemist, made a case for taking large daily supplements of 1-2 g to prevent colds, and even higher doses (4-10 g) to combat existing infections. The normal daily requirement is less than 100 mg.

However, other investigators have been unable to duplicate the results of Pauling's vitamin C studies and medical opinion remains, for the most part, steadfastly opposed to his theory.

Some recent evidence does, however, suggest that there may be some justification for Pauling's claims that vitamin C stimulates the body's immune response, even though the effect is not considered strong enough to warrant using the vitamin in treating the common cold.

HELP FOR SINUSITIS

Why do I seem to get sinusitis after every cold? Can I avoid it?

Sinusitis is an inflammation of the membranes of the sinuses, the air-filled cavities in the bones around the nose, eyes and cheeks. It often develops after a cold when mucus fails to drain away properly and the infection then spreads from the nose into surrounding areas. As mucus collects in the sinus cavities the membranes swell, causing symptoms of headache, facial pain, and sometimes fever. Some people also lose their sense of smell.

Unfortunately, once you have had sinusitis, the membranes become much more susceptible to repeated infections. As a result, you may not be able to avoid the problem completely, and attacks may recur whenever you catch a cold or have an allergy attack.

Even though it often arises as a complication of a cold, sinusitis is usually not caused by the cold virus but rather by a secondary bacterial infection. Treatment includes antibiotics to fight the infection along with oral and nasal decongestants to reduce inflammation and drain the sinuses.

When sinusitis is the result of an allergy, antihistamine drugs may temporarily reduce swelling and help you to breathe more easily. But both decongestants and antihistamines should be taken with care. Used too often, decongestants can have a 'rebound' effect, which cause nasal passages to become even more congested. Long-term use of antihistamines can dry the sinuses excessively and make mucus thicker and harder to expel.

Home treatments to try include inhaling steam or using a steam vaporiser to promote drainage, drinking warm liquids, and taking hot steamy showers.

Hints for healthy hair and nails

BLEACHING AND BLOW-DRYING

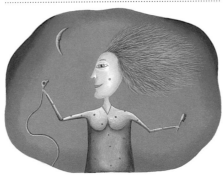

I bleach my hair once every three months. Am I causing any serious damage? What about blow-drying?

You could be, but you would probably know about it. Hair is quick to show damage and rapidly loses shine and condition when subjected to harsh treatment.

Repeated bleaching with hydrogen peroxide preparations can be harmful and may lead to rough, dry, brittle hair, with split ends. If you want to continue bleaching, keep a watch on the condition of your hair and stop if it seems to be deteriorating – or ask your hairdresser about changing to an alternative bleach. Snip the ends off every couple of weeks to prevent split ends.

A blow-dryer will not damage your hair as long as you keep the nozzle at least 6 in (15 cm) away from your head, and do not train it too long on any one spot. A properly functioning dryer heats air to no more than 85°C (185°F) – a temperature well below the 149°C (300°F) it takes to damage hair.

Conditioners can also offer some protection. Choose according to hair type and special needs. Cream rinses act on the surface to neutralise static electrical charges and make hair more manageable. Protein conditioners lubricate and add lustre and body.

WASHING YOUR HAIR

How often should I wash my hair?

There are no hard-and-fast rules about this at all. It really depends on how greasy your scalp is, what sort of environment you live and work in, and what sort of activities you engage in. If you work in heavy industry or work up a sweat at the gym every evening, every-day washing may not be too much. If you have a dry scalp and work in an office, every three or four days may be enough. If your hair is dry, however, try not to shampoo it more than once or twice a week – overwashing will strip away protective oils.

When you do shampoo, try to use the smallest amount you need (one teaspoon is plenty). If washing leaves your hair 'squeaky clean' you are doing it too often or using too much shampoo each time.

REMOVING UNWANTED HAIR

Hirsutism runs in my family and is making my life a misery. Is there any way of getting rid of facial hair permanently?

Heavy face and body hair is a much more common problem for women than is often supposed, so you are by no means alone. In a few cases – usually accompanied by irregular periods – there is a medical cause which needs treatment by a doctor. But in many more there is no underlying disorder. The problem is more common after menopause and it does tend to run in families.

The only method of removing hair permanently is electrolysis, available from qualified beauticians, which uses an electric current to destroy the growing part of the hair. It also destroys the surrounding cells so that hair cannot grow there again. Fine hairs disappear after one treatment; coarser strands may need several, but will grow progressively finer until they disappear. Because only a few hairs can be treated at a time, electrolysis is usually reserved for facial hair. The treatment can be painful and may make surrounding skin temporarily red and sore. It can be expensive if numerous visits are necessary.

Bleaching, although its results are not permanent, is effective for a light growth of dark hair and can be used on the face or body. It may, however, irritate the skin, so always do a patch test first.

PERSISTENT DANDRUFF

I just can't seem to get rid of my dandruff. What is causing it, and is there anything I can do?

Believe it or not, the exact cause of dandruff is still unknown, although some experts do believe it is a reaction to yeasts on the scalp.

For a moderate case of dandruff, the best advice is to avoid scratching and irritating your scalp and use an over-the-counter antidandruff shampoo once or twice a week. The condition should improve after a few weeks of treatment. If it persists, consult your doctor, who may refer you to a specialist dermatologist. You may also be given a prescription for a stronger antidandruff preparation. Sometimes what appears to be dandruff actually turns out to be psoriasis, ringworm or an allergy, in which case the doctors will prescribe appropriate treatment.

There are several different antidandruff shampoos available over the counter. Some contain a mild detergent to treat scaling

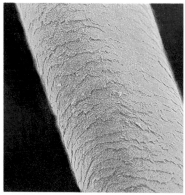

Healthy hair In top condition, the scaly outer shell, or cuticle, of each hair lies flat and smooth along the whole length of the shaft.

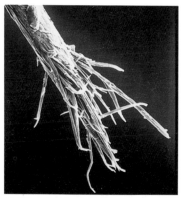

Split ends Excessive shampooing, dyeing and styling can all make your hair brittle and cause damage like this dramatically split end.

skin. Others have antimicrobial agents such as pyrithione zinc or coal tar to reduce yeast growth. Twice-weekly applications of selenium sulphide shampoo can also help, but don't use these products within 48 hours of dyeing or having a permanent wave.

SHAMPOOS AND CONDITIONERS

The number of different shampoos and conditioners available today is completely bewildering. What should I be looking for?

Consumers today have a choice of hundreds of different shampoos and conditioners, with additives ranging from extracts of tar to egg, beer, herbs, cucumber and a variety of perfumes, chemicals and colourings. Few of these do much good, since hair shafts are not living tissue, and the best advice is probably to use a simple, mild shampoo that will not dry out your scalp excessively. Baby shampoo is ideal, or look for a shampoo that has a pH value of 5 – close to the natural acidity of the scalp.

Conditioners are usually made of oils or waxes that are not water soluble and that leave a coating on your hair after rinsing. Applying a conditioner after shampooing will make your hair shine, stabilise the acidity and add body. However, the effects of added shine and body are only temporary and superficial: hair is dead and cannot be repaired or revitalised. Even so, conditioners do offer some protection from damage by smoothing down the outer layer, or cuticle, sealing in moisture and filtering ultraviolet rays. 'Two-in-one' products contain shampoo and conditioner and can make hair care easy. But they may not be suitable if you want chemical treatments – they contain silicon that is thought to build up an impermeable layer.

Dyeing hair safely

Scientists have been investigating the link between chemical hair dyes and cancer for decades. The latest evidence suggests that there is a risk, but it is tiny. Those who use dark hair dyes regularly for many years have a *slightly* increased risk of very rare cancers.

The chemicals under suspicion are phenylene diamines – found in both semi-permanent and permanent hair dyes. The only products that don't contain phenylene diamines are completely natural ones such as henna and sage leaves.

It is important to note that the risk only exists if the chemicals are absorbed into your bloodstream. To prevent absorption through your scalp, use foil or wear a rubber scalp cap through which hair is pulled. Try to reduce the intensity of the colour, and make sure you dye your hair in a well-ventilated room to avoid breathing in fumes from the chemicals.

WHAT FINGERNAILS SAY ABOUT YOUR HEALTH

Before undergoing surgery, women are asked to remove their nail polish. If a patient's lips are covered by an anaesthesia mask, it is the nails that the anaesthetist will examine – specifically the colour of the nail beds – to ascertain whether the patient is receiving enough oxygen. A skilled diagnostician can learn things about your health just by looking at your nails. Below are some of the most common disorders of nails, and the clues they provide to your general health. If a worrying one seems to apply to you, see your doctor.

Grooves

Fine grooves running across all your fingernails may reveal that you suffered a serious illness a few months earlier. Illness often slows nail growth and produces ridges in the nail root that are pushed outwards as the nail grows. The ridges grow out with time.

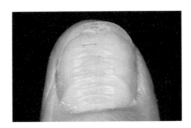

Deformed, spoon-shaped nails

Misshapen, backward-bent nails may indicate iron-deficiency anaemia. If so, it might help to eat iron-rich foods such as green vegetables, red meat and nuts, especially almonds. But make sure you see your doctor before taking supplements.

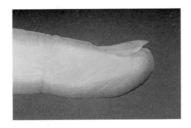

White flecks

Contrary to popular belief, white flecks are *not* due to vitamin or mineral deficiencies, but are caused by a minor injury, such as a knock, to the matrix which is the growing part of the nail. No treatment is necessary: the flecks will grow out in time.

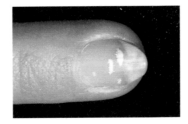

Pale nails

Anaemia is sometimes a cause and, if the nails are whitish, a kidney or liver condition is also a possibility. See your doctor for a diagnosis. Once the underlying condition has been treated, the nails should regain a healthy colour.

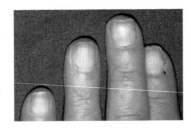

Blue nails

A disorder known as cyanosis is to blame, which arises when blood is not properly oxygenated in the lungs. Cyanosis happens most in low temperatures and may be a symptom of generally poor circulation, or of some heart or lung disorders.

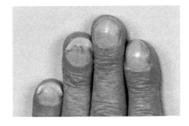

NAIL-BITING

How can I stop my daughter from chewing her nails to the quick? No amount of nagging seems to help.

Nail-biting is learned as a response to anxiety. Depending on your daughter's age, psychological methods as suggested on pages 178 and 179 may help most. If she is very small these will not be suitable, however, and it may be best to leave the issue for now – children often grow out of the habit.

Your daughter could also try one of the bitter-tasting over-the-counter preparations sold in chemists, or look for ways to keep her hands busy, such as knitting. Remember that nothing will work unless she *wants* to stop – perhaps buying a pretty ring would inspire her, or having a manicure.

SPLIT AND CHIPPED NAILS

I've always been proud of my long, strong fingernails, but recently they have begun to split and chip. What is causing this and what can I do to stop it?

The main cause of brittle nails is thought to be ordinary tap water and household detergents. Nails are porous and can absorb water when immersed. The water evaporates later but the process, when repeated hundreds of times, can do some damage to nail condition. Soaps, detergents and added ingredients in bathing and cleaning products make matters worse still.

You cannot entirely keep your hands out of water, of course, but always avoid soaking them for longer than necessary and wear gloves for cleaning chores and washing up.

Nail polish and polish remover can also cause problems. If you do wear polish, use an oil-based remover and apply moisturiser regularly to hands and nails (without polish).

HANGNAILS

The skin around my fingernails tends to peel off in thin strips that can be very painful. What causes this condition?

These dry strips of skin that partly split off from the area beside a fingernail are called hangnails. They are usually caused by excessive dryness, a bad manicure or tiny injuries.

To avoid infection, hangnails should be cut off (never pulled) not too close to the base. Prevent future problems with regular moisturising and good general hand care.

Protecting your skin

SENSIBLE SUNTANNING

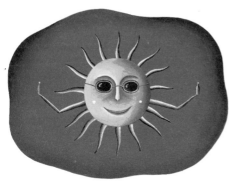

We are going to Greece this summer, and my daughter is determined to acquire a deep and enviable suntan. How can I make sure she doesn't burn and, more importantly, how do we minimise our risk of skin cancer?

If your daughter has very fair skin, she would do best not to sunbathe at all. Of course, it is not realistic to suggest going to Greece and spending the entire holiday in the shade! She should be aware, though, that her skin will not necessarily go dark brown however long she spends in the sun. Just as some people are blonde and some red-headed, so some people achieve a deep brown tan, and others no more than a gentle gold.

Remind your daughter that if she does burn, she will *have* to stay out of the sun and won't end up with the even tan she wants. This threat should encourage her to be sensible and to follow your advice.

There are also certain precautions that all the family should take, whatever their skin types, to prevent burning and minimise the risk of skin cancer:

● The commonest cause of sunburn is overexposure on the first day. Expose your skin to the sun for gradually increasing amounts of time, ideally starting with only half-an-hour or so on the first day, and building up to no more than a couple of hours a day. The sun is strongest between midday and about 2 pm, so sunbathing is best avoided during these hours.
● Do not assume it is 'safe' to sunbathe when there is a light cloud cover: 80 per cent of the sun's ultraviolet rays, which are responsible for sunburn and an increased risk of skin cancer, can penetrate cloud.
● If you are in the sun, you *must* use a protective lotion or cream, even if you are trying to develop a tan. Many experts feel that anything lower than factor 15 is inadequate. Remember that most suntan lotions and creams are easily washed off and need re-applying regularly – always after swimming and at least every two hours otherwise.

TANNING SALONS AND PILLS

I want to get a head start on my tan before I go on holiday. How safe are tanning salons? What about tanning pills?

Dermatologists take a dim view of tanning salons. The ultraviolet rays of an indoor sun lamp are actually *more* intense than the sun's own rays. You can be overexposed in a matter of minutes rather than hours. And that overexposure is at an unacceptably high price: rough, wrinkled skin and possibly a heightened risk of skin cancer.

Your eyes also are at greater risk in a tanning salon. If you go to one, you need to wear goggles that protect against ultraviolet rays, not just sunglasses, and avoid ever looking directly into the lamps.

Tanning pills contain a pigment that accumulates below the surface of the skin (as well as throughout your body). Taking the pills for a certain number of days causes enough pigmentation to build up to produce a noticeable colour – more an unnatural orange than a realistic tan. To maintain the colour, you must keep taking a minimum dosage of the pills.

Some people get dry, itchy skin from taking tanning pills; others may experience side effects such as nausea, cramps and diarrhoea. Doctors are also concerned that the pills, taken in large amounts, may cause liver damage and eye problems.

If looking tanned is important to you, the safest route is to use an artificial tanning lotion that you rub onto your skin. Several brands are available from chemists and cosmetic counters in department stores. Such lotions produce a fairly realistic colour, and are a safe alternative to excessive sun exposure. Remember, however, that they do not protect against sunburn. When you go out in the sun, you must apply a protective lotion.

Treating mild sunburn

Sunburn symptoms can range from skin that turns pink and feels hot to skin that becomes red, swollen, blistered and very painful. Relatively mild sunburn can be treated at home.

● Apply calamine lotion or a sunburn cream to soothe the burned skin.
● Do not use antihistamine creams; they have little effect and may cause allergies.
● Leave blistered skin exposed to the air.
● Take aspirin or paracetamol to relieve the pain, but do not give aspirin to children under 12 years of age.
● Stay out of the sun until the symptoms have disappeared.

CAUTION As with any type of severe burn, severe sunburn – where the skin is blistered – should be treated by a doctor, who may prescribe a steroid cream to relieve the symptoms.

SKIN CANCER ALERT

I've noticed that a dark-coloured mole on my shoulder has grown in size. Is this a sign of skin cancer?

Not necessarily, but it could be, and you should see your doctor immediately. Most skin cancers are curable if they are discovered and treated at an early stage.

Other symptoms that warrant a check-up include: a change in colour or shape of a mole or nodule; bleeding, itching, inflammation or crusting of a mole; or moles with a notched edge or multicoloured surface.

There are three main types of skin cancer:

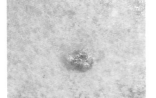

Basal cell carcinoma

The most common type of skin cancer, it starts as a fleshy bump, usually on the head, neck or hands. Left alone, the bump bleeds, crusts over, and then bleeds again. Untreated, a basal cell carcinoma slowly continues to grow, destroying the tissue directly beneath it, but not spreading to other parts of the body. It should be treated at the earliest stage.

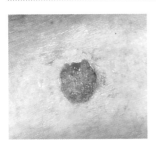

Squamous cell carcinoma

This cancer usually develops on the face, particularly around the mouth, or on the rims of the ears. It begins as a small bump or a red, scaly patch and grows more quickly than the basal cell carcinoma, above. Without medical treatment, such growths may spread to other parts of the body, and can occasionally be fatal.

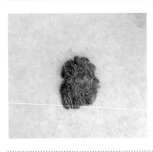

Malignant melanoma

The most dangerous form of skin cancer, a melanoma is curable if caught early enough, but may be fatal if the tumour has spread by the time you seek medical help. Malignant melanoma often, though not always, starts in or near an existing mole or dark patch of skin. It may grow in size, become lumpy, bleed, change colour or begin to itch.

Depending on the type of cancer and whether or not it has spread, skin cancer can be removed by surgery, electrodesiccation (drying up the tumour with a high-frequency electric current), cryosurgery (freezing) or radiotherapy. All of these treatments are suitable for basal cell carcinomas, and each has a cure rate of about 95 per cent. Squamous cell carcinomas and malignant melanomas are both removed surgically.

SUN PROTECTION

Exposure to the ultraviolet radiation in sunlight over many years can have harmful effects: premature ageing and an increased risk of developing skin cancer.

Sunshade creams

These opaque creams provide the strongest protection. They contain zinc oxide or titanium dioxide which block out almost all ultraviolet radiation. Sunshades are best for small sensitive areas such as the nose and lips.

Sunscreens and sunblocks

Sunscreens and sunblocks contain chemicals which partially block ultraviolet rays, allowing you to stay in the sun longer without burning. These lotions and creams are graded by 'sun protection factors' (SPF) of up to 20 or more according to how much protection they supply. The 'factor' represents the number of times by which the sunscreen reduces the effect of the sun's rays on your skin. So a factor six product reduces exposure to one-sixth, and means you can stay in the sun six times as long for the same amount of ultraviolet radiation. Sunscreen needs to be reapplied regularly every two hours and after swimming.

Regular application

Some people are sensitive to an ingredient used in many sunscreens, para-aminobenzoic acid (PABA), so there are many products now that do not contain PABA.

Whether you are very fair or dark, always apply a sunscreen of factor 15 or higher to exposed parts of your body when you go out into the sun for any length of time – winter or summer. Apply it 30 minutes before going out, and reapply it every two hours (sweat can remove sunscreen) and after swimming. Be sure to keep babies and young infants in the shade.

CURING WARTS

My daughter keeps her hands spotlessly clean, yet she still suffers from warts on her fingers. How can she get rid of them?

No one knows why some people get warts and others do not. Certainly personal hygiene plays no role. Warts are minor local infections caused by the papilloma virus. They are mildly contagious, particularly where no immunity to the virus exists. That is why children and adolescents are more likely to develop them than adults are.

Left alone, warts will often disappear within about two years. Common warts – the type your daughter has – can be treated with an over-the-counter acid compound that dissolves successive layers until nothing remains. Other methods of removal, such as freezing with liquid nitrogen or surgical removal, require a visit to the doctor.

Plantar warts or verrucas, which grow on the soles of the feet (see page 149), and genital warts (page 258) both require professional medical attention.

LIVING WITH ACNE

My teenage son is very self-conscious about his acne. What causes the problem and what is the best possible treatment?

Nature is unkind to teenagers. Just when good looks become a major concern, acne is likely to strike. But the distressing condition ranges beyond adolescence. It is in fact the commonest of all skin disorders, and many adults suffer from it too. In general, though, acne improves slowly over time, and often clears up by the end of the teenage years.

Likely causes

Acne breaks out when sebum (an oily substance produced by glands in the skin) plugs up pores around hair follicles. Trapped bacteria can then multiply easily and the pores become inflamed and infected. The cause of the change in sebum secretion at puberty is uncertain, but it is probably linked to a surge in the production of male hormones. Outbreaks are therefore generally worse in boys; although girls secrete male hormones too, it is in smaller quantities and so they generally suffer less. There may also be a genetic factor at work: acne tends to run in families.

Prevention and treatment

Alas, there is no cure for acne, but various treatments, used regularly, can improve the condition. Your son will need to follow a strict skin-care regimen for several months before he sees any benefit.

To prevent the build-up and spread of bacteria, he should wash his face gently with a mild soap twice a day and avoid touching his face if possible. Most importantly, spots should not be squeezed or picked; that could worsen the condition and lead to scarring. Regular shampooing will prevent oily hair

from aggravating the condition. As for diet, reasearch has shown that it makes little difference: avoiding oily foods will not in fact mean fewer spots.

Chemists sell many anti-acne preparations such as Acnegel, Acetoxyl and Quinoderm that act by unblocking pores. A doctor may prescribe a six-month course of antibiotics, which not only kill bacteria in the skin but also seem to reduce inflammation and sebum production. Tea-tree oil applied directly to spots may reduce infection. Ultraviolet light – either from a sun lamp or from sunshine – may also help, although strict safety measures must be followed to protect the eyes and prevent overexposure.

Adult acne

For many people, acne persists into adulthood. Where antibiotics have failed, an anti-androgen drug called cyproterone acetate, which restricts the production of sebum, has proved successful. Available on prescription, the drug acts in a similar way to the contraceptive pill, and may have similar side effects (see page 260). Manufacturers recommend that it should not be taken for longer than 18 months at a time.

WHICH DEODORANT?

What is the difference between an antiperspirant and a deodorant? Is one better than the other?

Antiperspirants do not prevent sweat from being produced – they reduce the amount. Their active ingredient is aluminium chloride, which reacts with proteins in your sweat to form a gel that partially blocks the sweat glands.

Deodorants contain mild germicides to kill the bacteria that feed off skin secretions and create the odour, and usually contain a perfume too, to mask the smell of sweat and germicide. But unless they also contain an antiperspirant, they will not actually reduce the amount of sweat.

As aluminium salts are the active ingredient in antiperspirants, there has been some concern about a possible increased risk of Alzheimer's disease (see page 441). While there is no clinical evidence that aluminium causes Alzheimer's, people suffering from the disease have been shown to have high levels of the metal in their brains. However, many manufacturers of antiperspirants argue that because the aluminium in their product does not penetrate deep into the skin, it will not enter the bloodstream.

DO'S
— AND —
DON'TS

for healthy skin

Do apply plenty of moisturiser to all exposed areas of skin as regularly as possible, particularly the hands, neck and face. A good moisturiser slows down the rate of dehydration by acting as a barrier to water loss.

Do use mild soaps with a pH level of 5 or less, particularly for your face. Harsh cleansers strip the skin of sebum, a naturally occurring protective oil, allowing moisture to escape more quickly.

Do apply moisturiser all over your body after having a bath. The longer the bath and the hotter the temperature, the more dehydrated your skin is likely to be.

Do wear clothes that are made from natural fibres, such as linen, cotton and silk, that allow your skin to 'breathe'.

Do eat plenty of fresh fruit and vegetables, pulses, grains and fibre as the basis for a fine healthy diet that will improve your skin.

Do apply a sunscreen of factor 15 or higher sunscreen to exposed parts of your body when you go out in the sun.

Do drink at least six to eight glasses of water every day to help keep your skin hydrated.

Don't use foamy additives in your bath which, again, remove sebum from the skin. Use bath oils instead.

Caring for your back

Head and neck
Keep your head upright, with weight centred at the top of the spinal column. Don't strain or tense your neck muscles.

Upper body
Hold your shoulders well back to open up the chest and rib cage. Don't tense your shoulder muscles or throw your chest forward unnaturally. Try to lift gently up from your hips.

Pelvic region
Gently pull your stomach muscles in and tilt your pelvis forward. Don't hold your breath or make a forced effort to suck in the abdomen. The stance should feel natural and relaxed.

Legs
Keep your legs straight when standing, but don't lock your knee joints. Bending your knees slightly helps you to tilt your pelvis forward and makes it easier to pull in the stomach muscles.

Feet
Distribute your weight evenly on both feet, adjusting your balance so that you have slightly more weight over the ball of the foot and the toes than over your heel.

BACK pain and back problems affect more otherwise healthy people in Britain than any other condition. While there is no certain way of preventing or curing back problems, there is a great deal you can do to protect yourself and to keep any troubles to a minimum.

The most common back problems arise from causes such as bad posture, excess weight, weak abdominal or back muscles, or strain due to lifting or bending awkwardly. By practising the exercises and techniques on the pages that follow, you can counteract and maybe even prevent them.

Before assuming that back pain is due to simple overstrain, however, it is wise to get a specialist opinion. Severe or persistent pain, in particular, may be a symptom of a more serious injury or a medical condition that needs treatment. See your doctor if rest and home therapy do not relieve pain within a few days, or if pain shoots down the back of either leg or is accompanied by other symptoms such as fever, dizziness or pain in the abdomen. Ask your doctor for a home visit if back pain immobilises you for more than two days.

But prevention is better than cure. Start by taking an honest look at your posture and identifying areas for improvement.

THE IMPORTANCE OF POSTURE

The spine is an intricate structure made up of 24 roughly circular vertebrae stacked on top of each other, with discs of cartilage in between. You can get some idea of the potential instability by trying to construct a similar column out of 24 children's bricks. A healthy back, however, is both stable and supple, with strong muscles and ligaments to keep it upright.

To minimise back strain, your aim should be to maintain the natural concave curvature of the upper and lower back. Hold your head erect and straight (habitual tilting is often unconscious and can strain the neck). Stand with weight evenly over both feet.

If you find it difficult to adopt a good posture without straining try the dancer's trick of imagining yourself suspended by elastic from the crown of your head. Good posture will usually then come quite naturally.

THREE COMMON FAULTS

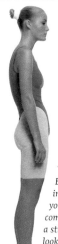

SLUMPING

This is how many people stand. By slumping the top of your body into your hips and hunching up your shoulders, you are compressing your spine and putting a strain on your muscles. It does not look attractive, either.

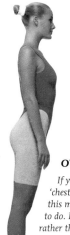

OVER-ARCHING

If you were brought up in the 'chest out, stomach in' tradition, this may be what you have learned to do. By tipping the pelvis backwards rather than forwards, you over-arch your spine, throwing your weight off balance and straining your back.

UNBALANCED

It is easy to over-compensate for poor posture by pulling your shoulders right back and thrusting the upper half of the body forwards. This posture unbalances and strains the whole body. You won't be able to keep it up, anyway – it is too uncomfortable.

THE RIGHT POSTURE FOR WORKING AT A DESK OR A KEYBOARD

If your job requires you to sit at a desk or use a keyboard for long periods of time, it is vital to adopt the right posture, to avoid placing unnecessary strain on your back. The chair you use is important too. You should be able to adjust the height of the seat, and the angle and height of the backrest. The chair should also be able to swivel, so that you do not have to twist your spine when turning sideways or reaching behind you. (For further information specifically about computer screen safety, see page 335.)

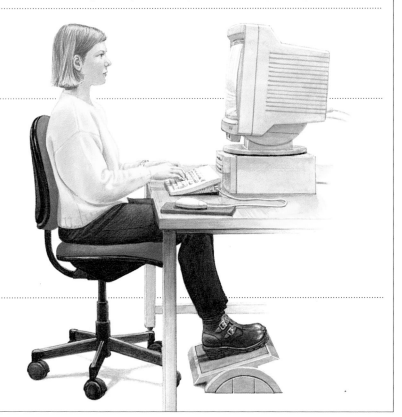

Head
Keep your head erect and poised vertically straight above your pelvis. If you work at a visual display unit your eyes should be level with the top of your screen to prevent neck strain from looking upwards.

Shoulders and arms
Hold your shoulders well back, but keep them relaxed and down (raised shoulders are a sign of tension). If you work at a keyboard, make sure you are sitting close enough to it for your upper arms to be vertical, and your lower arms approximately horizontal.

Back
Keep your lower back pressed flat against the back of the chair seat – a well-designed chair will give you lumbar support at the small of the back. Never sit tilted forwards on the very front of your seat. If you need to turn to the side, use the swivel action of the chair rather than twisting your spine.

Feet
Aim to keep your feet flat on the floor. If they do not reach comfortably, use a footrest. In either case, your thighs should be horizontal and parallel to the floor. If you have to tip forwards to rest your feet on the ground your back will come under constant strain.

EXERCISES FOR A HEALTHY BACK

One of the best things you can do for your back, whether you have pain now or want to prevent it in future, is to keep active. Joints need movement to stay lubricated and smooth, and ligaments and muscles have to be stretched to retain flexibility. Practised for just ten minutes every day, the exercises below can help to prevent many back problems, and may relieve existing back pain. They are suitable for both men and women, and for people of all ages. They are also extremely safe: however, as with any activity, stop immediately if you feel pain.

PELVIC TILT

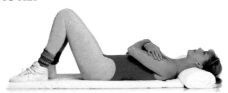

1 Lie on a mat on the floor, supporting your neck with a pillow or rolled towel. Bend your knees and place your feet flat on the floor. Relax arms across your chest or by your side.

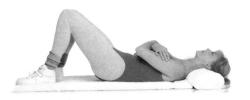

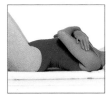

2 Gently squeeze your stomach and buttock muscles and tilt the pelvis up. Press the small of the back against the floor – do not arch as in the inset (right). Hold for 2-3 seconds and relax. Repeat 5 times.

SINGLE KNEE HUG

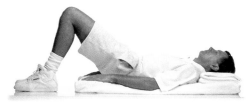

1 Lie on your back on a mat with a small pillow under your head. Adopt the pelvic tilt position, with feet flat, knees bent, pelvis tilted up and back pressed against the floor.

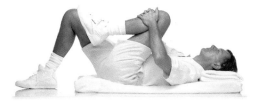

2 Clasp one knee and draw it towards your chest. Hold for 10 seconds, lower to the ground, rest and repeat with the other knee. Repeat 10 times.

LYING HAMSTRING STRETCH

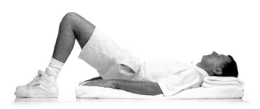

1 Lie on a firm, comfortable mat on the floor, with a pillow or rolled towel under your neck for support. Adopt the pelvic tilt position with your knees bent, feet flat on the floor, pelvis tipped upwards and back flat against the floor. Let your arms lie relaxed on either side of your hips.

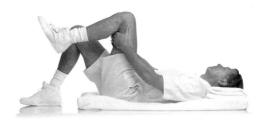

2 Grasp behind one knee with both hands. Draw the knee slowly up towards your chest but, unlike the knee hug, allow the leg to straighten as you pull it forwards. Do not pull farther than feels comfortable and keep the movement smooth, avoiding any sudden, uneven or bouncing motions.

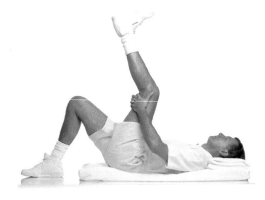

3 Straighten the leg, still grasping behind the knee. Hold for a few seconds, then gradually start to bend the knee again and return slowly to the starting position. When the foot is flat on the floor, slide the leg out straight, relax, return to the starting position and repeat with the other leg. Do 5 repetitions.

PROTECTING YOUR BACK IN EVERYDAY ACTIVITIES

Good bending and lifting technique is vital if you are to protect your back from strains, aches and pains. The methods described on this page are recommended by experts and can help anyone, whether or not they currently have back problems, to prevent trouble in future.

However strange some of these techniques may feel at first it is well worth getting into the habit of using them, as even one awkward movement can be enough to cause a strain. Being constantly aware of your back and how you are using it is the key to looking after yourself.

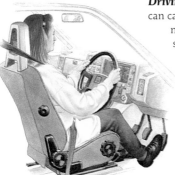

Driving A long stint at the wheel can cause an aching back or stiff neck. Before you set off make sure your driving position is comfortable. Bring your car seat forward so that you can depress the clutch without straining. Sit so that your knees are comfortably flexed and your lower back is well supported. Take regular breaks on a long trip.

Digging Using a spade is the most demanding job in the garden. Do a few minutes of warm-up exercises before you begin (see pages 78-79), use a lightweight spade and try to keep your back straight by bending your knees while lifting the soil. Rest your forearm against your thigh and use it as a lever. Take a break every 10 to 20 minutes.

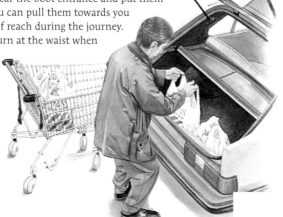

Loading and unloading a car boot Maintain a correct lifting posture at all times: that is, bend your knees and lift with a straight back. Place the heaviest items near the boot entrance and put them on a sheet so you can pull them towards you if they slip out of reach during the journey. Never twist or turn at the waist when lifting heavy objects out of the boot. Instead, lift the object and turn round by moving your feet.

Carrying heavy loads If you have a lot to carry when out shopping, do not put everything into one large shopping bag. Carrying all the weight on one side can strain your back, neck and shoulders. Instead, spread your purchases evenly between two bags and carry one in each hand. Your shoulders should be level and not raised. Take rests when you need to, and put your shopping down.

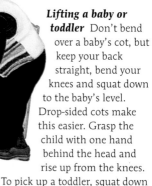

Lifting a heavy object Never stoop down and hunch your back when lifting an object such as a tea chest or packing case. Squat as close as you can to the object with your feet about 12 in (30cm) apart. Rise up using your knees and leg muscles, and keeping your back as straight as you can. If you have to walk with the load, carry it close to you. If possible, avoid wearing tight clothing, especially at the waist.

Lifting a baby or toddler Don't bend over a baby's cot, but keep your back straight, bend your knees and squat down to the baby's level. Drop-sided cots make this easier. Grasp the child with one hand behind the head and rise up from the knees. To pick up a toddler, squat down to the child, keeping your back straight. Use your leg muscles to rise.

WHAT IS CAUSING THE PAIN IN YOUR BACK?

Many people suffer from back pain at some time in life. In the majority of cases pain is due to strain or poor posture rather than to any serious underlying disorder. This is referred to as non-specific back pain and usually disappears with rest. But in some cases of back pain it is important to see a doctor. This chart is intended as a rough guide. As a general rule, be sure to seek immediate medical advice if pain is severe, or is associated with weakness in a leg or problems with bladder control.

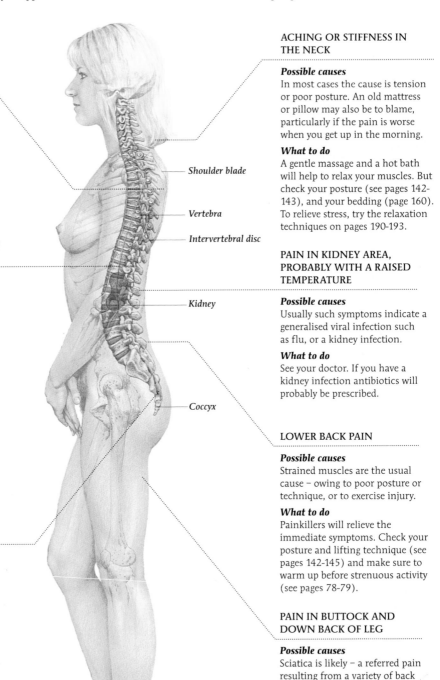

Shoulder blade

Vertebra

Intervertebral disc

Kidney

Coccyx

PAIN OR TENDERNESS IN THE FLAT OF THE BACK OR THE SHOULDER REGION

Possible causes
The symptoms probably indicate fibrositis – an imprecise term used to describe pain and tenderness in muscles, particularly in the back. It is often worse in cold, damp weather and may be associated with feeling generally unwell.

What to do
See your doctor.

VERTEBRAL PAIN AND SUDDEN INABILITY TO MOVE

Possible causes
A prolapsed, or 'slipped', disc is the classic cause. The discs between vertebrae are composed of a hard, outer layer and a soft, jelly-like core, and allow for cushioning and flexibility of movement. When a prolapse occurs, part of the soft centre bulges out through a weakened area of the outer layer. If the bulge presses on a nerve, pain can be intense.

What to do
See your doctor.

PAIN OR TENDERNESS AT THE BASE OF THE SPINE

Possible causes
Pain in the region of the coccyx (the bones at the bottom of the spine) is usually caused by falling and striking the coccyx against a hard surface, or by subjecting it to prolonged pressure – by habitual slouching when sitting down, for example.

What to do
Take painkillers and rest lying down. See your doctor if there is no improvement after a few days.

ACHING OR STIFFNESS IN THE NECK

Possible causes
In most cases the cause is tension or poor posture. An old mattress or pillow may also be to blame, particularly if the pain is worse when you get up in the morning.

What to do
A gentle massage and a hot bath will help to relax your muscles. But check your posture (see pages 142-143), and your bedding (page 160). To relieve stress, try the relaxation techniques on pages 190-193.

PAIN IN KIDNEY AREA, PROBABLY WITH A RAISED TEMPERATURE

Possible causes
Usually such symptoms indicate a generalised viral infection such as flu, or a kidney infection.

What to do
See your doctor. If you have a kidney infection antibiotics will probably be prescribed.

LOWER BACK PAIN

Possible causes
Strained muscles are the usual cause – owing to poor posture or technique, or to exercise injury.

What to do
Painkillers will relieve the immediate symptoms. Check your posture and lifting technique (see pages 142-145) and make sure to warm up before strenuous activity (see pages 78-79).

PAIN IN BUTTOCK AND DOWN BACK OF LEG

Possible causes
Sciatica is likely – a referred pain resulting from a variety of back problems, but most commonly from a prolapsed disc pressing on the spinal root of a nerve.

What to do
See your doctor.

Looking after your feet

CHILBLAIN PAIN

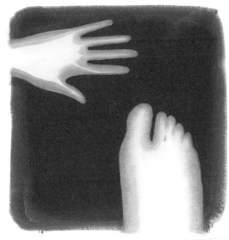

Chilblains make my life a misery in winter. Is there any way to prevent them?

People with poor circulation are often susceptible to chilblains, usually after exposure to the cold. These reddish-blue swellings that itch and burn occur when blood vessels shrink so much that the skin's supply of blood and oxygen is reduced. Chilblains usually break out on toes and fingers, but may affect other parts of the body, such as the buttocks.

The best way to prevent chilblains is to wear warm clothing – especially on your hands, legs and feet. Do not smoke, as nicotine reduces the blood circulation in the skin. If you have poor circulation, take regular exercise to stimulate the blood flow. You should never scratch chilblains; it only makes them worse. As a cure, you could try a form of hydrotherapy: bathe your feet in warm water for about three minutes, then dip them in cold for one minute. Repeat for about 20 minutes morning or evening, always finishing with cold. If the chilblains seem particularly severe, see your doctor.

ATHLETE'S FOOT

In hot weather, the skin between my toes cracks and blisters appear on my heels. What causes this and how do I cure it?

You probably have athlete's foot, a fungal infection that attacks the skin between and under the toes, causing itching, cracking, peeling and occasionally blisters. The fungus thrives on moisture, which explains why you suffer most in hot weather when your feet sweat more. Athlete's foot is easy to pick up from the damp floors of sports centre changing rooms and from wet walkways around public swimming pools. But there is no direct connection between the condition and sports. Anyone – regardless of whether or not they are athletic – can pick it up almost anywhere.

Chemists stock a wide variety of non-prescription foot powders and creams to treat the condition. If it persists, see your doctor who may prescribe a stronger topical antifungal preparation.

To prevent outbreaks of athlete's foot, make sure you wash your feet frequently and dry carefully between your toes. Change your socks and footwear at least once a day, particularly if your feet are very sweaty. Make sure that you go barefoot whenever possible, except in public places where reinfection could occur. Choose socks made from natural fibres such as wool and cotton, which allow the skin to breathe.

CORNS AND BUNIONS

I have suffered from corns and bunions for as long as I can remember. Is there a cure or will I have them for life?

Corns – small areas of thickened skin on the toes – are almost always caused by ill-fitting shoes and are very common. They are easily cured by wearing more comfortable shoes. Meanwhile, to ease any discomfort, soften your feet by soaking them in warm water, and use a file or pumice stone to rub away the top layers of hard skin.

A bunion, by contrast, is a bony protrusion from the outside edge of the joint at the base of the big toe. Bunions tend to affect people with an inherited weakness in that part of the foot. Poorly fitting shoes – especially those with high heels and narrow pointed toes – can make the bunions worse. Always make sure that your shoes fit properly, and allow plenty of room for your toes (see page 148).

If you have a bunion that has become troublesome, consult a chiropodist who may recommend felt pads to ease the inflammation and may even suggest a visit to your doctor. If your foot is seriously affected, surgery may be advised.

Cutting your toenails

The correct way to cut your toenails is straight across. This way, you will not damage the skin at the corners of the nails, and you will prevent an ingrowing toenail. Ideally, you should cut your toenails every three to four weeks.

High-heeled shoes

Wearing high-heeled shoes all day over a long period of time can lead to several health problems:
- Your calf muscles may become artificially shortened, which means that if you switch to low heels, you may rupture those muscles or the Achilles tendon anchoring them to the bones of the foot.
- If you have a weak base joint on a big toe, bunions may develop. Wearing high heels will intensify the problem, as the foot is pushed forward into the narrowest part of the shoe, and stress on the toe joint increases.
- Back pain may develop owing to the constant jarring of the feet.
If you want to wear high heels during the day, change into a flatter pair whenever you can – perhaps at lunch – and as soon as you get home.

WHAT TO LOOK FOR WHEN YOU BUY A PAIR OF SHOES

In supporting the weight of the body, the feet have to take a considerable amount of strain. To cope with this they have a complex structure of bones, muscles, sinews and nerves. Each foot contains 26 small, very delicate bones – the highest concentration in the human body. To keep the bones in their correct position and provide elasticity, ligaments and muscles abound, outnumbering the bones four times over. The resilience and spring of the foot are enhanced by the arches.

In an average lifetime your feet could walk the equivalent of four times around the Earth, so it makes good sense to look after them. Making sure that you wear shoes that fit properly is the primary way to prevent problems with feet. If your shoes are too tight or too narrow, they may cause bunions, corns or calluses. If shoes are too loose or big, they will fail to support the foot correctly and may cause blisters. Follow the tips below when buying new shoes.

Walk of life Left to right: at six months the foot is mostly cartilage; by two bones have begun to develop; at eight the bones are large and strong; not until the age of eighteen are the foot bones fully formed.

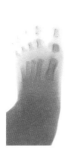
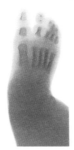
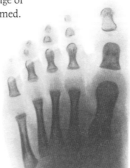
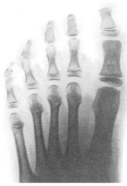
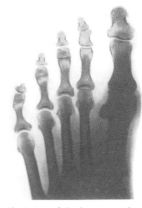

Adult's shoes
● A shoe should be wide enough to allow the toes to lie naturally, and at least ½ in (1.3 cm) longer than the foot so that you can move your toes freely.
● The shoe should fit snugly at the heel and instep so that it is not necessary to bunch up your toes to stop your foot from slipping forward.

● Walk around in the shoes inside the shop before buying them. Shoes that feel comfortable when you are sitting may pinch when you are walking.
● Remember that feet tend to swell in hot weather, so avoid shopping for summer sandals on a cold day.
● Avoid wearing shoes with a higher than 2½ in (6 cm) heel. Anything more can strain the joint of the big toe and cause a bunion. It also puts pressure on the ball of your foot, which may lead to arthritis in the joints.

Children's shoes
● The toe area should be square-shaped, not pointed, to allow plenty of room for growing feet.
● There should be at least ½ in (1.3 cm) in growing room in the toe.
● The back of the shoe should support the heel and, ideally, should be padded at the top for protection.
● The soles of shoes should be light, flexible and non-slippery.
● All children's shoes should have some form of fastening. Slip-on shoes are not suitable: to stay on the foot, they would have to be unduly tight.
● Because children grow in spurts, their shoe size should be checked every two to three months during their first few years.
● Do encourage children to go about barefoot as much as possible. Walking barefoot is one of the best ways to exercise the feet.

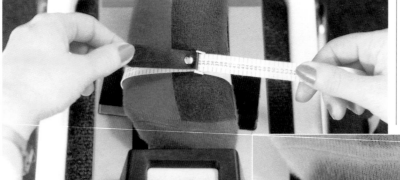

Perfect fit For the first few years of a child's life, shoe size should be checked every two to three months. The foot gauge, which measures both the width and length of the foot, is a vital aid for correctly fitting children's shoes.

PLANTAR WARTS

I have a small hard lump on the bottom of my foot that is painful to walk on. What is it and is it treatable?

You most probably have a plantar wart, commonly known as a verruca. This hard, rough-surfaced outgrowth is caused by a virus, usually picked up from floors in public swimming pools and communal showers. Because of pressure from the weight of the body, the wart is flattened and forced into the skin of the sole, sometimes causing discomfort or pain when walking.

Treat plantar warts daily with a topical wart preparation available from chemists. To relieve any discomfort, wear a foam pad in your shoe. If self-treatment doesn't cure the problem, see your doctor who may remove it under local anaesthetic.

TREATING BLISTERS

My new shoes have given me a blister. What is the best way to treat it?

Blisters caused by friction usually heal within a week. No first-aid treatment is necessary unless the blister breaks or is likely to be damaged by further friction. In such cases, wash the affected area with soap and water and protect it with an adhesive bandage.

Do not burst a blister deliberately unless it is causing severe pain. Opening the skin increases the risk of infection.

If a blister bursts by itself, expose it to the air as much as possible, but keep it covered with a bandage if there is a risk of dirt getting in. See your doctor if a blister becomes infected to the point of having a swollen, tender or inflamed area around it.

INGROWING TOENAIL

What can I do to cure a very painful ingrowing toenail?

An ingrowing toenail usually results from cutting the nail incorrectly (see page 147), from wearing tight-fitting shoes or from poor personal hygiene. As you have discovered, it is a painful condition in which one or both edges of the nail begin to grow into the surrounding skin, eventually leading to infection and inflammation.

For temporary relief from pain, bathe your foot once or twice daily in a strong, warm salt solution. After bathing, cover the nail with a dry gauze dressing. If self-treatment does not provide relief, see a doctor, who may prescribe antibiotics to control infection. In some cases, the edge of the affected nail may be removed under local anaesthetic.

HELP FOR FLAT FEET

Both my children have flat feet, and I'm concerned that it may cause them problems in later life. Are there any preventive measures that I should take?

The best advice is to make sure that your children's shoes fit well, and that they have plenty of opportunity to exercise growing feet and legs. Everybody begins life with flat feet. Only when a child begins to walk, and ligaments and muscles in the foot strengthen, do the bones rise to form an arch. Some people, however, remain flat-footed all their lives, though they almost always function perfectly well.

Adults may find that arch supports, available from shoe shops, improve foot comfort, but they will not restore arches to normal. Orthotics (arch supports moulded to an individual's foot) may be prescribed by a podiatrist. They help the foot to function more efficiently. Exercise, good posture, weight control and well-fitting shoes are more important.

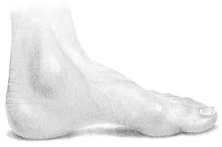

Normal arch Most people's arches form gradually, as supporting ligaments and muscles in the soles of the feet develop.

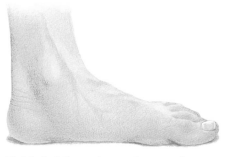

Flat feet Fallen arches are due to weak ligaments and muscles in the soles of the feet, but the condition is seldom cause for concern.

Treating digestive troubles

HEARTBURN AND ANTACIDS

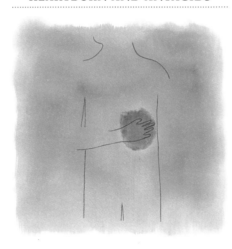

I often get attacks of heartburn and have to take antacids. What causes the condition, and can taking too many of these drugs do any damage?

Heartburn, despite its name, has nothing to do with the heart. The underlying problem is the slackness of the muscles at the base of your oesophagus (food pipe), allowing acid and other digestive juices to flow back into the oesophagus. That in turn may be caused by eating too much rich food, smoking or drinking excessively.

Antacids work by neutralising the acidity of your stomach with alkaline ingredients. And exceeding the recommended dose can, indeed, harm your health.

Most of these drugs contain magnesium or aluminium compounds that have a long-lasting effect, or sodium bicarbonate which provides short-term relief. Excessive use of antacids that contain magnesium may cause diarrhoea, while those containing aluminium may cause constipation. If you must take antacids, it is better to take a balanced preparation containing both magnesium and aluminium. Excessive use of sodium bicarbonate products may result in flatulence and retention of fluids.

Antacids can also mask the symptoms of more serious conditions, such as an ulcer. See your doctor if you experience stomach pain for more than two weeks, or earlier if pain is severe. In addition, antacids may affect the absorption of other drugs, so if you are on medication, do consult your doctor before taking antacids. Far better than treating the symptoms, of course, is preventing the problem. As a starting point, try following the advice outlined in the panel, left.

REDUCING WIND

My husband has a terrible problem with wind. Is there anything he can take to cure this embarrassing problem?

Whether it is expelled through the mouth (by belching) or through the anus (as flatus), wind originates in the upper digestive tract.

Belching expels air that has become trapped in the stomach, usually after eating or drinking too quickly. Some people also have a habit of swallowing gulps of air when they talk. The expelled air rises up through the throat, passes the vocal cords and makes a sound as it escapes.

Peppermint oil, available from chemists, may control this problem, but it would be better to take steps to prevent it. Your husband should try to eat more slowly and chew his food more carefully. If belching remains a persistent problem, he should consult his doctor: it may be a symptom of hiatus hernia or chronic indigestion.

Flatus, by contrast, is usually caused by a failure of the digestive system to break down certain foods (particularly high-fibre beans and vegetables), leaving a residue that ferments in the bowel. Certain species of bowel bacteria also produce more gas than others (see page 21). Not everyone is affected in the same way or by the same foods. Sufferers can find out which foods are causing the trouble by experimentally omitting the most likely candidates from their diet one by one.

Charcoal tablets, available from chemists, can sometimes provide fast short-term relief from flatus by absorbing gas in the gut.

INDIGESTION – OR ULCER

Every so often I experience dull pains in my stomach. How can I tell whether these are caused simply by indigestion or whether I might have an ulcer?

Ulcers are sores that form in the lining of the stomach, duodenum (the first part of the small intestine) or oesophagus (food pipe). Distinguishing between ulcers and indigestion is often a matter of recognising a pattern of symptoms over a period of weeks.

Like the occasional attack of indigestion, ulcers may produce a gnawing, aching or burning sensation in the abdomen just above the navel, but ulcer pain is likely to recur several times a day, every day, for weeks at a time. Sometimes the pain begins when the stomach is empty but eases or stops altogether after eating or drinking. Sometimes the reverse happens: the pain starts immediately after eating.

If the ulcer is advanced, the pain may become severe and be accompanied by blood in the stools (recognisable as a black tar-like substance), extreme weakness, fainting or unusual thirst – all of which are symptoms of internal bleeding.

If you suspect that your symptoms are those of an ulcer, see your doctor. He or she may recommend investigations such as an endoscopy (see page 232) or an X-ray of your digestive tract. For that you may need a barium meal: barium, a metallic element, is opaque to X-rays, so it provides an image of the tract on the X-ray film. Such tests are essential for diagnosing severe or persistent abdominal pain. (For further information on ulcers, see page 354.)

PERSISTENT PILES

What can I do to cure persistent piles and to stop them from recurring?

Straining too hard during bowel movements as a result of constipation is the commonest cause of piles or haemorrhoids. These are swollen and distended veins either inside the rectum or around the anal opening. The best solution is to increase the amount of fibre in your diet and to drink more water, which should make your stools easier to pass.

Taking hot baths can often cure a mild haemorrhoid problem and prevent its recurrence. Regular exercise also helps by increasing blood flow in the veins and decreasing pressure on the rectum.

For immediate relief, try over-the-counter haemorrhoid creams and ointments. Most of them contain a local anaesthetic to numb the affected area and relieve itching. Be cautious, however: repeated use can actually increase the irritation. Other products contain soft paraffin to soften the skin and relieve inflammation and irritation. But beware: prolonged use may soften the skin too much and lead to infection. If self-treatment doesn't bring any relief, see your doctor.

THE FACTS ABOUT REGULARITY

Bowel habits vary from person to person and depend on your diet, the amount of fluid you drink, how physically active you are and whether you are taking any medication. Genetics has a role too: patterns occur within the family. It is important to recognise significant changes in your regular pattern, and to see a doctor if these changes persist.

What is 'normal'?

Most people have a bowel movement at least once a day. But for some, once every three days is normal. Going a day or two beyond your usual pattern is not generally a cause for concern. If constipation lasts for more than a few days, or if it is accompanied by abdominal pain, a sudden unexplained loss of weight and bloating or stools that are very hard or that contain traces of blood, consult your doctor immediately.

Curing constipation

One of the most common causes of constipation is ignoring your bowel needs. The longer you neglect a bowel motion, the lazier your bowels become. It is, therefore, important to go to the toilet as soon as you feel the urge, and give yourself enough time there.

For the occasional bout of mild constipation, the most effective remedy is to increase the amount of fibre in your diet. Eat more vegetables, fruits, and wholegrain breads and cereals. Make sure you drink more fluids, and try to take more exercise.

Laxatives

These drugs are designed to produce a soft, easy-to-pass stool. Excessive use may cause diarrhoea; prolonged use may cause the bowels to become dependent and can lead to permanent damage. Stimulant laxatives, such as Bisacodyl, castor oil, senna or Epsom salts, because of their strength, produce a bowel movement that may then be followed by a bout of rebound constipation. They are therefore not helpful in the treatment of long-term constipation.

If you do occasionally need to use a laxative, the best choice is a bulk fibre type such as bran, methylcellulose or ispaghula husk. Stop use as soon as regularity is restored.

What is a histamine blocker drug?

Now available over the counter, histamine (or H_2) blockers can help to heal peptic ulcers, but must be used with care.

Whereas antacids merely neutralise acidity in the stomach, histamine blockers actually reduce the secretion of acid.

Doctors have expressed fears that H_2 blockers are such powerful weapons against indigestion that if used indiscriminately they may mask the early symptoms of cancer, or perhaps persuade patients to neglect ulcers. In Denmark, however, where H_2 blockers have been available over the counter for several years, there has been no detectable increase in ulcer complications or any increased delay in diagnosing cancer.

CAUTION Histamine blockers have been known to cause side effects such as reversible impotence in men, muscle and joint pain and hypersensitivity, but these are very rare.

MILD DIARRHOEA

I sometimes suffer from mild bouts of diarrhoea lasting for a few days. What could be causing this and what is the best way to treat it?

If it occurs infrequently and for short periods of time, diarrhoea is generally not a cause for concern. In fact, it is often part of the digestive system's effort to rid itself of an irritant or infection. Mild cases of diarrhoea are best treated by avoiding food, and drinking more fluids than usual; if necessary, try an over-the-counter medication such as a kaolin mixture, which will absorb water and harmful toxins.

CAUTION Persistent diarrhoea can cause dehydration, especially in babies and the elderly, and may be a signal of serious intestinal disturbances. As a rule, adults should see a doctor if symptoms last for more than four days, or are accompanied by blackish stools, severe abdominal pain or signs of dehydration. Young children should be taken to see a doctor if they have had diarrhoea for more than half a day.

Controlling your weight

FACT
—— OR ——
FALLACY?

'Dieting makes you fat.'

Fact Diets often make no attempt to change eating and exercising patterns. A further concern, especially about very low-calorie diets (those that recommend less than 800 Calories a day), is that your body adapts to the plumeting calorie intake by reducing its metabolic rate. When you return to normal eating, your body no longer needs as many calories as it did before you started dieting. It simply stores the excess as fat. So in the long-term, low-calorie diets can indeed, make you *gain* weight.

WHY WEIGHT MATTERS

Why is it unhealthy to be overweight? Is weighing too little equally bad for you?

Although it is possible to be overweight or underweight without developing a major disease, too much deviation from the recommended range does increase your risk of having health problems.

Being slightly underweight does not seem to present any major danger to health. On the other hand, obesity (generally defined as being 20 per cent or more over the acceptable weight range for your height and age) is associated with a greater risk of heart disease, high blood pressure, gallstones and diabetes. The extra weight that bones and joints have to bear can also aggravate osteoarthritis of the knees, hips and lower back. Excess fat around the chest and under the diaphragm may interfere with breathing and create a tendency to bronchitis.

However, if you find it difficult to lose weight and keep it off, don't despair. It may actually be healthier to maintain a weight a bit above the one recommended for you than to lose and regain extra pounds in an endless – and stressful – cycle.

HORMONAL IMBALANCE

My brother is convinced that being overweight is due in his case to a hormonal imbalance. Could he be right?

Hormonal disturbances *can* cause obesity, but only as part of recognisable medical syndromes, such as Cushing's syndrome, in which the pituitary gland and the adrenal glands malfunction. An underactive thyroid gland can also result in a depressed metabolic rate. In spite of what many people believe, there is only very rarely a glandular cause for obesity. The more probable reason for your brother's weight gain is simply eating too many fatty and sugar-rich foods and not doing enough exercise.

Weight patterns often tend to run in families. Family members may share similar lifestyles and eating habits, and may also share a dislike for exercise. Eating a healthy, low-fat diet and an increase in regular physical activity will help him to achieve and maintain a healthy weight. (See the slimming advice, opposite.)

KEEPING WEIGHT OFF

After months of dieting, I've finally reached my target weight. How can I make sure I stay slim now that I'm ready to go back to normal eating?

Congratulations on reaching your goal. What you need to do now is continue to eat a healthy, balanced diet for the rest of your life, and make sure that you keep physically active (see page 63).

Foods high in fat and sugar such as cakes, puddings, cream, chips, pies, mayonnaise and butter need not be banned for ever, but should not be part of your daily diet either. Keep a check on how often you eat these high-calorie foods. They can easily tip the scales. For example, compared with skimmed milk, half a pint (285 ml) of whole milk can add 95 Calories, while a mere one ounce (30 g) of cheese after each evening meal adds up to 805 Calories by the end of the week.

EAT LESS OR EXERCISE?

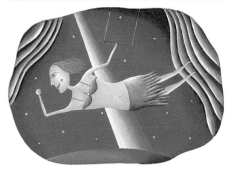

What is the best way to lose weight: eating less or taking more exercise?

Doing both. Exercise can help with losing weight (see pages 94-96) but is not effective on its own. You need to walk about 50 miles (80 km) to use up a single pound of body fat. Eating less will make you lose weight but unless you also take exercise your metabolic rate will slow down and you won't get the maximum benefit.

The easiest way for most people to eat fewer calories is to cut down on foods that are high in fat or sugar. Instead, eat more vegetables, fruit, wholegrains and pulses, which are filling and nutritious but not fattening.

Accept that losing weight will be a long-term process. Aim to lose 1-2 lb (½-1 kg) per week. There is no miraculous crash diet to take off large amounts of weight in a few days. Even if you ate nothing at all for a week – which would be highly dangerous – you could lose only 5 lb (2.3 kg) of body fat.

REDUCING CALORIE INTAKE

I have been very overweight all my life. I love food – and plenty of it. However, my doctor has told me that I must lose at least three stones. How can I do it?

The most likely reason for being overweight is that over a period of time you have eaten more than your body needs. The best way to achieve a safe, lasting reduction in weight is through a change in way of life that includes a well-balanced, low-fat diet (see page 38) and regular exercise.

This sounds easy in theory, but tackling the problem of overeating and changing habits can be difficult. Severely obese people may also find it difficult to exercise because of their size. However, you can increase your activity in many ways, for example taking more walks and using the stairs more often. The important thing to remember is that it

has taken you a lifetime to establish these eating and exercise habits, so it will take a long time – and strong motivation – to change them. The following suggestions may help:

● Eat only when you are genuinely hungry, not just because it is lunch or dinner time.
● Finish swallowing each mouthful before putting more food on the fork.
● Do not combine eating with activities such as reading or watching television – it is easy to eat too much without noticing.
● Do not keep fatty foods in the house.
● Shop for food as soon as possible after a meal, when you are less likely to be hungry and tempted to buy on impulse.
● Consider joining a weight-loss club. They help many people to remain motivated.

Most women will lose weight safely at the rate of about 1 to 2 lb (½ to 1 kg) a week on a diet of 1200 to 1500 Calories (kcal) a day when accompanied by increased exercise. Men will lose weight safely on 1500 to 1800 kcal a day. Before you embark on a reduced-calorie diet, buy a calorie-counter book and an accurate set of kitchen scales, and keep a written record of everything you eat.

SUCCESSFUL SLIMMING

I am no good at counting calories and weighing out portions – but I do need to lose some weight. Are there any simple guidelines I can follow, such as skipping meals or avoiding some foods completely?

Eating should be a pleasurable experience, and the best way to lose weight is to choose a diet that you enjoy and that fits in with your way of life. Anything else is unlikely to last.

While counting calories does work for some, it is almost impossible to keep up permanently, so you are right to seek a simpler method of weight loss. Skipping meals, however, is not a good idea. It will only make you more hungry and lead to overeating.

A better approach is to choose low-fat but filling meals, such as pasta, rice or potatoes with a large salad – and a low-fat dressing – or vegetables served with a little lean meat, fish, a boiled or poached egg, seafood or pulses. A wholemeal sandwich with a low-fat filling such as prawns, lean ham or cottage cheese and salad will satisfy your appetite without piling on too many calories. Watch out for ready-made sandwiches which may contain a lot of butter, margarine or mayonnaise. You should also restrict your intake of alcohol and sugary foods, which supply calories without other nutrients.

How useful are diet pills and products?

Taking diet pills may help you to lose weight – at least in the short term – but they can have serious side effects.

● Most over-the-counter diet pills contain a diuretic drug. All these drugs do is increase your output of urine, so that you lose water from your system temporarily. This can also cause loss of essential minerals. What it does not do is help you to lose fat.
● Diet pills based on bran and other types of fibre that swell up when eaten may make you feel full, but will not burn extra fat. They have also been known to cause blockages in the throat or intestines if consumed with inadequate quantities of liquid.
● Appetite-suppressing drugs are not a long-term solution either, and have many side effects. The drugs most commonly used to suppress appetite are similar to amphetamines and have many disadvantages, such as disturbed sleep, depression and weight gain when you eventually stop taking them. They can also be addictive.
● Diet foods and drinks may help you to eat fewer calories and less fat, but it will still be your overall calorie intake that counts. The best way to lose weight – and keep it off – is to exercise regularly and choose a low-fat, low-sugar diet.

ARE YOU OVERWEIGHT, UNDERWEIGHT OR JUST RIGHT?

What is considered a healthy weight depends on your build. To measure your frame, measure your wrist where it is narrowest, just below the joint. For women, a measurement of less than 5½ in (14 cm) indicates a small build, 5½-6½ in (14-16.5 cm) a medium build, and above 6½ in (16.5 cm) a large build. For men, a measurement under 6½ in (16.5 cm) indicates a small build, 6½-7 in (16.5-18 cm) a medium build and above 7 in (18 cm) a large build. When you have calculated your frame size, use the table below to find your ideal weight range.

An alternative method of assessing your weight is by means of the body mass index (BMI). The BMI is calculated by dividing your weight in kilograms (1 lb = 0.45 kg) by your height in metres squared (1 ft = 0.3 m). For example, a woman who is 5 ft 5 in (1.63 m) tall and weighs 10 stones (64 kg) would multiply 1.63 by 1.63 and then divide 64 by the result (2.66), giving her a BMI rating of 24.

A BMI of 20-25 is generally considered normal, 25-30 overweight, and over 30 obese. A result under 20 is underweight.

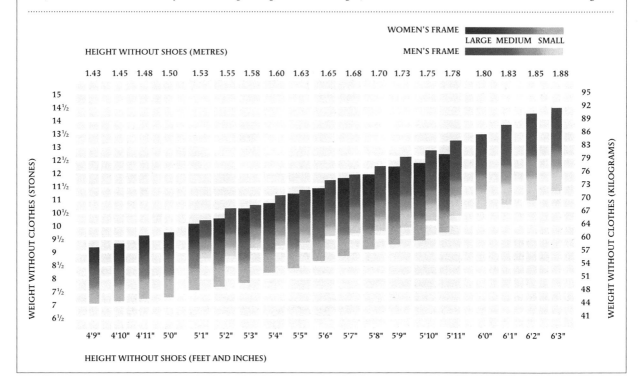

Sensible drinking

HOW MUCH IS SAFE?

We are always being told to drink alcohol only in moderation but what does this actually mean? Why are women advised to drink less than men?

People vary widely in the amount of alcohol they can drink and in the effects it has on them. Nevertheless, current guidelines from the Department of Health suggest that a safe limit (from the point of view of long-term health) is probably about ten pints of mid-strength beer or large glasses of wine a week for men, and two-thirds as much for women (see panel, right). In addition, the allowance should also be spread out over the week, not consumed in one or two binges. If you can, avoid drinking on an empty stomach (to reduce hangover symptoms and slow down alcohol absorption).

Alcohol has a stronger effect on women for several reasons. Firstly, women generally weigh less than men and have proportionately less water in their bodies, so alcohol is less diluted in the blood. There is also evidence that women's stomachs are not as well supplied with enzymes that break down alcohol. Women who are pregnant should take special precautions (see page 267).

The best and safest advice for all drinkers is to keep within the official guidelines, avoid bingeing, and to try to drink alcohol with a meal rather than on its own. It is also a good idea to have some alcohol-free days and, of course, don't drink and drive.

ADVANTAGES OF ALCOHOL?

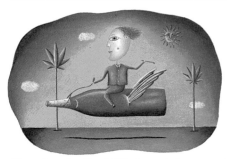

I keep hearing it said that a certain amount of alcohol is actually good for you. Is this true – or is it just wishful thinking?

Yes it does seem to be true, although no one really knows why. Scientific studies and statistical surveys show that light to moderate drinkers are less likely to die early than either complete abstainers or very heavy drinkers. Up to two units of alcohol a day (see panel, right) has been shown to lower the risk of developing heart disease by 20 per cent.

Various theories have been put forward to explain this: some researchers believe alcohol encourages the body to produce compounds known as high-density lipoproteins (see pages 364-365) which play a role in preventing cholesterol deposits in the arteries. Another view is that antioxidant substances (see pages 40-41) found in particular in red wine may be responsible for protecting the heart. The well-known relaxing effects of alcohol could also help by relieving stress.

The findings should not encourage anyone to drink, or to drink more. Heavy drinking can damage the brain, the liver, the digestive tract and the stomach. Cirrhosis of the liver and pancreatic cancer are diseases common in persistent heavy drinkers. Smaller quantities of alcohol can also cause obesity and raised blood pressure which is associated with an increased risk of heart disease and stroke.

DRINKING AND DRIVING

How much alcohol can I drink if I'm going to drive?

There is no amount of alcohol that is 'safe' to drink if you are driving. Even the smallest drink will adversely affect your judgment and self-control to some extent. According to British law, however, the blood/alcohol limit is 80 mg of alcohol per 100 ml of blood, or 35 µg of alcohol per 100 ml of breath. As a rough guide, this amounts to about four units in two hours for a man, and to about three units in two hours for a woman. You cannot rely on this alone, however. The concentration of alcohol in the bloodstream depends on a number of other factors too:

● Body weight: the heavier you are, the higher your tolerance of alcohol.
● Percentage of body fat: the higher your ratio of fat to lean tissue, the slower alcohol will be broken down and absorbed into your bloodstream.
● How much you have eaten: the fuller your stomach, the longer it will take for alcohol to enter the circulation.
● The nature and time of your last meal. Fatty or oily food slows down the absorption of alcohol and the rate at which the stomach empties. If you have a rich meal, the effects of alcohol will take longer to become apparent.
● Your personal reaction to alcohol. The way you react to 80 mg of alcohol might be quite different from someone else. In general, young people and women tend to have a lower tolerance to alcohol because they have fewer enzymes to break it down.

Low-alcohol drinks

Despite what some people think, there is a limit to how many low-alcohol drinks you can consume without becoming drunk. After an evening spent drinking low-alcohol beer your judgment and reaction time will certainly be affected enough to make driving dangerous. If you want to drink and drive, choose 'alcohol-free' beverages instead.

The alcohol content of low-alcohol drinks must be no higher than 1.2 per cent – as opposed to about 4 per cent in mid-strength beer. In practice, this means that every three to four low-alcohol pints has an effect equivalent to one mid-strength pint.

CALCULATING THE UNITS OF ALCOHOL IN DRINKS

Department of Health advice suggests weekly limits of 21 units of alcohol for men and 14 for women. Use the table below to help you to check your units. Alcohol-free beer does not appear as alcohol content is tiny (0.05 per cent).

TYPE	STRENGTH	MEASURE	UNITS PER MEASURE
Beer and cider	low (1 per cent)	Pint (570 ml)	0.6
		Can (440 ml)	0.5
		Bottle (330 ml)	0.4
	mid (4 per cent)	Pint	2.3
		Can	1.8
		Bottle	1.3
	top (9 per cent)	Pint	5.2
		Can	4.0
		Bottle	3.0
Wine	11 to 12 per cent	Bottle (750 ml)	8.3 - 9.0
		Glass (125 ml)	1.4 - 1.5
Spirits	40 per cent	Single (25 ml)	1.0
	50 per cent	Single (25 ml)	1.3
Fortified wine (port or sherry)	20 per cent	Glass (50 ml)	1.0

HANGOVER ADVICE

Besides avoiding alcohol, what are the best ways to prevent and cure a hangover?

Prevention is, of course, better than cure. One of the surest methods to avoid a hangover is to take care not to drink on an empty stomach. Some people swear by a glass of milk before drinking, since it slows alcohol absorption. If you follow this advice, drink moderately and alternate alcoholic drinks with soft drinks, you should avoid most symptoms.

The effects of a hangover are due primarily to dehydration. If you have failed to take proper precautions, start drinking water as soon as possible – you will probably need a pint (570 ml) or more to replace lost fluid. Eat a light snack, such as a slice or two of dry wholemeal toast, to settle your stomach and boost blood sugar, and so help to reduce weakness, dizziness and trembling. A gentle walk in the fresh air should make you feel better too, if you can face it.

Chemists also sell tablets of activated charcoal, which can help by absorbing substances called congeners that irritate the stomach lining and are found in some wine and spirit colourings and additives. Take several tablets as directed on the pack before going to bed.

Advice for smokers

What is in tobacco smoke?

Each puff delivers a dangerous cocktail of chemicals, including:

Tar

Over 1000 chemicals are found in tar, including a variety of irritants and at least 60 known carcinogens. Tar condenses into a sticky sludge in the lungs.

Nicotine

One of the most addictive drugs known, nicotine is absorbed rapidly from the lungs into the bloodstream, and reaches the brain in about seven seconds. Nicotine raises heart rate and blood pressure, and is associated with an increased risk of heart disease.

Carbon monoxide

This poisonous gas reduces the amount of oxygen in the blood. This is particularly dangerous for pregnant women and people with heart disease.

CUTTING DOWN

I've managed to cut my smoking from a whole pack to two or three cigarettes a day. Have I reduced my risk of developing heart disease and lung cancer proportionately?

Any significant reduction in the number of cigarettes smoked per day will improve your health, but not proportionately. People who smoke 1 to 14 cigarettes a day run eight times the risk of dying of lung cancer as non-smokers. Medium smokers (15–24 a day) run 13 times the risk, and heavy smokers (25 or more a day) 25 times the risk.

It does not follow that you can reduce your risk by cutting down only the number of cigarettes. The important factor is the amount of smoke that goes into your lungs. When smokers cut down they tend to compensate by inhaling more smoke from each cigarette. To the lungs, ten cigarettes a day at 20 puffs per cigarette is the same as 20 cigarettes a day at ten puffs per cigarette.

If you simply cut down the number of cigarettes you smoke rather than giving them up altogether, you are also more likely to resume heavy smoking whenever you feel stressed.

SIDE EFFECTS OF STOPPING

I've thought about giving up smoking for years now, but I'm terrified of putting on weight and becoming unbearable to live with. How can I avoid these side effects?

Unfortunately, you will probably gain a little weight when you give up smoking. Smoking increases your metabolic rate (the rate at which your body uses energy), so when you give up, your metabolic rate drops. Furthermore, many people find themselves resorting to food as a substitute.

However, most doctors agree that gaining a small amount of weight is much less harmful than smoking. To avoid putting on too much weight, try to eat healthy, low-calorie snacks such as fruit, vegetables and yoghurt. Exercising regularly will also help.

Withdrawal symptoms such as irritability, headaches and anxiety are temporary and should not trouble you for long. If necessary, try nicotine chewing gum or skin patches for short-term relief.

CIGARETTE SUBSTITUTES

Do nicotine replacement products work, and how effective are they?

Nicotine is not the most damaging aspect of cigarette smoking, but it is what makes smokers addicted, and giving up can cause both physical and psychological withdrawal symptoms. Nicotine replacement therapy (in the form of products such as skin patches, chewing gum and nasal spray) can help by preventing or alleviating the worst effects of withdrawal symptoms and allowing a gradual, controlled reduction in intake.

Most nicotine replacement products are available over the counter from chemists. Three main kinds are available:

NICOTINE PATCHES Worn like sticking plasters, patches release nicotine in a slow, controlled manner through the surface of the skin. They should never be used together with any other form of nicotine, such as gum, nasal spray or cigarettes. Patches can sometimes cause unpleasant skin rashes, and may not be strong enough to satisfy heavy smokers.

NICOTINE CHEWING GUM Before using gum, always read the instructions, as you need to adopt a particular chewing technique. Chewing gum is strong enough to help even heavy smokers, but some people find it unpleasant to take. Long-term use may also be addictive.

NICOTINE NASAL SPRAY The most recent nicotine replacement product, nasal spray comes in a bottle with a pump mechanism and offers faster absorption of nicotine than gum or patches. It is available on prescription but should be tried only if both patches and gum have failed. The effect is closest to that of a cigarette and there is a risk of addiction.

CAUTION Do not use nicotine replacement products if you are pregnant or are breast feeding a baby. If you suffer from persistent indigestion; or have a condition such as a peptic ulcer, pain in the chest, heart disease, epilepsy, diabetes or a thyroid problem; or if you are taking any medicines regularly, consult your pharmacist or doctor before using nicotine products.

PIPES AND CIGARS

How do pipes and cigars compare with cigarettes when it comes to health?

Because most pipe and cigar smokers don't inhale, they avoid the high risk of lung cancer and emphysema that cigarette smokers incur. However, neither pipes nor cigars are safe, and both types of smoking are associated with cancers of the lips, tongue and oesophagus. And like cigarettes, pipes and cigars can accelerate the development of heart disease (see page 363).

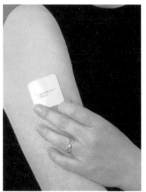

Smoking substitute Nicotine patches help to wean a smoker off the drug by relieving the withdrawal symptoms.

HOW TO GIVE UP SMOKING

No matter how long you have smoked, the risk of developing heart disease or chronic bronchitis decreases as soon as you give up. Motivation is the key factor in managing to stop successfully. Before you decide to try, ask yourself: 'Do I really want to give up?' If you are not sure, you will find it difficult to keep on when the going gets tough. Wait until you feel certain.

Step one
Analyse your smoking habits carefully. Make a list of every cigarette you usually smoke in a 24-hour period. Give yourself two or three weeks to study when and why you 'need' cigarettes. This increasing concern with the act of smoking is a good way to prepare for the task of giving up.

Step two
Make up your mind that there can be no turning back. List all the reasons why you want to stop, including all the good things that will happen when you have stopped. For instance, you will enjoy the taste of food and drink more, your morning cough may disappear and you will probably have fewer respiratory infections. Convince yourself that it is worth making the effort.

Step three
Name the day, circle it in your diary, and give up smoking completely on that day. Try to get family members or close friends to give up as well, so that you can support each other in the difficult early days. You may also find that it helps if you choose a time when your usual routine is changed anyway – just before going on holiday, for example.

Step four
Use any device that comes to hand as a cigarette substitute in the early days – chew gum or hold a pen or pencil if your hand feels empty without a cigarette. Use nicotine substitutes if you need help to overcome drug withdrawal symptoms. You could also try relaxation techniques (see pages 190-193) to ease tensions that smoking once relieved. Avoid situations that encourage smoking and make a point of sitting in non-smoking sections of restaurants and transport.

Step five
Enjoy not smoking! Don't forget that you will save a lot of money. Use the extra cash to buy yourself regular rewards.

Step six
Eat as much as you want during the first few weeks, provided it is healthy food. When you are feeling tense and restless (the result of overcoming an addictive habit) you may often want to eat, and you will probably gain a little weight. Remember that the first four weeks are the hardest. You can expect to lose your intense craving for tobacco after about eight weeks, and you should then begin to eat more sparingly.

Low-nicotine and low-tar products

Recent research suggests that both low-tar and low-nicotine cigarettes are less dangerous than others.

However, switching from ordinary cigarettes to low-tar, low-nicotine cigarettes will not benefit your health if you smoke more or more intensively. In fact, scientific studies have shown that smokers tend to compensate for reduced levels of tar and nicotine by smoking much more and inhaling more deeply.

If you are interested in these products, try them for a while, but keep a careful watch to see if your smoking habits do change.

Getting a good night's sleep

'You need less sleep as you grow older.'

Fact Older people take longer to fall asleep and wake more often in the night. They spend less time in deep sleep so are more easily disturbed, wake in the morning feeling less refreshed and are less likely to recall dreams. Conditions which disrupt sleep, such as diabetes, prostate trouble (which forces people to get up to pass urine), depression and snoring become more common. On the positive side, older people usually awaken more alert and take less time to become fully conscious.

CAUSES OF TIREDNESS

I'm often tired even though I get eight hours' sleep every night. What could be causing this? Would sleeping pills help?

Although seven to eight hours is widely thought to be the ideal length of time for a good night's sleep, the amount of sleep individuals need varies considerably, and you may be among those who need more.

To determine your own requirements, try going to bed an hour or even 90 minutes earlier for at least 10 days. Keep a diary, noting how refreshed you feel during the day and how your ability to carry out difficult tasks compares with the way you felt and performed before the experiment. You may be surprised to find a little extra sleep is all you need to revitalise your energy and spirits.

If extra sleep does not relieve your tiredness, you may have a sleep disorder that is undermining the quality rather than the quantity of your sleep. Or your fatigue may be a secondary symptom of some other problem – a viral infection, thyroid condition or depression, for example. Depression, stress and anxiety are, in fact, the most common causes of tiredness. But whatever the cause, sleeping pills, though they may help in the short-term, are not the solution. They do not give a natural night's sleep and can lead to dependency. To get at the source of the problem, see your doctor, who may ask you to keep a sleep diary for specialist analysis.

BREATHING DIFFICULTIES

Is it true that some sleepers have to wake up to breathe?

Yes. The condition is known as sleep apnoea and affects mainly middle-aged men who are overweight. Their throat muscles overrelax during sleep, causing tissue to sag and obstruct air flow. Sufferers stop breathing for an instant and partially wake up before starting again. As this can happen hundreds of times a night, sleep is severely disrupted.

As well as poor sleep, apnoea robs the body and brain of oxygen, and sufferers frequently show symptoms such as irritability, aggression and depression. They also have a greater risk of heart disease and high blood pressure. Treatments include weight reduction, surgery and a nasal mask that assists breathing.

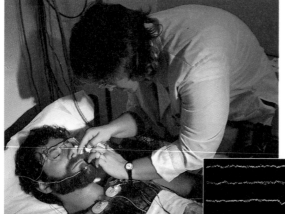

Wired for sleep When all else fails, a sleep clinic can investigate and treat poor sleep. Referral is through a GP.

WHAT HAPPENS WHEN YOU SLEEP AND DREAM?

Sleep is not a simple state of unconsciousness, but a series of stages that occur in regular cycles through the night, each cycle taking around 90 minutes. The stages fall into one of two categories: rapid eye movement (REM) sleep, during which the eyes are extremely active, and non-REM sleep, when the eyes are still. As you fall asleep, your body relaxes and brainwave patterns quieten down, breathing evens out, your pulse and temperature drop and the senses become less responsive. Gradually you pass through four progressively deeper stages of non-REM sleep before starting

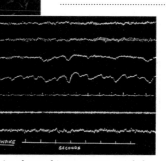

Awake An alert subject generates tightly compressed brain waves.

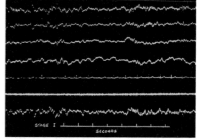

Stage one non-REM sleep Electrical activity slows down as sleep begins.

OVERCOMING INSOMNIA

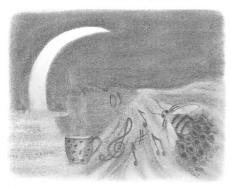

For weeks I have spent every night tossing and turning, unable to get to sleep. It is starting to affect my work. What can I do?

Most people put up with the occasional bad night's sleep without noticing any ill-effects. But if poor sleep goes on for weeks you may start to worry about whether it is affecting your health and to search for ways of getting better sleep.

Before trying any of the following techniques, see if you can accept the number of hours you do sleep as normal for you. You may need only five or six hours' sleep each night. Remember, the chief sign of insufficient or poor sleep is feeling tired during the day. If you don't suffer from tiredness during the day, you are getting enough sleep.

● Once in bed, try the relaxation techniques described on pages 190-191 to take your mind off worrying thoughts.
● Don't keep looking at the bedroom clock.
● Give up alcohol, smoking and caffeine – three causes of sleeplessness – and increase the amount of exercise you do during the day. But beware of evening workouts; they may keep you awake.
● Stay away from tea and hot chocolate, soothing as they sound. They contain caffeine, and will keep you awake.
● Avoid work, loud music, big meals, intense discussions and exciting television programmes late at night.
● Make the hours before going to bed as relaxing as possible to keep your mind off the day's problems. Take a warm bath. Listen to soothing music. Read a book.
● Save your bedroom for bedroom activities. Entering it should not make you think of the bills you haven't paid or the work you need to do the next day.

CURES FOR SNORING

My wife complains that I snore. Can I do anything to stop it?

There is, alas, no simple cure for snoring, but there are several things you can try.

The first is to change your sleeping position. You are most likely to snore if you are

to come up again through the same stages (in reverse order) into light sleep. Finally, you move into a period of REM sleep, when dreaming occurs. The eyes dart around (but stay closed) and brainwave patterns are similar to those of the waking state. Large body muscles enter a state close to paralysis – perhaps to prevent dreams being dangerously acted out.

Most people go through four or five sleep cycles a night, but both physical illnesses and sleep disorders can disturb the pattern or prevent you reaching the very deepest levels of sleep. Persistent problems may need referral to a special sleep clinic.

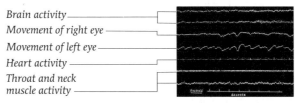

Brain activity
Movement of right eye
Movement of left eye
Heart activity
Throat and neck muscle activity

Sleep charts such as these record electrical traces from nerve and muscle activity picked up by electrodes placed on the body. The results appear as wave patterns on a monitoring screen.

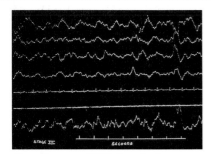

Stage three non-REM sleep Brain waves are more widely spaced as activity slows.

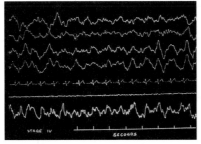

Stage four non-REM sleep The deepest level of sleep has broad, high waves.

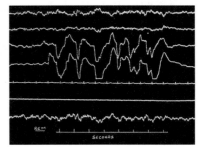

REM sleep Electrical activity is greatest in dream sleep, and eye motion dramatic.

lying on your back. Sleeping in that position leads to loss of tension in the muscles of the tongue and jaw, with the result that parts of the throat and soft palate vibrate as air is drawn in through the mouth and nose. Sleeping on your back also causes the tongue to slide backwards, constricting and speeding up the flow of air. If your husband protests that other sleeping positions don't come naturally to him, try sewing a pad of material or a small rubber ball into his pyjama jacket to make lying on his back uncomfortable.

A stuffy nose can also aggravate snoring. If that seems to be part of the problem, try raising the head of your bed by a couple of inches to allow the nasal passages to drain during the night.

Chronic snoring may sometimes be due to a sinus or respiratory problem. More often, it is associated with drinking too much alcohol or being overweight. If so, it is the causes that should be tackled.

PILLOW TALK

How important is it to sleep with a pillow, and what is the best type to buy?

The function of a pillow is to support your neck more than your head: never sleep with only your head on the pillow, or you may strain your neck and upper back muscles.

Whether you decide to buy a soft or a firm pillow is a matter of personal choice. But as a general guide, if you sleep on your side, try a firm pillow, which will give your head and neck extra support. If you sleep on your back, a medium-firm pillow will cradle your head and 'give' a bit more. And if you sleep on your stomach, choose a soft pillow to minimise the strain on your neck.

Pillows may be filled with synthetic fibres, foams or down and feathers. Polyester-filled pillows are the most popular, and are available in a variety of thicknesses and firmnesses. High-quality polyester-filled pillows are machine-washable, a quality that is vital for sufferers from asthma and allergies.

Down and feather pillows offer a luxurious feel, are extremely durable, and many wash well. The softness – and cost – of the pillow will increase in proportion to the percentage of down it contains. It is also worth noting that chicken feathers are straight and must be artificially curled – a treatment that eventually wears off.

Pillows made of foam and latex tend to be firm with a definite bounce to them. They can't be fluffed or plumped, but instead hold their shape very well.

For the healthiest possible sleep it is advisable to invest in quality pillows and replace them at least every two to three years. When they have lost their thickness and become lumpy, discoloured or misshapen, it is time to buy new ones.

CHOOSING A BED

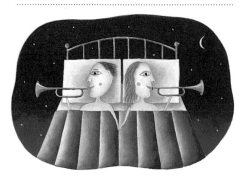

Our ten-year-old bed has finally become too uncomfortable to bear. What should we be considering when buying a new one?

'Try before you buy' is the golden rule when choosing a bed:

● If you are buying for two, both of you should lie down on the bed together. You may not have the same idea about what is comfortable, or how much support is needed.
● Take this test seriously. Don't just sit on the edge of the bed, or even lie flat on your back. Relax and adopt your usual sleeping positions. When considering the size of the bed, be aware that people who sleep on their side actually take up *more* room than those who sleep on their front or back.
● Check that the bed is made by a reputable manufacturer – preferably a member of the National Bed Federation.
● Make sure the bed is at least 6 in (15 cm) longer than you are – or than the taller partner – and at least 5 ft (1.5 m) wide if you are buying a double bed. The standard 4 ft 6 in (1.35 m) bed allows only 2 ft 3 in (69 cm) of space for each person – not much more than a baby's cot!
● Think of the mattress and base as a complete unit: the comfort of your mattress will depend upon the type and condition of the base. If you are buying a mattress on its own, try it out on a base similar to the one you have at home. Bear in mind that it would be a false economy to buy a new mattress for an old worn-out base: the base could damage the mattress, and even invalidate the mattress guarantee.

Women's health

TOXIC SHOCK SYNDROME

Several of my friends have stopped using tampons because of the 'toxic shock' scare. How much of a risk is this condition? Are sanitary towels really safer?

Toxic Shock Syndrome (TSS) is a serious illness caused by *Staphylococcus aureus*. These bacteria can grow from any vulnerable area, such as the site of a burn or viral infection; but the single most frequent association is with tampon use. TSS has a mortality rate of around 3 per cent, but even so the risk is tiny – about two deaths a year in Britain.

British tampon manufacturers now enclose warning leaflets about TSS, which stress the need to change a tampon every four to six hours, and never to leave it in place for longer than 12 hours. However, tampon-labelling has not yet been standardised in Britain, as it has been in the United States.

The risk of contracting TSS is virtually non-existent if you use the least-absorbent tampon for your needs and change it regularly. It is also a good idea to avoid using tampons at the beginning of your period, when 70 per cent of all cases of toxic-shock syndrome occur. However, if you want to eliminate completely the risk of contracting TSS in this way, use sanitary towels.

The symptoms of TSS resemble those of flu – high fever, aching muscles, sore throat, dizziness, vomiting, diarrhoea – but they also include a sunburn-like rash and a sudden, severe drop in blood pressure. A woman who suspects she has this syndrome should see a doctor or go straight to a hospital emergency department. Prompt treatment with antibiotics usually prevents serious consequences.

THRUSH INFECTIONS

I suffer from outbreaks of vaginal thrush regularly. What causes the infection, and is there anything I can do to prevent it?

The fungus that causes thrush, *Candida albicans*, occurs naturally in the vagina, and its growth is kept under control by the bacteria that are usually present there. If you have been taking a course of antibiotics, the drug may have destroyed too many of the bacteria; so allowing the fungus to multiply excessively. Symptoms of the condition include itching and soreness, accompanied by a white and sometimes thick vaginal discharge.

Other common causes of the growth of the candida albicans fungus include certain disorders such as diabetes; and the hormonal changes that occur in pregnancy or through taking an oral contraceptive. Although thrush commonly affects the vagina, it can also affect other areas of mucous membrane, notably inside the mouth, or moist skin.

The infection can be contracted by sexual intercourse with an infected partner. Infection of the penis is uncommon, however. It is more likely to occur in men who have not been circumcised.

There are several measures you can take to prevent recurring vaginal thrush infections. See the advice in the panel, right.

HEAVY PERIODS

I suffer from heavy bleeding during my periods, which often leaves me feeling completely exhausted. Is there any way to reduce my blood loss?

Some women have naturally heavier periods than others, but it is possible that excessive blood loss is due to a hormone imbalance, use of an IUD (intrauterine device), small non-cancerous growths in the womb known as fibroids, or an infection of the womb or uterine tubes. So to be safe, it is best to see your doctor.

Treatment depends on the severity of the bleeding, how old you are, whether or not you want to have children, and any underlying disorder. Hormone treatment may be prescribed to reduce the amount of bleeding, especially if you are very young. If the condition is severe, a hysterectomy (removal of the uterus) may be considered.

PREMENSTRUAL SYNDROME

What causes premenstrual syndrome, and is there anything I can do to eliminate, or at least lessen, the symptoms?

Up to 90 per cent of women suffer from premenstrual syndrome (PMS) at some time during their life. It begins at or after ovulation and continues until the onset of your period. For some, the symptoms must be endured for up to half of every month. Problems include

---

DO'S AND DON'TS

for preventing vaginal thrush

Do use sanitary towels, not tampons.

Do make sure you wipe from front to back after using the toilet.

Do tell your doctor that you are prone to thrush, particularly if you are prescribed antibiotics or the contraceptive pill.

Don't wear tights, nylon pants or tight jeans or trousers.

Don't use perfumed toilet preparations such as soaps and bubble baths; and don't use vaginal deodorants.

Don't use disinfectants in the bath.

Don't use strong detergents, particularly biologicals, when laundering linen and clothes, especially underwear.

Don't use soap if there is irritation; wipe the vulva with baby oil instead.

Don't take antibiotics unless absolutely necessary.

Don't bath, wash or shower more often; it will give only temporary relief.

A herbal remedy for thrush

As well as over-the-counter medication, vaginal thrush can be treated with a herbal extract known as tea-tree oil, which many women have found helpful.

An ancient Aboriginal remedy, tea-tree oil was considered such an important antiseptic that during the Second World War leaf-cutters were exempted from national service in order to continue producing it for the Australian Army. Nowadays it can be bought at most chemists and health shops.

To use the oil, add one teaspoon to a pint (570 ml) of water and use as a daily douche. Alternatively, dampen the tip of a tampon with water, sprinkle on three to four drops of tea-tree oil, insert and leave in place for an hour or two.

physical complaints such as water retention and swollen joints, breast tenderness, weight gain, skin problems, fatigue and headaches. There can also be psychological or emotional symptoms such as irritability, poor concentration, reduced sex drive, insomnia, tearfulness and depression.

Many theories have been put forward to explain PMS. Hormonal changes that occur throughout the menstrual cycle may be an influence: an imbalance between the levels of oestrogen and progesterone has been suspected, though not proved guilty. Similarly, deficiencies of vitamin E, vitamin B_6 and magnesium have also been cited as a cause, but scientific proof is lacking.

There are a number of measures you can take to relieve the symptoms of PMS: eat less salt to discourage fluid retention; try not to drink large quantities of tea and coffee, as caffeine can interfere with the body's ability to absorb essential nutrients and may aggravate skin problems. Relax by taking gentle exercise such as yoga, or by having a warm bath. If symptoms are severe, your doctor may prescribe progesterone or oestrogen in various forms, or a combination of the two, to restore hormone levels to normal.

COPING WITH CYSTITIS

Occasionally I suffer from a painful burning sensation when urinating. The condition often lasts for a week or so. What have I got and can it be cured?

You most probably have cystitis – inflammation of the bladder lining – usually the result of bacteria from the anus passing through the urinary tract. Other possible causes are thrush (see page 161) and bruising during sexual intercourse (see page 257). Symptoms vary from mild to very severe, sometimes disappearing within hours, sometimes dragging on for weeks. Many sufferers experience only a single bout; others tend to have numerous repeated attacks.

There are various over-the-counter treatments to try. If they relieve the symptoms only briefly, or not at all, see the doctor. And consult your doctor immediately if any of these complications arise: the urine becomes cloudy or blood is present; you develop a temperature; groin or stomach pain becomes severe or you start getting back pain; there is an unusually heavy vaginal discharge. If an infection is present, your doctor will probably prescribe a course of antibiotics.

Bouts of cystitis can often be cut short by taking the following steps immediately:

● Drink 1 pint (570 ml) of water as soon as you feel an attack of cystitis coming on. This will flush the bacteria out of the bladder.
● Make sure you go to the lavatory as often as you can, even if you pass only a small amount of urine.
● Try using hot-water bottles wrapped in towels to relieve pain in the lower back or pelvic region.
● Take a teaspoon of bicarbonate of soda dissolved in a glass of water every three hours. This makes the urine less acidic, and thereby stops bacteria breeding and relieves the burning sensation.
● Do not eat citrus or sour fruit, and avoid foods containing vinegar, and animal proteins such as eggs, fish, meat and cheese: they all make urine more acidic and painful to pass.

CAUTION People who have high blood pressure should consult their doctor before taking bicarbonate of soda.

Tests for men and women

A TEST FOR MEN

How common is testicular cancer? How often should I examine myself, and how is the examination done?

For men between the ages of 15 and 40, particularly those who have an undescended or partially descended testicle, testicular cancer is one of the most common types of cancer.

Early warning signs include a slight enlargement of one of the testes. There may be no pain, although a dull ache in the abdomen or groin is a common warning sign.

There is no way of preventing the disorder, but you should examine your testes regularly once a month to ensure early detection of any lump. The exam takes no more than three minutes. After a warm bath or shower, when the skin around the scrotum is most relaxed, roll each testicle gently in both hands. If you find any hard nodules, see your doctor immediately. The lump may be benign, but only a doctor can determine whether it is. In either case, the treatment is usually simple and highly successful.

Cure rates for malignant prostate tumours are high: with early detection, 95 to 97 per cent of patients are treated successfully, and even in cases where spreading has occurred, 85 per cent of patients respond well to further treatment. If surgery is necessary, and a testicle has to be removed, it should have no effect on sexual potency or fertility.

EXAMINING YOUR BREASTS

Why is it so important to examine your breasts? How often do I need to do it, and when is the best time?

From about the age of 20, all women should start examining their breasts once a month. Premenopausal women should pick a time about two or three days after a period, when

---

HOW TO DO A MONTHLY BREAST CHECK

Paying attention to your breasts, especially during day-to-day activities such as bathing and dressing, can alert you to a difference in size or shape, the emergence of over-prominent veins, discharge from the nipple or a dimpling of the skin. If your breasts are naturally lumpy, it is helpful to compare one breast with the other. The great majority of these changes are completely harmless, but consult your doctor *immediately* if you find an abnormality of any kind.

1 Strip to the waist and face a mirror in a good light. Look for any changes in the shape of either breast, for any puckering or dimpling of the skin, and for any changes in the condition of either nipple. Put your hands behind your head and look again. Turn sideways for another look and then lean forward and check again.

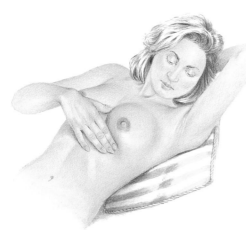

2 Lie flat with a cushion or folded towel under your left shoulder blade. Keeping your right fingers flat, work round your left breast, pressing firmly as you go and gradually spiralling from the outermost part towards the nipple.

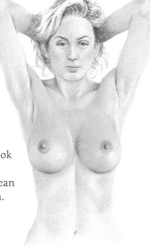

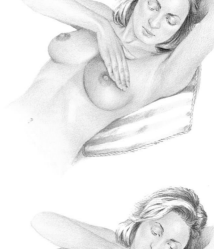

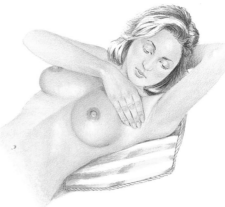

3 Make sure you check carefully underneath both of your breasts. Again, working with your fingers flat against the skin, you should be feeling for any lumps, thickenings or bumpy areas which seem to be unusual.

4 It is also important to check the whole armpit area (where the lymph glands are) for unusual lumps or thickenings. Using each hand in turn, press the opposite armpit, then move your fingers down towards the breast.

An end to smears?

Long waits and inaccurate smear-test results may soon be a thing of the past. A team of Australian doctors has developed a computer-aided device – called the Polarprobe – which detects pre-cancerous and cancerous cells in the cervix by means of light waves and electrical energy.

The probe looks like a large pen, and is connected to a computer. It is inserted into the vagina and moved across the cervix to check for abnormalities.

Unlike the traditional cervical smear test, where cells are physically scraped from the cervix and sent to a laboratory for testing, the Polarprobe operates on the principle that there are different blood-flow levels in cancerous and non-cancerous tissue. It produces its results within minutes. And on a test of 2000 Australian women, the device has so far proved over 90 per cent correct in its diagnoses, quite outclassing the current method of smear testing.

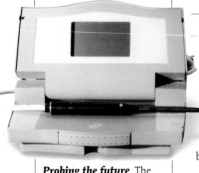

Probing the future The computer-aided Polarprobe is set to revolutionise cervical check-ups.

their breasts are least likely to feel tender, swollen or lumpy. Postmenopausal women can choose a date that is easy to remember, such as the first day of the month or the first Monday in the month.

If you detect a new lump, a discharge from your nipple, or a significant change in the shape or appearance of your breasts, see your doctor immediately. Very few symptoms will indicate a serious disorder such as cancer, but all should be reported. The success rate for treatment is much higher if problems are detected and reported early. (For breast self-examination see panel, page 163.)

CERVICAL SMEARS

I'm about to have my first cervical smear examination. What should I expect?

From the patient's point of view, a cervical smear involves nothing more than a quick internal examination about once every three to five years. The doctor will insert an instrument called a speculum into the vagina to allow a clear view of the cervix. A wooden or plastic spatula is then wiped across the cervix to collect a few cells – you may feel a little discomfort, but many women notice nothing. The speculum is removed, and the smear test is complete. The cells are then sent to a pathology laboratory for analysis.

Postmenopausal women should still have regular tests on the NHS until they are 65. Smears are not necessary if you have had a hysterectomy, unless you have had cancer.

The time taken for results to come back varies. In theory, no smear result should take more than a month. In practice, however, you may have to wait as long as about eight weeks. Results arrive by mail at your doctor's surgery. You should get a copy of them in the post too, or you may be asked to phone for them.

POSITIVE RESULTS

What happens if the results are positive?

A positive or 'abnormal' smear may simply be an early warning sign indicating that cells are changing or have changed on the surface of your cervix. It does not necessarily mean that you have cancer. There are four stages of abnormality: borderline, mild, moderate and severe.

If your smear result indicates borderline or mild changes, it may be repeated within six months. Borderline and mild changes usually clear up without treatment. Even with more severe changes, only half will become

cancerous even if left completely untreated. When cancer develops it is almost 100 per cent curable provided the cell changes are detected early enough and treated promptly.

With moderate or severe changes, you will be referred for a colposcopy, which involves examining the cervix with a lighted binocular microscope. The procedure takes only 20 minutes and the doctor may remove a small piece of tissue for laboratory analysis. The results take a week or two to arrive and if necessary laser treatment is then offered.

Self-help

If you have a slightly abnormal smear and you smoke – stop. Smoking damages the changing cells on the cervix and makes them more vulnerable to attack by viruses.

It is now almost certain that men pass on some agents, such as the genital herpes virus or genital warts, that increase the risk of cervical cancer. So the more sexual partners you have, the greater your risk of contracting the disease. If you think you may be at risk, consider using a barrier contraceptive, such as a condom or diaphragm, as these protect the cervix from infection (see also page 257).

HOW ACCURATE ARE SMEARS?

I have a cervical smear regularly, but I'm worried because they have been the subject of some controversy. Why are the results not always accurate?

There are a number of reasons why a cervical smear test does not always give an accurate result. Sometimes a smear is not taken properly. For example, it may be that the material scraped from the cervix was insufficient, or taken from the wrong site. In such cases you will usually be asked to come in for a repeat smear. A faulty finding of abnormal results may also arise from misinterpreting the natural changes that the cervix undergoes at various stages of reproductive life, for example, at puberty, in pregnancy, during menstruation and at the menopause.

Having a smear test every three to five years is adequate for most screening purposes. Although there are some fast-growing cancers that occasionally develop between routine smear tests this is unusual and slow development is much more common. The vast majority of problems, if caught at the stage when they are still only mild or moderate cell abnormalities, are easily treated. Always see a doctor for an examination and possibly an early smear if you have abnormal bleeding, particularly after intercourse.

Medicines and remedies at home

SAFE STORAGE OF MEDICINES

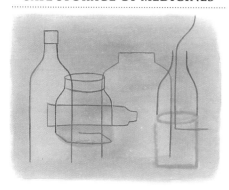

What safety precautions should I be taking when storing my medicines?

Treat all medication with respect, whether standard over-the-counter remedies or powerful prescription drugs. The best place to store medicines, including seemingly harmless preparations such as cough mixture and iron tablets, is in a wall cabinet well out of the reach of children. It is also important to store them under conditions that ensure their effectiveness; improperly stored medication can become inactive or toxic. Consult your doctor or pharmacist if you are unsure about where to keep particular preparations. Otherwise, follow these suggestions for safe storage:

● Most medication should be kept at room temperature in a dark, dry place. The bathroom, despite its popularity, is one of the worst places to keep certain medicines, such as glyceryl trinitrate tablets for angina, because a warm, humid atmosphere may reduce their effectiveness.
● Always keep medicines in their original containers so that you don't forget what they are and can check the label for directions.
● Keep medication away from direct sunlight, even when it is in a darkened container. Sunlight may cause it to deteriorate, to the point where it loses almost all its effectiveness.
● Pharmacists are required to supply childproof caps for medicines that are taken orally. So if you suffer from a disorder such as arthritis, and would have difficulty opening such bottles, ask for a lid that is easier to remove.

● Some medicines need to be stored in the fridge. But don't refrigerate medicine unless actually told to by your pharmacist. And never let liquid formulations freeze.

EXPIRY DATES

Do medicines such as milk of magnesia and aspirin ever 'go off', or is it safe to keep them indefinitely?

The length of time for which medicines stay safe and effective varies greatly. Some last for only a few days while others retain their potency for years. Either way, most drugs are marked with an expiry date, which should not be exceeded.

Provided they have been stored in a cool, dry place, away from direct sunlight, milk of magnesia and aspirin can be kept for up to two years. Medicines in the following categories, by contrast, should be safely disposed of, as by being returned to a pharmacist.

● Tablets or capsules more than two years old or any that are chipped, cracked, powdery or discoloured.
● Hardened, discoloured or separated ointments or creams.
● Thickened or discoloured liquids.
● Cracked, leaking or hard tubes.
● Capsules that have softened, cracked or stuck together.
● Medicines with a changed odour, such as aspirin or paracetamol tablets that smell of vinegar.
● Eye drops that have been opened for more than 28 days.
● Medicines that have expired.

CHOOSING A PAINKILLER

There is such a confusing variety of over-the-counter painkillers available today. What are their differences, and which is the best to keep around the house?

Although dozens of pain-relief products are available for sale over the counter, the active ingredient is almost always one of just four drugs: paracetamol, aspirin, codeine or ibuprofen. All four relieve mild to moderate pain, and all but codeine will reduce fever. Aspirin and ibuprofen also have an anti-inflammatory effect, and can be used for the treatment of arthritis and other inflammatory conditions. Ibuprofen is effective against menstrual cramps and soft-tissue injuries such as sprained tendons and strained muscles.

Some preparations contain a mixture of analgesics and other drugs such as antacids, antihistamines or decongestants. Caffeine is sometimes added to counteract the sedative affects of painkillers such as codeine – with questionable results. Such combinations are no more effective pain-relievers than single-ingredient medicines and may increase the chance of adverse reactions. Single-ingredient preparations are also usually less expensive.

Standard aspirin can irritate the stomach, but buffered or coated aspirin may protect against that side effect. Buffered aspirin is released in the stomach in just the same way as standard aspirin, but contains chemicals that counteract acidity and irritation. Coated preparations do not release aspirin until they have reached the small intestine.

CAUTION
● Avoid taking aspirin for seven days before surgery, as it thins the blood.
● Do not give aspirin to children under 12.

It has been linked to Reyes syndrome (see panel, page 288).
● Do not take ibuprofen if you are allergic to aspirin; you are probably allergic to both types of painkillers.
● Do not take ibuprofen if you have a long-term kidney disease.
● Do not take paracetamol if you have liver or kidney trouble.
● Do not take standard aspirin or ibuprofen if you tend to suffer from indigestion or stomach ulcers. Instead, choose a buffered or coated variety.

DISPOSING OF DRUGS

Our medicine cabinet is full of old prescription drugs. What should we do with them?

Dispose of all the medicines. Some may have become ineffective or even dangerous if they have been stored for a very long time. Never throw them in the rubbish bin or flush them down the lavatory. Take them to your local pharmacy or hospital pharmacy department for safe disposal.

Alternative cures for headaches

There are a number of things you can do to relieve a tension headache, if you would rather not take painkilling drugs.

Often the best remedy is to lie down in a dark room with a cool cloth over your forehead. Getting someone to give a gentle massage to tight neck muscles, or taking a hot shower, may also provide some relief.

If tension headaches are a regular part of your life, see your doctor, who may be able to help you to identify the source of the tension and resolve it in some way. For self-help try the relaxation techniques described on pages 190-193. Practised regularly they can help to prevent tension.

TYPES OF HEADACHE

Most headaches are not a sign of a serious underlying problem. However, if a headache is accompanied by symptoms such as visual disturbances, vomiting, confusion or loss of memory, numbness in some part of the body, lack of coordination, slurred speech, or high fever and a stiff neck, you should seek medical attention immediately.

Tension headache
This is the most common type of headache. Pain is caused by a tightening of the muscles of the neck, face or scalp, and is usually triggered by emotional stress (worry, anxiety, depression) or physical stress (sitting in a stuffy room or working too long in the same position). The pain often feels like a band of dull, steady pressure around the head. The most important thing is to avoid or to find ways of dealing with the stresses and strains that cause tension headaches. Most tension headaches respond to aspirin or other over-the-counter analgesics. Warmth or massage on the neck and scalp may help.

Cluster headache
These headaches tend to affect men more than women, do not seem to run in families, and are rare. Characterised by a piercing pain in one eye or on one side of the face, cluster headaches may occur a few times a day for weeks or months, and then disap-

pear. They often start in the middle of the night. The pain is continuous rather than throbbing. The eye fills with tears, the nose gets blocked on the affected side and then starts to run. The cheek may swell too. These headaches require medical attention. The doctor may prescribe a drug such as pizotifen, which is thought to block chemicals that act on the blood vessels in the brain. Taken before going to bed, this drug may prevent an attack from occurring.

Migraine headache
Characterised by a sharp throbbing pain, often on one side of the head and often associated with nausea, migraines affect more women than men and tend to run in families. For more information on preventing and treating migraines, see pages 368-369.

Other common headaches are triggered by various factors: too much caffeine or alcohol; certain foods, food additives, and drugs; and even orgasm.

WHAT YOU NEED FOR A FAMILY FIRST-AID KIT

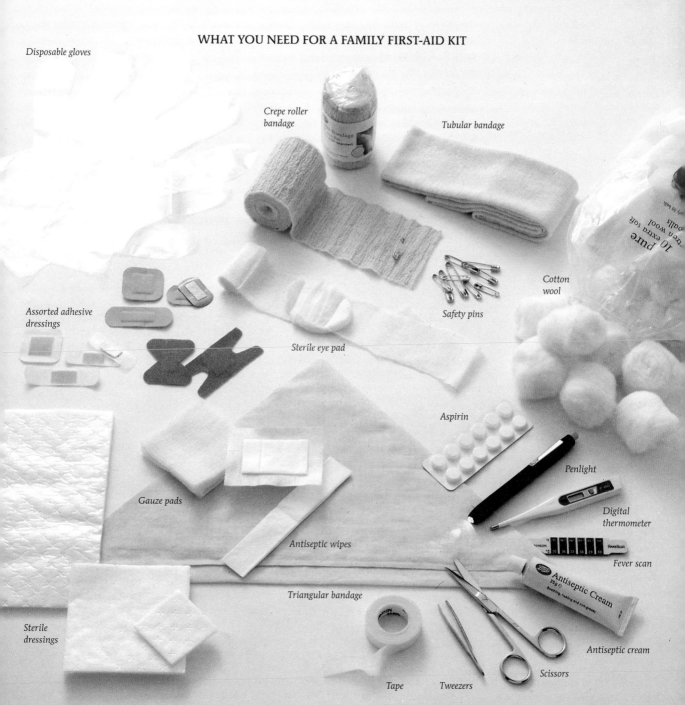

Disposable gloves

Crepe roller bandage

Tubular bandage

Cotton wool

Assorted adhesive dressings

Safety pins

Sterile eye pad

Aspirin

Penlight

Gauze pads

Digital thermometer

Fever scan

Antiseptic wipes

Triangular bandage

Sterile dressings

Antiseptic cream

Tape   Tweezers   Scissors

Accident insurance More than 35 per cent of all accidents occur in the home, according to the Royal Society for the Prevention of Accidents, and each year more than one million of these result in a visit to the local doctor or hospital. Even so, the majority of accidents can be dealt with fast and effectively in the home if you have a well-stocked first-aid kit.

First-aid kits can be bought ready-made from chemists, but it will probably work out cheaper if you make up your own from the items shown above. All of the medicines and materials should be kept in a sealed plastic box and stored well out of the reach of children. Do not keep first-aid materials in unsealed containers in the bathroom or kitchen; they may deteriorate in the damp air. It is a good idea to attach the address and phone number of your doctor and local hospital on a piece of paper to the inside of the lid. You may also want to keep a copy of *Reader's Digest Good Health Fact Book* with the kit, so you can, if necessary, consult the emergency procedures on pages 447-467.

Consider keeping an additional first-aid kit in the car and, if you are travelling abroad, carrying a basic first-aid kit with you – see pages 170-171 for more information.

WHICH THERMOMETER?

Which thermometer is more accurate: the digital type, the old mercury and glass one or the skin thermometer?

Mercury and digital thermometers are both about 98 per cent accurate. The chief difference between them is that many people find the more expensive digital design easier to use. Digital models bleep or buzz when the temperature reaches a maximum and display the results on a liquid crystal screen. A mercury thermometer must be shaken down to base level before it is used. Once inserted, it takes about three minutes for the mercury to rise to the correct level.

An electronic digital thermometer needs a new battery about every two years. A mercury thermometer won't run down, but sometimes the column of mercury breaks up after a time, rendering the thermometer useless. Mercury thermometers are also easily broken, making them unsafe for babies, and results are hard to read if your eyesight is poor.

Strip thermometers, or skin thermometers, are pressed against the forehead for about two to three minutes to obtain a reading, and use heat-sensitive chemicals that change colour as temperature varies. They last about a year and are slightly less accurate than mercury or digital instruments because they are affected by external factors such as room temperature.

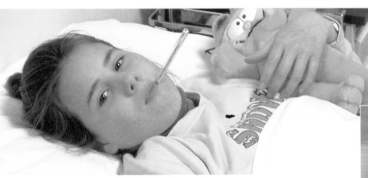

Mercury thermometer This tried and trusted instrument is accurate provided you leave it in long enough and have good eyesight. Don't leave a young patient unattended – breakages are common and can be dangerous.

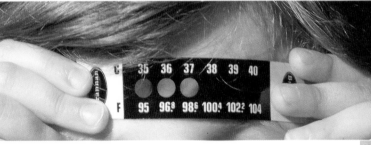

Strip thermometer Small, paper-thin and durable, strip thermometers are convenient for travelling. The results are not quite as accurate as with other types, and they are not reliable after more than a year.

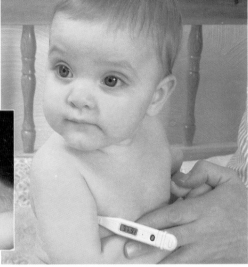

Digital thermometer A more expensive option, but digital thermometers are accurate, easy and very safe.

Holiday health care

TRAVELLER'S DIARRHOEA

I will be travelling through South-east Asia for two months. How do I avoid the dreaded 'traveller's tummy'?

Most cases of traveller's diarrhoea are caused by bacteria in contaminated water, milk and uncooked food. To avoid having your coming holiday spoiled by the common but unpleasant symptoms, take basic precautions:

● Before you leave, ask your doctor for prophylactic tablets to guard against stomach upsets. Take one tablet twice-daily throughout your holiday.

● Boil your water – even water for cleaning your teeth. Take tincture of iodine with you in case this is not always possible. A few drops added to a glass of water is a safe and effective method of sterilisation.

● Avoid ice unless you know it has been made from boiled water.

● Avoid high-risk foods such as shellfish, raw or under-cooked meat, raw seafood, egg products, cream, mayonnaise, fresh fruit, vegetables, salad ingredients and desserts. Ice cream should also be treated with caution and should never be bought from a street vendor.

● Avoid any food that is not covered. It could be contaminated by flies.

● Boil milk, or avoid it altogether.

It is also wise to take electrolyte salts with you (available from chemists), just in case your precautions fail. If you do develop vomiting or diarrhoea, dissolve the salts in boiled water according to instructions and drink in copious quantities to restore the right chemical balance of body fluids. You can make a rough equivalent by adding a pinch of salt to a jug of orange squash. Otherwise, just drink plenty of boiled water, soft drinks or tea.

Seek medical advice if: diarrhoea persists for 12 hours in a child or for 48 hours in an adult; you are in a cholera or typhoid area; the patient becomes feverish or dehydrated (sunken eyes and wrinkled skin are signs).

MOTION-SICKNESS

Our 12-year-old son suffers badly from travel sickness, which makes family holidays very difficult to arrange. Is there any way of overcoming the problem?

Motion-sickness is caused by a discrepancy in what the eyes see and what the inner-ear balance mechanisms feel. Most of the preventative measures are designed to make sure your eyes receive visual signals of motion; one or two try to prevent the inner ear being affected more than necessary.

All types of travel can cause nausea. Almost anyone is susceptible, but children between three and twelve years old are most vulnerable, so your son may find that things start to improve. In the meantime he could try some of these tips.

In the car

● Sit in a front seat and concentrate on watching the road ahead, trying to anticipate the car's movement. Keep windows and air vents open, unless driving in heavy traffic.

● Young children should be positioned safely on a booster cushion or safety seat (depending on their age) so that they have a good view of the road ahead from the back of the car. Don't let them read, write or draw. Instead try playing games that involve looking out ahead, or distracting them with songs or tapes.

● Eat sensibly before and during the trip. Avoid very rich food. Adults should also avoid alcohol.

● The driver can help by taking bends gently and accelerating and decelerating gradually.

● Don't read in the car.

● Stop at least once every hour, get out of the car and breathe some fresh air.

In the air

Ask your travel agent for seats over the wings where the plane is most stable. Tilt your seat back, close your eyes and keep your head still against the headrest.

At sea

Outside, stay on a low deck away from galley smells and fumes, and fix your eyes on the horizon. Inside, find a seat at the spot where the ship moves least (usually a low deck near the middle). If you start to feel ill, lie down, close your eyes and keep your head still.

Prevention and treatment

Pharmacies sell a variety of motion-sickness pills over the counter. Adults and children over five can take cinnarizine, and those over ten can use the prescription drug, hyoscine for car travel. Hyoscine is administered via a patch applied behind the ear before setting

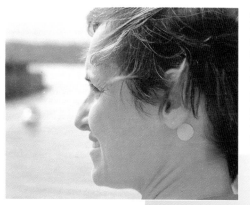

Slow release remedy
Wearing an adhesive patch impregnated with the drug hyoscine is an effective way of controlling motion-sickness, particularly on long journeys. The patch is applied behind the ear and works for hours. Despite its usefulness, side effects are common, including drowsiness, dryness in the mouth and blurred vision.

Applying pressure
Elasticated wristbands are now sold in seaports, airports and at chemists as a motion-sickness cure. They work on the Chinese principle of pressure points and incorporate a plastic bump that presses on a particular part of the wrist.

out, and works by blocking symptoms in the central nervous system where they begin.

You may also want to try traditional remedies such as ginger tea (pour boiling water over a few slices of fresh, peeled ginger root) or ginger biscuits. A Chinese approach called acupressure has shown proven results. Press in the middle of the inner wrist three finger widths above the crease where the wrist joins the hand, line with the middle finger. Wristbands work on the same principle.

BEATING JET LAG

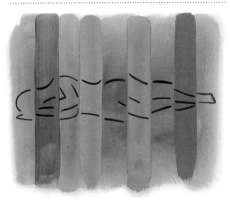

As a long-distance business traveller, I am regularly affected by jet lag. Is there anything I can do to lessen its effects?

Fatigue and feelings of sluggishness are completely normal after an east-west air journey that crosses any of the world's 24 different time zones. Such travel has the effect of disturbing the body's natural 24-hour cycle, the so-called circadian rhythm.

Jet lag generally dissipates over a few days as your body gradually gets used to the light and dark cycle of the new locality. However, there are some things you can do to speed up adjustment and minimise bad effects.

● If you are heading east, try going to sleep earlier for a few days before the trip. On the other hand, go to sleep later if you are travelling westward.
● During the flight make sure you drink plenty of water and other non-alcoholic beverages to prevent dehydration. Avoid alcoholic drinks – they can be dehydrating and have a stronger effect in low-pressure conditions. Eat lightly.
● Try to break a long flight with a stopover.
● Plan your trip so that you arrive at your destination in the early evening and then try to get to bed early.
● Spend some time outdoors, preferably in sunlight, on the first few days of your stay.

HOLIDAY FIRST-AID KIT

What should we include in the family first-aid kit when we travel abroad this summer?

Holidays are all too often marred by unexpected ailment or illness, so packing a first-aid kit is always a wise decision.

The items below are essentials for any kit, no matter where you are travelling:

● Sterile non-adhesive dressings – five pads 5 cm x 5 cm, and three pads 10 cm x 10 cm. Apply with surgical tape or a bandage and use for cuts, grazes and minor burns.
● Gauze swabs – two packs each with five 7.5 cm x 7.5 cm swabs. Use these to clean wounds or swab blood, or as an eye pad. Apply with surgical tape or bandage.
● Surgical tape – 2.5 cm x 5 m.
● Crepe bandage – 7.5 cm x 4.5 m.
● Fabric plasters – 24 in assorted sizes.
● Scissors – the blunt-ended first-aid type.
● Antiseptic dry powder or spray – to prevent infection in wounds.
● Antiseptic wipes – one pack of ten. Use them for cleaning small cuts and grazes.
● Adult painkillers – one 24-tablet or 24-capsule pack each of aspirin, paracetamol and ibuprofen.
● Children's painkillers – one pack of 24.
● Thermometer – a strip or digital thermometer is preferable because it won't break in your suitcase. A thermometer is especially important if you are travelling with children as it can help you to decide when to call a doctor. A child's temperature higher than 39° C (102° F) warrants medical attention.
● Insect repellent and insect bite medication.
● Anti-diarrhoeal medicine.
● Tweezers.

Personal medication
If family members are on medication, make sure you take supplies to last the trip. Keep medicine on you rather than in your suitcase in case your luggage goes missing.

Emergency travel packs
In some less-developed countries, blood for transfusions is not adequately screened for infectious agents such as HIV and hepatitis B, and the sterility of medical equipment is not guaranteed. The best advice if you are travelling in such areas is to avoid medical or dental treatment involving surgery, blood transfusion or injection if at all possible.

Another precaution you may wish to consider is that of taking your own emergency medical kit containing sealed, sterilised equipment such as syringes, needles and suture materials. In any emergency, hand the sealed kit to the doctor or nurse treating you so that you know the equipment used on you is safe. Personal kits are advised for travellers going to destinations including Goa in India, the Kenyan coast, sub-Saharan Africa, Egypt outside Cairo, rural Thailand, Mexico and Central America outside tourist resorts, and for most of South America. They are available from chemists and at private travel centres.

IMMUNISATION TO ENSURE A SAFE HOLIDAY

If possible you should ask your travel agent or doctor about immunisation at least two months before you are due to leave. Some immunisations take time to become fully effective, and some cannot be given at the same time as others. If you are taking children with you, it is important that they have had their full course of normal childhood immunisations. If you need antimalarial medication, your doctor will be able to advise on the best type, including varieties available over the counter in pharmacies. Although certain immunisations are free on the NHS, you may have to pay for others.

DISEASE	RISK AREAS	MEANS OF INFECTION	IMMUNISATION
Tetanus	Worldwide.	Skin-penetrating wound.	Three injections over eight weeks.
Yellow fever	Africa, South America.	Bite from infected mosquito.	Single injection.
Typhoid	Everywhere except Australia, New Zealand, North America, Europe.	Contaminated food, water or milk.	One injection or four doses of oral medication over eight days.
Cholera	Africa, Asia, Middle East	Contaminated water or food.	Two injections, seven to twenty-eight days apart.
Polio	Everywhere except Australia, New Zealand, North America, Europe.	Direct contact with infected person; contaminated food and water.	Three drops taken orally.
Hepatitis A	Most parts of the world.	Contaminated food or water.	One injection or a skin-scratch vaccine.
Hepatitis B	Worldwide.	Sexual contact with infected person; injection with infected blood or needle.	Three injections over six months.
Malaria	Africa, Asia, Central and South America.	Bite from infected mosquito.	Course of tablets beginning a week before travel and ending four weeks after return.
Rabies	Many parts of the world.	Licks, bites or scratches from any animal.	Pre-exposure vaccine if you are going to a remote, high-risk area.
Diphtheria	Main risk is in countries of the former USSR, and in developing regions.	Airborne bacteria.	If not immunised, three injections a month apart. Low-dose adult vaccine must be boosted every five years.

STAYING MENTALLY HEALTHY

To make the most of life you need a healthy mind and outlook as well as a fit body. Learn to handle stress, to think more positively and to develop yourself and your relationships with others, and you will enjoy a greater sense of personal fulfilment.

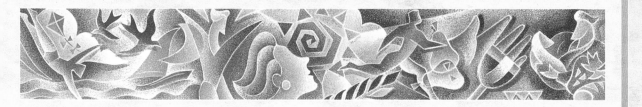

How stressful is your daily life?

Stress in itself, and in moderation, is not a bad thing. Having to meet demands and face challenges can be stimulating and good for your self-esteem. But when stress goes on relentlessly day after day, or makes you feel powerless to control your life, it can threaten your health. Tick the boxes below to see if you are at risk.

1 In the evenings, how often do you go over the events of the day and worry about them?

a) Every day. ☐
b) Occasionally. ☐
c) Never. ☐

2 Do you ever lose interest in sex for any length of time because of tense situations at work or at home?

a) Frequently. ☐
b) Occasionally. ☐
c) Never. ☐

3 How often do you wake up during the night with your heart beating fast, and feeling worried?

a) More than once a week. ☐
b) Occasionally. ☐
c) Never. ☐

4 How frequently do you resort to alcohol in an effort to take your mind off a problem?

a) Regularly. ☐
b) Only under extreme pressure. ☐
c) Never. ☐

5 How often do you lose your temper?

a) Nearly every day. ☐
b) Occasionally. ☐
c) Almost never. ☐

6 Which of the following phrases best describes the way you feel about your job?

a) I would leave tomorrow if I could. ☐
b) It pays the rent. ☐
c) I look forward to getting to work every day. ☐

7 How frequently have you felt that you no longer have any control over your life?

a) Much of the time. ☐
b) Occasionally. ☐
c) Never. ☐

8 How do you react when another driver pulls out in front of you, forcing you to stop?

a) Shout, swear and gesticulate. ☐
b) Curse under your breath. ☐
c) Stay calm. ☐

9 How do you respond to problems you encounter either in your work or in your personal life?

a) Feel angry or upset but say nothing. ☐
b) Try to forget about them. ☐
c) Talk about them. ☐

SCORING

Award yourself nothing for every (a) answer, 1 point for every (b) answer, and 2 points for every (c) answer. Add up your score.

13 to 18: You seem to have devised good ways of keeping stress under control.

6 to 12: You are probably managing to relax some of the time but experiencing high levels of stress at other times, especially at work. Try listing the day's priorities in advance to help you to gain control of your workload.

5 or less: Everyday life may be taking a heavy toll on you. Try to work out the major sources of stress and draw up a plan for controlling them. Build time into your weekly schedule for leisure and exercise – they are a necessity, not a luxury. Whatever your stress level, you can benefit from the relaxation advice on pages 190-195.

Wellbeing from within

HEALTH AND HAPPINESS

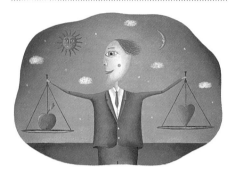

What is mental health? Is it the same thing as being happy?

No one is happy all the time. Rather than a state of constant bliss, mental health is more like a balancing act that requires the processing and integration of constantly shifting emotions and moods, negative as well as positive.

The root meaning of the word *health* is wholeness. Mentally healthy people continually work at balancing and developing all aspects of themselves – physical, mental, emotional and, in many cases, also spiritual. They feel generally purposeful, in control of their lives, committed to the work they do, supported by and supportive of the people around them.

Psychologists believe that the events of our lives, even the most devastating hardships, have less influence on our mental health than does the way we respond to them. Survivors of traumatic events – concentration camp prisoners, victims of terrorist kidnappings, lost polar explorers – often report triumph over pain, fear and desolation through the deliberate conditioning of their minds. Open-minded, hopeful attitudes seem to conquer adversity.

Negative, rigid and inflexible attitudes not only decrease ability to cope with the unavoidable stresses of life but can also prevent people from enjoying success and happiness to the full when they come.

An uninvolved, defeatist outlook on life may even be harmful to your physical health. In a study of elderly nursing home residents in the United States, it was found that those who allowed every decision (what to watch on television, for example, whether to go out to the cinema with friends, or whether to go out for an evening meal) to be made for them were twice as likely to fall ill and die as those people who made their own choices.

THE ROLE OF PERSONALITY

Are some personalities more likely to develop certain illnesses than others? Does being impatient or competitive, for example, make you more likely to develop heart disease or a stomach ulcer?

There is no simple answer to this question. It used to be thought that having a so-called Type A personality – hard-working, impatient, demanding – was indeed a risk factor for some stress-related illnesses. Now, however, it appears that there is some good news for Type As: some of the characteristics associated with forceful, ambitious personalities appear to be assets, rather than detriments, to health. While hostile, aggressive Type A behaviour is certainly still a risk factor for heart disease, doctors now make distinctions between Type As who are angry and socially isolated and those who despite other Type A characteristics are able to develop supportive relationships in families and with friends.

Having a Type A or a more easygoing Type B personality seems to have less of an impact on your wellbeing and mental health than whether or not you are a psychologically 'hardy' person with a well-developed sense of identity, who feels in charge of life, enjoys it and sees changes as opportunities rather

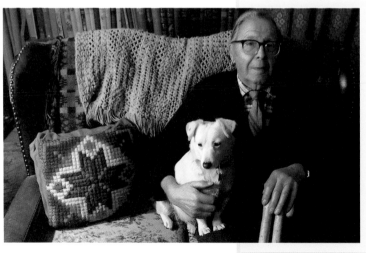

Man's best friend As researchers have found, dogs (and all pets) really are good companions.

than threats. Such people are also less likely to develop stress-related illnesses such as ulcers and high blood pressure.

People who do develop ulcers and similar illnesses, however, do not necessarily lead more stressful lives than anyone else, but they do appear to react to their problems more negatively. They may also find it more difficult to give expression to their true feelings, which remain bottled up until they erupt in the form of physical symptoms or emotions like anger or depression. Unlike more hardy types, so-called pressure-sensitive people do not see themselves as in control of their lives. Easily overwhelmed, they tend to be emotionally dependent and often feel exhausted, helpless and hopeless. They are also more likely to become depressed.

Fortunately, hardiness is something that anyone can work at acquiring, whatever their personality type. Face life with a positive attitude, maintain a variety of interests, express your true feelings (see panel, left) and nurture friendships and family relationships, and you will be well on the way.

DO'S AND DON'TS

for talking about feelings

Do try to be open about your own feelings.

Do try to draw others out if you think there are issues that need to be discussed between you.

Do ask how others feel about things, not just about events or facts.

Do try to be a good listener – give others time to respond and don't assume you already know what they are likely to say.

Do show interest and appreciation when someone is open with you, even if you don't always like what they say.

Do remember that it takes courage to talk about feelings, especially vulnerability or self-doubt. Be as supportive as you can.

Don't dispute what someone feels.

Don't criticise. If you have suggestions to make, phrase them positively and try to direct them at specific actions and behaviour, not directly at the other person.

EXPRESSING EMOTIONS

They say that women are more comfortable talking about their emotions than men. Is this really true? Is it a good thing?

Women and men experience similar feelings but often differ dramatically when it comes to showing them. In one study, participants were asked to write descriptions of themselves. Although men and women revealed about the same amount of information, the women's revelations were much more intimate. Despite social changes it still seems that women express feelings more readily.

There appear to be two exceptions however: anger and sexual arousal. In scientific experiments, when presented with situations designed to annoy them, men became angry but women said they felt hurt, disappointed or sad. When played erotic tapes, almost half the women denied being at all aroused, while all the men reported a sexual response. Social expectations, it seems, still make some men suppress sadness and some women suppress anger and sexuality.

Psychologists believe that such limitations are bad for both sexes. Men may be damaged by losing touch with softer emotions; while women suffer from 'personalising' the difficulties they encounter and blaming themselves unduly. Such different viewpoints often make it hard for men and women to communicate with each other.

CLASSIFYING DISORDERS

What is mental illness? What is the difference between psychosis and neurosis?

Human beings think, feel and behave in a huge variety of different ways. What is considered normal differs widely from person to person and culture to culture. Behaviour and mental processes have to be more than unusual to be considered a sign of disorder – they have to be destructive (to the person or to others) or to interfere significantly with the person's ability to function in society.

Psychosis and neurosis are two main groupings of mental disorder. Psychoses are serious illnesses, such as schizophrenia or paranoia, that involve loss of contact with reality and extreme abnormality of feelings, thoughts and actions. Psychotic patients are unable to cope with daily life and require intensive treatment, sometimes in hospital.

Neurosis is a general, rather vague term for nonpsychotic mental disorders that leave

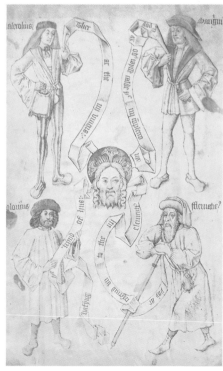

The four humours Since antiquity, attempts have been made to categorise mental traits according to a theory of types, or humours. This 15th-century manuscript shows (clockwise from top left) the four dispositions: melancholic (depressive), sanguine (confident), phlegmatic (unexcitable) and choleric (irritable). More sophisticated type theories are still in existence today.

the person's sense of reality intact but are still highly disruptive in daily life. They include depression, panic and anxiety attacks, compulsions, phobias, hypochondria and physical symptoms, such as blindness or paralysis, without a physical cause.

Mental illness is also categorised as either organic – connected with a brain disorder such as a stroke or tumour – or functional – affecting mental functions but without a physical cause. Psychologists also recognise

so-called personality disorders – such as a psychopathic or schizoid (highly eccentric) personality. In some ways, these are more like learning or developmental problems than mental illnesses.

In addition, it is known that after severe stress, mentally healthy people can temporarily show symptoms of illnesses such as depression and anxiety. This is not the same as having such an illness, since the cause is clear and the condition resolves naturally.

Developing yourself

STRENGTHENING YOUR MEMORY

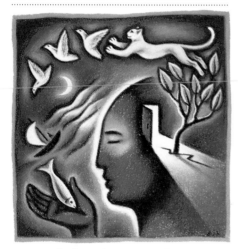

I seem to be becoming more and more forgetful as time passes. Is there any way of improving my memory?

This is a very common experience. Usually the problem arises with short-term memory as the mind tries to process and discard non-essential information as quickly as possible. Here are some tips to try.

● Learn to recognise situations where your memory lets you down and make a special effort to concentrate. You cannot expect to recall what you don't take in properly in the first place.
● Try not to rely on diaries, notes and lists, but make a point of committing things to memory instead. The more you practise remembering, the better you will get. If you keep a shopping list, read it through but don't take it to the shops with you – exercise your memory instead.
● Look for patterns when you have several items to remember, as for example, by

grouping a mental shopping list into meat, groceries and fresh produce, or by noting that you have three things to buy at the supermarket and three at the local shops.
● Recite to yourself the words you want to remember, accenting any rhythm or rhyme.
● Say things out loud to yourself or tell them to others while they are still fresh in your mind. There is nothing like having to reproduce information to make it stick.
● Try to visualise the objects or situations you want to remember, or try to imagine a name or a word written down, to involve your visual as well as your aural memory.

EFFECTIVE SELF-ASSERTION

I often let people walk all over me and then feel angry when it is too late. How can I learn to assert myself more effectively?

Standing up for your rights prevents hostility from building up. It also saves you from turning anger inwards against yourself. However you have been behaving it is never too late to start expressing your feelings and asserting yourself. If a troublesome situation has gone on for a long time, you can start by saying something like, 'I've been concerned about this for quite some time and...' or 'I've been meaning to talk to you about...'.

Being assertive does not mean you have to change your whole personality – just start taking responsibility for your feelings and express them. Focus your comments on how the situation makes you feel, not on blaming the other person. 'I'm angry...' or 'It really upsets me...' will get a better response than the more aggressive 'You make me cross when...'. When you have explained your point of view, offer a constructive suggestion about how you would like to see the situation improved.

Assertiveness training

Classes in assertiveness teach ways to defuse anger before it builds up and to improve communication with others. These are some of the basic strategies they recommend.

● Experiment with simple assertions first. Try telling a waiter your plate is cold before asking for a promotion at work or tackling your mother about treating you like a child.
● Use body language to help you. Make eye contact. Stand straight and tall, with your head up. Don't smile nervously or giggle when telling someone you are angry. Don't whisper or mumble – speak clearly.
● Choose a good time and a private place.
● Don't spend so much time worrying about the words to use that you put off speaking up. Expressing yourself imperfectly is better than missing your chance.
● Remember to listen to what the other person is saying. Don't focus so much on what you are getting off your chest that you miss the apology that was all you wanted anyway.

Are you a slave to habits?

Some habits (nail-biting, head-scratching) are harmless; others (compulsive eating, smoking) cause health problems. Some simple methods can help to weaken all of them.

● Learn how to relax. When you are tempted by, say, a fattening snack, sit down, close your eyes and practise the breathing and relaxation techniques described on pages 190-192. Take a few deep breaths. Remember that the urge will pass.
● Practise meditation, daydreaming, visualisation or some other form of mental relaxation.
● Reward yourself for small victories over your bad habit.
● Keep a sense of humour about the problem.
● List and analyse the reasons you want to stop smoking or drinking, for example, and any reasons you don't. Get a clear view of what the habit means to you and start thinking and talking of yourself as an ex-smoker or drinker.
● Avoid situations associated with your habit. If watching television is when you bite your nails, take a walk or read a book instead, or try doing exercises or knitting to keep your hands busy.
● If you cannot break your habit, at least limit the damage as far as possible. If you have to eat snacks, for example, make them healthy.

VALUING YOURSELF

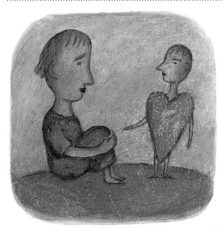

Friends tell me that I constantly put myself down, and it's true that I don't feel very confident. What causes low self-esteem? What can I do to build myself up?

Consciously or unconsciously we are all constantly talking to ourselves, sending private messages about who we are and how likely we are to get what we want and need. If the messages are more negative than positive, they can have the effect of lowering anyone's self-esteem. People caught in such a trap are in effect programming themselves to fail by giving themselves messages such as, 'I don't expect to get the job' or 'no one will want to talk to me at the party'. They go on to behave in accordance with what they expect to happen, so making it more likely that they really will fail, and reinforcing their destructive negative views.

To break the vicious circle, you need to change your way of thinking. Avoid seeing things as black or white with no room for grey areas, as this makes it hard to regard yourself as anything but either perfect or hopelessly inadequate. Be suspicious of the words *always* and *never*, which reflect the belief that you are fated to repeat the same mistakes over and over. We all know people who can listen to a litany of compliments and nevertheless fix on a single less-than-glowing comment. They sift through praise searching for criticism. Many of us have been trained from early on to discount successes and highlight failures. When we achieve something we undermine it, but when we fail we punish ourselves.

If this sounds familiar, try revising your internal conversations. The first step is to listen to yourself. The next time you are feeling unconfident, ask yourself what you are thinking. What was the last thought you had about yourself? Get a notebook and write down these thoughts, along with your feelings about them and some information about the situation that triggered them. Identify words like *all, nothing, always* or *never* and edit them out. Think through what is really true about the situation. If you made a mistake at work, is that really what you always do, or are you normally very competent? Revise your message to yourself by writing it out in your notebook. Then practise sending yourself more realistic and positive signals by consciously altering your interior monologues.

To build up your self-esteem, you must not only revise your thinking, but also act on the positive new messages you are sending yourself. If a colleague is undermining you at work, for example, or a partner constantly criticising, you will need to find ways to alter the situation by talking to them or changing aspects of your own behaviour. Don't expect everything to improve overnight, either. For most people building confidence is a lifelong process. Set yourself realistic goals and credit yourself for small changes along the way.

CONTROLLING YOUR TEMPER

I tend to lose my temper very easily and then regret it afterwards. Can a hot temper be controlled?

As natural as it may feel, a hair-trigger temper is not something you are born with, like red hair or freckles. It is a habit you have learned, and it can be unlearned.

In a provoking situation, the body reacts by releasing various hormones that heighten the emotional state. As hormones flood your system, your feelings are uncontrollably intensified, but how you interpret and respond to these feelings is determined by you, depending on the circumstances of the moment and on the habits you have developed. One man will react to a ball thrown through his living-room window by rushing out and shouting at the first child he sees. Another will find out who is to blame and talk calmly about paying for the damage.

No matter how hot your temper is, you can learn how to respond constructively and appropriately to anger.

● Think before you act. Count to ten before saying or doing anything in anger.
● Take a few deep breaths the next time you feel your temper starting to flare up.
● Try putting yourself in the place of the person who is making you angry. Maybe this

is a bad day for him or he is in pain or has personal problems you are unaware of.
● Develop a sense of humour. Few things are so serious there isn't a funny side.
● Reduce your general level of tension through yoga, meditation, exercise or the other anti-stress measures on pages 190-195.

BREAKING BAD HABITS

I'm incapable of getting anywhere on time. What can I do to change?

People who are always late may be expressing unconscious hostility. By making others wait you are in effect telling them that your time is more valuable than theirs. If this is creating difficulties in your business or social life think about why you are angry and how you could express your feelings in a more direct, positive way. What you are doing at the moment not only leads to missed appointments and disappointed or irritated friends and colleagues, but probably makes you feel constantly anxious and distracted yourself. Begin by recognising that everyone has bad habits and that, while it may not be easy, they can be changed. The first step should be a small, practical one. Perhaps you might sit down at a time when you can relax and jot down the experiences of a typical day. Analyse your schedule. Are you trying to accomplish too much? Are there any activities you could drop? Are there things you could do faster, or more efficiently? Are there small intervals of time that could be used for something practical?

Develop a habit of promptness one day at a time. Make your first goal a fairly easy one – getting to work on time or a little early, for example. Be realistic about accomplishing your goal and reward yourself for achieving it. If you fail or find you slip back into old habits, don't be put off – start again.

It will also help to seek out support. Find another friend who is also often late and make a bet, such as whoever turns up late for lunch pays the other's bill.

Sleep, dreams and hypnosis

WHY DO WE DREAM?

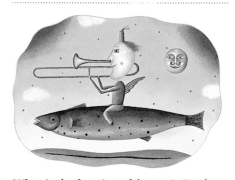

What is the function of dreams? Do they really mean anything or reveal deep-seated, unconscious emotions?

Sigmund Freud, the founder of psychoanalysis, called dreams the 'royal road' to the unconscious mind and believed that by interpreting them he could help his patients to discover and understand their deep, hidden drives, desires and emotions. So-called dream work continues to form an important part of the work of many psychologists, psychotherapists and counsellors. However, there are also many sceptics – including psychologists – who believe that dreams have no meaning. Despite numerous theories, few facts are known about the role of dreams and whether or not they have any health effects on body or mind.

What is known is that most dreams occur during light REM (rapid eye movement) sleep, when the nervous system is extremely active. REM sleep seems to help the mind to process information acquired during the day. This may explain why dreams so often reflect the day's events, albeit in a highly distorted or bizarre form.

Sleep and dreams may also have the effect of placing daytime experiences in perspective, helping us to cope better with problems and to come up with new ideas for dealing with them. If you have a problem to solve, the old adage 'sleep on it' may indeed be the best advice.

THE MEANING OF NIGHTMARES

Are nightmares a sign of some kind of emotional disturbance?

Not necessarily. New research shows that people have frightening dreams more often than they think they do (on average, once every two weeks) and that the frequency of bad dreams bears no relationship to waking levels of anxiety. Younger people have more

Recording dreams

If you are interested in dreams, but have trouble remembering them, the techniques below may be helpful.

● Keep a dream diary by your bed. Write down what you remember as soon as you wake in the morning and also if you wake during the night.
● Repeat to yourself before going to bed, 'I am going to remember my dreams tonight'.
● Read over the previous night's dreams before turning out the light.
● If you want to re-experience a particular dream, try to relive it in your imagination before going to sleep. Imagine how it might develop.
● Relate your dreams to someone else while they are still fresh in your mind. Explaining to a third party often brings back forgotten details.

troubled dreams, and frequency tapers off
with age. From the age of eight until the late
twenties, people report ten times as many
nightmares as in midlife. Children younger
than eight are more prone to night terrors –
dreams that cause panic so vivid that they
wake up screaming. There is nothing wrong,
but such children need comforting.

Also distinct from the occasional bad
dream, and more troublesome, are chronic
nightmares. These dreams are often lifelike
and detailed, with richly observed colours,
sounds, pains, tastes and smells. Dreamers
may become someone else in their nightmares or even another species of animal.
They have dreams within dreams and, once
awake, it often takes them a long time to
shake off the dream. In extreme cases it can
take the dreamer 30 minutes or more to
work out whether he is asleep or awake.

The latest theories pinpoint a personality
type associated with chronic nightmares –
so-called thin-boundaried people. They are
unusually open to outside influences and
are also more than usually introspective and
vulnerable. Often artistic and imaginative,
they do not deal with negative emotions as
quickly as most people but allow fears and
angers to grow and become more intense.

In some extreme cases, the fluid emotional states of thin-boundaried people can
resemble schizophrenia. And a small but significant number of people who suffer from
chronic nightmares do show some symptoms of schizophrenia or have a family history of schizophrenia or, less frequently,
some other type of mental disorder. Despite
this, many cope perfectly well on their own,
and they do not necessarily need any form of
treatment. But if nightmares are often so
vivid that the dreamer wakes in terror and is
afraid to go back to sleep, or if fear of nightmares keeps a person from falling asleep,
therapy can help.

Another type of nightmare is the so-called
post-traumatic nightmare that occurs after a
particularly stressful or upsetting experience,
such as witnesssing an accident or being
assaulted. These are quite different from
chronic nightmares. They most often occur
during the first stages of the sleep cycle
(most other nightmares occur during the
early hours of the morning), and their content directly reflects what the dreamer has
been through. At first the trauma is re-
enacted in realistic detail but as the event
recedes in memory, the dreams become less
upsetting. This is thought to be a natural
healing process that slowly helps people to
get over a traumatic experience.

DAYDREAMING

*Our daughter seems to spend a lot of time
daydreaming. Is this unhealthy?*

Certainly not – provided it is not interfering
with her concentration at school and she is
happy and well-adjusted in other ways.

Once considered a waste of time, daydreaming is now thought to be emotionally
healthy, useful for stress relief by taking our
minds off problems, and also a practical way
of dealing with problems creatively.

Psychologists believe that the two sides of
the brain have rather different functions,
with the left side generally believed to control logical thinking, reason, mathematical
and scientific abilities, and the right in
charge of emotions, intuition and artistic
expression. When you daydream, the theory
goes, you are getting in touch with the right
side of the brain and so drawing on imaginative abilities that you may be suppressing
most of the time in daily life.

Your daughter sounds as if she is one of
those who by nature favours right-brain
thinking. Nevertheless, pay her some special
attention and make sure that nothing is
troubling her. Unless this is recent or
unusual behaviour, there is probably nothing to worry about. If there are any problems, you will almost certainly notice other
signs, such as poor schoolwork, difficulty in
forming friendships or general withdrawal.

CAN HYPNOSIS CURE?

*I sometimes see advertisements in which
hypnotists claim to offer help with
overeating, smoking and other problems.
Does the treatment work and is it safe?*

The kind of problems hypnotherapists deal
with all tend to involve a large component of
anxiety. They may be habits and addictions
(such as compulsive eating or smoking,
where anxiety wells up if food or cigarettes
are avoided for long) or aversions (such as
phobias, where the patient becomes anxious
if he or she *cannot* avoid something). Some
patients also turn to hypnotherapy for help
with pain control during childbirth or dentistry, or for help with conditions such as
asthma and migraine.

The idea behind hypnotherapy is to help
patients to achieve a deeply relaxed state in
in which they can come to understand and
control their behaviour, and become more
receptive to positive suggestions. As treatment progresses, self-help techniques such

as autosuggestion and self-hypnosis may be taught to help patients to cope on their own. Success rates are hard to measure and some people are more susceptible than others, but many doctors and psychologists do accept that hypnosis can significantly reduce anxiety, relieve pain and play a part in treating many conditions. Provided you consult a reputable, trained therapist, it is considered safe. Don't go by advertisements, but instead contact the British Society of Medical and Dental Hypnosis, 151 Otley Old Road, Leeds LS16 6HN, or the British Society of Experimental and Clinical Hypnosis, Psychology Department, Grimsby General Hospital, Scartho Road, Grimsby DN33 2BA.

Friendship, love and marriage

WHY FRIENDS MATTER

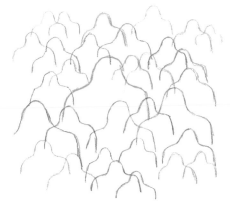

I've always enjoyed being by myself. Is having a large number of friends a necessary component of mental health?

People do need people. A time and place for solitude exists in everyone's life, and a quiet walk in the woods or a meditative afternoon on a deserted beach can be delightful, but too much isolation is not good for either your mental or your physical health. The true loner, the hermit who habitually prefers only his own company to that of others, is a rare individual.

A solid network of family and friends can help you to deal with stress and make it less likely that you will suffer from depression, anxiety or other mental health problems. A rewarding social life has also been found to increase longevity and lower the risk of developing cancer, heart disease and other major illnesses.

On scales of psychological satisfaction, friendships generally rank lower than stable marriages as a source of happiness but higher than work or leisure pursuits. Friendships are usually strongest in childhood, from adolescence until marriage, and again in old age, when retirement and bereavement can decrease other social attachments.

Psychologists believe that the reason women usually adjust better than men after divorce or the death of a spouse is largely the result of their broader social networks.

Exactly how friendship influences mental and physical health is not completely clear. One theory is that friends act as buffers, protecting one another from stress and nurturing one another's self-esteem.

LOVE OR INFATUATION

My daughter and her boyfriend are talking about getting married, but I'm worried that this is infatuation rather than true love. Is there a way to tell?

Only your daughter can decide whether this is the relationship for her. However, there are points you could look for or gently raise in conversation.

● Do your daughter and her boyfriend have similar backgrounds and attitudes?
● Do they like doing things together and share some of the same interests?
● Do they share similar views about relationships, marriage and children?
● Have they discussed their common goals?
● Would they be friends even if they were not in love?

Talk to your daughter about her intention to marry. Remind her that, as time goes on, romantic love must deepen into something stronger and more flexible. Differences ignored during the 'in love' phase may surface later to cause deep rifts. The issues can be as superficial as sharing housework or as serious as beliefs about how to bring up children. After the first flush fades, what often counts in a marriage is the degree to which partners share interests, beliefs, goals and commitments. Considering these now and building them up could well prevent boredom or disillusionment setting in at some time in the future.

181

DO'S AND DON'TS

for a healthy marriage

Do discuss joint hopes and plans.

Do agree 'ground rules' for everyday practicalities and chores, but remain flexible.

Do combine shared interests and friends.

Do keep up some separate pursuits.

Do share everyday affectionate gestures.

Do try to express your thoughts and feelings honestly.

Do accept your partner's right to feelings and opinions that differ from your own.

Do listen carefully and make sure you understand what your partner has to say about an important issue.

Do state what you want rather than complaining or accusing.

Do deal with problems as they arise.

Do set aside regular time to be together.

Don't let certain problems dominate the relationship.

Don't let courtesy slip just because you are married to each other.

Don't get out of the habit of talking to each other about things other than domestic issues.

Don't criticise sexual performance in a row.

Don't expect a partner to read your mind.

Don't make assumptions about your partner's beliefs, emotions or experiences.

Don't drag up events from the past or settled issues in arguments.

ATTRACTION TO OTHERS

I love my partner very much but still find myself attracted to other people from time to time. Is there something wrong with our relationship, or with me?

It is quite normal for men and women in stable, long-term relationships or marriages to find people other than their partner attractive and sexually stimulating. Indeed, many have sexual fantasies about film stars, people they see in the street or even friends and colleagues. It does not usually mean that they have any intention of being unfaithful or that there is anything wrong with their relationship. These fantasies are simply a harmless way of experiencing something different. However, if a particular person becomes the focus of your fantasies, or if you are strongly tempted to *act* on your feelings, it could be that aspects of your relationship need attention.

SURVIVING AN AFFAIR

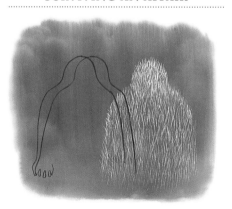

Can a marriage ever be the same after one of the partners has had an affair?

No. Even if an affair remains undiscovered, the deceit involved will inevitably have changed the relationship. Equally, the discovery of an affair is usually a shattering emotional experience. But even though most people consider infidelity the greatest potential threat to a relationship, statistics show that more couples stay together than part after an affair.

Most infidelity stems from a serious desire to leave the marriage or a desperate protest at aspects of the relationship that are causing unhappiness. A couple's willingness to deal with the underlying issues is the crucial factor in determining whether the relationship survives or not. If both partners want to mend the rift, they must discuss what happened, and go on doing so, perhaps for some time. Counselling can often help couples to confront problems and feelings in a constructive way. Many counsellors advise their clients to set aside a time each week to talk about the affair, so that it does not intrude into every area of life.

If the problems can be dealt with, the marriage may emerge stronger than before, but it will never be the same: readjustment, rebuilding trust and becoming close again will take a long time. Also, the old marriage that has gone needs to be grieved for: after an affair, the partners are effectively starting a new relationship.

WHEN ARGUING NEVER STOPS

My partner and I seem to be arguing more and more. Is this a sign that our relationship is in danger?

This depends on how and why you argue. It may be simply that one partner is under pressure and has become irritable. Perhaps one of you overreacts to things the other says or does, because they act as subconscious reminders of past traumas. Alternatively, a major event, such as having a baby or moving house, may have revealed differences that you need to discuss, particularly if one partner is secretly unhappy but feels too guilty or confused to talk about it.

Sometimes one particular issue, such as money or jealousy, causes deep unhappiness and provokes constant arguments. Other couples begin to bicker when one or both of them starts to feel that the marriage has not lived up to expectations but does not know how to go about improving it.

If the arguments are about important issues that affect you both, you need to ask whether harmony between you is important enough for you both to work at finding a compromise. If you find that arguments about trivial issues become major rows or if you argue about everything – or, equally, about nothing in particular – then there are probably much deeper underlying reasons for the anger your flare-ups are expressing.

The first step is to see if together you can pinpoint a specific problem. If not, take time separately to think about what could be wrong. Try writing down your thoughts, and look for links with similar feelings in the past. Then set aside time to sit down and talk as calmly and frankly as you can. A period of relationship counselling (see opposite) may help you to work out and resolve any underlying problems between you.

MARRIAGE GUIDANCE

I've heard a lot of talk about marriage guidance, but know nothing about it. What exactly is it and who is it suitable for? Where is it available?

If problems in a marriage seem insoluble or you have reached the stage where one or both of you is questioning whether it is worth staying together, an expert counsellor can often help you to see the issues in a clearer light. The British marriage guidance organisation Relate estimates that more than half of all the couples they see stay together, and that those who do separate do so with less animosity.

You do not need to be married to get help. Some counsellors will see whole families together, while some people go for individual counselling. Individual sessions may be because the spouse will not go (although often the reluctant partner joins in later) or because the person wants to talk about relationships that have broken down or experiences in the past.

If necessary, couples can be referred to specialists for other types of help, such as psychosexual counselling.

A consultation usually lasts about an hour. Many problems can be resolved in six sessions or less, while more serious difficulties may take rather longer. All consultations are strictly confidential. Demand for counselling is high and in many areas counsellors have long waiting lists. Relate tries to offer an immediate 'crisis' interview even if you have to join a waiting list for regular sessions. Fees vary depending on the client's income and no one is turned away because they cannot pay.

Your nearest counselling centre can be found in the telephone book under 'Relate' or 'Marriage Guidance'.

THE EFFECTS OF DIVORCE

Everyone seems to think that divorce is easier on middle-aged men than on women, but I am finding it very stressful. Am I unusual?

You certainly are not. Divorce at any age is hard on men as well as women. Initially, both partners suffer largely from the loss of each other's emotional support. Following a divorce, women who have not had a career of their own but have devoted themselves to caring for the family are likely to have a harder time financially than men, and often find themselves worse off than when married. Women are also more often left with the responsibilities of caring single-handedly for the children.

When men are the ones to leave the family home, however, they too tend to find themselves worse off financially than before. Having limited contact with their children can be an equal source of suffering for men as for women, though it is not always recognised as such by society in general. In addition, men who are the sole breadwinners can find themselves with the financial burden of having to support two families if they want to remarry. This can create deep resentment and hostility and even undermine the success of the second marriage.

Men who initiate divorce tend to feel better, but most divorces are instigated by women. For some men it comes as a shock, particularly if they have not noticed signs of dissatisfaction. Many women do their emotional separating before the break-up, while men more often have to cope with acute feelings of loss afterwards. Women may also have stronger relationships with family and friends to help them through difficult times, and so tend to manage better emotionally as single people.

In most spheres – happiness, mental health, career success – marriage is very good for men, but less so for women. So despite appearances and assumptions, men generally have more to lose in a divorce. More men suffer mental health problems after divorce, with 63 per cent reporting symptoms such as despair, helplessness, mood swings, withdrawal and even suicidal thoughts.

Relationships in trouble

Many problems can be put right if couples become aware of them in time. These are some signs of trouble.

- Arguments – try to find compromises. If disputes persist, consider counselling.
- Possessiveness – abnormal jealousy or possessiveness indicates insecurity and a destructive desire for control. Underlying problems may need help.
- Infidelity – affairs are often a sign of marital unhappiness. The issues need to be discussed and time allowed for healing.
- A 'difficult' child – sometimes the real problem lies with the parents. Such families need professional help.
- Growing apart – developing as an individual as well as a couple is healthy. Not sharing your thoughts and experiences can mean trouble.

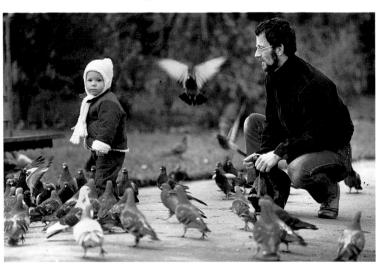

Staying in touch Ongoing contact with their children can help both parents get over a divorce, however they feel about each other. Normal pleasures such as a day at the park will build stronger ties than special treats or extravagant presents.

Coping with divorce

The stress of divorce is outweighed only by the death of a spouse, but there are practical ways to make coping easier.

● Keep channels of communication open and try to remain on at least polite and cooperative terms with your ex-partner.
● Obtain good legal advice early on – preferably from a member of the Solicitor's Family Law Association, P.O. Box 302, Orpington, Kent BR6 8QX. Members favour a non-hostile approach to divorce, especially where children are concerned.
● If you have children, put their interests first and agree amicable arrangements for regular access by the parent they will not be living with.

FACING LIFE ALONE

I'm in the throes of a messy divorce. Are there any ways to make it easier?

Divorce is extremely painful and is second in the ratings of life stress (see page 189). Most people experience very similar emotions to mourning – disbelief, anger and sadness – before they can accept what has happened and move on. These emotions accentuate the strangeness of living alone, made worse for most people by reduced social contacts as mutual friends take sides and shared activities are abandoned. Having to deal with domestic tasks which your partner used to undertake can create resentment, self-pity and feelings of inadequacy. If you have children or financial difficulties you may feel overloaded or exhausted. Loneliness, fatigue and stress tend to increase both brooding on the past and panic about the future.

Give yourself time and try not to contemplate the distant future too much until your divorce is a year or more behind you – it takes at least this long to adjust. Some tips that may help right now include:

● Find someone else in the same boat (about one in four households in Britain comprise a single person) to share the load.
● Contact a divorced or single parent group.
● Summon all your courage and enterprise to cope with problems in day-to-day living – each time you cope with a challenge it becomes less threatening.
● Don't be afraid to ask for help and support – draw in family and friends as much as possible in the early days.
● Get out of the house every day if possible, and meet people – through work, studying, hobbies, community and voluntary work, sports and leisure pursuits.
● Take up activities you can do at home – reading, needlework, mending motorcycles, but avoid resorting to extra television, which can make you lethargic and isolated.
● Confide in others.
● Don't pry into your ex-partner's new life.
● Make the atmosphere at home pleasant – redecorate, play music, cook good meals.
● Keep up your appearance, even if only you appreciate it.
● Give yourself treats, especially on special occasions such as birthdays and Christmas.
● Don't embark on a new relationship just because you are desperate for company.
● Mourn for what is gone, then put the past behind you and move on. Try not to see the marriage as a total failure just because it ended – try to remember the happy times.
● When you feel able, try to assess what went wrong and how you can learn from your mistakes.

Healthy attitudes at work

PROBLEMS WOMEN FACE

I've been accused of being abrasive at work, but my male colleagues are rewarded for the same behaviour. How can I reconcile my natural competitiveness with my employer's expectations of 'feminine' work habits?

This is a two-sided problem involving your behaviour and his. Accepting women in positions of authority can still be difficult for some men. Sexual stereotypes can be laid very early in childhood and overcoming them is not possible for everyone. Even today some men perceive ambitious women as tough, pushy and dominant, and their fears may go very deep. Unfair or not, it is realistic to recognise that as a woman you may, even in the modern world, find yourself judged by different standards from men.

The best policy is one of honesty coupled with tact. Be assertive but not hostile. Go after your goals calmly and directly. Camouflaging your ambitions or adopting a more traditionally feminine approach will not work. If you change your behaviour as a result of others' prejudices, you are more likely to reinforce them than change them.

Instead, you need to balance your image carefully. Take your employer's (and your coworkers') feelings into consideration and respond sensitively and respectfully to others' needs, but do not sacrifice your legitimate aims to them. If you have to criticise others, try to do so in a constructive, nonjudgmental way, directing your comments at the work rather than at the person. Make sure your employer knows that you are a valuable member of his team and is aware of the work you are doing.

Behaving like this is not being aggressive or abrasive, but should win you respect and professional recognition. If your employer continues to treat you differently from your

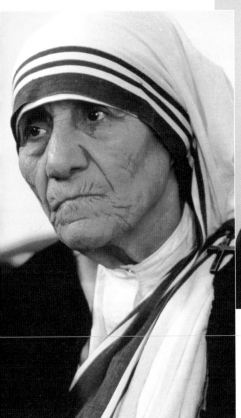

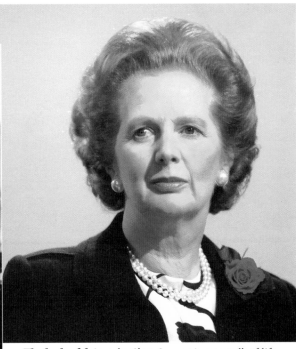

The look of determination Success in any walk of life depends on energy, drive and willpower to see things through. In their different ways, both Margaret Thatcher (above) and Mother Theresa (left) exemplify such qualities.

male colleagues, calmly point out the discrepancy to him. If he still does not change and the situation is holding you back, it may then be worth considering a move.

RESPONDING TO CRITICISM

My employer can be very critical and I sometimes find his comments difficult to take. Are there better ways to cope?

Criticism is never easy to take, particularly if you let it affect your self-esteem. It is easier said than done, but try not to take every critical comment to heart or let others' judgments sway you unduly. Remember, in the end your own judgment matters most.

Criticism is easiest to take when delivered privately in a respectful way. If it sounds like a parental telling-off or is done in public, it is much harder to concentrate on any value the advice has. But it can be done.

The way to use criticism constructively is to put aside all emotional responses and to concentrate on information that could be of use in furthering your own aims. Consider if there are rewards you will reap by changing. Then develop reasonable goals and take practical steps to achieve them.

COPING WITH FAILURE

I've been passed over for a job I expected to get and badly wanted. How can I use the experience constructively?

Don't label yourself a failure because you lost out on one promotion – the only people who never fail are those who never take chances. Pessimists see failure as defeat, but optimists see it as an opportunity to learn and to try again. Try to separate your emotional reaction to losing out from the reality of what occurred. If you analyse what went wrong, the incident could yield some valuable lessons: how to present yourself better, how to develop an argument, how to use the right timing to ask for and get what you want. The sooner you put your loss into perspective, the better you will feel.

● Be objective. If you lost the job because you lack a qualification or a particular skill, take steps immediately to acquire it.
● If your credentials are impeccable, how do you get along with others at work? Success in business can depend as much on politics, strategy and human relations as on ability.
● If you are not advancing fast enough, consider a change. Maybe another company would offer more opportunities to get ahead, or maybe a new line of work would suit you better.

If you lose your job

● Analyse what happened and what you can learn from it.
● Think of this as a chance to make changes you may have been afraid to try before.
● Take advantage of any services you are offered, such as counselling or aptitude testing.
● Keep up normal standards and routines. Don't eat, drink or smoke more than usual, or stop exercising. Don't avoid friends or watch daytime television.
● View the quest for work as a full-time job. If you have the use of an office, go to it every day. If not, set yourself up at home and keep regular office hours.
● Use the local library to look for advertisements in newspapers and other publications.

185

Help for workers

● The Equal Opportunities Commission will investigate claims of sexual and racial discrimination at work, and other forms of unfair treatment. Contact them at Overseas House, Quay Street, Manchester M3 3HN.

● Vocational guidance can help people unsure of the next step in their career. Advice can be obtained from CASCAID Unit, County Hall, Glenfield, Leicester LE3 8RF or from the Careers and Occupational Centre, Moorfoot, Sheffield, South Yorkshire S1 4PQ. Alternatively, you can get in touch with private careers counsellors through the British Association for Counselling (for address, see page 215).

SPEAKING IN PUBLIC

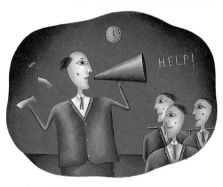

My fear of public speaking is beginning to affect my career. What can I do about it?

Almost everyone hates to speak in public. In one recent poll, public speaking surpassed flying, loneliness and even death as the experience people feared most.

With that in mind, here are some commonsense tips for effective and relatively painless public speaking.

● Practise in front of your friends or members of your family. Ask them to tell you when you are coming across effectively and when you are not.
● Record your next presentation on tape or video in advance, to hear or see yourself from the audience's point of view. Look out for special strengths you may be able to capitalise more on, and for weaker points where you may be able to improve.
● Keep your speech well organised and clearly focused on the important issues.

Make it short and simple and do not try to fit in everything you know. Remember that studies show audiences will absorb only one or two main points.

● The first few moments on stage are usually the worst. Clear your throat before you get up to talk. Take a few deep breaths to relax while you are being introduced. When you rise to speak, smile, thank your introducer and then wait. Do not begin to speak until everyone in the audience is giving you their undivided attention.
● Establish eye contact with three friendly looking faces – one towards the back of the room, one to your left, and one to your right. As you glance from one to another your eyes will sweep the room, giving everyone the impression that they are being spoken to personally.
● Use your hands to control anxiety. Moving slightly and making gestures will help you to relax, but try not to wave your hands in front of your face. Avoid clenching your fists or gripping the podium tightly.
● If you begin your speech with a joke, be sure it is actually funny. One of the fastest ways to alienate an audience is with a joke that falls flat. It is safer to start with an intriguing rhetorical question to arouse their curiosity.
● Consider your tone of voice. Clipped, staccato speech patterns can make you sound tense or authoritarian. If you end a sentence on a higher note you will seem to be asking for agreement – lower your voice to sound more sure of yourself. Concentrating on your voice can also help you to forget your nerves.

Dealing with stress

RECOGNISING THE SIGNS

What is stress and how do I recognise it?

The word *stress* is used to describe both external events that make demands on us, and the internal responses they trigger. Stressful life experiences range from trivial everyday annoyances (a rude driver cuts in front of you, or the baby tips over a carton of milk) to major life-altering crises (the loss of a job, a divorce, the death of a family member). Surveys suggest that a high percentage of the population feels regularly under stress.

Stress can be caused by any number of factors – changes in your life, either good or bad; personal problems; illness; lack of sleep; or overwork. Whether or not an event causes stress depends less on what the event is than on how well you feel able to cope with it. A small problem you are powerless to resolve may cause far more stress than a big issue that you know you can deal with.

Physical and psychological stresses are a fact of life. What matters are the amounts you face and the nature of your response. If your enjoyment of life is hampered by stress – if your relationships suffer, your sleep is disrupted, your appetite changes, your sense of physical wellbeing deteriorates – your body may be sending you warning signals that you are under too much stress.

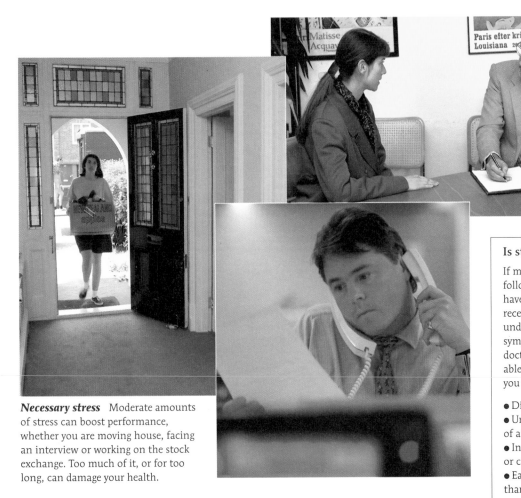

Necessary stress   Moderate amounts of stress can boost performance, whether you are moving house, facing an interview or working on the stock exchange. Too much of it, or for too long, can damage your health.

HOW THE BODY RESPONDS

What are the physical effects of being under stress? Can continuing stress cause health problems?

Certain stressful situations may set off what is known as the fight-or-flight response (see page 188). When it perceives a crisis, the brain sends out an alarm signal by means of chemical messengers called neurotransmitters. These signals from the brain trigger the production of hormones whose function is to put the body on the alert and prepare it to cope with trouble. Your pulse rate accelerates, your heart pounds, your knees may shake, and your stomach may become upset.

Some of the hormones that are released in response to stressful situations, especially adrenaline, also have the effect of stimulating the immune system. While moderate short-term stress may actually hasten the healing process, high levels experienced over an extended period deplete your supplies of stress-related hormones, slowing down the immune response and eventually making you more vulnerable to disease. Research into the functioning of the immune system is turning out to support the view that emotional states such as being under stress are indeed closely related to physical illness. Doctors have long suspected that stress is a contributing factor to such conditions as ulcers, high blood pressure, asthma and migraine. There is now increasing evidence that stress makes people more susceptible to infectious diseases and may even hasten the progression of some chronic and degenerative conditions such as rheumatoid arthritis.

The circulatory system is particularly sensitive to stress. In one recent study, cardiac patients were asked to speak publicly about personal habits that they considered to be faults. As they did so, the flow of blood in their arteries was measurably reduced (long-term diminished blood flow can be a cause of heart disease). Other studies show that newly widowed men face a significantly greater risk of heart disease. Along with the stress of bereavement, many of these men also suffered from loneliness and social isolation. Those who remarried, experienced a significantly decreased risk.

It is important to remember, however, that while stress may contribute to illness, it is rarely the sole cause.

Is stress a problem?

If more than a few of the following symptoms have affected you recently, you may be under stress. Report the symptoms to your doctor, who should be able to help, or advise you where to get help.

- Disturbed sleep.
- Unexplained feelings of anxiety.
- Indigestion, diarrhoea or constipation.
- Eating more or less than usual.
- Muscle tics.
- Carelessness or being accident prone.
- Tension in the neck or the shoulders.
- Difficulty in thinking clearly or in concentrating.
- Waking up tired.
- Irritability, tearfulness or sudden changes in your mood.
- Smoking or drinking more than usual.
- Withdrawal from other people.
- Feeling that you are unable to cope.
- Dry mouth or throat.
- Decreased sex drive.
- Continual aches, pains and minor ailments.
- Indecisiveness.
- Taking time off work or performing badly.
- Generally worrying about health.

FIGHT OR FLIGHT – THE NATURAL REACTION TO STRESS

When confronted by acute physical or psychological stress, the brain triggers a chain reaction that prepares the body to fight the perceived threat or to flee from it. Though essential to survival in life-threatening situations and often useful when dealing with challenges such as deadlines at work, the fight-or-flight response is less appropriate for dealing with more routine stresses. If triggered often enough, it can lead to serious health problems. These are some of the effects.

- The brain perceives some form of impending danger.
- Signals from the brain cause the adrenal glands to produce fight-or-flight hormones such as adrenaline and noradrenaline, which speed up heart and breathing rates and muscle response.
- Kidney function is reduced as less blood is available to the kidneys.
- Muscle fibres contract to prepare for sudden movement.
- The pupils of the eyes dilate.
- The salivary glands stop secreting saliva and the mouth feels dry.
- Skin becomes pale as surface blood vessels contract to direct more blood to muscles.
- Sweat production increases in order to counteract overheating.
- Heart rate increases to supply more blood to muscles.
- Blood pressure rises.
- Breathing rate increases to supply more oxygen to muscles.
- The liver increases its output of sugar and fat to fuel the muscles.
- Digestion slows or ceases.
- Tightened muscles stop urination and defecation.

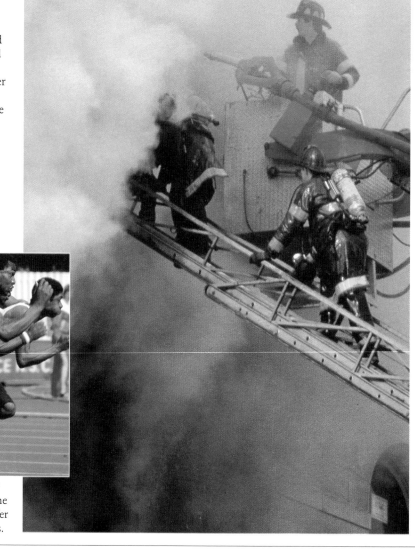

Hormones in action Physical activity helps to dissipate stress hormones – one reason why desk-bound executives suffer worse effects than firemen or sprinters.

AFTER A CRISIS

I have heard that people who have been through a harrowing event, such as an assault, accident or war, can suffer from a particular type of stress. What is this? Does it need treatment?

After a person has been through a shocking or life-threatening experience, he or she may well develop debilitating psychological or physiological symptoms – collectively known as post-traumatic stress disorder (PTSD). Research suggests that even a single incident of overwhelming terror can alter the chemistry of the brain and trigger subsequent adrenaline surges during which victims experience anxiety attacks, mental confusion, frightening flashbacks and other symptoms.

Most people are aware of the problems soldiers face in readjusting after a war ends, but post-traumatic stress has also been observed in survivors of earthquakes, fires and other disasters; people who have suffered major accidents; and in victims of violent assaults. The most severe cases arise when the threat to life or safety was overwhelming and when all sense of personal control was lost.

Whether a particular person develops PTSD seems to depend, at least partially, on the strength of the support he or she receives from others. Rape victims who are criticised or feel rejected by a spouse or partner are more likely to develop PTSD than those who

Someone to talk to Specially trained women police officers can offer counselling to victims of rape and other harrowing experiences.

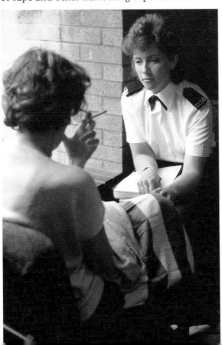

feel supported. People whose responses to a traumatic event are very defensive, especially those who deny the significance of the trauma or who refuse to talk about it, may also be at greater risk.

Time alone does help most people to overcome PTSD, and counselling or psychotherapy is also often effective. Drug companies are currently working to develop medicines that can reduce PTSD symptoms. If drugs can help sufferers to sleep better or to feel less anxious, psychologists hope counselling or psychotherapy for emotional problems may become even more effective. Cognitive and behavioural types of therapy (see page 212), in which the patient repeatedly relives the traumatic event, have proven useful in relieving PTSD symptoms in rape victims.

MEASURING STRESS

The Holmes-Rahe stress scale was devised by two American researchers. A score of more than 150 points for the past year means you have a 50 per cent chance of developing a stress-related illness in the near future. If you score more than 300 the chance increases to 90 per cent.

Death of a spouse or partner	100
Divorce	73
Marital separation	65
Serving a jail sentence	63
Death of a close relative	63
Serious illness or injury	53
Marriage	50
Loss of job	47
Marital reconciliation	45
Retirement	45
Change in family member's health	44
Pregnancy	40
Sexual difficulties	39
New baby or family member	39
Significant change in financial state	37
Death of a close friend	36
Changing line of work	35
More domestic arguments	35
High mortgage	31
Foreclosure of mortgage or loan	30
More or less responsibility at work	29
Child leaving home	29
Friction with in-laws	29
Outstanding achievement	28
Spouse starting or ending work	26
Starting or completing education	26
Trouble with employer	23
Change in working habits	20
Moving house	20

Help for the victims of crime

Being physically, sexually or emotionally harassed or assaulted can cause profound distress, especially for people who feel they have no one to turn to. No victim has to cope alone, however – help is available from many different sources.

Domestic violence
In an emergency, dial 999. At other times, contact your local police station and ask for the Domestic Violence Unit, which will have specially trained staff available to help. Calls are treated confidentially and women can ask to speak to a female officer if they wish.

Malicious telephone calls
At the time, keep calm, show no emotion and never reveal any details about yourself. Replace the receiver immediately. Report calls to the police and if the problem persists contact British Telecom on 150 for advice.

Violent crime and rape
Contact the police immediately. The Rape Crisis Centre also operates a helpline on 0171 837 7509.

Victim support
To be put in touch with a support group in your area contact the National Association of Victim Support Schemes, Cramer House, 39 Brixton Road, London SW9 6DZ.

Learning how to relax

STRESS evolved as an important aid to survival. It is a natural mechanism that triggers fight-or-flight responses when danger threatens. But the very same responses that once protected our ancestors from physical danger can actually be harmful in the modern world – where few problems can be dealt with either by head-on aggression or by running away.

We cannot easily change the challenges that we face in day-to-day life, but we can change the way we react to them. Stress experts advise that we start by learning to live 'in the moment' – that is, being aware of and improving our state of mind in the present. Since almost all feelings of anxiety are directed at past or future events, this is an effective way of reducing stress.

The simple but effective techniques on the pages that follow have been designed to give quick relief from stress, or for use as part of a daily relaxation routine.

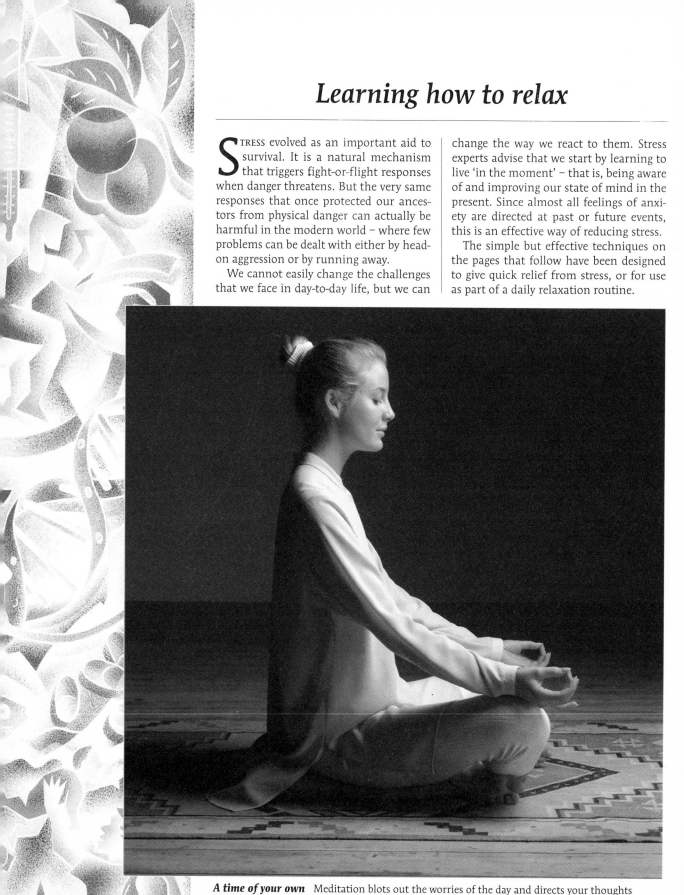

A time of your own Meditation blots out the worries of the day and directs your thoughts inwards. Choose a quiet room where you won't be disturbed and wear loose, comfortable clothes.

CONTROLLING YOUR BREATHING

Breathing patterns are directly related to the stress response and can both indicate and influence your emotional state. In particular, emotional stress leads to shallow breathing from the chest, which makes anxiety worse and reduces your energy level. In order to ensure the correct exchange of oxygen and carbon dioxide in the lungs you need to learn to breathe more deeply – and to use the diaphragm instead of the chest muscles.

To practise diaphragmatic breathing, lie flat with one hand on your chest and one on your abdomen. Breathe slowly through your nose, keeping your mouth closed. As you inhale, allow the air to push your abdomen up so that your hand rises. Hold each in-breath for a couple of seconds, and as you exhale feel your abdomen deflate and your hand fall. The hand on your chest should be almost stationary. Repeat a few times. You can also try this exercise sitting and standing up until it becomes natural.

RELAXATION TECHNIQUES

Muscular tension commonly occurs when stress makes the nervous system overactive. Similarly, learning to relax your muscles will help to relax your mind. It will also reduce your heart rate and blood pressure. There are two main techniques, and both are easily learned. Practise them either lying down or sitting in a straight-backed chair with your feet flat and your hands resting in your lap. Spend about 15 minutes on each – preferably after work or just before going to bed.

Progressive muscular relaxation (PMR)

Close your eyes and direct your attention to each part of your body in turn. As you do so, tense the muscles of the area and hold for five seconds, then release and totally relax the muscles. Concentrate on the sensation of warmth and heaviness you will experience for about ten seconds.

Start with your feet: clench up your toes, then tense your calves by pointing and then flexing your feet. Move on up the legs, tightening the thigh muscles, the buttocks and the abdomen. Continue by clenching your hands, flexing your arms, shrugging up your shoulders, and then moving your chin up and down. Finally, screw up your face, open your mouth and eyes wide, and then let go. Now be alert to your breathing, making sure that it comes from the diaphragm. Be aware of your deep state of relaxation, and enjoy the sense of stillness.

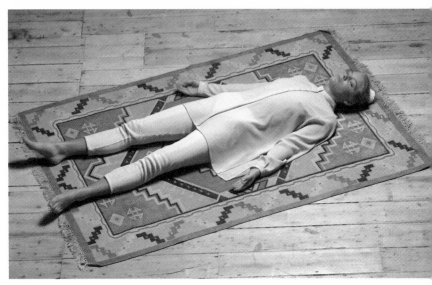

Draining away tension Use the so-called corpse position for practising muscular relaxation. Keep head, neck and back in alignment, feet about 18 in (45 cm) apart, and hands upturned and held slightly away from the body.

Deep muscular relaxation (DMR)

Use the same routine as for PMR, but without tensing. Focus only on relaxing by directing your attention to each set of muscles in turn, feeling them become weak and heavy.

HOW MEDITATION HELPS

Meditation techniques allow you to achieve a deep state of calmness and serenity while remaining alert. It also causes your oxygen requirement, breathing rate, heart rate and blood pressure to drop, and your muscles to relax. It is particularly beneficial for people with high blood pressure, chest complaints such as asthma, and muscular pain. It can also help against insomnia, as brain wave patterns during meditation are similar to those of sleep. Practised regularly, it can also lead to a more relaxed general view of life. There are numerous different techniques, including so-called mindfulness meditation and visualisation.

'Mindfulness' meditation

The idea is to relax the mind by concentrating on one aspect of the present moment. One way of doing this is to sit either cross-legged on the floor or upright in a straight-backed chair with your feet placed flat on the ground, hands in your lap, head straight and eyes closed. Begin with a few minutes of muscle relaxation and slow, diaphragmatic breathing. Then quieten your mind either by sliently repeating to yourself a simple sound known as a mantra – 'ohm' or 'one' is often

Massaging for stress

Massage is one of the oldest therapies known to man and has been practised since at least 3000 BC as a way of improving physical and mental health.

The best way of finding a practitioner is through personal recommendation or at the suggestion of your doctor. Do not simply take a name from an advertisement as treatment from an unqualified person could be harmful.

Equally, before attempting to give anyone a massage, it is advisable to learn the correct techniques from a qualified practitioner.

For further information and the names of therapists in your area, contact The London College of Massage and Shiatsu, 21 Portland Place, London W1N 3AF.

used – or by concentrating on the sensation of breath passing through your nostrils. Do not try to make your mind blank; instead focus on what you are doing.

Inevitably, you will notice that your attention drifts and that thoughts and images stream through your mind. Try not to get involved in these; just notice them and then return to concentrating on your mantra or breath. This is part of the process of 'letting go' and living in the moment, and it aids stress relief by helping you view life in a more detached and accepting way.

Practise meditating twice a day (morning and evening are good times, but avoid meditating immediately before you go to bed or just after a heavy meal). Start with 5-minute sessions and build up gradually to about 20 minutes. As you get used to the technique, you will find you can meditate almost anywhere as a form of instant stress-relief.

Meditating with mental images

Sometimes it is helpful to focus on a specific positive image during meditation – a technique called visualisation. This is especially useful if you feel upset or lacking in energy.

Sit upright in a chair and start with a few minutes of muscle relaxation and breath awareness, as with mindfulness meditation. Now focus on some deeper breathing, slowly bringing the breath right up into the chest (it may help to do this to a count of ten). As you exhale slowly (also to a count of ten), try to visualise your worries as a grey colour and imagine yourself expelling them with the air. And as you inhale slowly, see a clear bright colour – golden yellow, orange, green, anything you wish – filling your whole body up with energy.

Another good technique is to try to visualise your breath as clearing away stresses and worries, and then to imagine a pure white light streaming into you from above through the crown of your head. Mentally draw the light down into your solar plexus and then imagine it radiating out of yourself to form a protective bubble or cocoon of light all around you.

Alternatively, imagine yourself in beautiful surroundings – a forest or in the mountains, for instance. Try to imagine the details of the scene as vividly as you can – smells, textures and sounds as well as sights – and on how good it feels to be in the setting.

To enhance visualisation, repeat silently to yourself positive phrases such as 'I am full of energy and light' or 'I feel calm and serene'.

Practise any of the above techniques in isolation or in combination for 5–20 minutes or use them for one or two minutes whenever you feel lacking in energy or under pressure. You can also incorporate them into your mindfulness meditation routine.

USING BIOFEEDBACK

It is also possible to learn to control bodily stress responses such as muscle tension by using specialised types of machinery known as biofeedback instruments. The equipment does not affect the body in any way, but simply lets you monitor responses such as brainwave patterns, muscular tension, temperature or the electrical responsiveness of your skin. By practising effective relaxation techniques such as diaphragmatic breathing

Focusing your thoughts Sitting in a straight-backed chair is a comfortable way to meditate. Choose a chair low enough for you to have the soles of your feet flat on the floor. Keep your eyes closed or lowered, and rest your hands in your lap.

and meditation while you are connected up, you can actually see the results and learn to relax more effectively, or to control conditions such as anxiety or high blood pressure.

For further information or help in finding a biofeedback therapist in your area, contact the Institute for Complementary Medicine, 21 Portland Place, London W1N 3AF. There are no officially recognised qualifications, but some therapists are attached to hospital psychological departments.

Mind over matter The glow of a light bulb lets a biofeedback patient monitor his blood pressure level while he practises relaxation techniques aimed at reducing it. The dimmer the bulb, the lower the blood pressure reading and the more effectively the patient is relaxing.

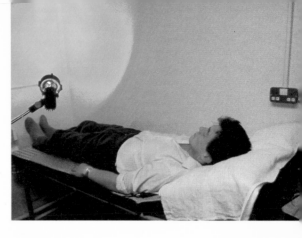

EXERCISES TO REDUCE STRESS AT YOUR DESK

Aches in the neck, shoulder and back are common office ailments – the result of poor posture and mental tension. The simple exercises below are designed to help and can be done as often as you like during the day. If some worrying thought or emotion is making you tense, anxious or irritated, you may also find it helpful to try a technique known as the quieting reflex, which takes just a few seconds. Close your eyes and focus on the worrying thought. Say to yourself: 'I now release this thought.' Breathe in slowly and gently, imagining air being drawn in through your feet and up to your head. Breathe out, imagining air flowing down from your head and out through your feet. Feel your body become warm and heavy.

SHRUGGING OFF YOUR CARES

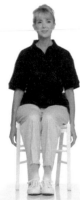

1 Sit comfortably in a chair, with your feet flat on the floor and your arms hanging loosely down at your sides.

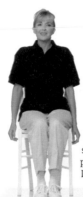

2 Take a deep breath and raise your shoulders slightly so they are parallel to the floor. Don't tense the neck.

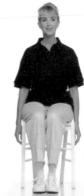

3 Gently lower your shoulders, exhaling as you do so, until you have returned to your starting position.

WAVING GOODBYE TO TENSION

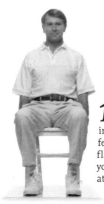

1 Sit comfortably erect but relaxed in a chair with your feet slightly apart and flat on the floor. Let your arms hang loosely at the side of the body.

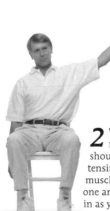

2 Without raising your shoulders or tensing your neck muscles, slowly raise one arm, breathing in as you do so.

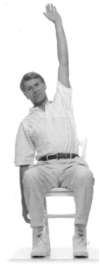

3 Reach right up to give a gentle stretch. Slowly lower the arm and exhale as you do so. Repeat with the other arm.

MAKING LEISURE PART OF YOUR LIFE

Free time is not an optional extra or a luxury but an essential part of life. However hard you work and whatever your other commitments, it is vital to have time for your own interests. Leisure broadens your experience of life. It enables you to step back and reflect on your work, your relationships and your way of life. It is also an ally in the fight against stress – it keeps worries in proportion and it reinvigorates you so that you deal with them better. Because it can take so many different forms, leisure can also help you to lead a richer, better-balanced life and to express different aspects of yourself. If you work at a desk all week, get out and do something active; if you spend your days looking after others, make time to be alone.

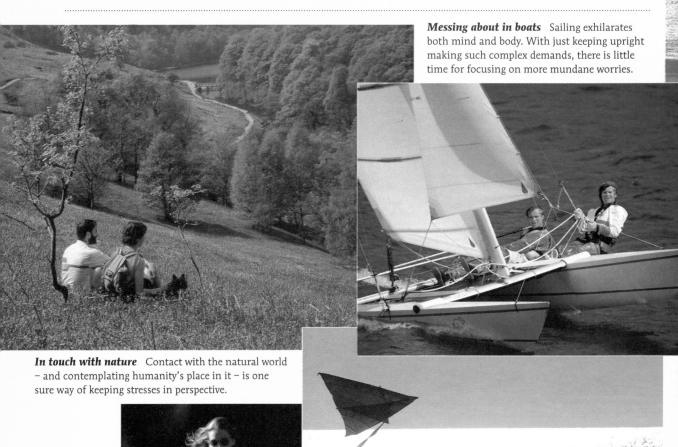

Messing about in boats Sailing exhilarates both mind and body. With just keeping upright making such complex demands, there is little time for focusing on more mundane worries.

In touch with nature Contact with the natural world – and contemplating humanity's place in it – is one sure way of keeping stresses in perspective.

Child's play Adults have a lot to learn from children when it comes to coping with stress. Simple activities such as flying a kite are often the most fun, especially in company. Kites get you out into the open air too.

Body in balance Roller blading may not suit everyone but we all do need to find some way of expressing ourselves physically and using the body to its full capacity – for rhythm and poise as well as fitness.

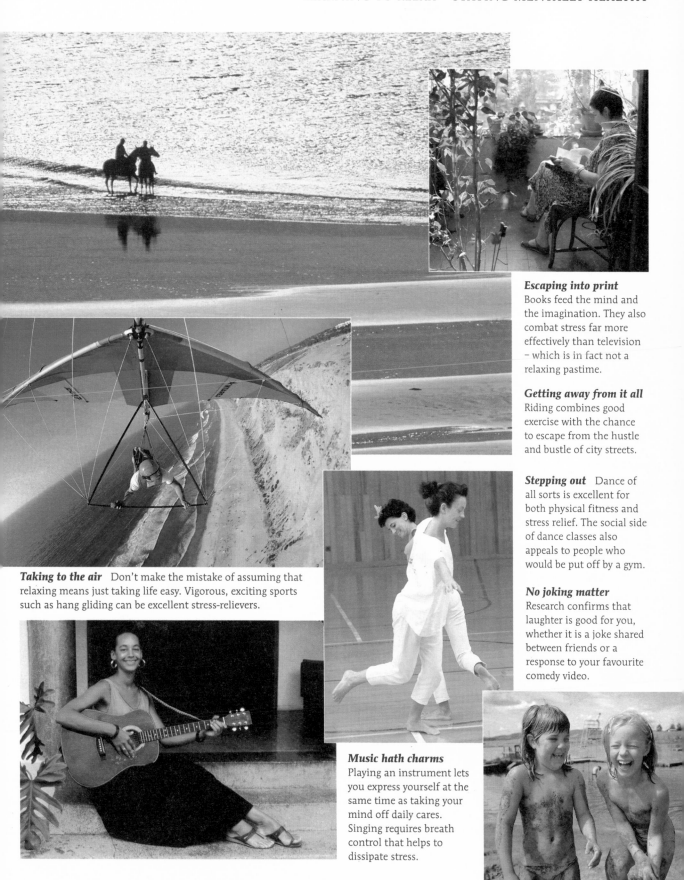

Escaping into print
Books feed the mind and the imagination. They also combat stress far more effectively than television – which is in fact not a relaxing pastime.

Getting away from it all
Riding combines good exercise with the chance to escape from the hustle and bustle of city streets.

Stepping out Dance of all sorts is excellent for both physical fitness and stress relief. The social side of dance classes also appeals to people who would be put off by a gym.

No joking matter
Research confirms that laughter is good for you, whether it is a joke shared between friends or a response to your favourite comedy video.

Taking to the air Don't make the mistake of assuming that relaxing means just taking life easy. Vigorous, exciting sports such as hang gliding can be excellent stress-relievers.

Music hath charms
Playing an instrument lets you express yourself at the same time as taking your mind off daily cares. Singing requires breath control that helps to dissipate stress.

Mourning and grief

COMING TO TERMS WITH LOSS

What is grief? Is it a form of depression?

Grief is an unavoidable human emotion, a natural response to a central experience of life and not necessarily a symptom of depressive illness. In reaction to a major loss, such as the death of a partner, it is a normal and essential part of coming to terms with and surviving the devastating event.

Studies suggest that although each experience is individual, grieving generally passes through several distinct, identifiable stages. Some people go through the stages once only, others return to certain stages more than once, or repeat the cycle a second or even a third time.

No two bereavements are exactly the same but given the right conditions of patience, support, respect and a listening ear most people will manage to work out their grief according to their own needs. There is no set time scale for this and relatives and friends need to accept that the process may be lengthy. Nor does grief ever leave people unchanged. It should not be viewed as something to be 'got over', but as a fundamental experience that alters life for ever. At first, the bereaved person is preoccupied with the person who has died and with recalling and evaluating the past. Sometimes the grieving person tries to hold on to the loved one by holding conversations with him, wearing his clothes or undertaking the things he used to do. While some of this behaviour may seem bizarre to others, it is a natural part of the grieving process and should always be treated sympathetically.

In the second stage, the pain becomes more pronounced as the bereaved person starts to accept the fact of loss. Anger, despair, emptiness and thoughts that life is really not worth living predominate. Grief colours every experience, and memories can cause overwhelming pain. In the third and final stage, the person returns to normal functioning and behaviour. Friendships and activities that were ignored during the second stage become important again, and the constant pall of grief gradually lifts.

NOT SHOWING YOUR FEELINGS

When my father died, my mother showed few signs of emotion. Is this normal or even healthy?

A stoic response to death, especially to the death of someone so close as a husband, may not be a good sign. Your mother may not feel able to deal with the loss or may be unconsciously unable to accept that your father is gone. Her unresolved

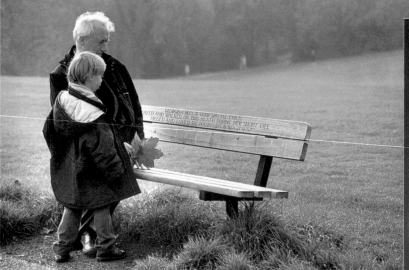

Remembering helps When someone close dies, memories become intensely painful – and immensely important. Revisiting favourite places, recalling happy times and just looking at photographs can all help with the healing process.

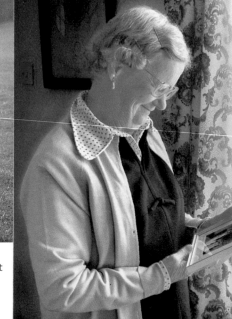

grief may present problems later on. If you can get her to talk about your father, perhaps her memories will bring tears and allow her to proceed with the process of grieving.

Suppressed emotion is only one possible sign that the mourning process may not be proceeding normally. Hysterical grieving – screaming, fainting or developing psychosomatic symptoms – can also be an abnormal reaction to loss. Overreaction and underreaction must be judged in terms of cultural background, however – what seems extreme in one culture may be normal in another.

Other danger signs include hyperactivity that leaves no time for mourning, fury at a doctor or hospital, and self-destructive acts (giving away treasured belongings or signing contracts for bad business deals). Idolising the deceased as a saint or denigrating him as a villain may also signal unresolved grief.

AN END TO GRIEF

How long does grief usually last?

Every experience is different, but research shows that although four out of five people emerge from the most acute stages of mourning after about three months, it usually takes two years to come to terms with the death of someone close. Most bereaved people benefit by returning to work or other normal activities in three to six weeks, even though the loss continues to be felt. And depending on the intimacy of the relationship, the period of intense bereavement varies. Widows and widowers, for instance, remain at increased risk of death for a year after the death of their partner. The families of murder victims and suicides similarly suffer extended periods of bereavement.

Getting in touch with others

If you or someone you know needs help in coming to terms with bereavement or would like to talk to others who have been through it, contact these societies.

● CRUSE – Bereavement Care, CRUSE House, 126 Sheen Road, Richmond, Surrey TW9 1UR.
● Compassionate Friends, 53 North Street, Bristol BS3 1EN.

When depression strikes

DIAGNOSING THE PROBLEM

What's the difference between being depressed and just being a bit low?

Every normal person feels sad at times. There are life events – marital problems, the loss of a job, the death of a loved one – that will temporarily depress anyone. Psychiatrists draw the line between normal sadness and clinical depression when gloomy feelings are particularly intense and predominate for weeks instead of days. Very often there are also disturbed patterns of behaviour such as eating and sleeping. Clinical depression often begins as the kind of normal unhappiness everyone experiences from time to time. When the person starts to realise that the feelings are not lifting, help should be sought.

Depressive symptoms are very common, affecting about 20 per cent of the population at any one time. Severe depressive illness is rarer but still quite common – 2 per cent of men and 4 per cent of women suffer from it. Depression is highly treatable, but it is also often misunderstood. Because we so often speak about depression when we are referring to perfectly normal, short-term experiences, many people who actually need help fail to get it. Instead they assume that it is up to them to cope alone. Casual references to anxiety also confuse the issue. The anxiety experienced by about two-thirds of

clinically depressed people involves deep inner distress, dread, fear, foreboding and physical symptoms such as palpitations, sweating, rapid pulse and stomach upsets.

A PHYSICAL ILLNESS

My brother has been down in the dumps lately, but his wife says it's all in his imagination. Is she right?

No. Many people believe that depression can and should be willed away. But this is wrong and grossly underestimates the suffering caused by this illness.

Signs that depression has a physical component abound. Scans of brain activity, recordings of brainwave patterns and chemical activity in the brain show marked differences from normal in certain depressed patients. Some of the most compelling evidence is the fact that drug treatment affords relief in most cases, strongly suggesting a biochemical cause.

Severe depression that responds to treatment with antidepressant drugs is thought to be caused by reduced levels of certain excitatory neurotransmitters – chemical messenger substances that can alter mood by stimulating brain cell activity.

Even when depression has a primarily psychological basis (childhood traumas such as incest are at the root of some cases) it can be as real a physical condition as diabetes or

Are you depressed?

A surprisingly wide range of symptoms can point to depression.

● A pervading feeling of sadness all or most of the time for more than two weeks.
● Loss of motivation.
● Loss of interest in activities that you normally enjoy.
● A sense that nothing matters any longer or means anything.
● Suicidal thoughts.
● Restlessness.
● Difficulty concentrating.
● Sleep problems, particularly waking in the early hours.
● Decreased libido.
● Loss of appetite or, more rarely, increased appetite, especially in the evening or at night.
● Unexplained physical symptoms such as head, neck or back pain, tightness in the throat, blurred vision, nausea, muscle cramps, painful urination, indigestion or constipation.

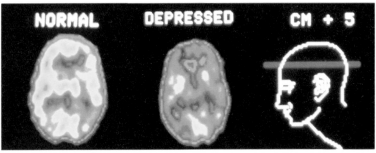

How depression affects the brain A scan shows lower than normal activity in a depressed brain. Red and yellow areas are using most glucose – the brain's fuel – and blue and green ones least. The red line (right) shows the plane of the scan.

FACT
— OR —
FALLACY?

'Creativity is linked to manic depression.'

Fallacy No link has been proved between artistic achievement and any particular mental illness. Writers and artists such as Vincent Van Gogh, Edgar Allan Poe and Ernest Hemingway may have been manic depressive – but so have many people from all walks of life. Artists' manic phases may just be more noticeable if they correlate with bursts of intense creativity.

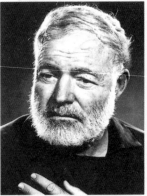

Ernest Hemingway
Manic phases may have fuelled his intense creative periods.

heart disease, and just as debilitating. The real danger of ignorance is that serious depressive illness may go undiagnosed and untreated. And untreated depression can deepen, with thoughts of suicide sometimes turning into real attempts.

Even if one episode of depression subsides without treatment, the condition cannot be counted as cured – at least half will experience recurrences. When treatment is given, it is usually highly effective, but seeking help first requires people to overcome the stigma attached to the problem.

HOW TO FIND HELP

What should I do if I get depressed?

If your depression continues unabated for two to four weeks, talk to your family doctor, who may prescribe antidepressant medication or refer you to a counsellor, a psychologist or a psychiatrist.

Depression is a highly treatable disease; at least four out of five of those who seek treatment get significant relief in a matter of weeks from drug therapy, psychotherapy or a combination of the two. Many people who are mildly depressed will improve quickly with only short-term, goal-orientated counselling. Such limited therapy works best for temporary depression that is triggered by specific events – treatment does not delve into childhood experiences but focuses strictly on the present.

Vigorous exercise can also sometimes ease a mild, short-term case of depression. But jogging will not cure a major depression. Neither will alcohol, nicotine or food.

Some depressed people resort to drugs such as cannabis or cocaine, but while such drugs can mask depression temporarily or blunt its sharpness – as with alcohol – in the long run they seriously exacerbate the problem. Depressed smokers not only damage

their health but have a harder time giving up cigarettes than other smokers do.

Support groups can often help sufferers by making them realise that they are not the only ones to go through such terribly dark periods. One such organisation to get in touch with is Depressives Anonymous, 36 Chestnut Avenue, Beverley, North Humberside HU17 9QU. Most people with major depression, however, will need medical or psychotherapeutic help. For serious or persistent symptoms, always see a doctor.

HAVING SHOCK THERAPY

I was surprised to hear about someone having shock treatment for depression. How much is it still used? Is it safe?

Highly criticised in the 1950s and 1960s, shock therapy – or, more accurately, electro-convulsive therapy (ECT) – has now widely re-established its credentials with mental health professionals treating depression. The treatment consists of applying electric current via electrodes placed on the temples for a fraction of a second. The patient has a convulsion similar to an epileptic seizure.

About 20 000 patients undergo ECT each year in Britain – primarily the victims of severe depression. Its use in young patients is controversial and is usually avoided, but it is generally thought safe for adults. Even so, some groups and therapists still oppose ECT, believing that other methods of treatment can be as effective and safer.

ECT patients are anaesthetised and given muscle relaxants before treatment to prevent the jerky movements that in the past could cause fractures. Oxygen is also administered during treatment and new techniques used to prevent memory loss. In unilateral ECT, for instance, electrodes are not attached to each temple but one is attached to the right temple and one to the top right half of the head to avoid transmitting current through the brain's left hemisphere, where verbal memory is centred. Brief-pulse therapy uses the lowest effective electrical current administered for the shortest possible time.

Curiously, doctors are still not sure how ECT works. The prevailing theory is that electrically induced seizures produce changes in brain chemistry. Despite some critics who maintain that memory loss is still possible, ECT remains, at present, the only hope for some patients with severe depression. Until other treatments are developed, it is likely to continue as a part of psychiatric practice, but a carefully controlled one.

MANIC DEPRESSION

A relative has been diagnosed as manic depressive. What exactly is this condition and what sort of help is available?

Manic depression (technically called bipolar disorder) is a mental illness in which moods swing from severe depression to elation and hyperactivity. Manic periods are marked by raised self-esteem, uncritical self-confidence, grandiose ideas and bursts of intense energy. The person may go on spending sprees or sexual escapades, or start up unrealistically ambitious projects. These episodes do not usually last as long as the depressive parts of the cycle and may begin and end abruptly after a period of a few days to a few weeks.

Manic depression is rare. While as many as one in five women and one in ten men experience unipolar depression at some time, only about 1 per cent of the population ever suffers a bipolar disorder. Manic depression is equally common among men and women and is apt to recur if not treated. Lithium salts are highly effective in controlling manic depressive mood swings, and your relative will probably find that sensible use of medication controls the problem. He or she may also wish to contact the Manic Depressive Fellowship, 8-10 High Street, Kingston upon Thames, Surrey KT1 1EY.

Food and your mood

Changes in eating or drinking habits can be a sign of depression. Watch out for these.

- Compulsive eating.
- Losing your appetite.
- Continually craving sweet or starchy foods.
- Weight loss or gain.
- Increasing reliance on caffeine-containing or alcoholic drinks.

REAL LIVES

BACK FROM THE BRINK – HOW A MODERN-DAY SAMARITAN SAVED A LIFE

Having walked out of his job some months before, and with his marriage in serious trouble, Ken Poursain had nothing left to live for, or so he felt. He was standing on the Clifton Suspension Bridge, looking down into the Avon gorge, while planning his jump.

He scrambled over the railing. Sheer despair was driving him on – this was his way out, his release from the grip of severe depression. It was a condition reaching all the way back to a miserable childhood, and intensified by a car accident six years previously. Some 15 per cent of people with major depression die by suicide, and Ken was about to join the statistics.

'Right, here we go then,' he thought. Suddenly a voice called out, 'Life's too precious'. He turned. Running towards him was a young woman, arms outstretched.

Angela Stratford rushed towards the man on the bridge, pushing onlookers out of her way, and bypassing a police cordon.

For three and a half hours, as traffic was brought to a halt, and police and crowds looked on, they talked. They talked about God, they talked about their pets, Angela even joked about taking a bungee jump from the bridge with Ken some day. She stroked his hands, apparently having won his confidence. But his behaviour was still volatile: he would start shouting at the police negotiators, for instance, or lean precariously out over the gorge in a renewed suicide threat. As Angela persisted in her efforts to comfort him, he would once again calm down.

Finally he said, 'I thank you from the bottom of my heart for everything you've done, but you've got to let me go'. She did. She had given all she could. She had shown, to an inspiring degree, just how we really can do something to help in a crisis. But the last move was up to Ken alone. Slowly, shakily, Ken Poursain climbed over the railings, and into the arms of the young woman who had saved his life.

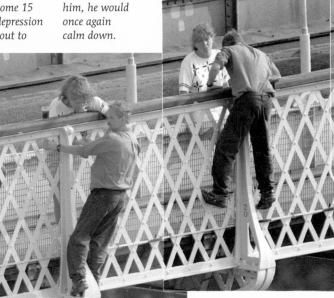

Safe return *When Angela Stratford encouraged Ken Poursain to climb back onto the Clifton Suspension Bridge, she helped him to give life another chance.*

What to do if suicide is threatened

Never ignore the risk – some people who make threats are serious.

- Listen.
- Don't argue, criticise, disapprove or try to solve the person's problems.
- Suggest calling the Samaritans, a minister of religion or a doctor.
- Don't leave the person alone. If you can't cope, take him to a hospital or contact his GP.

RECOGNISING SUICIDE RISK

Is there any way of telling if someone is in danger of committing suicide?

The person most likely to commit suicide sees himself in an unbearable and hopeless predicament. Death seems preferable to continuing to live under such circumstances. Lacking self-esteem, the potential suicide sees no way out of his crisis; he feels not only hopeless, but helpless as well. Alcoholics, drug abusers, the terminally ill and the chronically depressed are all at increased risk of suicide.

Someone contemplating suicide may or may not give clues to his intentions, but those who do should always be taken seriously. Watch for these signs.

- Social withdrawal – the person becomes increasingly withdrawn and socially isolated, often after a traumatic event or stressful period, such as financial loss, divorce, bereavement or chronic illness.
- Talk of suicide or death – contrary to popular belief, people who say they want to take their own lives may actually do so. Repeated threats or the revelation of specific plans should never be ignored.
- The giving away of valued possessions.
- The return of a cheerful or calm demeanour after a period of depression – once the decision to commit suicide has been made the person may feel a sense of relief at having finally found a way to resolve his problems. The risk of suicide is greater when a person seems to be recovering from a deep depression.

Anxiety, phobias and obsessions

FEELING AGITATED

I occasionally find myself becoming very agitated for no apparent reason. What could be causing this?

You may be experiencing a panic attack – an intense burst of anxiety accompanied by such physical symptoms as heart palpitations or chest pains, dizziness, numbness of the hands or feet, trembling, sweating or a choking sensation.

Fear and a sense of unreality may be overwhelming. Sometimes flashes of bright light may alternate with a clouding of vision. If the attack occurs in public, the victim may feel an urgent need to rush home.

Panic attacks usually begin suddenly and unpredictably; when they recur, the condition is called a panic disorder. Some people suffer panic attacks for a brief and limited period, and then their anxieties vanish as mysteriously as they started.

Others with long-term panic disorders may go on to develop other anxiety-based disorders such as agoraphobia (the fear of open spaces – literally, fear of the marketplace, the streets and even the park). Afraid to set foot outside of their home in case a panic attack overwhelms them in public, these people can eventually become completely housebound.

The causes of panic attacks are not yet fully understood. There is increasing evidence that an individual's patterns of thinking play an important role, in particular a tendency to anticipate disaster.

High blood levels of adrenaline and other stress hormones have also been recorded in people who suffer from panic disorder and some researchers now believe that a sudden release of such hormones could be what triggers a panic attack.

Another possibility is that improper functioning of the autonomic nervous system, which regulates blood supply, could be to blame for the fainting spells, dizziness, palpitations and feelings of anxiety characteristic of panic attacks.

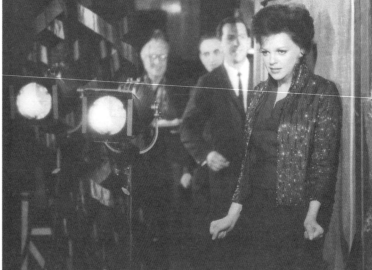

Stage fright Nerves affect even the most experienced performers – as Judy Garland's clenched fists and tense expression show. In moderation, anxiety can lead to a better performance. If it gets out of hand, however, the results can cripple a career.

TREATMENT FOR PANIC ATTACKS

Can my panic attacks be treated?

No sure cure exists, since no one knows exactly what causes panic attacks, but several treatments are being used successfully. The most effective psychological approach combines techniques from cognitive and behavioural therapy (see page 212) that focus on the patient's physical sensations and on the way they are interpreted. Panic attacks can also be treated with antianxiety or antidepressant drugs that alter the way neurotransmitter chemicals act in the brain.

People prone to panic attacks are urged to eliminate coffee, tea and other caffeinated drinks from their diets. Regular exercise provides a healthy outlet for anxiety and can help to soothe tensions. You might also try some of the relaxation techniques described on pages 190-193.

FROM FEAR TO PHOBIA

What are phobias? How do they differ from normal fears?

Phobias are fears that are extreme, irrational – without a real threat – and disruptive. A fear of tunnels is not a phobia if it merely makes you eager to reach the end. On the other hand, if you start mapping out routes for avoiding tunnels you could be developing a phobia. If you find yourself cancelling meetings or inventing reasons to stay at home, the phobia needs treatment.

Phobias are of two types. Simple phobias involve single objects or situations, such as heights, snakes or enclosed spaces, and usually the victim is aware of the problem. More disabling complex phobias combine several fears and often intense panic attacks as well. Agoraphobics, for instance, may fear not only leaving the house but also heights, enclosed spaces and germ contamination. Victims of such conditions are less likely to realise that their behaviour is abnormal.

OVERCOMING A PHOBIA

Are there any effective treatments for overcoming a phobia?

Yes, although they are not always needed. Many people suffering from mild, simple phobias never seek treatment. Some conquer their own fears over time; others don't, but manage to find ways of coping. People who do seek treatment find that simple phobias

involving a single object or situation, such as fear of spiders or of flying, are often quite easy and quick to cure.

The most common treatment takes the form of controlled, gradual exposure to the feared object or experience. A therapist (or, in the case of a child, a parent) accompanies the phobic person and helps to ease him or her into situations ranging from, at first, the least distressing level of contact to, eventually, the most anxiety-provoking. People with complex phobias – especially agoraphobics – can also benefit from exposure therapy, usually with the help of both a partner or friend and a therapist. Antianxiety or antidepressant drugs may be used in conjunction with exposure therapy to reduce the severity and frequency of panic attacks that are often associated with phobias.

Information on self-help programmes and other forms of therapy is available from the Phobics Society, 4 Cheltenham Road, Chorlton cum Hardy, Manchester M21 9QN.

What phobics fear

Phobias affect more than one in ten people at some time in their life. These are some of the commonest fears.

- Public speaking.
- Heights (acrophobia).
- Snakes (ophidiophobia).
- Dogs (cynophobia).
- Enclosed spaces (claustrophobia).
- Thunder (brontophobia).
- Lightning (astraphobia).
- Darkness (nyctophobia).
- Flying (aerophobia).

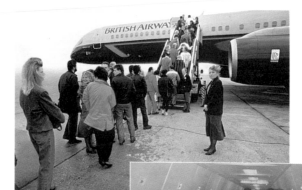

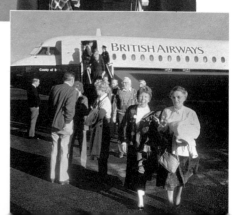

Flying without fear
Aerophobics can take a one-day confidence-building course at either Heathrow or Manchester airport. The course is run by British Airways pilots and a psychologist, and aims to help nervous fliers to understand and control their fear. Participants learn about flying and practise relaxation techniques before taking a short flight. Airline staff escort them on board (above) and show them to their seats (centre). When they emerge (below), about 95 per cent feel confident enough to think of flying again.

How obsessions and compulsions differ

Obsessions and compulsions frequently occur together.

● Obsessions are intrusive ideas that recur and persist, or thoughts that cannot be ignored, and may also include impulses almost impossible to control.
● Compulsions take the form of repetitive actions based on an obsession or on complex rituals. Normal behaviour, particularly hygiene and cleanliness, may be carried to excess.

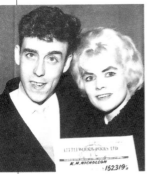

Compulsive spenders
After they won the pools in 1961 the Nicholsons could not stop spending.

COMPULSIVE HAND-WASHING

I have a colleague who is obsessively neat and always seems to be washing his hands. Is this what is meant by a compulsion?

It is never a good idea to make amateur diagnoses, particularly when it comes to mental health, but it does sound as if your colleague may indeed be suffering from an obsessive-compulsive disorder – a condition that affects around a million people in Britain.

Once in a while most people have fleeting urges to check that the cooker has been turned off or that the front door is properly secured. When you were a child, you may have lined up your toy soldiers in a precise order and become upset if anyone disturbed them. Imagine such feelings vastly magnified and constantly felt, and you will gain an idea of what it is like to have an obsessive-compulsive disorder (OCD).

OCD sufferers may constantly wash their hands or pull their hair or disinfect their houses. An obsessive-compulsive may stop his car every few blocks to convince himself he has not run over anyone. Or he may feel compelled to leave work repeatedly to make perfectly sure that he has not left a cigarette burning in a wastepaper bin at home.

Psychotherapy has not been very successful in treating OCD. Although in the past the condition has been linked by some psychologists to childhood conflicts or emotional traumas, such as overly rigid toilet training, the evidence is mounting for a physiological cause. Brain scans, in particular, have shown physical aberrations in some people with OCD. Treatment for OCD generally focuses on finding ways to control anxiety levels. Some success has also been achieved with antidepressant drugs which increase the production of the chemical serotonin in the brain.

AFRAID OF ILLNESS

What is the dividing line between a normal concern for health and hypochondria? Is there any way of telling when someone is really ill and when their symptoms are all in the mind?

Like all phobias and anxiety-based disorders, the distinction between normal and abnormal health worries is mainly one of degree. Hypochondria, or correctly hypochondriasis, is a chronic, excessive fear of illness and injury. The hypochondriac is so concerned about sickness that he magnifies normal bodily sensations in his mind until they feel like aches and pains. Hypochondriacs may in fact have more sensitive nervous systems than most people do, and normal aches and pains may feel more ominous to them. The symptoms they report are often bizarre and don't follow the pattern of a known illness. Because hypochondriacs visit doctors frequently, they usually have a good grasp of medical terminology and can sound very expert on the subject of illness.

Anxiety and depression are often the root of a hypochondriac's problems – the obsession with physical illness can be a way of avoiding the need to face emotional difficulties. Like everyone else, hypochondriacs do get sick from time to time and it is very difficult – even for doctors and psychiatrists – to distinguish a genuine disease from one presumed to be imagined.

Problems children face

CHILDREN UNDER STRESS

Some children seem to have such difficult lives. Are they at risk from stress and depression in the same way as adults?

Sadly, yes. Children lead stressful lives today, and often suffer the consequences both emotionally and physically. Each year thousands of children live through their parents' divorces, and millions more watch parents fight the losing battle of an unhappy marriage. Some inner city children face risks an adult would have difficulty handling, just to get to school each day. And affluent children are subject to increasing pressures to compete and do well.

Even so, children can remain cheerful and resilient, even in the face of critical family problems such as alcoholism or divorce. Those who fare best lead busy lives and are involved in activities such as music and sport that give plenty of opportunity for displaying talents and being rewarded for achievement. Being able to form deep, satisfying relationships with other children and adults, both in and out of the home, also appears to have a protective effect.

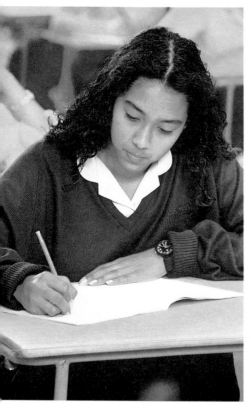

Under pressure Examinations are intensely stressful, especially for high-fliers. Today's youngsters are increasingly showing similar signs of stress to those observed in adults.

Recognising the signs of stress

It is not always easy for parents and teachers to know when children are under stress, but there are some signals to watch for.

- Bad behaviour and unusually poor schoolwork are often a sign that something is wrong.
- When a child suddenly becomes quiet and withdrawn, forsaking activities that normally interest him, he may be exhibiting symptoms of depression. Children as young as eight may become pessimistic, lose interest in play and refuse to talk about things that are bothering them. By 12, a depressed child may have physical symptoms such as sleeping problems, loss of appetite, and stomachaches. A depressed 17-year-old may have nightmares and thoughts of suicide as well. The risk of depression increases with age – one study found that 17-year-olds were four times more likely to be depressed than eight to twelve-year-olds. Given the increase in teenage suicide (see page 204) getting professional help immediately is essential.

BUILDING CONFIDENCE

My 15-year-old daughter has always been shy and shows no signs of coming out of her shell. Is there anything I can to do to help her to be more confident?

Shyness is a common childhood experience, and teenage girls in particular are apt to be self-conscious. The importance of being popular at this age and the budding of sexuality can further escalate insecurities.

You can help your daughter to cope with this difficult stage by encouraging activities such as sports, music, dancing or group holidays with other youngsters, and by inviting her friends to the house or on outings. Looking attractive always bolsters confidence, so encourage fashionable haircuts and stylish dressing. Breaking free of shyness is not accomplished overnight, so don't try to force your daughter. Respect her natural inclinations and support step-by-step changes. In any case, most teenagers quite naturally step into independence the moment they go off to college or take a summer job.

THE DANGERS OF CULTS

I've heard rumours that a cult group in our area is trying to recruit local youngsters. How can I protect my children, and should I inform anyone about my suspicions?

You are quite right to be concerned – cults can be extremely dangerous, particularly to young people, and it is a good idea to inform both the teachers at your children's school, other parents and the police so that they can keep an eye on the situation. Assistance and information is also available from the Cult Information Centre, BCM CULTS, London WC1N 3XX.

Talk to your children about your suspicions and explain that cults are dangerous because they try to destroy people's power over their lives and their ability to think for themselves. Teach your children to be suspicious of over-friendly strangers, people with instant answers to difficult questions and groups that pressurise individuals to join them or to conform once they have joined.

Remember, too, that cults are trained to exploit people who are vulnerable. No child should have to wrestle alone with a problem such as exam stress, loneliness or bullying. Teenagers can be particularly at risk since this is a stage when fitting in feels vitally important and when identity is being questioned. The promise of group acceptance and

DO'S AND DON'TS

for helping children through examinations

Do give regular meals and healthy snacks to keep up their blood sugar levels.

Do encourage some regular periods of exercise and relaxation, however brief.

Do make sure children get enough sleep.

Do take an interest in their work and talk about it.

Do offer to help with drawing up a revision timetable.

Do encourage other members of the family to be considerate.

Do make sure there is a comfortable, quiet place to work.

Don't add pressure by expressing hopes or fears about results.

Don't give extra coffee or tea – stimulants such as caffeine can contribute to stress.

Don't let children skip their meals or rely on highly sugared or salted snacks. Nutrition needs to be better, not worse, when you are under special pressure.

Help for children with problems

Young people and those concerned about them can obtain information and assistance from these sources.

● ChildLine operates a 24-hour telephone helpline on 0800 1111, and offers confidential counselling to children.
● The National Society for the Prevention of Cruelty to Children (NSPCC) runs an all-hours Child Protection helpline on 0800 800 500, offering advice to anyone concerned about a child's welfare.
● The Children's Legal Centre, 20 Compton Terrace, London N1 2UN provides legal advice on issues affecting young people.

a clear sense of belonging may be irresistibly attractive. Make sure you know what is going on in your children's lives and thoughts, be there to give help when it is needed, and make sure your children have other trustworthy adults to turn to as well – teachers, relatives, friends or counsellors.

DRUG-PROOF CHILDREN?

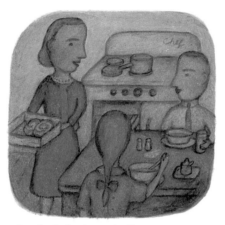

What is the best way to discourage my children from experimenting with drugs?

Few parents sit down to talk about drugs unless they have to – generally when it is too late and someone in the family is suspected of using them. Then children may be lectured or ordered to 'say no', without being given ammunition to help them resist peer pressure and without an informed explanation about the dangers of taking drugs.

The best way to help your children to make sensible decisions about cigarettes, alcohol and drug abuse is to set a good example yourself and to make sure they know the facts about drugs and the damage they can do (see pages 207-211). Make sure you understand how drugs and alcohol can interfere with children's physical and emotional development so that you can explain these things clearly to them. Find out, too, what schools are teaching children about drugs.

Contact the organisers of any parties your children go to and ask them what antidrugs measures are planned and who will be in charge. Do not let your children go if you get an unsatisfactory reply, and inform other parents of the situation.

Parents who hope to help their teenagers to avoid drug problems cannot be hypocrites. Examine your own use of alcohol, nicotine and prescription drugs and be prepared for honest discussions about your attitudes to both legal and illegal intoxicants.

TEENAGE SUICIDE

There have been lots of headlines lately about teenage suicides. Is suicide in any way 'catching'?

Obviously, suicide is not contagious in any literal sense. However, if a friend's or classmate's suicide brings the possibility of self-destruction closer to home, or makes it seem more like a reasonable solution, then it could precipitate suicidal thoughts in the mind of a teenager who is already looking for a way out of a difficult situation.

For the past 20 years or so, the alarming rise in the rate of teenage suicide has mirrored the rise in the divorce rate, and many experts are drawing conclusions about the damaging effects of divorce, particularly on adolescent boys (among whom the rise has been greatest).

Studies show that sons of absent fathers have a harder time trying to control their impulses – and an inability to control aggressive impulses is a hallmark of male suicidal behaviour. Research also shows a statistically significant higher incidence of separation and divorce among parents of teenagers who attempt and commit suicide.

Four to five times more teenage boys actually *commit* suicide than teenage girls do; however, four to five times more girls than boys *attempt* to take their lives.

Parents who are separated or divorced cannot change this basic fact, but they should always keep in mind the importance of remaining close to their children, whether living with them or not, and of carefully maintaining open channels of communication with their teenagers.

Families in which both parents work significantly more than 40 hours a week may create a dangerous environment too. Sons (both nursery-school age and adolescents) are more likely than daughters to show adjustment problems in homes where both parents work.

The overwhelming bulk of evidence discovered by the research indicates that the absence – whether physical or emotional – of supportive and caring adults can put a child's wellbeing in jeopardy.

Why sons are more vulnerable remains something of a mystery but it may be that when family troubles arise, relationships with the father are more likely to be damaged or disrupted than those with the mother. The absence of a strong, respected father-figure may be particularly difficult for boys to come to terms with.

Eating disorders

SPOTTING ANOREXIA

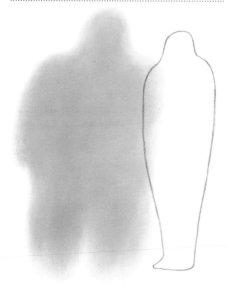

My young niece, an aspiring ballerina, has put herself on a radical weight-loss plan. Is it possible that she's becoming anorexic?

The profession your niece has chosen puts her at higher risk for developing an eating disorder such as anorexia nervosa. Her age and sex do, too. The vast majority (90-95 per cent) of anorexia victims are female, and many of them begin to exhibit eating problems during early adolescence. Statistics are difficult to come by, but anorexia is not common, probably affecting less than one in a hundred young women.

Whether your niece is actually developing anorexia depends in part on her body image. Anorexics, however, do not see their body in realistic terms. However they look to others and whatever they weigh, they believe themselves fat and overweight. And anorexia is more than just dieting. Like other eating disorders, it is a lived-out expression of much deeper emotional or psychological turmoil.

Considering the following questions may help to establish whether your niece is at risk. Does she often talk about herself as being fat even when she is far from overweight? Are her eating habits extremely restrictive – does she, for example, limit herself to fewer than 900 calories a day? Does she exercise constantly? Has her weight dropped considerably below the normal range? If you think she is in danger, talk to

her about your concerns. If she is not receptive, talk to her parents. If they are worried too, get her to see a doctor, preferably one who specialises in eating disorders.

WHAT HAPPENS IN BULIMIA

What is bulimia? Is it a form of anorexia, or a completely separate illness?

Both conditions stem from deep-seated anxiety and have much in common. However, they are not the same. Anorexics compulsively starve themselves and are usually extremely thin. In severe cases, they can lose a quarter or more of their weight and require a period in hospital to keep them from literally starving to death. Bulimics, in contrast, binge on high-calorie food and purge themselves afterwards, usually by making themselves vomit or by taking laxatives. They may be thin, of normal weight, or even fat.

Bulimics feel guilty about their binges and try to keep them secret, making their condition hard to detect. Some signs include disappearing to the lavatory after every meal, mood swings, gradual withdrawal from social life, secretive behaviour and the use of large amounts of laxatives. As the condition develops, tooth enamel can become eroded from brushing after vomiting has exposed teeth to stomach acids. If weight drops low enough, menstrual periods may stop.

Both anorexics and bulimics tend to be young women in their teens or twenties, but they can be older and men too can be affected. The distinction between the two conditions is sometimes clouded by the fact that half of all anorexics binge and purge when they are at very low weight, and bulimics may alternate periods of bingeing with periods of strict dieting. It is also not uncommon for people to go from one condition to the other – in most cases from anorexia to bulimia.

Anorexics and bulimics alike see themselves as fat even when they are extremely underweight. In their relentless pursuit of thinness, they often take to exercising obsessively. Their blood pressure and pulse rate will be low, and they may develop an irregular heartbeat. Gastrointestinal problems are also common. Bulimia is much commoner than anorexia, although the incidence of both disorders appears to be increasing.

Treating eating disorders

Many techniques have been tried to help anorexics and bulimics to build up a healthier relationship with food. Some of the most successful include:

● Rewards for eating or gaining weight.
● Individual or group psychotherapy.
● Family therapy.
● Self-help – contact the Eating Disorders Association, Sackville Place, 44 Magdalen Street, Norwich, Norfolk NR3 1JU.
● Drug treatment for related disorders such as clinical depression.

Fighting alcoholism

CAUSES OF THE PROBLEM

What causes alcoholism? Can the problem be inherited?

Inherited factors possibly play a part in some cases of alcoholism, but it is now widely believed that any person, regardless of his or her genetic background, personality or environment, is at risk of developing a dependency on alcohol if he or she drinks heavily for a prolonged period.

Nevertheless, there is evidence that a *tendency* can be inherited. Studies of twins and adopted children have shown that heredity can play a more critical role than environment in determining the development of alcoholism. Children of alcoholics tend to tolerate greater amounts of alcohol when they begin drinking and are apt to start drinking at a younger age. Later their reactions change – they become more sensitive to alcohol than others, and they show worse physical effects after being intoxicated. Such children are between four and six times more likely to develop drinking problems than others. Much new scientific research is being devoted to identifying a genetic basis for alcoholism. In one recent study, a gene associated with dopamine, a neurotransmitter chemical that plays a part in pleasure-seeking behaviour, was located in the brains of 77 per cent of alcoholics, compared with only 28 per cent of non-alcoholics. Exactly what role the gene may play in the development of alcoholism is unclear. One suggestion is that by activating the release of dopamine, it could affect the degree of pleasure felt when an individual drinks alcohol, and may lead to a craving for more alcohol to stimulate the release of more dopamine.

However, no single biological explanation for the development of alcoholism is entirely satisfactory. Social and cultural factors can lead people to abuse alcohol whether or not they are genetically predisposed to the disease. And the way families pass on a tendency toward alcoholism may not be entirely biological but may also stem from particular patterns of family relationships, as well as from the way alcohol is used and drunkenness is regarded in the home.

HELP FOR PEOPLE WITH DRINKING PROBLEMS

Alcoholism can be treated in many different ways, depending on the severity of the problem and the individual circumstances and personality of the patient. The first step is acknowledging that a problem exists. Thereafter, it is a matter of choosing the right type of help.

Self-help
For all types of assistance and advice, contact the national alcohol helpline on 01345-320202, or get in touch with Alcohol Concern, Waterbridge House, 32-36 Loman Street, London SE1 0EE. Alcoholics Anonymous runs groups across the country – look in your telephone directory for the local branch, or contact the head office at PO Box 1, Stonebow House, Stonebow, York YO 1 2NJ. Families can contact Al-Anon, 61 Great Dover Street, London SE1 4YF.

Drug therapy
Doctors can prescribe disulfiram (Antabuse) which causes nausea, flushing and other unpleasant symptoms when alcohol is drunk. This works well for highly motivated people able to cope with withdrawal symptoms. Medication is generally taken daily.

Psychotherapy
People who drink excessively usually need to tackle the problem psychologically as well as physically. Doctors can refer patients to counsellors or psychotherapists on the NHS. Many specialist agencies also offer treatment. Contact Alcohol Concern (above) or ACCEPT, 72-74 Fulham Road, Hammersmith, London SW6 5SE.

Detoxification programmes
Severe addiction to alcohol may need treatment in hospital or a special clinic to help with withdrawal symptoms and to provide long-term rehabilitation. The length of stay varies depending on individual needs, and is normally followed by a period of outpatient treatment to prevent a relapse and help with any difficulties. Referral is generally through a family doctor or a counsellor.

ARGUING ABOUT ALCOHOL

My husband and I argue a lot about his drinking. He says it's no problem. I'm afraid he may be becoming an alcoholic. How can I tell who's right?

In most people, the development of alcoholism is insidiously gradual, hard to trace and easy to ignore. Alcoholism affects thousands of families in this country, and while families react to drinking problems in different ways, there are some signs that commonly indicate the existence of a problem. Ask yourself these questions – if the answers are affirmative, your husband may indeed have a drinking problem.

● Do you and your children find yourselves tiptoeing around your husband when he has been drinking? Most families of alcoholics live in a constant state of insecurity – family members never know whether it will be a pleasant day or whether alcohol will make life miserable for everyone.
● Do tension levels in your home rise when your husband starts to drink? Are you afraid to talk about his drinking habits?
● Does your husband miss work frequently after evenings of heavy drinking?
● Has he been involved in traffic offences or fights when he drinks?
● Does he begin to drink in the morning, try to hide his drinking, feel guilty about drinking bouts, or make promises to stop?
● Has he tried to stop drinking and been unable to?

The very fact that you and your husband argue frequently about his drinking habits may in itself be a sign that alcohol is becoming a problem. Try to find a good time to talk calmly to your husband, avoiding arguments and criticism if you can. Suggest he speak to his doctor or contact an organisation such as Alcohol Concern (see panel opposite) for referral to advisory and helpline agencies.

CONSIDERING FRIENDS

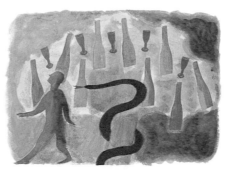

How dangerous is it for a recovered alcoholic to have the occasional drink? Should friends refrain from drinking in his or her presence?

Although some people with drinking problems do find that they can keep them under control while continuing to drink socially, most of the evidence suggests that total abstinence is the only really safe approach, particularly for anyone struggling with a severe dependence on alcohol.

In the first few weeks it would clearly be kinder for friends to avoid drinking in front of a recovering alcoholic. Gradually, however, the person will need to get used to facing situations where alcohol is being consumed and where the urge to drink has to be controlled. If you know someone is a recovered alcoholic, don't offer them alcohol but, equally, don't avoid it completely yourself. It will not help the person to feel that others are behaving abnormally in their presence.

Alcohol and the mind

Despite being so much a part of our culture, alcohol is a dangerous drug with powerful effects on both mind and brain, including:

● Lowered activity in the central nervous system. In large amounts, or in combination with drugs such as sedatives, the effect can be dangerous.
● Diminished inhibitions.
● Forgetfulness.
● Weakened judgment.
● Drowsiness.
● In large amounts: slurred speech, staggering, memory loss, eventually coma and even death.
● Prolonged heavy drinking: dependence, permanent memory damage; hallucinations and convulsions when alcohol is withdrawn.

Overcoming drug dependency

ADDICTED OR DEPENDENT?

Sometimes you hear about people being 'dependent' on drugs. What does this mean – is it the same as being addicted?

Mood-altering drugs affect the brain in ways still not fully understood. Why some of these drugs become addictive is an even more complicated matter. The language itself can be quite confusing, with the term addiction increasingly being supplanted, at least among professionals, by the term dependence. The newer term avoids the difficult issue of distinguishing between physical and psychological dependence (the term addiction can properly be used only when there is physical dependence).

There are two aspects to physical dependence: tolerance – the need to take ever larger doses in order to achieve the same level of intoxication – and withdrawal symptoms – painful or distressing symptoms that occur when the drug is denied. Some drugs, such as heroin, give rise to both; some to one or the other; and some to neither. Drugs that do not produce true physical dependence such as cannabis may still cause psychological dependence – a state in which the user has a compulsive emotional need for the substance. However, since both types of dependence have a biochemical basis in the brain, the distinction between the two terms is blurred. Whether the drug is nicotine, alcohol or heroin, breaking a drug dependence can be a difficult, sometimes painful, process. The first step is recognition that a problem exists, followed by detoxification, either abrupt or gradual, depending on the drug and the user.

Withdrawal symptoms, when they occur, also vary from drug to drug and user to user in both kind and severity. In the worst cases, such as heroin, withdrawal can cause severe physical symptoms and should be undertaken only under expert medical supervision (see page 210). In addition to medical help, rehabilitation measures can include psychotherapy to deal with any underlying or contributing behavioural or psychological problems, personal counselling and membership of support groups.

The vicious spiral of drug abuse and its cost to individuals, their families and society at large have heightened scientific interest in finding medical treatments that can facilitate withdrawal from drugs, or eliminate the desire for them. Antabuse and methadone were two of the first and best-known drug

treatments, and are still used for overcoming dependence on alcohol and heroin. More recently new antidepressant, anticonvulsant and antianxiety drugs have been yielding promising results in animal trials. Although such drugs may one day help to win the battle against addiction completely, today relapses remain common among recovering addicts, and it may take several attempts before a dependency can be broken.

PERSONALITY AND ADDICTION

Why is it that some people who take drugs become addicted while others don't seem to? Is there really such a thing as an addictive personality?

Although human beings have used mood-altering substances since their earliest history, no one yet fully understands why one person can remain a casual user while someone else will become dependent.

Scientific research is building up knowledge of the various ways in which psychoactive drugs interfere with the workings of the brain. But biochemical descriptions alone only partially explain the process by which an individual develops a dependency on drugs. The same is true of personality and environment. The concept of an addictive personality is a controversial and not very useful one. It suggests, on the one hand, that 'weak-willed' people are to blame for their drug problems and, on the other, that they are not responsible for their behaviour.

While the tendency to abuse drugs may be encouraged by psychological traits such as low self-esteem as well as certain environmental factors, such as poverty, family upheavals, and social and peer-group pressures, it remains a fact that people from all walks of life and of different psychological types become habitual drug users.

Three overlapping factors appear to affect anyone's reaction to intoxicants: the nature of the drug, the nature of the user and the setting in which drug use takes place. The kind of drug – in particular, its potential to cause physical or psychological dependence – interacts with an individual's biological and temperamental make-up and with his or her background and environment to determine whether that person will become an addict. The availability of any drug and whether its use is condoned or condemned in a particular social setting also play a critical role in determining how widely it will be used and what its use will mean to those who take it and to those around them.

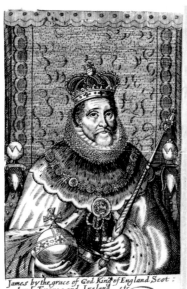

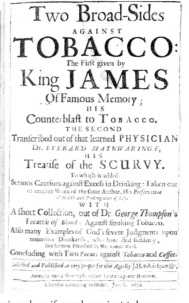

Monarch with a message James I campaigned vociferously against tobacco – which he rightly viewed as a dangerous drug. Like modern antidrugs campaigns, his tract did not convince everybody, and tobacco use soon became widespread.

SPOTTING THE SIGNS OF DRUG ABUSE

In addition to well-known, socially acceptable drugs such as nicotine and alcohol, dozens of other substances are used recreationally for their mind or mood-altering properties. They include both medical drugs such as tranquillisers and sleeping pills, over-the-counter glues and other solvent-based products, and so-called street drugs such as cannabis and cocaine. Not all users come to harm or experience dependency, but there are real risks and, in a small minority of cases, they can be grave. This table outlines the potential effects and signs of use of some common drugs.

DRUG	EFFECTS AND DANGERS	SIGNS OF USE
DEPRESSANTS		
Barbiturates Taken orally as sleeping pills, capsules or liquids; sometimes injected.	Reduced tension and anxiety, slowed heart rate and breathing, lethargy. Overdose can lead to coma, brain damage or even death. Risk of HIV and other infections if injected with shared needles.	Slurred speech, drowsiness, lack of interest. Person may stagger or appear disorientated.
Benzodiazepines Usually swallowed as tranquilliser pills or capsules such as diazepam, nitrazepam and temazepam.	Relaxation, reduced anxiety, slowed physical and mental functioning, depression. Blunted perception of pleasure and pain. Tolerance can lead to need for increased dosage.	Drowsiness, poor concentration, increased aggression. Normal inhibitions are reduced or disappear.
Solvents Inhaled as vapours from glues, lighter fuels and cleaning fluids.	Euphoria, giddiness, confusion, loss of appetite. Outbreaks of bad temper. Overdose is easy and can lead to organ damage or death from asphyxiation or heart failure.	Changed behaviour and personality. Dilated or constricted pupils, bloodshot eyes, swelling around eyes, nasal discharge. Breath and clothes frequently smell of solvent fumes.
STIMULANTS		
Amphetamines Swallowed as tablets (including 'ecstasy'); occasionally inhaled as powder or injected in solution.	Quickened pulse, nervous exhaustion, insomnia, depression, dizziness, palpitations, paranoia. Risk of infection if injected with shared needles. Ecstasy occasionally causes sudden death.	Hyperactivity, dilated pupils, staring or prominent eyes, bad breath, mouth ulcers, flushed skin.
Cocaine Inhaled or injected as cocaine hydrochloride powder; smoked as 'crack'.	Euphoria, enhanced self-confidence, racing pulse, loss of appetite, agitation, anxiety, depression. Dependence, damaged nasal passages, risk of infection if needles shared. Overdose may cause seizure or heart failure.	Nasal discharge, weight loss, behaviour or personality change.
PAIN RELIEVERS		
Opiates Smoked, inhaled or injected as heroin; injected or swallowed as methadone, codeine or other narcotic drugs.	Euphoria, lethargy, stupor, unconsciousness, shallow breathing, loss of self-control. Diminished reaction to pain and anxiety; feelings of contentment. Dependence frequently develops. Risk of HIV and other infections if needles shared.	Constricted pupils, speech slow and slurred. Inhalation causes nasal rawness or redness, injection leaves needle marks.
DRUGS THAT ALTER PERCEPTION		
Cannabis Smoked or swallowed as dried leaf, resin or oil.	Euphoria, relaxation, giddiness, mood swings, dry mouth, hunger, loss of coordination and sense of time, drowsiness. Panic, confusion and paranoia with large doses.	Talkativeness, mood swings, bloodshot eyes. Increased appetite.
LSD (lysergic acid diethylamide) Swallowed in various forms.	Hallucinations, disturbed sensation, muscle rigidity, paranoia, panic, depression, tolerance. Flashbacks and psychological problems from 'bad trips' are possible.	Unpredictable or violent behaviour, dilated pupils.

How do drugs influence mood?

Drugs that affect the way you feel do so by altering the level and activity of messenger substances, or neurotransmitters, that carry signals from one brain cell to another.

● Stimulants such as cocaine bind to receptor sites for the neurotransmitter dopamine, preventing its reabsorption into nerve cells. The resulting increase of dopamine levels in the brain produces the euphoria characteristic of a cocaine high.
● Heroin and other opiates imitate the action of natural pain-killing neurotransmitters called endorphins. When heroin is available to the brain, endorphin production is suppressed. If drug use suddenly stops, the brain is left without a buffer against pain; the result is distressing withdrawal symptoms.
● Depressants such as alcohol and some sleeping pills may enhance the action of the inhibitory neurotransmitter GABA. Alcohol also seems to affect several other neurotransmitters.

SMOKING CANNABIS

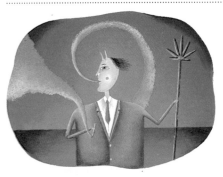

What, if any, are the long-term effects of smoking cannabis?

To date, most studies looking at chronic and heavy use of cannabis have failed to produce clear evidence of any physical or psychological damage. However, possible connections between long-term, heavy use and various health problems are still suspected, including chromosomal damage, birth defects in babies, impaired immune system responses, lower levels of testosterone in men and menstrual irregularities in women.

In the short term, there is evidence that memory loss and anxiety reactions occur in some users. Schizophrenics and people who are clinically depressed are more at risk and may experience worse symptoms.

Because cannabis smoke is inhaled very deeply and held in the lungs for several seconds, smoking four cannabis cigarettes is potentially as damaging to respiratory capacity, and as carcinogenic, as smoking a pack of 20 cigarettes.

Even so, cannabis is a very widely used drug. Intoxication creates a mild sense of euphoria, with effects usually lasting from two to four hours. It tends to relax users, making them feel sleepy, dreamy and often extremely hungry.

Apart from the possible physical risks, driving under the influence of cannabis is also a hazard, since intoxication can impair judgment, slow reaction time, and impair visual tracking (the ability to follow moving objects accurately with the eyes).

It was once thought that cannabis led people inevitably on to harder drugs. While it is true that many users of heroin, cocaine and psychedelic drugs did begin by smoking cannabis, experts now believe that this has more to do with the nature of drug culture than with any pharmacological effects of cannabis. Before cannabis, most drug users very probably smoked cigarettes and drank alcohol, but this does not mean that these things led them on to cannabis. Nevertheless, the use of any mood-altering substance for non-medical, recreational purposes is not advisable, especially for young people, whose emotional responses and sense of identity are still developing.

GIVING UP HEROIN

What makes heroin so addictive? Is there any way of helping people to give up the habit without suffering terrible withdrawal symptoms?

Like other drugs derived from opium, heroin effectively mimics the action of natural mood-enhancing, pain-killing brain chemicals known as endorphins. If it is taken long enough, the body may stop producing endorphins and, if the supply of heroin is then also stopped, the effects on body and mind can be (but by no means always are) agonising. Symptoms range from sneezing, cramps, chills, tremors and vomiting to – in the absence of treatment – seizures, coma and sometimes death. Because of these risks, giving up heroin should never be attempted except under medical supervision.

Despite this, it is the policy in some countries not to provide relief treatment for patients in withdrawal clinics. This is the source of most of the horrific tales of suffering when people try to give up. In Britain, however, efforts are made to control symptoms and to minimise discomfort. This is accomplished either with a programme of gradual reduction or by substituting less harmful drugs such as methadone, which is then slowly withdrawn. Under these conditions, symptoms may be no worse than a bad case of flu. The more difficult aspect of treatment, and the real test, comes with preventing relapses in the weeks that follow.

HELP FOR DRUG USERS

Where can drug users go for help in overcoming their problem?

Provided they feel comfortable about it, drug users are probably best advised to speak to their doctor, since he knows their medical history and background and may have some insight into the problem. Although they do not always treat drug addiction themselves, doctors are the best source of information about local drug centres and programmes where specialist help is available. If necessary, they can also refer patients to psychiatrists or psychiatric nurses. People who feel reluctant to speak to their own doctor may find it easier to contact an agency such as one of these:

● Release, 388 Old Street, London EC1V 9LT provides help with all drug problems and refers callers to drug projects in their area.
● Narcotics Anonymous operates a helpline on 0171 498 9005.
● Resolve helps with solvent abuse and can be contacted on 01785 817 885.
● Cocaine Anonymous, on 0171 284 1123, can help with cocaine or crack dependency.

● People who find they cannot give up prescribed tranquillisers can get help from the Council for Involuntary Tranquilliser Addiction, Cavendish House, Brighton Road, Waterloo, Liverpool L22 5NG.

Help is also available from several sources for families of people with drug problems.

● Adfam – call 0171 638 3700.
● Families Anonymous – contact them on 0171 498 4680.
● Parent Line – mothers and fathers can call the helpline on 01268 757 077.

Coping with schizophrenia

WHO GETS SCHIZOPHRENIA?

How common is schizophrenia and what causes this illness?

About one person in a hundred is afflicted by a schizophrenic illness at some time in their life. There are many more people, however, who are affected in terms of disrupted relationships and family life.

Although the disease can begin at any time, it usually first appears during late adolescence or early adulthood. Roughly equal numbers of men and women are affected.

The symptoms can be alarming and, more than any other type of mental illness, reflect the popular conception of insanity. Victims lose contact with reality and become increasingly difficult to relate to. Classic symptoms of schizophrenia include bizarre conversation and behaviour, disturbed thoughts and perceptions, disordered thinking, a lack of energy, hearing voices or seeing visions, inappropriate emotional responses and signs of agitation or even violence.

No one knows exactly what causes schizophrenia. While drugs can control its symptoms, no cure exists. Enlargement of brain ventricles and excessive sensitivity to the neurotransmitter substance dopamine have been observed in some studies of schizophrenics but it is not known how these might be related to the illness.

While heredity appears to be a factor in certain cases, inheriting a tendency to schizophrenia does not on its own guarantee that the disease will inevitably develop. When it does, some complicating external factor is often found to be involved, such as a viral infection, a particularly traumatic event or a prolonged period of stress.

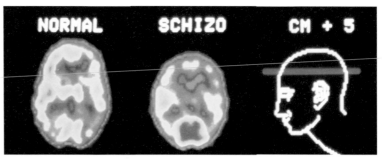

The effect of schizophrenia Colour-coded PET scans show a different pattern of activity in the schizophrenic brain. Blue and green areas are using less glucose, yellow and red more. The plane of the cross-section is indicated on the right.

HELP FOR A SCHIZOPHRENIC

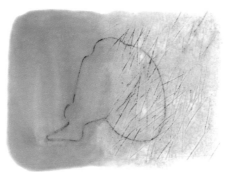

Our son has schizophrenia and although he is on medication his behaviour is seriously disrupting our home life. Would he and the rest of the family be better off if he were placed in a long-stay hospital?

Schizophrenia is very hard on families, but with the right type of treatment your son can almost certainly be helped to reach a stable state that will allow him to continue living a relatively independent life, either as part of the family or in sheltered housing of some sort. Before you do anything else, try to make sure that your son actually is taking his medication: stopping is one of the commonest causes of relapses. The next step is to discuss your son's medication with his psychiatrist. If you wish, you are also entitled to ask for a second opinion about his diagnosis and treatment at this stage.

As your son is clearly not managing well at home at the moment, it is possible that he will need a period of drug treatment in hospital – probably lasting several weeks or even a few months – to stabilise his condition.

Once this is achieved his psychiatrist and social worker will be able to advise you on longer-term living arrangements.

While schizophrenia is extremely distressing for everyone in the family, you can take heart from the fact that only a tiny number of cases cannot be controlled by drugs.

For further help, you may wish to contact the National Schizophrenia Fellowship, 28 Castle Street, Kingston upon Thames, Surrey KT1 1SS, or SANE, 2nd Floor, Worthington House, 199-205 Old Marylebone Road, London NW1 5QP.

How to get help

How drugs can help the mind

Many psychological symptoms can be helped with medication.

● Antidepressants raise levels of certain neurotransmitters and stimulate brain cell activity. They include tricyclic antidepressants, monoamine oxidase (MAO) inhibitors and a newer group of drugs (SRIs) such as fluoxetine and paroxetine which appear to have fewer side effects. Antidepressants are sometimes also given for anxiety attacks and eating disorders.
● Antianxiety drugs, or minor tranquillisers, relieve tension but can be addictive. Benzodiazepines such as temazepam also promote drowsiness and can be used against insomnia. Beta-blockers are used when there are physical symptoms such as palpitations. They are not addictive.
● Antipsychotic drugs, or major tranquillisers, are used to control some serious mental and behavioural disorders.
● Antimanic drugs such as lithium help against manic depression.

TREATMENT ON THE NHS

What sort of help is available on the NHS for people with mental, emotional or behavioural problems?

Many different types of treatment and help are currently available. If you are feeling anxious or depressed, have problems with a relationship or are suffering from stress, visit your doctor. He or she may offer a prescription for a drug with psychological or mood-altering effects or refer you to someone more specialised in treating your particular problem. A growing number of doctors have counsellors attached to their practice these days but as demand often exceeds supply you may have to join a waiting list or be offered only a limited number of sessions. However, treatment is free of charge. Many people find it extremely helpful to have someone sympathetic to talk to about their concerns.

Some find a great release in just being listened to, others in learning to express deep, hidden emotions or in exploring a difficult situation and working towards improving it. Longer-term psychotherapy is also available for more in-depth analysis, although waiting lists are often long – up to twelve months in some areas.

Patients with a specific behavioural problem, such as a phobia or eating disorder, can be referred to a clinical psychology unit. For problems with a physical basis, patients may be referred to a psychiatrist instead. Psychiatrists approach mental problems from a medical point of view and are expert at diagnosing and treating chemical imbalances in the brain, mainly by means of drug therapy. Neurologists and neurosurgeons treat brain disorders such as tumours and injuries.

There are large overlaps in the work of all these professionals, but your doctor should be able to refer you to the kind of service best suited to your needs.

CHOOSING AN APPROACH

What are the main schools of psychotherapy and how do they differ?

Most psychotherapists today do not follow a single rigid approach, but combine elements taken from several, adapting them to the needs of individual patients. Nevertheless, they often have a basic training in and orientation towards one of the major approaches. Before signing up with a therapist, it is as well to check that you are in sympathy with his or her fundamental outlook and that it is suitable for the kind of help you want.

Behavioural therapy
Practitioners focus on changing or eradicating unwanted aspects of behaviour, such as phobic reactions or addictions. Treatment is short-term, and specific, measurable goals are set. It is less suitable for probing the deeper questions of life.

Cognitive therapy
The emphasis is on altering thought patterns that underlie particular feelings and behaviour. Therapy is intensive and short-term, and aimed at problems such as depression and oversensitivity to criticism.

Counselling
The aim of counselling is to help people to come to terms with a crisis in their lives or to improve their lives or relationships in practical ways. Counselling is short-term,

goal-directed and often specific – as in bereavement counselling, marriage guidance or vocational guidance.

Humanistic or existential therapy

There are wide differences among these therapists, but all aim to help the patient – or client – to take responsibility for his life and to realise his full potential. Therapy may be short or long-term, depending on the needs and goals of the client.

Psychoanalysis

Therapists use deep and intensive analysis of the past to help patients to understand their hidden motives and desires. The relationship with the therapist is central and therapy may continue for years. It is most suitable for people who want to engage in personal discovery or who have personality problems.

Making your choice

Whatever sort of therapy you want, look for a practitioner you trust, like and feel relaxed with. Start by making a trial appointment and don't be pressured into signing up if you have any doubts. Ask about the therapist's training and qualifications, whether he has had therapy himself, how therapy will help you, how long it will take and what it will cost. To find a therapist, contact the British Association for Counselling, 1 Regent Place, Rugby CV21 2PJ or The British Psychological Society, St Andrew's House, 4 Princes Road East, Leicester LE1 7DR for information.

JOINING A GROUP

Are there any advantages to group therapy over individual therapy? Are self-help groups effective?

Group therapy allows people to see how they are viewed and accepted by peers. In groups, people can act out family relationships and relive childhood experiences from an adult perspective. Groups also encourage empathy. By listening to others' stories, people learn more about their own problems and how to cope with them. Hearing the pain others endure, people better understand their own suffering and learn to put it in perspective. Group therapy is particularly helpful for those who have problems with interpersonal relationships, and it often works well in conjunction with individual therapy. Group sessions are also less expensive than individual therapy.

The healing power of talking to others with similar problems also explains the proliferation of self-help groups. Across the country, people meet to support each other through cancer, phobias, bereavement, rape, incest, single parenthood, depression and many other problems.

Most experts recommend that self-help groups be used to complement rather than as a substitute for psychotherapy, at least during an acute crisis. And after individual therapy is finished, groups can help to consolidate the gains.

Do-it-yourself treatment

For people without serious problems, but who want to enrich their lives, some everyday activities can be as effective as any kind of therapy.

Exercise
Sports and physical activity build confidence, improve health and make you feel and look better. Exertion also promotes the release of brain chemicals called endorphins, giving a safe natural high.

Artistic expression
Painting, writing, singing, playing a musical instrument, dancing and acting can all help you to express and develop yourself.

Talking
A friend you can really confide in performs many of the same functions as a professional counsellor. See page 176 for advice on how to talk about your feelings.

Self-development
Never stop learning. Foster old interests and new pursuits. When something arouses your curiosity, follow it up.

Giving to others
Everyone needs to be needed. However busy you are, try to make time for voluntary work of some sort. If free time is limited, perhaps you could occasionally offer professional services free of charge to a good cause.

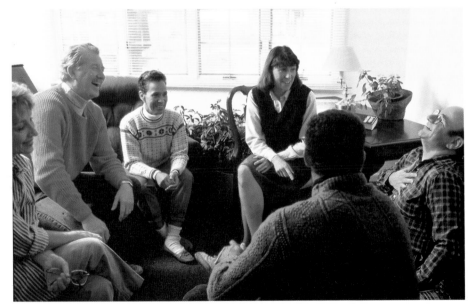

Helping one another Group therapy sessions are growing in popularity. Under the eye of a trained therapist, members enact their experiences and talk about their problems. As well as receiving treatment, participants benefit by seeing that they can contribute to healing others.

USING THE HEALTH CARE SYSTEM

*Being on the receiving end of medical care
should not be a baffling experience - study after study
shows that informed patients make faster progress when being
treated. They talk to doctors more easily, use the health
care system well and make wiser decisions.*

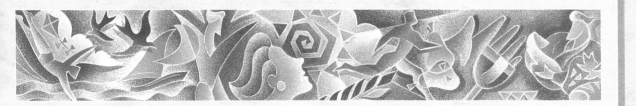

Are you getting the best from your doctor?

Good medical care needs open communication and a good relationship between doctor and patient. Here is a quick test to help you to assess your own situation.

In each case, tick the box that applies most closely to your doctor and practice. Then check your score to see how well you and your doctor are getting on.

1 Generally, if you phone first thing in the morning, can you expect to get an appointment with your own doctor on the same day?

a) Almost always. ☐
b) Sometimes. ☐
c) Very seldom. ☐

2 Do you ever come away from a consultation with questions that have not been answered?

a) Almost never. ☐
b) Occasionally. ☐
c) Frequently. ☐

3 How would you rate the answers and explanations your doctor gives to your questions?

a) Very good – they are both informative and useful. ☐
b) Fair – he tells me what to do but doesn't always say why. ☐
c) Poor – I sometimes feel unsure what advice I have been given. ☐

4 Does your doctor tell you why a drug is being prescribed and warn you about possible side effects?

a) Always. ☐
b) Most of the time. ☐
c) Rarely. ☐

5 Which statement most closely reflects your attitude to visiting your doctor?

a) I don't go for every cold, but I do go whenever I feel worried or doubtful. ☐
b) I see my doctor as soon as possible whenever I notice any symptoms. ☐
c) Only if it becomes an emergency. I prefer to let things sort themselves out. ☐

6 Have you ever had to complain about your doctor?

a) No, there has never been any reason. ☐
b) No, but I have thought about it. ☐
c) Yes. ☐

7 How many of these subjects has your doctor spoken to you about and, if necessary, offered advice on: smoking, exercise, alcohol consumption, hereditary illness, diet?

a) 4 or 5. ☐
b) 2 or 3. ☐
c) 1 or none. ☐

8 What are the other practice staff like?

a) Friendly and efficient. ☐
b) Businesslike but too busy to be really helpful. ☐
c) Difficult to deal with. ☐

SCORING

Award your doctor 2 points for every (a) answer, 1 point for every (b) answer, and nothing for every (c) answer. Add up your score.

13-16: You seem to be getting an excellent service from your doctor. You are probably a good patient too, asking questions and taking an interest in your own health care.

7-12: Your doctor is probably providing a good basic service but it sounds as if he or she may not always explain things properly. Make sure you don't leave the surgery until you are happy about your treatment.

6 or less: You may not be getting the most from your doctor. Remember, doctors are often under pressure and if patients don't speak up they will not know what is wrong. Good communication depends on you as much as your GP.

Choosing a family doctor

GETTING A RECOMMENDATION

We have recently moved to a new town and need to find a family doctor, but without knowing anyone in the area we feel lost. What should we do?

A personal recommendation is always helpful, so even though you have not yet made friends in the area try asking neighbours, parents at a child's school, the local chemist or even shop assistants. At least this may reveal any names that should be avoided.

If your enquiries don't produce a firm recommendation, call the local Family Health Services Authority (FHSA) – it will be listed in the *Yellow Pages* under 'Health Authorities and Services' – and ask for a list of local practices. Make a shortlist of practices near your home and visit the most promising, following the guidelines in the panel (right).

When you have made your choice, contact the practice and ask to join the list. All they will need are your family medical cards. If their list is full, you can either wait for the list to open again or approach your second choice. If no practice will accept you, which rarely happens, contact the FHSA, which is obliged by law to find you a doctor.

INITIAL CONSULTATIONS

I have just signed up at a new practice and have been asked to come in for an initial consultation. What is this for, and am I obliged to go?

When a patient joins a new surgery's list, most doctors like to take the opportunity to arrange a simple health check and learn something about the person's way of life.

This is usually performed by the practice nurse and is made up of two components – a physical check-up concerning blood pressure, weight and a test for diabetes, followed by a discussion or questionnaire about your personal history, habits, way of life and immunisation record.

Women may also be asked about contraception and any pregnancies, and may be encouraged to take part in screening programmes for cervical and breast cancer. The initial consultation is not compulsory, but it is very much in your interests to make sure you attend. Not only does it help with the

prevention and possible early diagnosis of problems, but it is also a good opportunity to get to know the practice staff in a relaxed way, rather than when you are ill.

APPOINTMENTS SYSTEMS

From the patient's point of view, is it better to choose an appointments-only practice or one that operates a first-come, first-served system?

It all depends on your personal needs. If you have a medical condition that has to be monitored regularly, such as diabetes or high blood pressure, then you will almost certainly want to find a doctor who operates an appointments-only system so that you can plan your time in advance.

If on the other hand you seldom need to see a doctor, you may prefer to register with a practice that runs on a non-appointments system. You will at least have the assurance that you can see a doctor on the day you want, even if it might mean waiting.

A good alternative may be to look for a practice that operates a combination of the two systems with, for example, a 'free for all' morning surgery and an evening surgery by appointment only.

In any case, even practices that run an appointments-only system should always be able to find a slot for a patient when the problem is really urgent.

DIFFERENT TYPES OF PRACTICE

I have the choice of registering with a National Health Service centre or with a traditional general practice. What are the pros and cons of the different types of system?

There is in fact very little difference between these two types of practice.

When health centres were first established back in the 1960s, they were intended to be places where different health professionals could work together – regardless of whether they were self-employed (as are GPs) or employed by the National Health Service (as are the country's midwives, district nurses and health visitors). At that time, most doctors used to practise singly or in small partnerships, and it was something of a rarity for

DO'S
— AND —
DON'TS

for finding a good practice

Do ask for practice leaflets.
Do ask about the partners' special interests and qualifications.
Do think about convenience. Will you need transport to get there? Is it on a bus route? Is it on the way to and from work?
Do talk to the staff at the reception desk.
Do ask for details of emergency calls and home visits.
Do ask how the practice operates its procedure for appointments.

Don't judge a practice by appearances. The quality of the doctor is much more important than the quality of the waiting-room carpet.

FACT
— OR —
FALLACY?

'Doctors can remove difficult patients from their list.'

Fact But it usually only happens to abusive or violent patients. Fears have been voiced that fundholding doctors may try to remove patients requiring expensive treatment (see page 248) but there is no evidence that it happens.

Why register?

People who don't have a doctor cause problems for both themselves and the health service.

● Hospitals are not obliged to treat minor ailments a GP could deal with. If they do, they give minimal supplies of drugs and dressings.
● Medical care is about prevention too. People without a doctor miss out on screening and other vital services.

a medical practice even to have a nurse of its own. Nowadays, however, nearly every GP practice has at least one practice nurse and many can offer additional services such as counselling and physiotherapy, regardless of whether they are based in a health centre or in a more traditional type of surgery.

The premises from which a practice operates is just one of the factors to consider when deciding where to register. It is also advisable to find out about staff and their qualifications, any special clinics that the practice runs and the appointments system they operate before you finally make up your mind whether a practice is right for you.

Finally, don't overlook the human side. Find a doctor whom you like, trust and can talk to easily – vital factors in the success of any medical treatment.

CHANGING WITHIN A PRACTICE

After years of being treated by our long-standing family GP, my daughter wants to transfer to another doctor at the same practice. Can she do so without upsetting the family's relationship with the GP?

Any patient over 16 years of age has the right to change doctors within the same practice or to join the list at another local practice, provided the list is open. She should just ask – it is not necessary to give a reason.

It is highly unlikely that your family's relationship with your existing doctor will be affected in any way by such a change. He or she will almost certainly respect your daughter's desire for independence and should not be offended in any way.

Special services for special needs

Your doctor can refer you to many therapists for particular kinds of treatment, including:

● Audiologists – for hearing disorders.
● Chiropodists – for foot problems.
● Chiropractors or osteopaths – for back and neck pain.
● Community nurses – for mother-and-baby care, home care, psychiatric care and other forms of assistance.
● Counsellors – for marriage guidance and emotional and behavioural problems.
● Dentists – for tooth and gum care.
● Dieticians and nutritionists – for weight problems and diets.
● Geneticists – for help with hereditary diseases.
● Physiotherapists and occupational therapists – for rehabilitation after accident or injury.
● Speech therapists – for speech impediments.

Making an appointment

AM I WASTING MY GP'S TIME?

Some people seem to run to the doctor at every opportunity while others take risks by leaving it to the last moment. How can I tell when a visit is really justified?

A visit to your doctor is always justified if you have a genuine concern about your health and the way you are feeling. Your doctor would always prefer to reassure you than to tell you that you are seriously ill.

Although nine out of ten illnesses clear up in their own time and need no medical intervention, never delay reporting any of the symptoms listed on page 125. Other cases can be more difficult to judge. Be guided by common sense and self-knowledge and, if in doubt, make an appointment.

THE RECEPTIONIST'S ROLE

How much should I tell the doctor's receptionist when I make an appointment?

A doctor's receptionist has an extremely difficult job. He or she has to apportion a doctor's time according to the demands and medical needs of all the patients on the doctor's list. As demand usually exceeds supply, especially at short notice, appointment slots are frequently booked up days in advance. Even so, the receptionist can always fit in a new case that is genuinely urgent – but judging this requires some information from the

patient. While they are not medically qualified, receptionists who have been doing the job for years do know a surprising amount.

If you want a simple routine appointment, then there is no need to discuss your reasons with the reception staff, who will probably not be interested anyway. If, on the other hand, you want an urgent appointment it helps everyone if you are prepared to tell the receptionist the nature of the emergency. Few receptionists are the dragons of popular myth; they do the job because they like to help people. In addition they are sworn to secrecy about any information they acquire in the course of their duties.

SEEING YOUR OWN DOCTOR

I'm often offered the choice between taking the first available appointment with any doctor or waiting longer to see my own doctor. Does it really matter if I sometimes see a different doctor?

The real question here is whether the quality of care that you receive is affected by seeing a succession of different doctors.

In most cases the answer is a straightforward 'no', although in a few circumstances it may be best to stick with the same doctor. Although all treatment is recorded on your medical card, continuity is generally desirable when you have a chronic complaint that requires monitoring or variations in treatment or drug dosage, or when you have a complex medical history that is well known by one particular doctor. In general, psychiatric problems also tend to benefit from a consistent doctor/patient relationship.

TELEPHONING FOR ADVICE

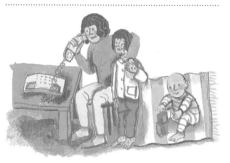

Is it a good idea to telephone my doctor for advice if I'm not sure whether I need to come in for a consultation or not?

The telephone can be extremely useful when it comes to dealing with straightforward problems and can save time for both you and your doctor. In rural areas some doctors set aside specific times for telephone consultations. Formal arrangements of this kind are less common in towns and cities, but most doctors will call back in an emergency in response to a telephone enquiry even if they cannot talk to you at the time of your call. You will probably have to explain the nature of your problem to the reception staff before a call back is arranged, and you will obviously have to wait by the telephone until you are contacted. The expected arrival of video telephones may in the future make full long-distance consultations a real possibility.

ALL-NIGHT SURGERIES

I've heard that there is a scheme to open all-night surgeries for treating emergency cases. How will this work? Will I be able to get a doctor to come and see me if I am taken ill at night?

General practitioners are self-employed, and have a contract with the government to provide health services to people on their list. This contract makes your doctor responsible for your medical care 24 hours a day, 365 days a year. In partnerships and group practices doctors can arrange a rota so that they are not on call every night, but doctors who work alone cannot do this.

Night calls have doubled in recent years, and increasingly GPs are finding that a night on duty means little or no sleep. It usually comes between two full days' work and it is not surprising that doctors sometimes feel too tired to give of their best. As a result doctors are increasingly employing night-time deputising services, even though these are a particularly expensive option. Also, deputising services are available only in well populated areas, and rural doctors still have to do all their own night work.

Many doctors now feel that the 24-hour-a-day clause should be removed from their contracts, and night cover run as a separate service within the NHS. One suggested way to provide this is by means of all-night surgeries run by different medical staff.

In one or two larger towns, GP practices have now banded together to experiment with this idea, and the results look promising. Unlike a deputising service, an all-night surgery can offer telephone advice and treatment on the premises as well as house calls when necessary. One such surgery claims that four out of ten night calls are dealt with on the telephone and, in a large percentage of the remaining cases, the patient is well enough to visit the surgery. Those who need home visits still get them.

THE PRACTICE NURSE

My doctor refers patients to the nurse for simple treatments – which means a new appointment and a second trip to the surgery. Could I simply make an appointment with her in the first place?

There are no general rules here. Every practice is different, and the activities undertaken by practice nurses vary greatly.

Until recently, nurses' duties and responsibilities were very restricted, and they did little more than dress wounds and remove stitches. But things have changed, and the 'nurse practitioner' now has an increasingly important role to play in primary health

Saving a doctor's time The nurse plays an important role in the surgery, doing routine work, such as blood pressure monitoring, that would otherwise take up much of the doctor's day.

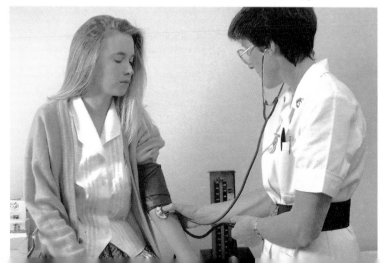

care. Previously, nurses could not prescribe drugs, but new regulations now permit district nurses and health visitors who have had special additional training to prescribe from a limited range of medicines.

These new rules do not apply to practice nurses, however, who can initiate treatment in only a very few circumstances.

In some surgeries, the practice nurse may do all routine cervical smears, run clinics for diabetes, asthma and hypertension patients, take blood, give initial health checks to new patients and administer routine innoculations. Nevertheless, all the nurse's work is under the direction and the responsibility of the employing doctor.

Ask at the reception desk if you feel that you have no need to see the doctor, but the general rule, unless you have been specifically told otherwise, is that you must always see a doctor first. The doctor then prescribes appropriate treatment from the nurse.

ASKING FOR A HOME VISIT

My father has difficulty walking even a short distance. Can he ask the doctor to visit him at home?

Unless home visits are absolutely necessary they are discouraged for two main reasons – time and the consulting environment. General practitioners have an extremely busy life, and good time management is critical to the successful running of a medical practice. On average, a surgery consultation takes from five to ten minutes whereas a home visit takes about half an hour. It is obvious that too many home visits can be disruptive and interfere with the service offered to other patients. The other problem is the environment in which a patient is seen. A surgery is

well-equipped and organised to make examinations easy. Examining patients at home can often be awkward.

Difficulty in walking may be due to a wide range of medical problems from arthritis to heart disease, and from back injury to multiple sclerosis. The reasons for your father's immobility and the possible alternatives to walking to the surgery are all-important in determining if a home visit is appropriate. Whatever the problem, however, you can be assured your father will get a home visit if he really needs one. If it would merely be more convenient for him to be visited at home, however, his request may well be refused.

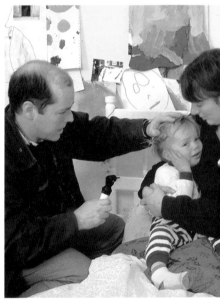

Doctor on call On a home visit, a GP uses an otoscope to examine the ear of a sick child. Despite their busy schedules, doctors will always find time to call at a patient's home whenever there is a real need.

Consulting your doctor

WHO DECIDES THE TREATMENT ?

I was once surprised to be asked by a doctor if I wanted a prescription for antibiotics. Isn't it up to the doctor to decide?

In this case, you will almost certainly have consulted your doctor about a respiratory infection and it is in this area that the use of antibiotics is in most doubt. The majority of coughs, colds, sore throats and flu-like illnesses are caused by respiratory viruses, and

antibiotics have no effect on viral infections. A small number of these infections, however, are caused by bacteria, and bacteria are susceptible to antibiotics. Like viral illnesses, nearly all bacterial infections will in time be overcome by natural defences, but there is evidence that recovery is quicker if antibiotics are used.

The doctor's problem is always to determine which infections are caused by which microorganism, and this is often impossible on clinical examination alone. The decision whether or not to prescribe antibiotics in such a case can be very difficult.

When asking if you wanted a prescription for antibiotics your doctor will have decided that you do not absolutely require one, and could have had several things in mind. He or she may have wanted to hear your opinion with a view to educating you about antibiotics and their uses, perhaps hoping to save you from unnecessary consultations in the future. Or your doctor may have wanted to know your preferences for getting better slightly more quickly as against relying on your body's own healing powers.

This is all part of an increasing tendency in modern medicine to encourage patients to become better informed about health, to take more responsibility for themselves, and to participate more in treatment decisions. No medical intervention is without disadvantages as well as benefits, and weighing up the pros and cons should rightly involve patients as well as doctors. Feel free to raise the issue with your doctor – most GPs would welcome more input from patients.

IMPROVING CONSULTATIONS

My doctor seldom explains anything, even when he gives me a prescription. As a result, I often find I have unanswered questions later on. Is there any way of making our meetings more constructive?

Doctors are highly trained to think in a particular way, and although the patient may not always realise it, the doctor is proceeding according to a set pattern. Understanding how he is thinking may help you to get more out of your time together.

The first part of a medical consultation is intended for you to present the history of your symptoms. Your doctor will want to know what they are, how badly they affect you and how long you have had them. In the case of an infectious illness, he will want to find out whether anyone in your immediate circle has had similar symptoms. With certain kinds of illness, the doctor may also need to know details of your medical history that could have a bearing on the current problem. Some doctors merely listen in this early consultation stage, while others may lead you through it by direct questioning.

While you are presenting your case the doctor will be drawing up a list of possibilities, or a 'differential diagnosis', in his mind. In the second part of the consultation the doctor takes charge, and will ask direct questions about your symptoms. Your answers

allow him to rule out some of the diagnoses he has been considering and narrow down the list of possibilities even further.

At this stage he will decide whether an examination is necessary in order to exclude some possibilities or to confirm the diagnosis he has come to. This is the time when your doctor should tell you what he thinks is wrong. If he does not, ask him. If he still has not reached a final diagnosis, he may want to arrange further investigations, such as blood tests, X-rays or urine samples. If he does not volunteer the information, ask him what he is hoping to establish by performing any suggested tests.

The final part of the consultation is given over to what needs to be done to treat your condition. This is called 'management', and your say should be important here.

Treatment may require drugs, hospital referral, physiotherapy, changing your diet or simply having a few days' bed rest. If your doctor does not tell you what he hopes to achieve by the course of action, you must ask. It is *your* body that is being treated, and you have every right to know.

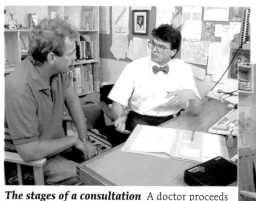

The stages of a consultation A doctor proceeds by listening to and then questioning his patient (above). Examination (right), diagnosis and, if necessary, prescription of treatment follow.

WITHHOLDING TREATMENT

My doctor told me to lose weight, but I haven't been able to. Now I feel somewhat guilty about going back to him. Could he refuse to treat me?

If your doctor has advised you to lose weight, it was probably for a good reason. Being overweight is not an illness in itself, but it does increase the strain on the body, making the heart and lungs work harder and exerting pressure on the joints. Even so, there is no need to feel embarrassed about going back to your GP. The very fact that you are finding it difficult to lose weight means it is a good idea to get further advice and possibly referral to a dietician. You should certainly not avoid your doctor – he will be quite used to this situation and cannot refuse treatment (nor will he wish to).

The only possible exception is if you were asked to lose weight in advance of an operation, in which case you may find that for medical reasons the procedure has to be postponed or even cancelled.

FEELING SHY

I know that doctors have 'seen it all before' but I still find it difficult to talk about personal complaints in the surgery. How can I overcome my embarrassment?

You are certainly not alone in this problem and your doctor will be used to dealing with it. If you can, explain how you feel; you may be pleasantly surprised at how sympathetic and sensitive he or she turns out to be.

Another approach is to write down the symptoms you find embarrassing or practise talking about them with a close friend. Or you might feel more comfortable with a different doctor – perhaps one of the same age, sex or background as yourself. Many women choose to see a woman doctor for intimate examinations such as cervical smears, even if they are normally quite happy with a male GP. Whatever the circumstances, it is well worth sorting out the issue; a relaxed relationship with your doctor will make consultations much more useful.

If your embarrassment stems from gynaecological or sexual matters, then a visit to a family planning centre or a hospital genitourinary, or 'special', clinic may be a good idea. You can simply walk in without an appointment, wherever you are, and your anonymity is guaranteed.

VOLUNTARY CHECK-UPS

I would like to know my general state of health. Will my doctor be able to give me a check-up without a special reason?

Usually not within the NHS – but if you really want one you can consider paying for a check-up as a private patient, or having one through a health insurance scheme.

The whole subject of screening for people without apparent symptoms arouses fierce controversy within the medical profession. Some doctors feel that checking people who are basically healthy is of little medical value.

There are many reasons for this, some very technical, but even well-established screening programmes such as those for breast and cervical cancer have respected opponents.

This aside, there are a couple of examinations which all doctors agree are extremely worth while, and which you will certainly be able to have. The first is a blood pressure check, and the second is a urine test for diabetes. Some people also have family or personal medical histories which make other screening tests advisable.

By all means see your doctor and discuss any particular health worries. If your condition indicates the need for further tests, rest assured that they will be arranged.

CHILDREN'S CHECK-UPS

How often does a child need a check-up? What health checks are done at school?

During the preschool years, children should receive check-ups at regular intervals from a health visitor or at a child health clinic. The exact timing may vary from area to area, but in general checks are done at about the ages of one week, six weeks, eight months, eighteen months and three years, and also before starting school. The purpose is to monitor the child's development, movement, vision, hearing and social skills. Once at school, children are seen annually by a nurse and also have two hearing checks.

All children should also be registered with a general practitioner, whose main role is to treat illness rather than to monitor development. If clinic or school check-ups reveal any problems, the child's doctor is informed so that suitable treatment can be arranged.

Getting a head start Height is just one aspect of school clinic assessments. Other tests are made for coordination, speech and sight.

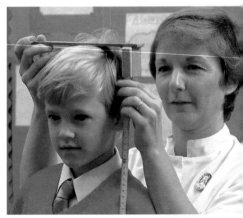

SPECIALIST CLINICS

What are the relative advantages and disadvantages of attending specialist clinics instead of seeing your own doctor?

Most hospitals run several specialist clinics for diabetes, high blood pressure, antenatal care and other common health problems. These generally need a referral from your doctor, so it is not an either/or option. There are two specialist clinics which you can consult without a referral, however – family planning clinics and genitourinary clinics. Family planning clinics provide contraceptive advice, medication and equipment, and genitourinary clinics are devoted specifically to the diagnosis and treatment of sexually transmitted diseases (STDs).

Although most doctors offer contraceptive services, some patients prefer to consult a specialist family planning doctor (usually a woman) for independent advice, or to take advantage of the special opening hours that clinics operate (lunchtime and after work, for example). Some people also prefer the anonymity of a clinic and a doctor they do not know. In addition, and unlike GPs, clinics can prescribe condoms free of charge.

As far as genitourinary clinics are concerned, diagnosis of STDs can be difficult and if you visit your doctor with symptoms (see page 218) he or she is in any case likely to direct you to visit a walk-in genitourinary clinic (probably at a local hospital) where any necessary tests can be done immediately.

SEEING A PHYSIOTHERAPIST

I hurt my shoulder playing tennis and other members of my tennis club have suggested that physiotherapy may help. How do I go about seeing a practitioner?

You can call a physiotherapist directly (you will find them listed under 'Sports Injury Clinics' in the *Yellow Pages*) and make an appointment for private treatment, or you can see your doctor first.

If you are unsure about precisely what is wrong with your shoulder, it might be best to start with your doctor – you need not necessarily have the same problem as others who found physiotherapy helpful, and the doctor may be able to suggest helpful exercises. Your doctor is better qualified to consider all the possibilities, make an accurate diagnosis and offer, or refer you for, appropriate treatment.

In any case, if you see a physiotherapist first, you may be sent back to your doctor if the therapist feels uncertain about diagnosis or treatment. If your doctor thinks that physiotherapy is needed, you can be referred on the NHS or, of course, go privately.

On-the-spot tests

More and more tests are now being carried out in the consulting room. Some give instant results; others have to go for laboratory analysis.

● Tests with immediate results include blood pressure, urine tests for diabetes, 'pinprick' blood tests for sugar count, simple tests of lung function, and sometimes a heart electrocardiogram.

● Tests that require laboratory analysis include blood sampling for cell counts, checking blood chemistry and clotting; swabs for infections; cervical smears; and urine tests for infections. Results of complicated tests may need to be explained at a second appointment.

Prescriptions and drugs

REPEAT PRESCRIPTIONS

Why do I have to repeat my prescription for ongoing medication every so often – and pay for it again? Is there a maximum length of time doctors may prescribe for?

In 1950 the total NHS drug bill was £20 million; in 1990 it was £3 billion – 150 times as much. It continues to increase every year.

This huge expenditure amounts to more than 10 per cent of total NHS resources, and not surprisingly controlling drug costs is a high priority. Research has shown that a large proportion of prescribed drugs are not used, and doctors are told that regular drugs (except for the contraceptive pill) should generally be prescribed in monthly quantities. This instruction is not legally binding, and in certain circumstances a doctor can prescribe larger quantities. Quite apart from the restraints on doctors' prescribing habits, there is another very sound reason for prescribing monthly amounts. Most drugs have a limited shelf life and the efficacy of out-of-date drugs cannot be guaranteed.

If you take a number of drugs on a regular basis and find the charges hard on your pocket, it may be worth investigating the prepayment scheme (see below).

A PRESCRIPTION SEASON TICKET

My parents are finding it difficult to afford all the various medicines they are supposed to take. I've heard that there is some sort of 'season ticket' scheme to help people in this position. How does it work?

Your parents may be entitled to free prescriptions (see panel, page 225) but if not, then the 'season ticket' scheme you mention could help them to diminish their medical expenses. Prices do change, but in 1995 the

---

DO'S AND DON'TS

for cutting the cost of prescriptions

Do check whether drugs can be purchased more cheaply over the counter.

Do ask if your condition will clear up without taking drugs.

Do check regularly with your doctor if long-term medication continues to be needed.

Don't assume you need a prescription. Studies show 80 per cent of patients expect one, putting doctors under pressure to provide it.

prepayment scheme was working out cheaper for patients who required six or more prescription items in a four-month period, or 15 items in a single year.

The cost of prepayment certificates tends to go up annually but as prescription charges also increase from time to time, certificates are likely to remain an advantageous option for many people.

Patients who wish to register with the prepayment scheme need to fill in Form FP95, obtainable from some doctor's surgeries or from a local social security or post office.

MEDICATION FOR TRAVELLERS

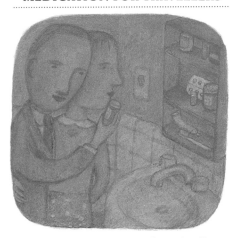

I am being sent overseas with my family on a two-year contract and am not sure what medical facilities will be available. Can my doctor prescribe enough medication to last the whole time? Will my wife be able to get a two-year supply of contraceptive pills?

Doctors in the NHS are not allowed to prescribe drugs for use abroad except over ordinary holiday breaks, so neither you nor your wife is entitled to NHS prescriptions to cover your overseas contract.

Your doctor may be prepared to give you a private prescription so that you can buy sufficient quantities of necessary drugs to see you through your overseas tour. This will depend on the shelf life of the drugs, the reasons you are on long-term drug therapy, how often your condition requires monitoring and where you are going.

He is likely to insist your wife has regular blood pressure checks while she is taking the contraceptive pill. Wherever your destination, it is essential to research your options before you go. If your employer does not provide private medical insurance while you are abroad, you will need to buy it for yourself and the family (see page 243).

Prescription checklist

If your doctor gives you a prescription, ask him or her these questions.

● Why is the drug needed and what is it supposed to do?
● What is the dose? How much and how often must you take it?
● When should it be taken – with food or at bedtime, for example?
● How long will the drug take to work and when can you stop taking it?
● Can you get a repeat prescription if needed?
● Are there any possible side effects? Could the medicine react with alcohol or other drugs?

USING ANTIBIOTICS

You hear such a lot about the overuse of antibiotics. What exactly are these drugs and how do they work? Do they cause any special problems?

Antibiotics are one of modern medicine's greatest lifesavers. Before their development – initially in the form of penicillin, discovered in 1928 – sore throats, chest infections, blood poisoning and dozens of other quite common bacterial infections could be fatal.

These days, dozens of different antibiotic drugs are used. Some work by killing off bacteria (bacteriocidal antibiotics) and others by halting their growth so that the immune system is better able to deal with them (bacteriostatic antibiotics).

Antibiotics are generally given only once an infection has developed, but they may also be prescribed as a preventative measure if the immune system is weak or if an infection would have serious consequences – in a patient with lung disease, for example.

Despite their huge potential for treating illness, antibiotics can be misused. Because they are so effective, some patients expect a prescription even when their body is quite able to fight off invaders without help. In the past some doctors have also been guilty of handing out antibiotics unnecessarily – although most now use them very judiciously (see pages 220-221).

As well as the possibility of side effects, which all drugs have, there is evidence that the widespread use of antibiotics is breeding

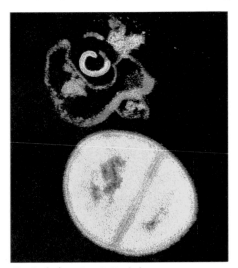

Bacteria in retreat *Staphylococcus aureus* faces an onslaught from antibiotics – below, a still intact bacterium about to divide; above, the remains after the drug has done its work.

stronger strains of bacteria, since these survive while weaker strains die. There are now some entirely drug-resistant strains of illnesses such as tuberculosis.

All this means that doctors are unlikely to offer antibiotics unless patients really need them. If they are prescribed, be sure to finish the course. If you don't the problem could flare up more virulently a second time and you may need more or stronger drugs.

DEALING WITH SIDE EFFECTS

How can I reduce the risks of side effects when I am taking medicine?

If you are offered a prescription for drugs, it is always worth asking your doctor whether other simple measures could avoid or reduce your need for medication – for example, reducing your alcohol intake and weight, and giving up smoking, if you have slightly raised blood pressure.

When you are given a new prescription, always make sure you know what time of day you need to take the medication, whether with food or liquid or on an empty stomach, and what you should do if you forget to take a tablet. Check how long you will be taking the drug and what the symptoms are of common side effects. If you are taking other medicines, including any over-the-counter types, ask the doctor whether there is any risk of bad interreactions between them.

Use all medicines with care, even over-the-counter ones, and follow the instructions exactly. Report any possible side effects to your doctor as soon as you notice symptoms. Inform anyone else who treats you, such as a dentist, about the drugs you are taking.

DRUGS THAT DON'T MIX

Which drugs are most likely to cause problems when taken together?

There are numerous ways that drugs interact with one another. Some effects are beneficial but others reduce the effectiveness of treatment. While doctors avoid prescribing bad combinations, over-the-counter medications are less easily controlled – be careful how you use them and consult a doctor if in doubt. These are some common problems.

● Alcohol, a drug in its own right, alters the effectiveness of many other drugs by slowing down digestion and absorption.
● Alcohol and aspirin both irritate the stomach – avoid taking them together.
● Some foods bind with drugs to form compounds that are difficult to digest, rendering medication less effective. Milk often has this effect, and iron pills and antacids can bind with antibiotics.
● Sedative drugs, such as alcohol and sleeping pills, can have a cumulative effect.
● People taking anticoagulants need to be careful of aspirin and antibiotics, which can promote bleeding.
● Antibiotics can reduce the effectiveness of the contraceptive pill.

Free prescriptions

Certain people are entitled to free prescriptions on the NHS.

● Old age pensioners.
● Children under 16.
● Students under 19 in full-time education.
● People with a current prepayment certificate (see page 223).
● People holding DSS exemption certificates.
● People with a current exemption certificate (Form FP92).
● Expectant mothers and those who have had a child in the last year.
● People with certain chronic conditions including an underactive adrenal, thyroid or parathyroid gland; or epilepsy requiring continuous treatment.
● People with disabilities that make it impossible for them to get about on their own.

Using your pharmacy

ADVICE FROM A PHARMACIST

I recently heard a radio programme where people were encouraged to consult pharmacists for advice about minor ailments. This sounds sensible, but how do I tell when I really need a doctor?

Many hours of a general practitioner's time are spent seeing people with minor illnesses which could quite safely be treated by a pharmacist. Most coughs, colds, minor injuries, skin rashes, stomach upsets and headaches really need no treatment at all and will get better on their own.

All that doctors can do is provide symptomatic relief from drugs generally available over the counter, such as painkillers, cough mixtures, laxatives, decongestants, expectorants, antihistamines, anti-inflammatories and low-dose steroid preparations such as hydrocortisone. All these can be supplied by a pharmacist without a prescription.

Pharmacists know a great deal about the use of drugs and about which medications are likely to work best in particular circumstances. You may also find that they have more time to discuss minor complaints than doctors with a queue of patients to see.

So even if you do need to see a doctor, there is no harm at all in talking to a pharmacist first. If your problem is minor you will probably get help immediately. And if there are signs that it could be more serious, you will certainly be advised to seek treatment from your doctor.

Complementary medicine in Britain

GONE is the sharp distinction that in the past existed between orthodox medicine, with its rigorous scientific approach to health and use of drugs and surgery, and so-called fringe or alternative treatments such as acupuncture, massage, herbal medicine and homeopathy. More and more doctors now incorporate diet, stress relief and even exercise into treatments they prescribe, while in hospitals nurses routinely offer massage, reflexology and aromatherapy alongside conventional types of care. And therapists themselves, instead of offering an alternative to orthodox treatment, prefer to refer to their skills as complementary – a *supplement* to but not a *substitute* for orthodox medical care. The 'holistic' view of treatment shared by complementary therapies sees health as a balance of mind, body and spirit, not as simply a matter of treating symptoms. While doctors may be sympathetic to such a view, few have the time to put it into practice. As a result, complementary medicine is likely to keep its place as a valuable part of health care.

ACUPUNCTURE

Traditional Chinese medicine views illness as an imbalance or blockage of energy in the body. Acupuncturists use tiny sterile needles inserted into the skin at specific points to stimulate energy pathways, or 'meridians', and so, they believe, restore good health. Acupuncture and other traditional Chinese therapies are not generally available on the NHS, but clinics attached to some leading hospitals do use acupuncture for pain relief.

Suitable conditions
Acupuncturists treat many problems, including arthritis, bronchitis, back pain, angina, asthma, insomnia, stress and ulcers. Success is widely claimed for pain relief, especially in muscle and joint conditions.

Seeing a therapist
Consultations normally last up to an hour. Patients should feel an improvement after six to eight sessions, though a complex problem such as asthma may require more. Treatment sessions cost around £30-£35 for an initial visit, and usually less thereafter.

Finding an acupuncturist
Contact The Council for Acupuncture, 179 Gloucester Place, London NW1 6DX for a

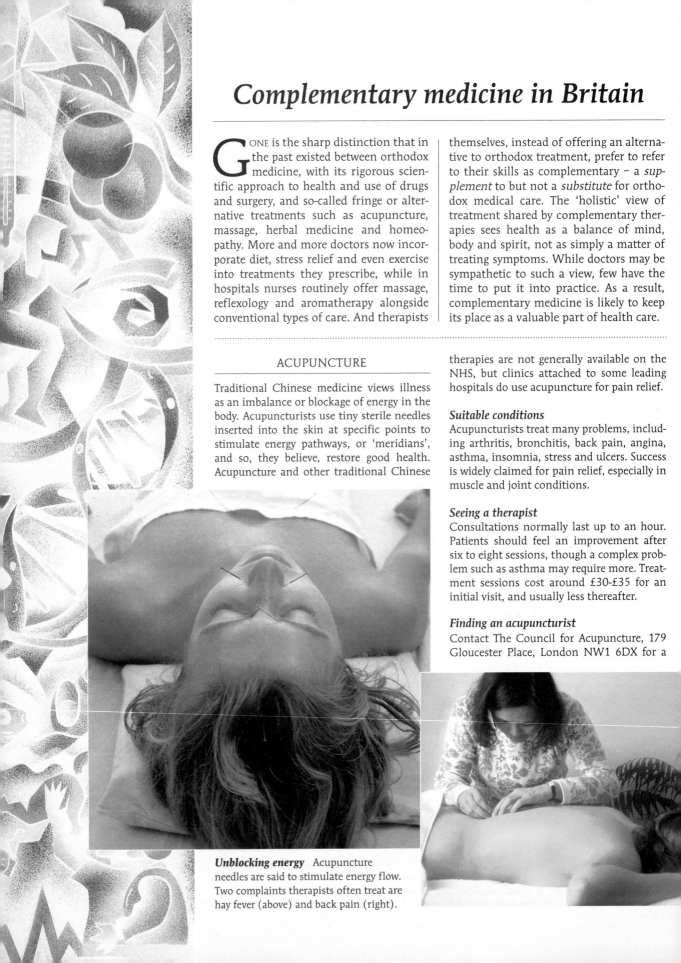

Unblocking energy Acupuncture needles are said to stimulate energy flow. Two complaints therapists often treat are hay fever (above) and back pain (right).

register of therapists, or look in the *Yellow Pages* under Acupuncture Practitioners. The letters MBAcA, FBAcA, LicAc, BAc or DrAc indicate a recognised qualification.

NATUROPATHY

Therapists aim to help the body to cure itself. They use a variety of techniques including diet, massage, water therapy, relaxation and breathing. Naturopathy is not available on the NHS, but sympathetic doctors will sometimes refer patients for private treatment.

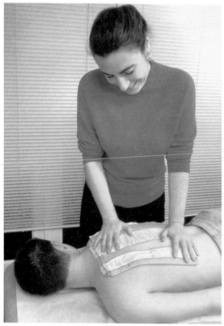

Nature cure   Treatments such as hot and cold compresses have been used for centuries and are still employed by modern naturopaths.

Suitable conditions

Naturopaths treat medical problems ranging from chronic conditions such as emphysema and arthritis to colds, rashes and allergies.

Seeing a therapist

Treatment varies according to the condition. It can involve long-term changes to diet and way of life as well as fasting or herbal remedies. Costs range from £30 to £50 for a first consultation, and less thereafter.

Finding a naturopath

A list of qualified practitioners is available for a small fee from the British Naturopathic Association, Frazer House, 6 Netherhall Gardens, London NW3 5RR. Members with the initials BCNO after their name have completed four years of full-time training.

HERBAL MEDICINE

Plants were man's first medicines, and are still among the most effective. Aspirin, digitalis, belladonna, quinine, morphine – the catalogue of plant-based cures is a long one. Modern herbalists, however, specialise less in such potent drugs than in remedies with a milder action suitable for minor complaints. Treatment is not available on the NHS.

Suitable conditions

Patients seek help for many ailments, particularly long-standing or recurrent problems such as arthritis, migraine and eczema.

Seeing a therapist

An initial consultation usually lasts an hour and subsequent appointments about half as long. You will probably be asked about your medical history, your eating habits and how much exercise you take. Remedies may be prescribed as pills, infusions, creams, teas or alcohol-based tinctures. Effects are usually very mild and emerge more slowly than with conventional medicines. Fees are about £30 for an initial visit, and £20 for subsequent visits. Treatment in London may cost more.

Finding a herbalist

A fully qualified herbalist will always have the initials MNIMH, FNIMH, FRH or IMH after his or her name. For a list of registered practitioners in your area, send a stamped, addressed envelope to The Honorary Secretary, National Institute of Medical Herbalists, 51 Longbrook Street, Exeter EX4 6AM.

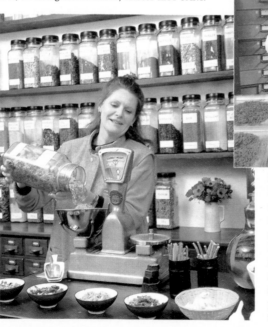

Plant power Both European herbalism (left) and Chinese (above) have an ancient and venerable history, and are still thriving. Patients should have no trouble finding a qualified practitioner of either type in Britain today.

HOMEOPATHY

Treatment is based on the theory that 'like cures like', and practitioners prescribe remedies composed of minute amounts of substances that in larger doses would actually cause similar symptoms.

Suitable conditions

Many kinds of illness are treated, ranging from the common colds, hay fever and headaches to eczema and depression.

Seeing a therapist

The first consultation usually takes an hour or a little longer, and involves assessing not only your symptoms but also your personality, appearance, state of mind, worries, fears and beliefs. Treatment is available both on the NHS and privately. Costs vary – £20-£50 is usual for an initial consultation, and about half as much for further visits.

Finding a homeopath

A medically qualified homeopath will usually be a Member or Fellow of the Faculty of Homoeopathy. Contact the Royal London Homoeopathic Hospital at Great Ormond Street, London WC1 3HR to find a practitioner. Alternatively, write to The Society of Homoeopaths, 2 Artizan Road, Northampton NN1 4HU, for their register of members. Initials indicating a recognised qualification are FFHom, LCH, MCH, MFHom or RSHom. You can also receive treatment at five NHS homeopathic hospitals – in London, Bristol, Tunbridge Wells, Liverpool and Glasgow.

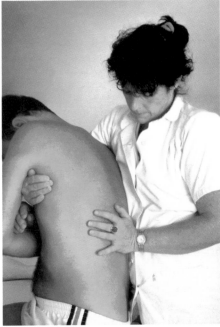

Hands-on treatment Manipulating a slipped disc is a skill osteopaths practise daily – and one that leads to many referrals from doctors.

Treatment can sometimes be obtained on the NHS, and some doctors now have their own on-going contracts with osteopaths.

Suitable conditions

Osteopaths will treat back and neck pain, tension headaches and sports injuries to the muscles or joints of the hips, knees, ankles, feet, wrists, shoulders or elbows. People with osteoarthritis may also benefit, as well as women with back pain during pregnancy.

Seeing a therapist

Treatment sessions last 20-30 minutes and are generally spread over a few weeks. Acute problems may need only a single session. Expect to pay £20-£50 for the first consultation, and £20-£40 for subsequent visits.

Finding an osteopath

Ask your doctor for a recommendation, or look in the *Yellow Pages* for the names of registered practitioners. Most osteopaths go through a four-year training course and will have the initials GCRO or GOsC after their name, or MLCON if they are also doctors. The names of qualified osteopaths can be obtained from the General Council and Register of Osteopaths, 56 London Street, Reading, Berkshire RG1 4SQ, and also from The London College of Osteopathic Medicine, 8-10 Boston Place, London NW1 6HQ.

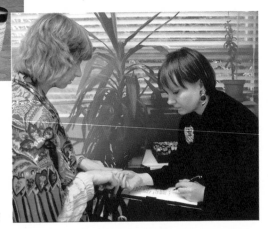

Seeing a homeopath
At the initial meeting (right) the homeopath pays detailed attention to physical signs and symptoms as well as questioning the patient for psychological clues. Medication is frequently prescribed in the form of small white sugar pills (above) made from extremely dilute concentrations of herbal or other remedies.

OSTEOPATHY

In this very popular complementary treatment, therapists use massage and manipulation to treat spinal, joint and muscular problems, such as arthritis and back pain.

CHIROPRACTIC

Therapists aim to relieve pain by manipulating the joints. Chiropractic technique is similar in many ways to osteopathy, but makes far greater use of X-rays and conventional diagnostic methods. Treatment is sometimes available on the NHS.

Suitable conditions

The overwhelming majority of patients are seeking relief from some form of musculoskeletal pain, especially in the back or neck. Whiplash injuries, headaches and sports injuries are also treated.

Seeing a therapist

Some patients report relief after a single treatment, while others experience aching and stiffness at first and need several sessions before noticing an improvement. Costs average £20-£50 for a first visit and £20-£40 for further consultations.

Finding a chiropractor

Contact the British Chiropractic Association, 29 Whitley Street, Reading, Berkshire RG2 0EG for a list of registered practitioners. Qualified therapists will have the initials MBCA or MCA or MIPC.

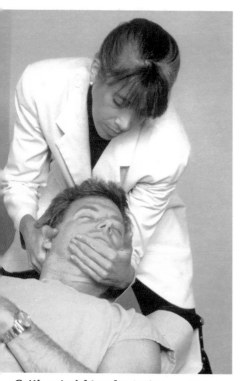

Getting straightened out Chiropractic may look uncomfortable but can bring immediate relief – for insistent neck ache, in this case.

OTHER COMPLEMENTARY THERAPIES

There are literally hundreds of other therapies in use today, both ancient and modern, local and foreign. Those below are some of the most popular.

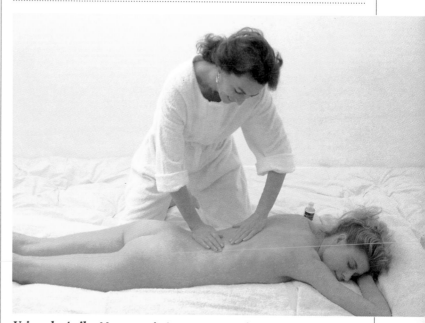

Using plant oils Massage techniques are a central part of professional aromatherapy treatment. Home treatment is also increasingly popular but it is important to use the highly concentrated plant essences with care.

Aromatherapy

Potent plant extracts known as essential oils are diluted for massage, added to baths, applied to the skin or taken internally.

Relaxation techniques

Meditation courses, tapes and breathing exercises help with pain, stress, insomnia and anxiety.

Massage

Treatment relaxes body and mind, and promotes healing by increasing blood flow to muscles and tissues.

Hypnotherapy

Practitioners treat problems by relieving anxiety. Hypnosis can also relax nervous patients and help with pain control.

Reflexology

Points on the feet and hands are said to correspond to other parts of the body. A wide range of complaints is treated by massage.

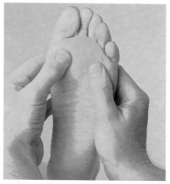

Reflex action According to reflexologists, massaging points on the feet can ease distant pains.

For further information

Most complementary therapies have their own official registering bodies. To contact such organisations or to find out more about obtaining complementary treatment, send a stamped, addressed envelope to: Institute of Complementary Medicine Enquiries, PO Box 194, London SE16 1QZ.

Symptoms that
can be referred to
a pharmacist

- Coughs, colds, sore throats and hay fever symptoms.
- Minor feverish illnesses in children.
- Muscular aches and pains, and headaches.
- Indigestion, heartburn and wind.
- Haemorrhoids.
- Short-term diarrhoea or constipation.
- Cold sores and mouth ulcers.
- Minor cuts, scrapes, bruises, bites and stings.
- Minor skin complaints and allergic reactions such as rashes, itching and blistering.

OVER-THE-COUNTER DRUGS

I recently found out that a medicine I was being prescribed was available more cheaply over the counter. Shouldn't the doctor or the pharmacist have told me?

More and more drugs which were formerly sold as prescription-only medicines (POMs) are now available over the counter in pharmacies. The medicines involved all have well-established safety records and seldom cause significant side effects.

It is part of government health policy to expand the list of over-the-counter medicines for two reasons. One is to save the NHS money; the other is to relieve the pressure on general practitioners in treating relatively minor complaints.

Most doctors are also keen to cut down on prescription costs and will usually tell you if they know that a drug is available more cheaply over the counter. However, there are now so many drugs involved that GPs cannot know the retail price of all of them. In addition, the relative costs also depend on how much medicine you need and for how long, which adds to the difficulty.

There is, however, an official list of medicines available under the NHS but cheaper over the counter. Most doctors and pharmacists will happily look up a drug if you ask them, but bear in mind that this is a favour rather than a right. There is no obligation to provide such information.

DO BRAND NAMES MATTER ?

Apart from the packaging, is there any difference between a brand-name drug and its generic equivalent?

Possibly, but they are probably very minor. The main difference is in the price, which can vary as much as tenfold for the same basic drug. Within the NHS there is a strong movement towards generic prescribing and in some cases the NHS will no longer fund more costly brand-name prescriptions. There is also an increasing tendency among members of the public to buy over-the-counter drugs such as aspirin and paracetamol in cheaper 'own brand' or 'no name' packaging instead of asking for branded medicines.

Despite this, some doctors worry that equivalent generic drugs are not quite identical. In theory, all drugs that are manufactured within European Union countries have to meet the same standards of purity and safety but in practice quality control does vary to some extent. Even so, there is no real evidence that poor quality drugs have ever been made available in Britain.

The other concern about generic drugs is that although the active ingredients may be identical, inactive 'carrying' agents such as colourings, bulking agents and fillers may be quite different. Very occasionally, this may affect drug absorption or uptake, or cause allergies. These are minor worries, however, and a British licence generally guarantees the efficacy and purity of generic preparations. There is in any case no doubt that generic prescribing will increase.

'NATURAL' REMEDIES

I know that there are strict rules governing the sale of conventional drugs, but how can I be certain that herbal remedies, homeopathic pills and other alternative medicines are safe?

At present, there are few guarantees or guidelines to give you other than to advise avoiding unnecessary medication and, if you do use alternative remedies, always to make sure you buy them from a reputable supplier. From time to time, proposals are put forward to bring 'natural' remedies more into line with the very strict licensing requirements imposed on orthodox drugs. There are some substantial problems with this approach, however, and it is unlikely that completely equal standards will ever be applied.

For a start, unlike multinational pharmaceutical corporations, the companies that manufacture complementary remedies are usually small. Few could afford to finance the extensive testing that drug manufacturers have to undertake. Even if they did, the results could take years to obtain, so many remedies would have to be taken off the market for a long period of time. Overall, the result of insisting on drug-standard research would probably be to drive many small companies out of business and deprive the public of their products.

In exceptionally rare cases a few natural remedies have been reported to cause side effects, but the vast majority have either been used for years, even centuries, without problems (the case with most herbal cures), or are considered harmless (homeopathic remedies are one example). The best advice is to consult an experienced and registered complementary practitioner (see pages 226-229) before taking any remedies. Ask your doctor's advice about proposed treatment, and report any side effects straight away.

Second opinions, referrals and tests

GETTING A SECOND OPINION

I would like a second opinion. Can I get this on the NHS and, if so, how do I do it without damaging the relationship with my own doctor?

Whether you want to see a second general practitioner or a second specialist, the first person to consult is your own family doctor.

Explain that you have some doubts about your current diagnosis or treatment regime and ask if you could seek another opinion. Your doctor has no obligation to arrange this for you, but most doctors will happily agree to such a request, particularly if you wish to see another GP. If this is the case, your doctor will probably suggest that you see another doctor in the practice.

If your doctor will not arrange a second GP opinion, and after discussion you are still certain that you want one, then you should question the value of your relationship anyway. It may not be worth as much as you thought it was, and you could consider transferring to another doctor to get a second opinion.

A second specialist opinion may be harder to arrange. If your doctor feels that the existing diagnosis is certain, that any specialist would recommend the same treatment and that there is no personal difficulty affecting the relationship between you and the consultant, then he or she may well try and dissuade you. If your doctor feels very strongly that you do not need a second opinion, you may even receive an outright refusal on the grounds that it would be a waste of valuable NHS time and money.

If you meet with such a refusal there is nothing much you can do except to consider changing your doctor or consulting a specialist privately. You have no automatic right to a second opinion on the NHS. Most requests, however, are successful.

CONFLICTING DIAGNOSES

What happens if a second opinion conflicts with the original diagnosis?

It is more likely that a second opinion will suggest an alternative type of treatment than an alternative diagnosis, but on some occasions a second diagnosis does emerge. On balance, the second diagnosis is more likely to be the right one, since the second doctor will have been able to take into account all the information used to reach the first diagnosis, and probably some additional information as well.

Nevertheless, on the rare occasions when diagnoses do conflict, the situation can be both confusing and worrying for the patient. In such circumstances, the only real solution is to discuss the matter in detail with your general practitioner. Don't start any course of treatment until both you and your doctor are completely happy with the diagnosis and the proposed plan of action. Treatment is seldom successful if either patient or doctor feels halfhearted or doubtful.

INSISTING ON A SPECIALIST

I would like to see a consultant about my condition. Do patients have a right to be referred, or is the decision entirely up to the doctor?

It is really the doctor's decision. Your doctor is, after all, a highly trained and experienced professional and should, ideally, have won the trust and confidence of patients. Family doctors are expert in all fields of primary care, including identifying symptoms that indicate a need for further investigations or specialist help. In general they know more about the natural history of ordinary illness than consultants, who are specialists in a narrower field.

Having said that, family doctors will usually not hesitate to refer patients to a consultant if there is the slightest chance that specialist help is needed. Most would far rather err on the side of caution than risk overlooking something serious.

Before you do anything else, however, you should talk to your doctor about your condition and explain why you feel unhappy with the current diagnosis or treatment.

You may well find that he or she can solve your problem or set your mind at rest without referral to a specialist. If not, and you continue to feel worried, you will very likely be referred. Or you could consider requesting a second opinion from a general practitioner, which is seldom refused. Another option, of course, is to make your own private appointment with a specialist.

**DO'S
—— AND ——
DON'TS**

for requesting a second opinion

Do ask for a second opinion if you think your treatment isn't working or if symptoms get worse.

Do ask for a second opinion if you are not confident that your doctor knows enough about your condition.

Do ask for a second opinion if you are not getting enough information from your doctor, or if you simply feel a need for confirmation.

Don't be put off by the thought of offending your doctor. This is very unlikely to happen.

Seeing a specialist Hospital consultants, such as this bone specialist, can help when conditions are too complex for a general practitioner to treat.

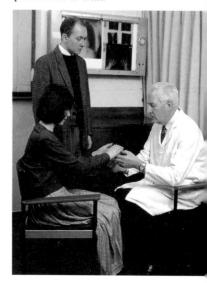

HOW TECHNOLOGY HELPS DOCTORS TO SEE INSIDE THE BODY

In 1895, while carrying out an experiment with the flow of electric current in a cathode-ray tube, the German physicist Wilhelm Röntgen happened to notice that a nearby surface coated with a barium-based compound was lit up by fluorescence, even though the tube was covered by black paper. Some sort of radiation was escaping through the black paper, crossing the room and being absorbed by the barium, causing it to fluoresce. Investigating further, Röntgen found that objects placed between the tube and the screen had the effect of casting shadows, showing that the rays could not penetrate some substances as easily as they could black paper. Röntgen had discovered the X-ray, and for his work was awarded the Nobel prize for physics. More than that, his discovery paved the way for a variety of sophisticated techniques that now help doctors to view the interior of the body with little or no risk to the patient. Today's high-tech scanning and imaging procedures are usually carried out in the radiology department of a hospital under specialist supervision. Their main application is still in diagnosing illness, but increasingly they are being used to guide doctors in carrying out therapeutic procedures as well.

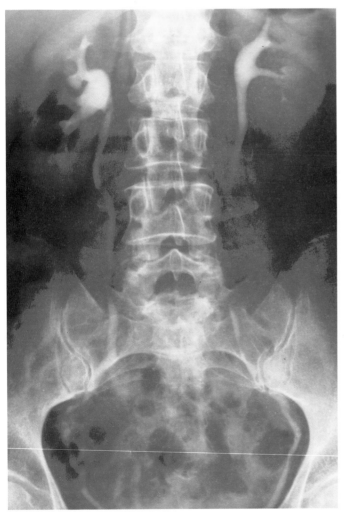

Contrast X-ray imaging Bone shows up naturally on an X-ray, but for blood vessels and internal organs to be seen a contrast medium generally needs to be introduced – a dye or other substance that is impervious to the rays. Here, an iodine-based contrast medium has been injected to show urine draining from the kidneys down the ureters towards the bladder. Contrast X-rays are widely used in diagnosis. As well as iodine, barium may be used – especially to highlight the digestive tract. Depending on the area, it is given either orally or as an enema. Special contrast mediums have also been developed for other organs.

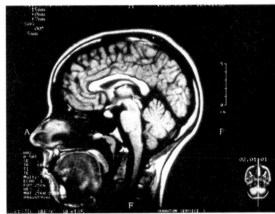

Magnetic resonance imaging (MRI) A powerful magnetic field used in conjunction with radio waves produces sectional images, such as this vertical brain scan. MRI can reveal extremely subtle abnormalities and is particularly useful for studying soft tissue encased in bone, such as the brain and spinal cord. It can also help to diagnose organ and joint disorders.

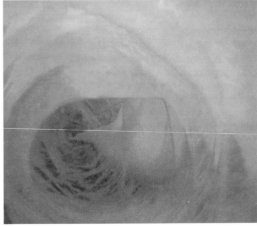

Endoscope imaging A flexible fibre-optic tube is introduced into the body, allowing doctors to view internal organs directly – in this case, the small intestine. Special attachments can be fitted to take tissue samples and to perform surgical procedures such as removing torn cartilage from a knee joint.

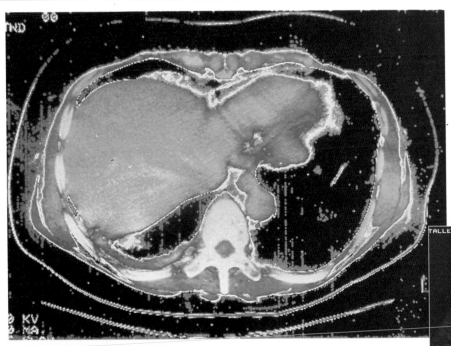

Computerised tomography (CT) scanning   This technique combines a series of X-rays taken from a source rotating around the patient with computer analysis to produce complex images in different planes. The scan on the left shows a false-colour cross-section of the abdomen. A vetebra of the spine shows up in yellow (lower centre), as do the bones of the lower ribcage. The large orange-coloured organ (left and centre) is the liver.

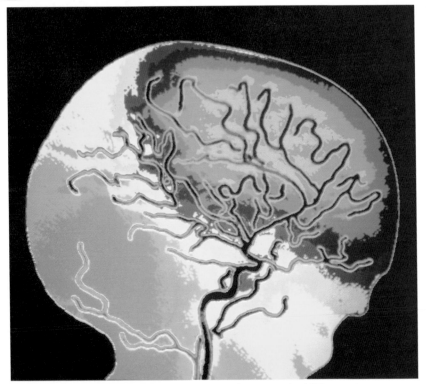

Angiography   Like ordinary X-rays, computerised tomography (CT) scanning sometimes needs to make use of a contrast medium. In the technique known as angiography, the contrast medium is injected into the bloodstream to show up blood vessels, such as the large carotid artery and its branches above. Expert radiologists are trained to interpret details on such scans, and can use them to diagnose conditions ranging from a blocked artery or aneurysm (arterial swelling) to a tumour or stroke.

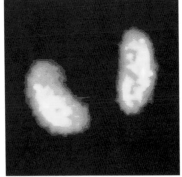

Ultrasound scanning   Not all scans use radiation. Ultrasound relies on high-frequency sound waves instead, building up a picture from the echoes, as ships do in depth-sounding the ocean floor. Medically, ultrasound is used mainly for foetal monitoring, and for diagnosing disorders of organs such as the liver, pancreas, kidneys and, as above, the gallbladder.

Radionuclide scanning   Radioactive substances are introduced into the body and a special camera used to detect emitted radiation. These kidneys show a normal, healthy pattern of emission.

Your rights regarding medical tests

Consent

Most patients receive simple tests from time to time from their family doctor, such as a blood pressure check. You are not asked directly to give consent – you are deemed to have given it by attending the doctor. But you can, of course, refuse any test you don't want, no matter what the circumstances. This applies particularly to procedures which might be regarded as invasive or intimate, such as giving blood or having a cervical smear. Your consent must be sought before your blood can be used for any other purposes such as additional anonymous HIV testing.

Intimate examination

Women patients may ask for a female chaperone during any test which requires intimate examination by a male doctor (such as a cervical smear). The doctor is not legally bound to comply with such requests, but most are more than happy to agree to anything that will help a patient to feel more relaxed.

Results

You have the right to be told the broad results of any tests – for example whether a blood test was normal – and you should be notified of any result that will require further action, such as more tests, or an abnormality that needs treatment.

CHOOSING A HOSPITAL

I have heard of patients being sent to hospitals far from where they live in order to get faster treatment. How does this work? Do patients have any say in the matter of where they go?

Assuming you are a National Health Service patient and that you are being referred to a hospital by a doctor, you may have a certain amount of choice. You should discuss this fully with your doctor who will be able to tell you exactly what options are open to you. These can vary greatly depending on where you live, and whether or not you belong to a fundholding practice.

The chances are that if your doctor is sending you for routine tests – such as X-rays, ultrasound examinations, electrocardiographs or blood tests – you will have no choice. Your doctor will probably have existing arrangements with the nearest hospital that has the necessary facilities. If, on the other hand, you are being referred to a hospital consultant for a specialist opinion or for surgery, the options may be greater.

In theory, doctors can refer patients to any consultant in the NHS who is prepared to see them, and not just to specialists who operate within their own district. With the emergence of the internal market in the new NHS, exercising this privilege can, however, be extremely complicated. For fundholding practices, the option to go farther afield generally depends on the state of the practice budget. For non-fundholding doctors, the option depends instead on whether the local district health authority will approve such an 'extra-contractual referral'.

In a nutshell, it all comes down to money. If you have private medical insurance or can pay for yourself, you have unlimited choice throughout the private sector. If, however, you are relying on the NHS, you can only ask your doctor or, alternatively, your local Community Health Council, about the various options that are available to you.

WHAT DO CONSULTANTS DO?

Every profession has its specialists, none more so than the medical profession. Medical experts are known as consultants and generally work within a hospital, although they often combine public and private work. Their background can be either as a physician or as a surgeon.

General physician

Treats most medical conditions but may also be an expert in one of the following medical specialties:
- Cardiology – heart diseases.
- Respiratory medicine – lung diseases (specialists may also be called 'chest physicians').
- Gastroenterology – disorders of the digestive system.
- Rheumatology – diseases of the joints.
- Endocrinology – hormonal disorders such as diabetes.
- Renal medicine – kidney diseases.
- Neurology – diseases of the brain and nervous system.

General surgeon

Treats conditions likely to require an operation and may also be an expert in one of these surgical specialties:
- Cardiac or vascular surgery – heart or blood vessel diseases.
- Thoracic surgery – diseases of the lungs and chest.
- Urology – urinary tract diseases.
- Breast surgery.
- Brain surgery.
- Ear, nose and throat (ENT) surgery.
- Transplant surgery – kidney, liver or heart transplants.
- Plastic surgery – repair and reconstruction of damaged or deformed features. Sometimes also cosmetic surgery.
- Obstetrics and gynaecology – dealing with pregnancy and female reproductive disorders.

Other specialists

- Paediatrician – treats most children's illnesses.
- Dermatologist – treats skin diseases.
- Orthopaedic surgeon – deals with bone diseases and fractures.
- Ophthalmologist – treats eye diseases.
- Radiologist – deals with all the medical aspects of X-ray diagnosis.
- Radiotherapist – uses X-rays in treating cancer.
- Oncologist – treats cancer.
- Geriatrician – deals with illness in elderly people.
- Psychiatrist – gives medical treatment for mental illness.

Treatment in hospital

EARLY WAKING

Why do you always get woken up so early in hospital?

Hospitals are at work every hour of the day and every day of the year. The routine work of the hospital – operations, outpatient clinics and so on – is performed in the working day, but accidents, emergencies and sickness in general are no respecters of office hours so, inevitably, hospitals have to operate their own schedules.

The hospital day starts early with the nursing day shift taking over from the night shift some time between 7 and 8 am. The first job of the day is preparing patients for surgery, which usually begins at about 8 am. Other essential business also has to be attended to before morning ward rounds, which often start at about the same time. Drugs have also to be administered and breakfast served.

Some patients need their temperature and pulse taken regularly, including through the night. Such a disturbed night followed by the noise and bustle of the ward in the early morning can leave patients feeling tired and badly rested. There is not much you can do about this except to catch up on sleep at other times of the day. Afternoons are usually quiet. Going to sleep earlier on in the evening will also help.

BEING SEEN BY STUDENTS

I am due to be admitted to a teaching hospital. Will I be treated and examined by medical students?

Medical students spend nearly three years of their training on hospital wards. In order to become competent doctors when they qualify it is essential that they get as much practice as possible with real patients in a real hospital environment. As they gain new clinical skills, medical students also take on more and more of the routine ward work and become increasingly involved in diagnosis and patient care, relieving some of the pressure on qualified doctors. Even so, all the work undertaken by medical students is directly supervised by more senior doctors who are also clinical teachers.

You will be certain to encounter medical students during the course of your stay in a teaching hospital. They will always identify themselves as students and there is no possibility of mistaking a student for a qualified doctor. You may be asked to allow students to examine you, but you have no obligation to agree to this. It is worth remembering, however, that without trained medical students, there will be no future doctors. They have to learn somehow.

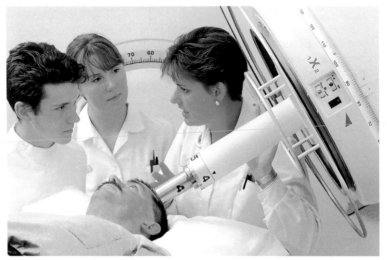

Tomorrow's doctors Medical students learn their skills on the job as well as in the lecture room and the laboratory. No amount of book learning can replace clinical experience.

CHILDREN IN HOSPITAL

My five-year-old daughter has to go into hospital. How much shall I tell her in advance and how can I make the experience less upsetting?

Hospitals have changed a lot in the last few years. They have become much more 'patient friendly', and nowhere is this truer than in a children's ward. Gone are the days of tyrannical matrons and limited visiting hours.

Many children's wards now accommodate parents too, and parental participation in all aspects of hospital life is not just encouraged, but relied upon. Try to arrange a visit to the ward prior to your daughter's admission – you may be pleasantly surprised both by the welcoming atmosphere and the happy faces of the other children you see.

It is also important to find out as much as you can about your child's condition and any tests or surgical procedures she will face. Ask your doctor to explain anything that you are unclear about or any doubts you have. Be open and honest with your daughter and try

---

DO'S AND DON'TS

for parents of children going into hospital

Do emphasise positive aspects, such as the chance to make some new friends.

Do play hospital and nursing games at home.

Do demonstrate what will happen on a doll or a teddy. Practise bandaging or treating the toy with the child.

Don't show your anxiety or express misgivings.

Don't be dishonest or misleading but do give plenty of reassurance.

to answer any questions she raises as accurately as you can. Give plenty of reassurance, but be truthful if there is a possibility of pain or discomfort. Find out and tell her exactly when you can be with her and when she may have to be alone. Mention anything such as an intravenous drip that she may need, and tell her how long it will be before she can get out of bed and eat normal food.

Accept the fact that your daughter will be afraid – afraid of being separated from you and from the rest of the family, afraid of the operation and afraid of pain. Acknowledge any fears she expresses and give plenty of reassurance. Treating her worries as childish or trivial will only make things worse.

Most importantly, show plenty of love and attention. Listen carefully when your daughter speaks to others about going into hospital. Her words to a brother, sister, playmate, teacher or neighbour may give you insights into any particular fears or misconceptions that need to be dealt with.

SEEING YOUR CONSULTANT

Once I'm in hospital, who will I be able to ask about my treatment and progress, and how often will I see my consultant?

The nursing staff on the ward will be able to answer many of your questions about routine tests, treatment and procedures, and especially about the practicalities of what happens when – when you will receive medication, for example, and what sort; how you should expect to feel; or how long you may spend having an X-ray or scan.

If you have a specific medical enquiry, the junior doctor taking care of you will usually visit the ward at some time every day, and you can ask the nurse to let him or her know that you would like a word. For any urgent problem, the nurses can call a junior doctor to see you – either your own or the duty doctor on call.

Sometimes a consultant will make a point of visiting a patient specially – before an operation, for instance. In general, however, your main contact is likely to be on the ward round. Most consultants make a regular tour around all their patients, usually with a retinue of junior doctors and nursing staff in train to keep them informed of the patients' progress. This may happen weekly, or more often, and is a good time to raise points and ask questions of your consultant. If you want to see him or her between ward rounds, or individually, ask the nurses or the junior doctor if they can arrange it.

ILLNESS FROM TREATMENT

I've heard that many people develop new illnesses while in hospital, as a result of infection or the side effects of the treatment itself. How much of a risk are these illnesses and is there anything that patients can do to protect themselves?

Hospital is not a normal health environment in the sense that those who are in hospital are there precisely because they are less healthy than the rest of the population. Despite the best precautions, hospitals contain types of bacteria that are particularly resistant to antibiotics, and people who are already ill are more vulnerable than the general population. It is not uncommon for patients to develop new infections after they arrive in hospital – pneumonia owing to prolonged bed rest after a stroke, for example, or a urinary infection after having a bladder catheter inserted. Strict hygiene procedures are followed to minimise the risk of such complications, but the possibility can never be totally eliminated owing to the nature of illness and the nature of hospitals. Most cases, however, are easily treated.

Other complications arise directly from medical treatment – these are termed iatrogenic illnesses. They occur because no form of treatment is completely effective and also completely beneficial – even the safest drug can cause side effects and any form of surgery will also have some effect on healthy tissue. The benefits of treatment always have to be weighed against possible risks and doctors are specifically trained to do this.

A doctor should always discuss the risks of a course of treatment with you before encouraging you to go ahead. In most cases the potential problems are minor and can be offset by some simple precautions.

● If drugs are prescribed, make a point of asking about possible side effects.
● Report any side effects or new symptoms as soon as you notice them.
● Follow dosage instructions precisely. Don't try to catch up on missed pills, don't take medication for longer than instructed and, equally, don't stop before the course is finished – unless your doctor agrees.
● Before having an operation, try to get as fit as you can. Lose weight if necessary and take as much exercise as your condition permits. Keep your alcohol intake low and avoid smoking, or at least cut down, as far ahead as possible. Afterwards, get mobile and independent as soon as you can.

Having an operation

COUNTDOWN TO SURGERY

I'm about to go into hospital for an operation. What will actually happen?

Hospital procedures vary slightly, but most follow a similar basic pattern.

Admission
You will probably be admitted either the night before or on the morning of your operation. A nurse will show you to your bed and give you admission forms to complete, including details about illnesses, operations and any drug allergies. Routine tests such as blood pressure and temperature will follow, and usually examination by a junior doctor.

Surgeon's assessment
The surgeon will visit to check your condition, answer your questions, obtain formal consent and, if necessary, mark the site.

Visit from anaesthetist
A specialist check ensures you are fit for anaesthesia and allows premedication to be prescribed if needed.

Overnight fast
If you are having a general anaesthetic you will usually be asked not to eat or drink anything from the evening before the operation.

Premedication
If prescribed, relaxant tablets may be administered a few hours before the operation.

Anaesthetic
Shortly before surgery, you will be taken to the anaesthetic room and put to sleep, usually with an injection in the back of the hand. Once unconscious, you may be transferred to a gas anaesthetic administered via a mask over the face. An artificial airway will be inserted down your throat and connected to a ventilator to help with breathing.

Operation
The anaesthetist monitors you continuously while the surgeon performs the operation.

Recovery room
After the operation you will be taken to a recovery room to wake up. Then you will be returned to the wards.

Post-operative care
You may wake up with a drip in your arm, or find a catheter has been inserted to drain urine. After big operations there is sometimes a drainage tube for the wound. If you have had major surgery, you may spend a period in intensive care, particularly if you need assistance with breathing or artificial feeding. The wound will be dressed regularly until the stitches are removed – usually within five to ten days. Nursing staff will keep a close watch on your general condition and on indicators such as blood pressure and temperature. If necessary, special help such as physiotherapy may be offered.

OVERCOMING ANXIETY

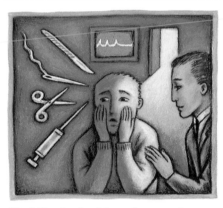

My father is about to undergo a minor operation and although it is a simple, routine procedure, he is becoming extremely anxious about it. How can I stop him from worrying so much?

Going into hospital can be very stressful, particularly to those who have had no previous experience of hospital life, and who have little acquaintance with doctors, nurses and other hospital workers. It is natural to experience fear and anxiety when confronted with the unknown, especially in connection with surgery. Newspapers are full of alarmist stories of operations going wrong, of surgeons removing the wrong limb or organ, and of people dying under anaesthetic.

But it is only because such occurrences are so rare that they hit the headlines. Although every operation carries some risk, either from the surgery or the anaesthesia, minor operations are extremely safe. A considerable

---

Badges take over from nurses' belts

There was a time when hospital patients could tell the status of the nurse looking after them by the colour of the belt around the waist – red for a staff nurse, blue for an assistant nurse, green for an enrolled nurse and white for a student nurse. Such nurses also usually wore the traditional blue and white chequered dresses (the deeper the blue, the more senior the nurse).

But times are changing. Many hospitals now have their own style of uniforms and their own system of colour coding with nurses' belts.

Generally, however, all nurses in British hospitals today wear a badge displaying their name, nursing rank and, in most cases, an identifying photograph.

Fact But it is exceptionally rare, so much so that when it happens – usually to women who have been given an extremely light anaesthetic for a Caesarean section – it makes front-page news.

In general, the lighter the anaesthetic administered, the smaller the risk of complications and the more rapid a patient's recovery is likely to be. It is up to the anaesthetist to balance the dose administered against the patient's level of unconsciousness.

Not all senses are equally affected by anaesthesia – hearing, for example, is often the last of the senses to go. Despite being oblivious to the actual operation, patients sometimes recall details of conversations going on at the time in the operating theatre.

Very rarely, a patient may be sufficiently aware to remember some hazy sensation during an operation, such as a feeling of pressure or of pulling. The chance of finding yourself fully conscious, however, or of feeling any sensation of pain is virtually nil.

amount of research has been done into the state of mind of patients and the outcome of surgical procedures. Time and again results have shown that the patients who do best are those who exhibit a realistic degree of anxiety, and who are well informed about their surgery. Such people tend to experience less pain, need fewer drugs and suffer fewer postoperative infections.

Many hospitals produce leaflets explaining what to expect. Try to get hold of one of these for your father. His doctor and consultant should also be able to answer any questions that are troubling him, and to set his mind at rest generally – if necessary, make an appointment to talk through any fears.

DIFFERENT ANAESTHETICS

What are the main differences between local and epidural anaesthetics and general anaesthetics, and how are the different types used?

General anaesthetics are used to induce and maintain unconsciousness while a painful or distressing procedure is performed. Most combine sleep-inducing properties and pain-killing effects, and sometimes they include a muscle relaxant.

Local anaesthetics prevent sensation and movement at a specific place in the body but do not interfere with consciousness. They are suitable for less invasive procedures, supplementing general anaesthesia, relieving pain from illness and for use when a medical condition, such as a weak heart, might make general anaesthesia unsafe. There are many types of local anaesthetic. In addition to drugs (mostly derived from cocaine), heat, hypnosis and acupuncture have all been successfully used for controlling pain at particular sites.

Epidural and spinal anaesthetics come somewhere between local and general anaesthesia. They do not interfere with consciousness, but block pain throughout the lower half of the body and are technically referred to as regional anaesthesia.

Even though anaesthetic drugs and techniques have improved greatly over the past few years, drug hangovers following general anaesthesia are not uncommon. Local and regional anaesthetics are generally simpler and safer. Improvements in surgical methods and the development of new techniques, mean that many procedures are now much less painful than before and no longer need general anaesthesia. Even complicated operations can sometimes be done with local or

regional pain relief and a sedative drug such as Valium. To avoid side effects, doctors will usually employ the lightest anaesthetic that is suitable. Even so, if you are having surgery it is always worth asking about the options.

NEW TECHNIQUES

I have heard that conventional operations can often be replaced by less traumatic procedures such as laser or keyhole surgery. Are these options available on the NHS and do they reduce the time spent in hospital?

Technological advances have indeed brought about a revolution in medical practice over the past few decades. The key innovations include ultrasonics, fibre optics, lasers, new scanning and imaging techniques, improved anaesthetics, and the increasing miniaturisation of medical instruments.

One result has been a boom in the use of new high-tech surgical techniques, especially the minimally-invasive type. Operations that once involved weeks of recuperation can now be performed as day cases or with much shorter hospital stays. Kidney stone removal, for example, is now often a day case operation owing to the use of ultrasound. Such innovations *are* available to NHS patients, although the cost of equipment and a limited number of trained staff mean that they are not always easily obtainable.

Fears have also been voiced that training may not keep pace with new techniques, and that not all surgeons who use them are properly qualified. However, as training programmes increase and expertise and clinical experience develop, it is hoped that such worries will become a thing of the past.

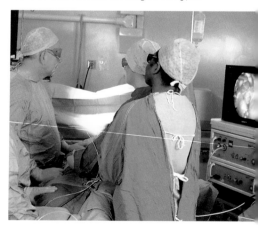

Laser surgery A video monitor guides a surgeon as he removes a gall bladder by laser. Such procedures are revolutionising medicine and reducing hospital stays dramatically.

CONSENTING TO SURGERY

I am due to have a major operation and am worried about signing the consent form. What exactly am I agreeing to? What will happen if I don't sign?

Most consent forms are worded to the effect that you agree to have a particular procedure performed, that it has been explained to you, and that you also give permission for any other necessary measures to be taken during or after the operation when you are not conscious and able to give verbal agreement.

This final clause is probably what is worrying you. In fact, the surgeon is very restricted in what he may do. The clause applies only to measures that are absolutely necessary and that have to be performed immediately as a result of unforeseen complications.

Usually these involve life-threatening situations, such as excessive bleeding or a malignant tumour. Very occasionally, patients are unhappy about unanticipated extra surgery. In such situations, patients can complain or seek legal redress if they believe an action was unnecessary or negligent.

The consent form is a contract between you and the surgeon, who may refuse to operate if you do not sign. If you are worried about something specific, discuss the matter with your surgeon before admission. Some surgeons will agree a particular stipulation, such as avoiding a blood transfusion on religious grounds, provided you take full responsibility for the consequences.

THE DECISION TO DISCHARGE

What criteria are used in deciding when to discharge a patient from hospital?

Essentially it is in everyone's interests that patients leave hospital as soon as it is medically safe. Hospital beds are expensive to maintain, and a huge cost to the health service. As a result there is great pressure to capitalise on advances in medicine that can reduce hospital stays and maximise the use of every bed so that more patients can be treated and waiting lists reduced.

It is also in patients' interests not to stay in hospital longer than necessary. A lengthy period in the wards increases the risk of contracting an infection from another patient or developing a condition such as bedsores as a result of immobility.

The medical decision to discharge is in the hands of the consultant, who must be satisfied that acute medical or nursing care is no longer required. Patients who are not able to look after themselves must also have somewhere to go where help is available. In some cases, particularly for older or chronically ill people, discharge may be delayed if a suitable place cannot be found immediately.

DISCHARGING YOURSELF

Are patients entitled to discharge themselves from hospital if they feel that they are ready to leave?

Unless you have been compulsorily admitted to hospital under mental health legislation, you can leave whenever you choose – whatever doctors, nurses or anyone else says.

However, if you want to leave before medical staff think you are properly fit, you will probably face strong pressure to change your mind. If you insist, you will be asked to sign a form stating that you are discharging yourself against medical advice. Legally, you are not obliged to sign the discharge form, but there is no good reason not to do so.

Of course, quite apart from any immediate hazards of discharging yourself before the hospital staff think you are medically fit, you may find that future relationships with your doctors could be strained.

DO'S AND DON'TS
for leaving hospital

Do make sure you take adequate supplies of any prescribed drugs with you when you leave.
Do check that you understand the dosage instructions for any discharge drugs, and how long you should carry on taking them.
Do ask whether you need to see your GP or get a repeat prescription.
Do, if necessary, let your GP know that you are back at home.
Do encourage friends to visit you once you are at home again.
Do ask a relative or friend to prepare your home for you.

Don't forget to check for personal belongings before you leave, including any valuables in the hospital safe.
Don't worry if hospital transport does not arrive exactly on time to take you home.
Don't forget to leave a forwarding address if you have been in hospital for some time, in case mail arrives for you after you've left.

Looking after teeth and eyes

FINDING A GOOD DENTIST

Are there any tips patients should know about for finding a good dentist?

As with finding a family doctor, word-of-mouth recommendations and warnings can be very helpful. Ask around locally – you may even be given the chance to inspect the results of dentists' work. You can also obtain a list of dentists from your local Family Health Services Association, or look in your local *Yellow Pages*.

Unlike doctors, good dentists may earn a lot through private work, and the condition of the premises and equipment can sometimes give a clue to a dentist's popularity – although, of course, not all dentists put their

---

Dentistry is free . . .

● If you are under 18.
● If you are under 19 in full-time education.
● If you get certain social security benefits.
● For women expecting a baby when accepted or who had a baby in the past year.

Taking the pain out of dental treatment

If fear of pain puts you off seeing the dentist as often as you should, take heart – there are many ways around this common problem.

● Local anaesthetic – injection into the gum around the tooth. Highly effective and the commonest method of pain relief.

● Laser drills – still relatively rare, but likely to become more common in the future. They are less painful than conventional drills, but they cannot cut enamel or old fillings. Laser drills can be used in conjunction with a local anaesthetic.

● Sedation – sometimes given as an extra for anxious patients or when prolonged work is being carried out.

● Relative analgesia or gas and air – a mixture of nitrous oxide (laughing gas) and oxygen can relieve pain and tension. Good for children and adults who are nervous.

● General anaesthetic – increasingly rare, but often used in hospital dentistry, especially for wisdom tooth extraction.

● Hypnosis – limited availability, but effective when performed by a dentist qualified in hypnosis or a hypnotist specially brought in.

● Acupuncture – limited availability, but offered by some specially trained dentists or, if the dentist agrees, a practitioner can be brought in.

money into furnishings and the number of private patients varies from area to area in any case. Even so, it is always worth visiting surgeries before making your decision. If you are a dental coward, you might want to look for a dentist who has an interest in helping nervous patients. You may also want to ask the dentist about the various types of pain relief that are on offer (see panel, left).

Remember, too, that dentistry is a high risk area for the transfer of hepatitis B and other infectious agents, including the AIDS virus. So look for signs that the dental staff you will be dealing with take hygiene seriously. Gloves, masks and sterilising equipment should be well in evidence.

Finally, remember that you can always try out a dentist by arranging a routine check up. If you are not happy with the choice you have made it will be easy to change. Unlike changing your doctor, changing dentist does not require form-filling or the transferring of past notes – although your old dentist will always send copies of notes to your new one if requested to.

DENTIST OR DOCTOR?

What sort of mouth injuries should be seen by a dentist and what sort require a doctor's attention?

The decision depends on whether the mouth or lips of the victim are severely injured (for example, by deep cuts, gashes, embedded foreign objects such as pieces of glass, or persistent heavy bleeding) or whether the damage is mainly to the teeth.

If an injury such as a punch on the jaw has caused only minor cuts and bruising or a small amount of bleeding in the mouth, but at the same time has dislodged, broken or knocked out teeth, then a dentist should be sought as a matter of urgency.

After dental treatment, anyone injured in the mouth should see a doctor in case the wound needs stitching or a tetanus injection is required. If there is a fractured jaw, the patient may need referral to a specialist.

If a tooth has been knocked out completely, it may be possible for a dentist to re-implant it successfully – especially if it is a child's permanent tooth. But here minutes count, so get to a dentist with the tooth as quickly as you possibly can.

Never pick up a knocked out tooth by the root – hold it by the crown. Do not clean the tooth. Instead, place it in milk or, if possible, get the casualty to carry it inside the mouth, taking great care not to swallow it.

ORTHODONTIC TREATMENT

My teenage daughter is very self-conscious about her front teeth, which are a little crooked. Would orthodontic treatment help and, if so, how do we go about getting it?

Yes, if your daughter wants it, orthodontic treatment will certainly help. She will need to wear braces – probably for between six and eighteen months – and she may find them a little uncomfortable and difficult to get used to at first. Apart from this there are few drawbacks. Orthodontic treatment is now so common few youngsters feel self-conscious.

Start by consulting your daughter's dentist. If it is agreed that treatment will help, referral to an NHS orthodontist (or, should you wish it, a private one) will follow.

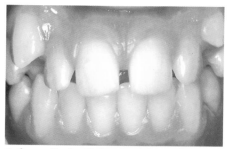

Before orthodontic treatment . . . The teeth of this 12-year-old were badly misaligned and unattractive. The orthodontist proposed removing four teeth and fitting braces.

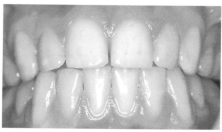

. . . and after The same teeth, now evenly spaced and growing normally without the need for further intervention. The whole course of treatment took under two years.

COSMETIC DENTISTRY

How effective is cosmetic dentistry for adults, and is it very expensive?

Depending on the problem, cosmetic treatment on teeth can be extremely effective, even on adults. It is important to remember, however, that changing the look of your teeth – like cosmetic surgery – will not change your life in other ways. Patients with unrealistic goals can find themselves disappointed. If you do seek treatment, consider it carefully first, and don't fall into the trap of imagining that a new look will necessarily make you happier or more self confident.

Prices for cosmetic treatments vary from dentist to dentist, so you may want to shop around. Even so, bear in mind that top class materials and skilled dentistry are not cheap and some procedures may cost hundreds or even thousands of pounds. Treatment may be available on the NHS if there is a health as well as a cosmetic reason, but it usually has to be paid for privately. These are some of the most common procedures:

TOOTH STRAIGHTENING Treatment from an orthodontist can straighten most misaligned teeth. Children and teenagers are generally treated on the NHS, but seldom adults.

REPLACING METAL FILLINGS Old amalgam fillings can be removed and replaced with white porcelain ones that are bonded to the teeth. Front teeth may be done on the NHS.

REPLACING TOOTH FACING If the front of a tooth is unsightly, a thin layer of enamel can be removed and replaced with a veneer.

CROWNS The whole surface covering of the tooth is replaced with a porcelain cap or a porcelain-bonded-to-gold cap to correct misalignment, damage or discoloration. Costs can run to several hundred pounds a tooth.

HAVING YOUR EYES TESTED

How often do I need an eye test? And how often should my children's eyes be tested?

Provided you are in good health, and have good eyesight and no reason to suspect any developing problems, every two years should be enough. If you wear glasses or contact lenses, or have an illness such as diabetes that could affect eyesight, or a family history of glaucoma, you may need more frequent tests – ask your doctor or optician. People who work at computer screens also have special requirements and rights – see page 335.

Apart from regular check-ups, you should make an appointment if you develop problems such as blurred vision, haloes around bright lights, difficulty seeing things close up or far away, or poor night vision. See an optician or doctor immediately if you experience double vision, pain in the eye or any loss of sight that comes in patches or appears as a curtain falling down across the visual field.

Children should start having annual eye examinations no later than two, especially if either parent has short or long sight, astigmatism or a squint, which could be inherited. The examination needs to be done by a qualified optician. The basic eye tests carried out by family doctors, health visitors and school nurses are not comprehensive.

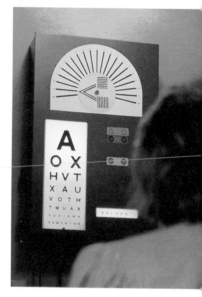

Eye testing Regular check-ups are essential to safeguard your eyesight. Some people are eligible for free tests on the NHS – doctors and optometrists can advise.

Health at work and on holiday

SICK LEAVE ENTITLEMENT

Is my employer required to continue paying my salary when I am ill? When do I need to get a doctor's certificate?

By law, provided you are earning enough to pay National Insurance contributions, your employer must pay you statutory sick pay (SSP) when you are ill for four or more days in a row (including weekends and holidays), for a maximum of 28 weeks. You do not have to be paid for the first three days, but many employers operate schemes that cover these too. If you are still unable to work after 28 weeks, you become eligible for Sickness Benefit or Incapacity Benefit.

The rate of SSP depends on your salary before you fall ill, and the money is paid in the same way as your salary – you do not have to register or do anything special to get it, except inform your employer that you are ill. If you are unable to let your employer know yourself, someone else may do it on your behalf. If you are ill for fewer than seven days your employer will probably ask you to fill in a self-certification form when you return. After seven days, you may need to provide a doctor's note. Find out what scheme your employer operates and take care to meet the requirements.

TIME OFF FOR APPOINTMENTS

Does my employer have to give me time off work for dental and medical appointments?

No – unless you are a pregnant woman attending for maternity care, when you have a right to time off for antenatal appointments during working hours. In all other cases, time off is at the discretion of your employer, although some large companies provide for it in employees' contracts. It is

DO'S — AND — DON'TS

for taking time off

Do stay at home if you have an infectious illness, even a cold.

Do have a proper rest if you stay at home. Don't end up doing chores.

Do consider a half day or working at home as an alternative to a day off.

Do let your employer know as soon as possible if you are not going in.

Don't be a martyr – if you are ill, don't force yourself to work.

Don't feel guilty if you are really unwell.

rare for such requests to be refused, but if an employer considers that someone is taking excessive or unjustified time off, he or she could deduct it from holiday entitlement.

INJURIES AT WORK

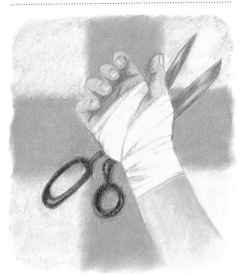

What happens when there is an accident at work? Does it have to be reported?

Accidents involving loss of life, severe injury, being in hospital for more than 24 hours or certain work-related illnesses, such as chemical poisoning or asbestosis, have by law to be reported to the authorities immediately by telephone, or within seven days in writing.

The same applies to accidents involving extremely dangerous situations – an explosion or a wall collapsing, for example – even if no one is hurt. In general, businesses that serve the public, such as shops and cinemas, must report accidents to the environmental health department of the local authority, while offices and factories report to the area office of the Health and Safety Executive. Employers must also keep a written record of any accidents, including a brief description of what happened, the names of all those involved, and the date, time and place.

STAYING AWAY FROM HOME

My elderly father is planning an extended stay in another part of the country. If he becomes ill, will he be able to see a local doctor? Will he need his medical records?

The NHS operates a scheme under which patients can, when necessary, see a doctor away from home. If your father becomes ill while he is away, he can ask a local doctor to take him on as a temporary resident. The doctor is paid for this arrangement, so it is not a favour and your father should have no trouble finding a doctor who will see him. In practice, he will become the new doctor's patient for the duration of his stay in the area, for any period of up to three months. After three months, he will be expected to register formally as a new patient.

There is no need for your father to take his records with him. In fact, it is almost always advisable for records to be kept by a patient's regular doctor so that they can be easily located in an emergency. If your father needs regular attention or treatment, such as blood tests or injections, he should ask his usual doctor to provide details in a letter that he can take with him. Similarly, if your father is at all forgetful, it may be wise for him to write, or to ask his doctor to write, a brief résumé covering his medical history, current complaints and details of medication.

TRAVEL IN EUROPE

Are British citizens entitled to free health care when visiting other countries in the European Union?

All British citizens are entitled to emergency medical treatment while they are travelling in a European Union member state. Sometimes treatment is free, and sometimes you may have to bear part of the cost. In some countries you may have to pay at the time and claim a full or partial refund later.

In order to claim this benefit, you must have on you a validated Form E111 to prove your eligibility. The form, together with a Department of Health information booklet for travellers, can be obtained from doctors' surgeries, travel agents and post offices. The booklet outlines the health care arrangements that apply in all EU countries and in many other destinations as well.

Form E111 must be validated at a post office. Once this is done it is valid indefinitely for short visits abroad. If you go to live outside Britain its validity ceases and you will need to register in the country you have moved to. It is worth remembering that few countries have health care systems as sophisticated as the NHS, and that Form E111 covers only emergency treatment for you and your dependants, and only in the foreign country. Repatriation is not covered. For further provision, you will need to make private arrangements (see 'Travel Insurance' , opposite). Travel agents, banks and insurance brokers can also advise.

VISITING REMOTE REGIONS

I am travelling with my family to some fairly remote places on holiday. Are there any health precautions we should take?

Start by seeking the advice of your doctor, travel agent and the consulates of the countries you are to visit. The Travel Advice Unit of the Foreign Office operates a health and safety information line on 0171 270 4129.

In particular, make sure your family have all necessary immunisations. Take out travel insurance and pack a travel medical kit (see page 170), including adequate supplies of any medicines. If any family members have special needs (formula milk for a baby, for example) find out what will be available and if necessary take your own supplies.

TRAVEL INSURANCE

How good are travel insurance schemes? Do they guarantee a certain standard of medical treatment or just a basic minimum? And if the local facilities are inadequate, will the insurance company meet the cost of getting me home?

As with most types of insurance, you generally get what you pay for in a travel policy. The only way to find out exactly what you are buying is to read the small print in the contract. Bear in mind, however, that no scheme can guarantee that a certain standard of care will be available at your destination – not even a 'basic minimum'. Even if you have a policy which allows for repatriation, you will have to rely on local facilities until help arrives. And you will also probably have to pay your bill on the spot and claim the money back when you get home.

If you have no repatriation clause, you may have your medical bills met, but again you are dependent on local skills and equipment for however long your recovery takes. This may not matter in New York or in the south of France but it could require careful consideration if you are travelling in developing countries. Travel insurance schemes are not designed only with health in mind, but also to cover eventualities such as loss of luggage, accidents and personal liability, legal expenses and delayed travel. However, most have generous provision for medical cover, including repatriation costs.

Some travel insurance policies specifically exclude activities such as driving and skiing that involve particular risks. If you want cover for these, you may have to pay extra for a better policy, or take out separate insurance. If you use a credit card to pay for your tickets, the card company may provide automatic cover – find out before buying more.

Medicines abroad

A few precautions are wise if you use medication and are travelling abroad.

● Check the generic name of any drugs before you leave home – brand names are seldom exactly the same abroad. Generic names are more likely to correspond, and even when they don't, doctors and pharmacists can often recognise them. Also ask your doctor if he knows what your medication is called in the country you will be visiting.

● Keep medication in its original, labelled container, so that customs officials can see what it is straight away.

● Ask your doctor if changes in weather or altitude could affect drug reactions.

Accidents and emergencies

MEDICATION IN A HURRY

What should I do if I need emergency medication after hours?

First, try calling your doctor's after-hours number to see if he can arrange a prescription. Alternatively, contact a hospital accident and emergency department. If there is no other option and the drug is urgently needed, a pharmacist may be able to supply it if you have had a prescription before.

DOCTOR OR HOSPITAL?

If I have an accident, should I go to my doctor, or straight to a hospital accident and emergency department?

It depends. In any crisis you must be guided first by common sense. The severity of your injury or condition, where you are, how far you are from the nearest hospital and the availability of your doctor must all be taken into account. If you are far away from home, a hospital accident and emergency department may be your only option. If you have serious injuries which you feel need urgent attention, you should generally get to a hospital as quickly as possible, no matter where you are – if necessary by dialling 999 for an ambulance to take you there.

However, if you live almost next door to your doctor's surgery but the nearest hospital is half an hour's drive away, it may make sense to try your doctor first – even if you end up going to hospital, he will be able to start treatment immediately.

If your injury is not serious and does not need immediate attention, your own doctor will offer rather more flexibility than that available in a hospital. For instance, you can ask for an urgent surgery appointment for, say, a wrist injury, or for a home visit if you

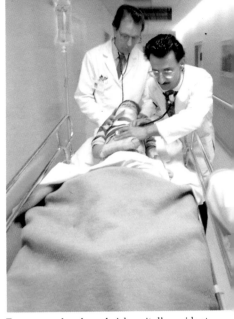

Emergency treatment A hospital's accident and emergency department is on 24-hour, year-round standby to treat urgent cases.

Why you may have to wait at A&E

People who arrive in a hospital accident and emergency department are treated according to the seriousness of their condition, not in order of arrival. The less critical your symptoms or injuries, the longer you may have to wait – especially if more serious cases continue to arrive. Try not to get impatient if you do have to wait – remember, you are one of the luckier ones.

---

are unable to travel to the surgery owing to a back problem. There are some emergencies, however, that need hospital treatment:

● Extensive burns, severe bleeding, severe injury or broken bones.
● Unconsciousness or serious injury after an accident.
● Head injury with loss of consciousness, loss of memory, subsequent vomiting or bleeding from the ears or nose.
● Suspected heart attack.
● Any other injury where you are worried about the patient's immediate condition.

Go to a GP with the following problems:

● Minor cuts and small burns or scalds.
● Minor head injuries without loss of consciousness or other symptoms.
● Any other injury which is not immediately serious but you feel needs a check-up.

At the end of life

HELP AND SUPPORT

What forms of help and care are available for patients who are terminally ill and for their families?

Both practical help and emotional support are available from several sources.

● Hospital care is suitable in acute crises and often continues through a final illness.
● Hospice care – see page 444.
● Macmillan nurses offer home care based on hospice principles – ask your doctor.
● Respite care – the patient is temporarily admitted to a hospital or hospice during crises, or to give relatives or carers a break.
● GP services such as home visits and community nursing.
● Social services for practical assistance.
● Voluntary agencies – doctors and hospital staff can put you in touch.

DEALING WITH A DEATH

What needs to be done when someone dies?

The procedure depends on where the death occurs. When someone dies at home, relatives suddenly find they have to cope with not only their own shock and grief, but with numerous practical arrangements, some of which require urgent attention. Deaths in hospital are easier on relatives, since much

of the organisation is handled by hospital staff. This is the procedure in each case.

At home
● Remove bedding or pillows, lay the body straight and, if you wish, close the eyes. Turn off any heating in the room. The undertaker will do the rest.
● Contact the deceased person's doctor, who will need to certify the death officially. Provided there is no reason to refer the death to the coroner (see opposite), you will be given a medical certificate of the cause of death.
● After the medical certificate of death has been issued, call an undertaker. He will wash and dress the body and guide you through the funeral arrangements, whether for cremation or burial. At this stage you may wish to consult other family members, or look up the dead person's will, to see if any preferences were expressed regarding the funeral. If cremation is chosen, the doctor will need to sign a special form. You may need to contact the deceased person's solicitor to find out about the will.
● If you are religious, contact your vicar, priest or other official who can offer both emotional and practical guidance.
● Make sure close relatives and friends have the chance to view the body and to say goodbye if they wish. Children can be given the same choice but should never be

pressurised into it and a parent or close adult should stay with younger ones.

● Once funeral arrangements have been made, you can ask the undertaker to take the body away or, if you prefer, you can keep it at home in a cool room until the funeral.

● Locate any insurance policies and pension plans that pay out on death.

● Take the medical certificate of the cause of death and the deceased person's medical card to the local registry office – the address is in the telephone book – to register the death. Make a copy of the death certificate for each insurance policy to be claimed on.

In hospital

● After a death in hospital or in a hospice, care of the body will be handled for you, the attending doctor will certify the death and staff will guide you through practical details.

● A minister of religion is often at hand, or you can call your own.

● Ask for some time and privacy for family members and friends to say their goodbyes.

● Decide on an undertaker, look up the will, locate any insurance policies and register the death as for a death at home.

DEATH CERTIFICATES

What is the purpose of a death certificate? How are the time and cause of death determined, and by whom?

The requirement for all deaths to be legally certified helps to ensure that any suspicious circumstances surrounding a death come to light, and provides official confirmation of death for purposes such as inheritance and insurance. It also enables official records to be amended and accurate up-to-date statistics to be compiled regarding issues such as population size and causes of death.

Legal certification

A patient is not legally dead until medically certified by a doctor. On rare occasions an expert such as a forensic pathologist may be needed to estimate the actual time of death (for example, if foul play is suspected). In most cases, however, the death certificate is simply given out by the registrar on receipt of the doctor's medical certificate of death, which specifies both the direct cause and any antecedant or contributory causes.

When a coroner becomes involved

In certain circumstances, a death must be referred to the local coroner who must be satisfied as to the cause of death before the death certificate can be issued. These situations include:

● If no doctor saw the patient within 14 days of death or attended the patient during the last illness.

● If there is uncertainty about the cause of death or the death occurred in suspicious circumstances.

● If the patient died as a result of unnatural causes such as an accident, violence or poisoning.

● If the death occurred in police custody, in prison or in a mental institution.

● If the death followed an abortion.

● If the death occurred under general anaesthetic, within 24 hours of the end of an operation, or within 24 hours of admission to hospital.

If, after seeing the records or talking to the attending doctors, the coroner concludes that the patient died of natural causes, he may allow the death certificate to be issued without any further action. If not, he may request that a postmortem examination be carried out in order to determine the exact cause (see panel, right).

When, and why, is a postmortem done?

Most postmortems (or autopsies) are performed at the request of the coroner – in Scotland, the procurator fiscal – in order to establish definitively the cause of death. Sometimes, however, the patient's own doctor may request a postmortem – either to investigate the cause of death or to assess the process of disease or the effects of treatment before death. Relatives can appeal against a coroner's request or refuse a doctor's, but most agree.

Doctors realise that the thought of a postmortem can be distressing for newly bereaved relatives, and do not ask lightly. However, the examination can yield valuable information, not only to doctors and medical researchers, but sometimes to relatives too. Very often, a postmortem can explain an unexpected death or reveal more about a hereditary condition.

Legal and ethical issues

SEEING YOUR RECORDS

I have heard that patients are entitled to see their medical records. How do I go about this – can I just call in at the surgery and ask to read them? What about records kept by hospitals and specialists?

The right of patients to see their medical records is set out in the Access to Medical Reports Act, that came into force in 1991.

Under the Act you are entitled to see any written medical notes or reports made about you after November 1, 1991. Under the Data Protection Act you must also be given access to *computerised* records, medical or otherwise – regardless of when they were made.

In order to view your medical records, you should make a written request to your doctor or to any private doctor who has treated you. In the case of hospital records, you should write to the health authority or to your own

Making a claim for medical negligence

Patients who feel their doctor has been negligent, or who have suffered some form of medical mishap, can claim compensation through the courts.

Many factors constitute medical negligence, including the failure of a doctor to attend a patient, the removal of a wrong limb, sterilisation or vasectomy that is not successful, bad reactions to drugs, accidents with anaesthetics, paralysis or gangrene from tight plaster casts, and foreign objects such as swabs left in the body after surgery.

Claims for negligence can be long and costly affairs, and obviously it is best for everyone if the need for them does not arise in the first place. For a doctor, this means spending time with the patient, being thorough with any examination and giving clear explanations in terms that are easily understood. It is up to the patient to cooperate with treatment, to ask questions if unclear about anything, and to raise objections sooner rather than later.

If a doctor fails to diagnose an illness, it is not necessarily a sign of negligence. However, the doctor does have to show that a 'reasonable degree' of skill was used in deciding what was wrong with a patient.

Further advice on complaining about health care appears on pages 248-249.

consultant. Putting your enquiry in writing legally obliges the record-holder to comply with your request. You can also see records kept by other health professionals such as nurses, physiotherapists or psychologists by following the same procedure.

The law requires that you must be shown your records within 40 days of requesting access (or 21 days for paper records made within the past 40 days), and you may either view the records where they are kept or ask for photocopies. For computer records you may be charged up to £10 for access, and for written records a charge of £10 may also be made, provided there have been no additions in the previous 40 days. Access to medical reports is otherwise free, apart from an unspecified 'reasonable' fee for photocopies.

Although the law grants you access to your own medical records, it gives you no right to those of your children without their explicit consent. In the case of very young children, your right to access is decided by the record-holder on the basis of what is in the child's best interest.

There is one provision in the Act that allows a doctor to withhold part of a record. This is when he or she believes that your physical or mental health might be seriously harmed if you have access. Doctors do not have to tell you if this is the case.

In practice, seeing your records is seldom particularly difficult. In many surgeries you can simply walk in and ask to look at them, although it is probably wise to telephone first to make arrangements for access.

TELLING THE TRUTH

Can a doctor ever choose not to tell a patient the truth about his or her condition, or to tell another member of the family instead?

A doctor has a duty to the overall wellbeing of his or her patient, and this includes a duty to mental, as well as physical, health. Breaking bad news is always difficult, and requires tact and diplomacy. Insensitive handling of a diagnosis of cancer which might prove fatal, for example, could easily lead a depressive person to take drastic measures.

In these circumstances, a doctor will frequently confide in a close member of the family in order to discuss a sympathetic and appropriate way of approaching the patient. Similarly in the case of young children, or mentally infirm patients, the family must be involved by the doctor. In general, doctors are much less secretive than they once were,

and prefer to lay all their cards on the table so that the future care of their patients can be properly organised. People with fatal conditions often achieve a great deal of spiritual peace as they come to terms with approaching death, and this is the result for which doctors aim. Doctors only withhold information after a great deal of thought, and usually only after discussion with their colleagues. They must also always be prepared to justify any decisions they make about non-disclosure of information.

TEENAGE CONTRACEPTION

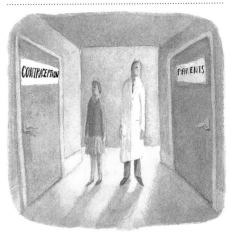

Could a doctor give contraceptive advice to my teenage children against my wishes or without even consulting me?

Sexual intercourse is illegal under the age of 16, and most parents would wish their children to remain sexually inexperienced until at least this age. Nevertheless, a minority of underage children do, and probably always will, participate actively in sexual relationships regardless of the law and the disapproval of their parents.

When it comes to giving advice about contraception to children under the age of 16, doctors are faced with an ethical dilemma. They have duties to the law as well as responsibilities to their patients.

In practice, most doctors will acknowledge that they cannot stop underage youngsters from having sex, and realise that if they fail to give advice, they may be exposing teenage patients to unwanted pregnancy as well as to HIV and other sexually transmitted diseases.

Generally speaking, a doctor will encourage a teenager to involve a parent in any decisions about contraception. But if the young person is unwilling to speak to a mother or father, most doctors will take a pragmatic approach and agree to give advice on sexual matters and contraception. Since the purpose of the law in this instance is to protect the vulnerable young, it accepts that doctors are similarly motivated, and does not prosecute for what could technically be seen as 'aiding and abetting a criminal act'.

Once children have reached the age of 16, they are legally entitled to receive contraception on the NHS, and in confidence.

UNCONSCIOUS PATIENTS

Who is legally responsible for making medical decisions for someone under anaesthetic or in a coma – the doctors or the family?

Medical responsibility for a patient who is unconscious depends largely on the circumstances in which consciousness was lost.

In the case of a surgical procedure or operation, the patient will have signed a consent form prior to administration of the anaesthetic. Although the forms are not standardised, they all contain clauses authorising the medical team to perform 'such further or alternative measures as may be necessary'. In effect, patients sign over both their own and their relatives' rights to make urgent decisions about treatment for as long as they are unconscious. Legal and medical responsibility is then vested in the consultant in charge.

After an accident or emergency, or in the case of a serious illness, a patient may be unconscious or in a coma when the doctor sees him for the first time. In such a case, the doctor will always try to contact the next of kin. In the interim, however, he is entitled to carry out any necessary emergency treatment, including surgery or the administration of drugs. This treatment should be no more than is immediately needed.

If a patient remains unconscious or is in a coma for a long period of time, further decisions about treatment may need to be taken. Responsibility then falls to the next of kin – though it is almost always exercised in consultation with the medical team.

More complex cases involve patients who are attached to life-support systems, particularly if signs of brain activity have ceased. Occasionally such cases are brought to court and then legal arguments tend to be about the definition of death.

The whole area is a medical, ethical and legal minefield, and is likely to become yet more complex if proposals on 'living wills' (see pages 443-444) enter the statute book.

REPORT FOR AN EMPLOYER

A prospective employer has asked for a medical report from my doctor. What is likely to be in it and can I ask to see it before it is sent?

It is quite reasonable for a would-be employer to ask for medical evidence that you are fit to take on a job you have applied for. But any doctor's report should confine itself strictly to issues relating to that.

The doctor should not give information about irrelevant conditions – a history of skin problems may be relevant to a job in a chemical plant, but is not likely to matter if you want to be a tax inspector. The report is intended only to reassure a future employer that you will not be a risk to yourself or to others, and that you are fit to do the job.

The rights of patients regarding medical evidence to others are set out in The Medical Reports Act. Under the Act, you have a right to see what is written about your health and to contest extraneous or false information.

Side effects and your right to be informed

By law, a doctor must obtain informed consent for any test or treatment proposed. This means that your consent has to be based on a reasonable understanding of what will happen and of any likely consequences. While it is hard to define exactly what constitutes a reasonable understanding, it is accepted that doctors have a duty to explain even complex treatment in broad terms.

Although doctors cannot detail every possible side effect of treatment – some of which will be very rare – you should always be warned about the most common or serious risks. In extreme cases, failure to do so may constitute medical negligence. Once your doctor has explained the procedure and any dangers, the decision whether or not to go ahead is yours alone. Adults are always free to refuse treatment.

The National Health Service

WHY AM I WAITING?

I thought NHS waiting lists were being shortened, but I'm told I will have to wait two years for my operation. Why so long?

The promise to cut hospital waiting lists was made in April 1993 as part of the Patient's Charter (see panel, page 248). Before then, some people found themselves waiting more than three years for a cataract operation, or hip or knee replacement. In this respect,

therefore, the waiting time has been cut – to no longer than two years from the time the consultant puts your name on the list.

There are three possible ways to shorten your wait: tell the hospital you are prepared to go on 'stand-by'; ask about waiting times at other local hospitals; and telephone the College of Health's National Waiting List Hotline (0181 983 1133). Remember that the NHS will generally fund treatment only in a hospital where your Health Authority or fundholding GP has a contract.

Your rights under the Patient's Charter

The Patient's Charter was drawn up in 1992 as part of the government's Citizen's Charter programme, and added to early in 1995. Under the Charter, you have the following rights.

● To receive health care on the basis of clinical need, regardless of ability to pay.
● To be registered with a general practitioner.
● To receive emergency medical care at any time.
● To be referred to a consultant acceptable to you, when your doctor thinks it necessary, and to be referred for a second opinion if you and your doctor agree.
● To be given a clear explanation of any treatment proposed, including risks involved.
● To have access to your health records.
● To choose whether or not you wish to take part in medical research.
● To be given detailed information about local health services.
● To be admitted for treatment no later than two years after being placed on a waiting list.
● To be able to see a consultant within six months of referral.
● To wait no longer than one year for heart surgery.
● To be given hospital food prepared to a certain standard.
● To have any complaint about NHS services investigated and to receive a written reply from the chief executive or general manager.

FUNDHOLDING DOCTORS

My doctor is about to become a fundholding GP. What does this mean and what difference will it make to patients?

A fundholding practice takes over responsibility for its own budget. It 'purchases' medical services such as outpatient treatment, operations and tests from hospitals, laboratories and other institutions on behalf of the patients. Fundholders can enter into 'bulk buy' contracts for particular services (usually at the same local hospitals they used before) based on statistical estimates of their anticipated needs. While the money still ultimately comes from the government, doctors acquire considerable economic power to negotiate better services and wider choices for patients, while at the same time keeping a tight rein on spending.

Like other NHS changes, the introduction of fundholding practices has aroused fierce controversy. It is probably too soon to judge the system but two concerns in particular are regularly voiced.

Firstly, some doctors claim that there is now a two-tier health service, with patients of fundholding practices receiving preferential treatment to those of non-fundholding practices, which are still dependent on the arrangements of their Health Authority.

Secondly, it has been argued that fundholding doctors may be more reluctant to take on potentially expensive patients, such as those with chronic diseases, or may even try to remove them from their list. Doctors have been warned against such behaviour and told that it will be regarded as unethical.

TRUST HOSPITALS

What is involved in a hospital becoming an NHS trust? What differences, if any, will it make to the care patients receive?

Since 1991, NHS reforms have permitted hospitals to leave the control of the district health authority and run themselves as an NHS trust, or self-governing hospital. They still operate within the NHS but are managed like a commercial organisation, with a chief executive and a board of trustees at the top. NHS trusts do not receive direct government grants but finance themselves by selling medical services to fundholding doctors and district health authorities. They invest capital, decide their staffing levels and set charges independently. In theory, the best and most efficient hospitals should attract more business and thrive, enabling them to improve and increase the services they offer.

Like any institution, a trust hospital can get things wrong and overspend or even run out of money – and this is where patients can be affected. When the money runs out, wards close down, staff are lost and non-emergency operations cease. This is one of the reasons why waiting lists vary so much throughout the country.

Fears have also been voiced that the commercial spirit of NHS trusts may encourage them to concentrate only on more profitable areas of medicine such as cosmetic surgery and obstetrics while neglecting some other branches. It is still too early to say whether this will be a real problem. In any case, district health authorities remain responsible for ensuring a complete range of services.

COMPLAINING ABOUT CARE

My husband is unhappy about medical treatment he received. How should he go about complaining?

The best course of action depends on why your husband is unhappy, who was responsible and what he is hoping to achieve. If possible, he should start by deciding what he wants – probably one of these.

● Action to sort out an immediate problem.
● Action to ensure the problem does not happen again.
● An acknowledgment of what happened.
● An apology or explanation.
● An improvement in services for the benefit of other patients.
● Disciplinary action against the person responsible.
● Compensation.

Whatever he wants to achieve, your husband should make his complaint as soon as possible, and definitely within 13 weeks if it concerns a GP, six months if a dentist and one year if a hospital. If he leaves it longer, his complaint may not be considered. Provided he feels able to, he should start by talking or writing directly to the person involved or by approaching the person's immediate superior, explaining the problem and what he would like done about it.

If the complaint concerns the actions of a senior practitioner, it is usually fair to give the person the chance to explain and, if possible, to put the matter right. If it concerns actions performed by a member of staff, the employer needs to know, especially if there could be legal or professional implications (doctors, for example, are ultimately responsible for a breach of confidence by a member of their practice staff). If your husband does not want to complain directly to the person involved or if he feels the matter is too serious for this, he can complain through official channels such as:

● The hospital general manager or chief executive if the complaint is about hospital staff or administration.
● His doctor or Family Health Services Authority for a complaint about general practice staff or practice administration.
● The Family Health Services Authority if the complaint concerns an NHS doctor, pharmacist, optician or dentist.
● The General Medical Council or General Dental Council if there is a suggestion of gross professional misconduct.
● The chief executive of the NHS if the complaint affects a breach of rights under the Patient's Charter – call the Health Information Service on 0800 665 544.
● Voluntary agencies such as the Citizens Advice Bureau or MIND.

Private medicine and insurance

CHOOSING A SCHEME

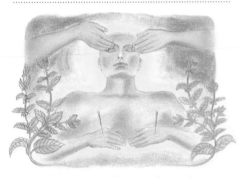

What factors should I consider in choosing a health insurance scheme? Do any schemes cover complementary treatment?

In making a choice you need to balance the benefits of a policy with how much you can afford to pay. Most schemes allow for special extras such as complementary treatment – but usually at an increased premium.

Costs vary enormously – among 16 companies that were surveyed in 1994, premiums for comprehensive family cover ranged from £55 to £284 a month. Since then, new budget schemes have been introduced by some insurers, which can cost much less. In general you get what you pay for, although not everybody needs the most inclusive type of cover. These are some points to consider.

● Is there a monetary limit on individual claims, or a limit on the amount you can claim annually? Is there a limit on the length of a course of treatment?
● Does the written information show clearly what is not covered, and are you happy with any exclusions?
● Does the policy provide full cover in all specialities, for all inpatient treatment including intensive care, all operation fees, all consultations, outpatient treatment, physiotherapy, radiology and pathology?
● Is there a good choice of hospitals, including the best in your area?
● Are the premiums competitive for the level of cover? Shop around if in doubt.
● Can you reduce your premiums by agreeing an excess – for example, paying the first £100 of any claim?
● Are there simple arrangements for settling claims? In the best schemes medical bills are paid directly by the insurance company.
● Can you get extra cover for special requirements. As well as complementary treatment you may want benefits such as accommodation for a parent if a child goes to hospital, home nursing or travel cover.

CALCULATING PREMIUMS

How are health insurance premiums set?

Unlike life insurance – where premiums vary according to factors such as sex, medical history, habits such as smoking, and your state of health – health insurance premiums are the same for eveyone of the same age buying a similar type of policy. The premiums do, of course, go up regularly in line with inflation.

Where health insurance policies differ is in the extent of cover they provide. Someone with a family or personal medical history of an illness such as heart disease will have that condition specifically excluded from the policy. Dental insurance, however, does vary with the state of your teeth and you may also need treatment done first.

Remember that policies are invalidated if you fail to declare a pre-existing condition.

Is it worth joining a private scheme?

When it comes to treating accidents and emergencies, NHS care is generally acknowledged to be among the finest in the world. Since you will be taken to the nearest hospital and treated by the first qualified person available, there is little advantage in belonging to a private scheme for the sake of emergency treatment. People who take out insurance usually want other benefits such as:

● Faster consultations.
● Consultations at more convenient times.
● More say in the choice of consultant.
● Shorter waiting lists for non-urgent treatment.
● More privacy in hospital.
● Treatment in a hospital closer to home.
● Better food and conditions in hospital. Schemes don't pay for everything, however. If you want private medicine in fields such as childbirth, dentistry or eye care you may still have to pay for it – or take out extra cover.

Fact It would not be financially viable, or fair to other clients (whose premiums would have to increase), if insurance companies offered policies to people with conditions such as advanced cancer in which there is a very high risk of having to pay out within a short time. Since those who die early have contributed fewer premiums, their claims are in effect paid for by those who survive longer. To avoid the risk of being refused later, it is best to take out insurance early in life and when you are in good health.

PAYING FOR PRIVATE SURGERY

I am considering paying to have my hip replacement done privately. How do I go about finding the best surgeon and at a price I can afford?

Strictly speaking, finding a surgeon is not up to you since you are dependent on your doctor's referral, even for private treatment. If you have a preference, however, most doctors will try to accommodate it. In any case, your choice may be limited by the number of private hospitals within the area or to which you are willing to travel.

You have probably already seen an orthopaedic surgeon and determined that you do need a hip replacement. If you were happy with the surgeon but simply do not want to wait until treatment is available on the NHS, call the secretary of the hospital department where he works and ask if he operates privately, and where. If not, unless you have another recommendation to go on, the best way to find a surgeon with a good reputation is to ask your doctor.

Finding out about operation costs is relatively simple. For a major surgical procedure, it is the price charged by different hospitals which you need to know.

If you have private health insurance, contact your company for a list of hospitals in various price brackets and check which of these your policy covers. If you have a preferred surgeon, telephone the hospital where he operates and ask how much the operation will cost. If you want to compare prices, telephone your nearest private hospitals and ask whether they perform hip replacements and also what they charge.

PRIVATE DENTAL SCHEMES

Are private dental schemes worth the money? What are the major types of schemes available and how do they work?

Private dental schemes are increasingly popular but only you can decide if joining one is worth it for you. Schemes are of three types.

Capitation schemes
You pay a monthly fee to the dentist, which covers most basic treatment, such as check-ups, fillings and X-rays. Special treatments such as crowns and bridges will usually cost extra. If you pay higher premiums, you may get additional cover. Fees vary according to the condition of your teeth and the type of cover – usually from £5 to £20 per month.

Patient insurance schemes
You pay a premium and claim back the cost of any dental treatment from the insurance company. Fees vary according to the level of cover, typically from £3 to £30 per month.

Corporate dental schemes
Some employers pay part or all of the cost of dental premiums. Usually you pay the dentist yourself and then claim the money back from the company policy.

Playing your part

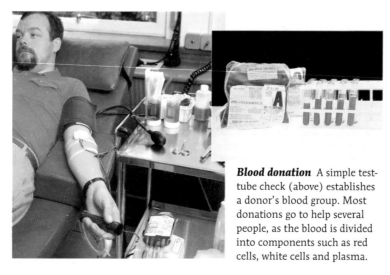

Blood donation A simple test-tube check (above) establishes a donor's blood group. Most donations go to help several people, as the blood is divided into components such as red cells, white cells and plasma.

GIVING BLOOD

I'd like to donate blood, but I'm a bit of a medical coward. What actually happens to donors? Does giving blood hurt or affect your health?

Many people feel a bit anxious about giving blood, but there is no need to. When you go along to a donor clinic for the first time, you will initially be asked for details such as your name and address. You will be given information to read about who should not give blood. If you have any doubts about your health or suitability to donate, you can ask to see a doctor in confidence. A tiny pinprick test will be done to make sure you are not anaemic and then you will be asked to fill in a questionnaire relating to HIV and other illnesses that can be transmitted in blood.

Once all the paperwork is complete, the donation is taken. Usually, there is no pain at all except a prick as the needle is inserted. The procedure takes six to eight minutes but you are advised to rest lying down for a further 15 minutes. You will then be offered a soft drink and biscuits, and be free to leave.

Donating blood is an entirely safe procedure. You cannot contract an infection or suffer any serious side effects from it. A few people feel a little faint afterwards but you can reduce the chances of this happening by drinking plenty of fluids before and after (preferably not alcohol or black coffee), and by having a light meal beforehand. Try not to smoke for two hours afterwards, and choose a day when you are feeling fit and well.

BEING A GUINEA PIG

My doctor has asked me to take part in a trial for a new arthritis drug. I'd like to help, but are there any risks?

All drugs carry some risk, whether you are taking part in a medical trial or not. New drugs undergo rigorous testing, first on animals and then on healthy volunteers, before they are tested on real patients. By the time a drug is ready for widespread clinical trials, common or serious side effects should have been spotted, and the drug's potential benefits should have been demonstrated to be greater than any possible hazards. Nevertheless, there is always a small risk that some extremely rare side effects may have gone unnoticed or that there are long-term effects which cannot yet be detected.

In some trials, new drugs are compared with placebos (inert substitutes) – in which case you must remember that you may not actually be receiving any medication at all. If your symptoms are severe, however, it is far more likely that the trial will either compare an established drug with the new one, or that additional medication will be given so that you receive increased treatment.

There are also real benefits to being in a trial. New drugs are intended to be better than old ones, so you could be receiving a safer and more effective treatment. Patients also tend to receive more attention as a result of being in a trial, so your condition will be monitored more closely, and you may get more chance to discuss it with interested medical staff. You will be closely watched for any side effects, which will be picked up early and dealt with. In general, patients in trials

do a bit better, irrespective of any new treatment they receive. They also gain by knowing they are helping to make life better for other people in the future.

DONATING YOUR ORGANS

What is the best way to register as an organ donor?

The best and most reliable way is by registering on the national computer database of organ donors. Registration forms are available from post offices, doctor's surgeries and some libraries, or by calling the Health Literature Line on 0800 555 777.

Alternatively, pick up and fill in a donor card from your doctor's surgery, and carry it at all times. Or, if you are about to apply for or renew a driver's licence, you will find an optional box to tick on the form.

Whichever way you choose to register, but particularly in the case of the second two options, make sure your relatives know.

HELPING SCIENCE

I would like to donate my body to science. How do I go about it and what will be done with my remains?

As well as donating your organs for transplant, there are various other ways of helping medicine after you die. If you have a rare or little-understood condition, ask your consultant whether research projects might benefit from tissues or samples – you might even be able to help in this way while you are still alive. If a postmortem is likely to produce useful scientific information and you would wish to consent, ensure that your next of kin knows. Remember, however, that undergoing a postmortem may mean your remains are unsuitable for anatomical dissection.

If you do wish your body to be considered for anatomical examination by medical students, you can arrange for it to be offered to a medical school. Bodies are preserved and used for teaching for up to three years, after which the school arranges and pays for cremation. Occasionally, the institution may wish to keep certain tissues longer for teaching, research or, if there is a rare condition, as museum specimens. If you wish to leave your body for anatomical examination, your relatives must know of your wishes and agree. Further details and a consent form – which should be kept with your will – can be obtained from the anatomy department of your nearest medical school.

Becoming involved

There are two ways to have your say in local health matters. One is through The Patients' Association, 8 Guildford Street, London WC1N 1DT, whose directory, *The Health Address Book*, details more than 1000 self-help groups. The other is through your Community Health Council (CHC), listed in the telephone book.

DO'S
— AND —
DON'TS

for medical research

Do take part if you feel able – ongoing research is the only way that treatment can be improved for future patients (and for you).
Do remember that it may also be in your own interests to take part.
Do ask any questions that you want to.
Do follow instructions precisely. If they are unclear, ask for details.
Do report any drug side effects promptly.

Don't feel you are obliged to take part just to please your doctor.
Don't cover up errors you make in following instructions. You could invalidate the results.
Don't take any additional medication unless the trial doctor agrees to it.
Don't get too enthusiastic if new treatments work well. You may not be able to continue after the trial.

SEX AND FAMILY LIFE

*Loving relationships and happy families
don't just happen - they need nurturing, openness
and information. From sex through pregnancy to birth
and the bringing up of children, knowing the facts
prevents problems and dispels anxiety.*

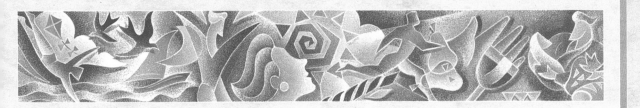

Are you well-informed about family life?

Nothing could be more natural – or more demanding – than having children and rearing them. Yet parents are not trained for the job and often don't know the facts that could help to make it easier. Try this quiz to rate yourself for basic parenting knowledge. In each case tick the correct box and check your score below.

1 Which of these steps is most important for women who want to conceive?

a) Losing weight if overweight. ☐
b) Eating plenty of meat and protein foods to build up her strength. ☐
c) Having her blood pressure checked. ☐

2 Which one of these statements about pregnancy is true?

a) Making love during pregnancy is a common cause of miscarriage. ☐
b) Liver is a good source of iron and vitamins for pregnant women. ☐
c) Older mothers adapt better to pregnancy than women in their 20s. ☐

3 What is the best way for a mother to lose weight after having a baby?

a) By exercising. ☐
b) By breast-feeding. ☐
c) By dieting. ☐

4 Which may not be good for a baby?

a) Feeding on demand. ☐
b) Being left to cry. ☐
c) Baby massage. ☐

5 What should you do if a child has a temperature of 38°C (100°F)?

a) Give half an aspirin. ☐
b) Give paracetamol and wrap the child up warmly. ☐
c) Keep the child cool and watch for further developments. ☐

6 At what age do children usually stop needing to sleep during the day?

a) 2 years. ☐
b) 3 years. ☐
c) 4 years. ☐

7 How can parents best stimulate a toddler's intellectual development?

a) By providing educational toys and games. ☐
b) By constantly trying to raise the level of play to the next stage. ☐
c) By praising all achievements, no matter how small. ☐

8 Which is the least constructive way of disciplining a child?

a) Ignoring bad behaviour but giving praise when the child is good. ☐
b) Making an issue out of bad behaviour so the child can see how upset you are. ☐
c) Explaining your reasons and offering alternative choices when you forbid the child to do something. ☐

9 Which child is more likely to have a learning difficulty?

a) The one who still can't tie his shoelaces long after all his classmates have learned to. ☐
b) The one with few friends. ☐
c) The one who bullies others or who gets bullied. ☐

SCORING

Award yourself 1 point for each of these answers: 1(a), 2(c), 3(b), 4(b), 5(c), 6(c), 7(c), 8(b), 9(a). Add up your score.

6 to 9: You seem to know a great deal about having and raising children – possibly the result of many years' experience. Carry on enjoying family life.

5 or less: Though love and not learning is what really makes a good parent, you may find that knowing a little more could sometimes smooth the path of family life.

Building better relationships

COMPATIBLE COUPLES

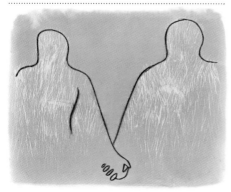

What is the best way of maintaining a good sexual relationship?

There is no single solution. A good sex life thrives on the same things that make up a good relationship – communication, love and concern for each other. It also helps if a couple are physically affectionate in general and show their feelings by gestures such as hugging, even when they are not contemplating sex. Contrary to popular belief, physical beauty and sexual athleticism have little to do with making someone a good lover. Most partners rate enthusiasm, openness and a sense of humour far more highly.

To enjoy sex to the full, a couple need time alone in surroundings where they can relax. It helps if both partners are unselfconscious and can talk about their likes and dislikes.

Arguments, resentment and unresolved differences – more than any other factor – are more damaging to intimate relationships. Try to talk about problems, possibly with the aid of a trained counsellor (see page 183) if the divisions are deep or long standing.

LESS FREQUENT SEX

After 25 years together, my wife and I seldom have sex, though we still love each other. Could there be something wrong with our relationship?

Not as long as you are both happy with the situation. For many couples sex is never the most important thing and its declining frequency over the years is not regretted – provided the relationship remains loving in other ways. However, even if nothing is said, a diminishing sex life can come as a severe blow to either or even both partners. Talk to your wife and find out how she feels about the situation – you may discover that you have simply lost the habit of doing the intimate things that lead to sex, or you may have settled into a routine and become bored without either of you even realising. Luckily, it is never too late to add new interest to your sex life (see panel, below right) if that is what you both want.

Physical problems such as pain and arthritis can also be a cause of diminishing sex in an otherwise happy marriage. All such difficulties can be treated, however, or ways found around the problem as, for example, by experimenting with different positions. Family doctors can generally offer good advice on what methods might work best for a particular couple.

TIME FOR EACH OTHER

My husband often works late and comes home too tired for sex. I miss the intimacy we once shared, but I don't want to put pressure on him. What should I do?

Try to discuss the subject with your husband when he's not tired and in a non-sexual situation, such as on a walk at the weekend. Tell him how you are feeling and ask how he feels, too. Fatigue may not be the only cause of his lack of interest: he may have worries about work or money. Or he may feel that you have drifted apart and spend too little time together for intimacy to flourish. Only you and your husband can decide how to tackle these issues, but whatever you do, talking and showing concern will help.

If the problem is straightforward exhaustion, simple measures will help most. When he comes home, let your husband talk about the day's events if he wants to, but don't insist if he'd rather be left alone. After he has unwound, he might feel more affectionate: try a massage or some other form of physical contact that creates closeness but doesn't necessarily lead to sex.

Sex doesn't have to be in bed at night, either. It might work better to set aside a special time, such as Sunday morning. Finally, remember that sex should be a pleasure, not a duty or a chore – for either partner. Share affection, intimacy and time, and sex will follow naturally.

DO'S
—— AND ——
DON'TS

to improve your sex life

Do make intimacy and affection a priority.
Do set aside time for sex.
Do be open about your feelings.
Do show consideration in general.
Do use lighting, perfume and music to create the right mood.
Do be sensual: share baths and back rubs; use touch to convey feelings.
Do share your fantasies and experiment if any appeal to you both.

Don't feel that physical contact must lead to sex.
Don't restrict sex to the ten minutes before you go to sleep.

DO APHRODISIACS WORK?

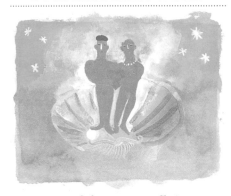

Do oysters and champagne really increase sexual desire, or are popular beliefs about aphrodisiacs just old wives' tales?

There is little scientific evidence to show that any so-called aphrodisiacs actually work. Most, such as royal jelly, vanilla pods and ground rhinoceros horn, will do no harm, except possibly to your purse. Some, however, including the notorious Spanish fly, or cantharis, made from dried blister beetles, are poisonous, and can be fatal.

Oysters may be of some benefit, but only if you have an inadequate diet. They are a rich source of zinc, and a lack of zinc may lead to a loss of libido. However, if your diet is already rich in zinc, getting more will not help. In any case, zinc is also found in liver, turnips and many equally unromantic foods. As for champagne, there is no proof that it increases sexual desire, although a few glasses might well reduce inhibitions and induce the same effect.

The root of the ginseng plant and chocolate have slightly better-deserved reputations. In scientific experiments some rats seem to have enjoyed the effects of ginseng, and chocolate is known to contain mood-enhancing chemicals. However, music, dancing, perfume and a romantic atmosphere are, it seems, more important than what is on the menu.

SEX DURING A PERIOD

Is there any reason why my partner and I should not have sexual intercourse during her menstrual period?

There is seldom any medical reason to abstain from sex during menstruation, provided you are both comfortable with the idea. Some experts believe that younger women, under about 20, may be slightly more vulnerable to infections of the cervix during their periods, and advise them to use a barrier contraceptive, such as a condom or diaphragm, at this time of their cycle.

Remember, too, that it is still possible to become pregnant during a period, although it is less likely than at other times of the menstrual cycle.

CAUTION Human immunodeficiency virus (HIV) can be transmitted in menstrual blood. Women who are HIV-positive must abstain from sex during their periods, as a condom will not protect their partner.

Help for sexual problems

LONGER LOVEMAKING

I often find that I ejaculate too quickly for my partner. Is there anything I can do to prolong our lovemaking?

Yes, there is. First, talk to your partner. Premature ejaculation is one of the commonest sexual problems and, while men are often worried by it, their partners may not be, particularly if other forms of stimulation are shared before and afterwards. Sex therapists also recommend the following techniques:

● First aid: Take a deep breath when close to climax. This can briefly shut down the ejaculatory reflex.
● Squeezing: Withdraw and squeeze just below the tip of the penis for 10 to 15 seconds when ejaculation is imminent. You could ask your partner to help with this.
● Stop-start: Ask your partner to help you with manual stimulation – and stop when you are close to orgasm. You should gradually be able to prolong the time taken to reach a climax.

Do not forget that premature ejaculation is generally the result of anxiety – about performance or about sex itself. Worrying too much about it, or trying too hard to overcome it, will just put pressure on both you and your partner, and may even add to the difficulty. If, after a few weeks' practice, the methods above have had no effect, see your doctor as there may be a deeper problem.

DEALING WITH IMPOTENCE

My husband sometimes fails to have an erection when we want to make love. I reassure him that it doesn't matter, but he becomes very upset. Surely this happens to all men at times?

Yes, it does. Failure to have an erection may be due to stress, fatigue, alcohol or even some common medications. As with many sexual difficulties, the anxiety it creates can itself become one of the major perpetuating factors.

The answer in most cases is to take the emphasis off intercourse, both when the problem occurs, and in the relationship generally. Reassure your husband and explain that kissing, hugging and other forms of intimacy give you pleasure whether or not they lead to sex. Make physical signs of affection part of your daily lives. As well as bringing you closer and being enjoyable, you'll find that if touching occurs more often and is not always equated with sex, what happens in the bedroom may not seem so important. In time, both of you will stop anxiously watching to see if the penis will 'perform' – and thereby make it much more likely that it will. And if your husband does still fail to have an erection occasionally, it won't matter nearly so much if your relationship is physically satisfying in other ways. You could also try making more use of other forms of stimulation, such as kissing or using your hands.

CAUTION Always see your doctor if impotence is persistent or worsening. It can sometimes indicate a physical disorder, such as diabetes or depression, that needs medical treatment.

PAINFUL INTERCOURSE

I find intercourse painful, and it's affecting my relationship with my husband. Should I see a doctor?

Definitely. There are many possible causes of pain during sex, and a woman who has this problem should always see a doctor.

If the pain occurs on penetration, it may be that there is not enough natural lubrication, possibly because you are not yet fully aroused. The problem is easily solved by spending longer on intimate foreplay and not attempting penetration until you feel really ready, and then very gently. Sometimes taking the contraceptive pill can reduce the amount of mucus and make the vagina dry.

This also tends to happen more after the menopause. The use of a lubricant such as KY jelly can often help.

Infections of the vagina and vulva can also make penetration uncomfortable and cause superficial pain, as can bruising during childbirth. In these cases, it is best to wait until the problem has cleared up before having intercourse. Infections should be seen by a doctor and may need antibiotics.

Pain can also be caused by vaginismus, a spasm of the muscles around the entrance to the vagina. The root of the problem is usually an upsetting experience in the past or fear that sex will be painful. Many couples are able to solve it on their own by adopting a slow, gentle technique, or by practising relaxation techniques. Medical treatment and counselling can also be highly successful.

Deeper pain during intercourse nearly always has a medical cause that requires treatment. Ovarian cysts, endometriosis and pelvic inflammatory disease are common culprits.

AVOIDING CYSTITIS

I often have an attack of cystitis after making love. Is there anything I or my husband can do to prevent this?

This is a very common problem. Cystitis – inflammation of the bladder lining – results from either bruising or infection of the urinary tract, and is often brought on by sexual intercourse. It causes discomfort in the lower abdomen, burning pain on passing urine and a frequent, urgent need to urinate. Women are much more at risk than men because of their shorter urethra – the tube through which urine is excreted – which leaves the bladder vulnerable to bruising, irritation and bacterial infections.

You and your husband can minimise the risk of infection by making sure that you always urinate and then wash before sex. If soap irritates the urethra, just use water. When making love, try to avoid being over-vigorous and don't use positions that feel at all uncomfortable. If you have a diaphragm that feels as if it could be pressing on the bladder, consider an alternative form of contraception. It will also help to urinate and wash immediately after sex, and to drink copious quantities of water to flush out any bacteria in the urethra.

CAUTION If an attack of cystitis does not clear up within 24 hours, see your doctor. Untreated bladder infections may spread to the kidneys.

Overcoming impotence and frigidity

The ability to become sexually aroused varies enormously among individuals and at different stages of life. Usually, a temporary lessening of desire is nothing to worry about, but occasionally it can indicate a medical problem, cause anxiety or threaten a relationship – in which case help may be needed. The best approach depends on the cause of the problem.

Troubled relationship
Only talking about the problem will help, with or without the aid of a counsellor.

Other sexual problems
See your doctor if you suspect a medical disorder, or a sex therapist (see page 258) if the problem is psychological.

Stress and emotional upsets
Time, understanding and gentleness will help. Ongoing problems may need counselling.

Illnesses and drugs
Conditions such as diabetes and hormonal imbalances can cause impotence. So can antidepressants, diuretics and antihypertensive drugs. Seek medical advice.

Heavy drinking
Drink less alcohol.

Pain
Consult your doctor.

SEEKING SEXUAL THERAPY

I've heard that there is such a thing as sex therapy that can help couples in trouble. What exactly does it involve, and how does it differ from marriage guidance?

The proper term for sex therapy is psychosexual therapy. It is suitable for any couple with specifically sexual difficulties – as opposed to the broader emotional and practical problems dealt with by marriage counsellors. Often sex therapists and marriage guidance counsellors work together. Typical problems dealt with by sex therapists include impotence, premature ejaculation, pain, lack of desire, inability to have an orgasm and confusion about sexual orientation. Psychosexual therapy can involve discussing the origins of the beliefs and attitudes to sex which may be causing problems in a relationship. The therapist may offer information and advice about sexuality and sexual technique, or suggest practical measures such as setting aside more time for sex. Specific sexual techniques may also be taught for particular problems.

It is a good idea to talk to your family doctor before considering sexual therapy. He or she may well be able to provide a simple solution to the problem and, if not, can always refer you to a sex therapist for specialised help. Alternatively, it could help to seek marriage guidance first, possibly from a Relate counsellor (see page 183). Other problems in the relationship will be dealt with first and then, if necessary, you may be referred to a sex therapist.

Sexually transmitted diseases

Warning signs

All sexually transmitted diseases are treatable, particularly if caught in their early stages. See your doctor or contact the genitourinary clinic of your local hospital if you notice any of the following symptoms.

● Sores, ulcers, warts, irritation, blisters or spots in the genital area.
● A burning sensation on passing urine.
● Genital discharge.
● Small white eggs and pinhead-sized insects in the pubic hair.
● Any genital symptoms accompanied by flu-like symptoms or by pain in the joints.

Protection for partners

If a sexually transmitted disease is diagnosed, sexual partners should be treated at the same time to avoid reinfecting each other. After treatment, a follow-up test is needed to make sure the condition has cleared completely.

WHO IS AT RISK?

How common are sexually transmitted diseases? Who is most at risk?

People with many sexual partners face the greatest risk of contracting a sexually transmitted disease (STD), and those whose partners have many partners.

In Britain, five STDs are particularly prevalent. The most widespread is non-specific urethritis (NSU) with about 150000 cases reported every year in Britain. Warning signs in men include mild burning when urinating and discharge from the penis. The equivalent condition in women is called non-specific genital infection and is usually symptomless unless there are complications in which case vaginal bleeding may occur. Both infections are curable with antibiotics, but if left untreated can cause infertility in both men and women. Women may also develop a condition known as pelvic inflammatory disease.

About 50000 new cases of genital warts are reported each year in Britain. Wart-like swellings appear around the genitals and sometimes the anus. They are easily cured if treated early, but tend to reoccur.

Gonorrhoea has become less common and is easy to cure in its initial stages, but can be difficult to detect. Genital herpes, while not life-threatening, is recurrent and, so far, incurable. Trichomoniasis is the fifth most common STD. It does not usually cause symptoms in men, but women experience a heavy vaginal discharge. It is easy to diagnose and cure with antibiotics. Other common STDs include crab lice, syphilis – now rare – and the human immunodeficiency virus (HIV). The important thing to remember is all STDs are treatable and most are curable *if* they are diagnosed and treated early enough.

MAKING SEX SAFER

What is safe sex? Can you ever be 100 per cent protected against AIDS and other sexually transmitted diseases?

Except for couples who are and always have been entirely monogamous and who are not at risk from other factors, such as sharing needles when using intravenous drugs, there is no such thing as safe sex. However, using a condom can considerably reduce any risk of infection – not so much 'safe' as 'safer' sex. It is essential to use condoms correctly (see panel, right), and to avoid other high-risk activities (see The Facts About AIDS, opposite). To make sure you get the maximum amount of protection from a condom:

● Buy only latex condoms with the BSI kitemark and a reservoir at the tip.
● Store condoms in a dark, cool dry place. Avoid keeping them in a wallet or hip pocket for any length of time – prolonged exposure to heat can cause them to deteriorate.
● Always inspect a condom for deterioration or perforations before use.

- Don't keep condoms past the expiry date.
- Don't use oil or petroleum-based lubricants such as vaseline as these may weaken the rubber. Use only water-based lubricants.
- Use a new condom for each act of intercourse, and any other sexual activities involving direct genital-to-genital contact.

CERVICAL CANCER

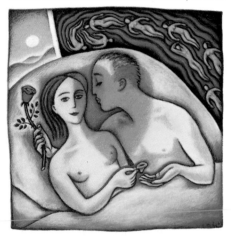

I have heard that having several sexual partners can increase a woman's chances of developing cervical cancer. Is this true?

Cervical cancer is virtually unknown among nuns, but common in prostitutes, which suggests that the number of sexual partners affects a woman's risk. However, some women who develop cervical cancer have only ever had sex with one man. It is now thought to be almost certain that men pass on some agents that increase the risk of this disease, and genital warts is the most likely candidate. A woman in a sexual relationship with a man who has genital warts has about a one in three risk of developing a precancerous condition of the cervix. Even so, not all women who get genital warts develop cervical cancer. In any case, the more partners a woman has, the greater the risk of exposure to the infection. In addition, the danger of a man carrying the responsible agent is increased by the number of sexual partners *he* has had.

Women who fear that they may be at risk from cervical cancer should opt for barrier contraceptives such as the male or female condom (see page 261) as these protect the cervix from infection. Fortunately, precancerous changes in the cervix are curable if caught early enough, which is why women are advised to have a cervical smear test every three to five years (see page 164).

LIVING WITH HERPES

Is there a cure for genital herpes?

There is no known way of eliminating the virus from the body. However, an antiviral drug called Acyclovir is very effective in reducing the severity of outbreaks when prescribed on a regular basis. Although cold sores and genital herpes are both caused by the herpes simplex virus, the types differ (HSV1 and HSV2 respectively) and one cannot cause the other.

The first attack of genital herpes usually occurs between 2 and 12 days after intercourse with an infected partner. Tiny cold sore-like blisters appear on the genitals and the surrounding area. These burst a day or two later and form ulcers, which heal during the following weeks. A sufferer is infectious whenever there are open or healing ulcers; however, they may also be infectious when sores are not present. After the first attack has settled down, the virus lies dormant in local nerve endings until stress, illness or some other factor triggers another attack.

During an attack, the area must be kept clean and comfortable to encourage healing. To prevent passing on the virus it is important to avoid intercourse.

THE FACTS ABOUT AIDS

What is the link between HIV and AIDS and how much of a risk is AIDS really?

AIDS (acquired immune deficiency syndrome) is the name given to the symptoms caused by the human immunodeficiency virus (HIV). Most people who have been exposed to HIV – indicated by the presence of antibodies in the blood – will develop AIDS eventually. It normally takes about ten years, but some people have remained healthy for much longer.

The HIV virus is not very resilient and can be transmitted only through direct contact with the blood or body fluids of an infected person. Most cases result from sexual intercourse, especially anal intercourse. In Britain, homosexual and bisexual men make up the largest group of AIDS patients, followed by intravenous drug users (owing to shared needles) and their sexual partners. Transfusions of contaminated blood products in the early 1980s were responsible for some AIDS cases, but this route of infection has been virtually eliminated since 1985, when new blood-screening techniques were put into practice.

How to use a condom

To be effective, condoms have to be used correctly.

- Put the condom on once the penis is erect but before it comes into contact with the woman's vaginal area.
- Squeeze all the air out of the reservoir at the tip of the condom.
- Keep the reservoir pinched between the finger and thumb while unrolling the condom over the penis.
- After ejaculation, encircle the end of the condom with finger and thumb to keep it securely in place and withdraw while the penis is still erect.

When should you use a condom?

Use a condom if you are uncertain about someone's sexual history, or if either partner:

- is not monogamous.
- is HIV-positive.
- has any other sexually transmitted disease.
- has shared needles to inject drugs.
- has had an operation or injection in a high-risk area of Africa, the Caribbean or the Far East.

If either partner is concerned about having a sexually transmitted disease, have a check-up at the genitourinary clinic of your local hospital before you stop using condoms.

Using contraception

CHOOSING A METHOD

How can I decide which is the best method of contraception for me?

There is no ideal, totally reliable and convenient method of contraception. Finding the method that will work best for you depends on many factors.

● How liable you are to side effects? The pill may not be advisable if you smoke or have high blood pressure. Some barrier methods can provoke cystitis.
● How important is avoiding pregnancy? Protection varies (see opposite page).
● Would the idea of an intrauterine device (IUD) trouble you? Would you mind taking artificial hormones every day?
● How regularly do you have sex? If it is occasional, condoms can be convenient.
● How much medical contact do you want? The pill, for example, requires regular visits.
● What method suits your personality? Not everyone can remember to take a daily pill.

Discuss these matters with your doctor or local family planning clinic. They will help you to decide what's best for you, carry out fittings and supply you with whatever you need. All forms of contraception are free on the NHS, and your local family planning clinic will supply free condoms.

PROS AND CONS OF THE PILL

Taking the pill sounds so convenient, but I worry about the possible side effects. What are the short and long-term risks?

Many women who take the contraceptive pill notice very few side effects, or none at all. Women who take oestrogen-containing pills, however, may experience weight gain, nausea, vomiting, depression, water retention and headaches. Such effects usually disappear after a few months but, if they persist, it may be necessary to change to a different type of pill or to an alternative method of contraception. The higher the oestrogen content, the more likely such side effects are, so doctors tend to prescribe low-oestrogen pills wherever possible.

A more serious adverse effect of the pill is a greater tendency to blood clotting which can increase the risk of leg vein and lung thrombosis, and high blood pressure which increases the risks of heart disease or stroke. However, for non-smoking women under 35 years old the risk of any of these is tiny – about one in 77000. It increases with age, smoking and obesity, to about 1 in 500 for smokers over 45.

Oestrogen-containing pills are also associated with a slightly higher incidence of breast and cervical cancer (if condoms are not being used), especially among women who take them for long periods when very young and before having their first child. Oral contraceptives may also exacerbate or trigger conditions such as diabetes, heart disease or gallstones in women prone to these conditions.

On the positive side, the pill protects against cancer of the uterus and ovaries and against conditions such as rheumatoid arthritis and endometriosis. Used wisely and under medical supervision, it is a convenient, reliable and safe method of contraception for most women. Your doctor will advise you further.

MISSING A PILL

What should I do if I forget to take a contraceptive pill?

It depends when you realise and what type of pill you are using. All oral contraceptives work best if you take them at the same time each day, and it is absolutely critical with the progesterone-only minipill. If you are more than three hours late with the minipill you are effectively starting all over again and you will need to use some other form of contraception for the next seven days to be safe.

Timing is more flexible with combined oestrogen-and-progesterone pills. If you are more than 12 hours late, take a pill as soon as you remember, and take the next pill at the correct time. Use an additional form of barrier contraception, such as condoms or a diaphragm, for the next seven days.

THE MALE PILL

How close are we to having a male contraceptive pill?

Not very. Despite several promising leads, research has yet to produce a male pill which is both safe and effective. This is difficult to achieve as such a pill would have to interfere

---

Which pill is best?

The standard pill gives fixed doses of the hormones oestrogen and progesterone. It is usually taken for 21 days followed by seven pill-free days. Various other options are also available.

● Low-dose pills have fewer side effects but are slightly less reliable.
● Every-day (ED) pills provide seven inactive pills instead of breaking your routine with pill-free days between packs.
● The minipill contains no oestrogen and is safer for some women.
● High-dose pills provide extra protection for very fertile women.
● Pills of different hormone content can help with problems such as acne or facial hair.
● Phasic pills which vary the hormone content are available for women who experience breakthrough bleeding with monophasic variety.

HOW DO DIFFERENT CONTRACEPTIVES PREVENT A PREGNANCY?

Artificial contraceptives work in several different ways. Barrier devices such as condoms, diaphragms and caps, physically prevent sperm cells from reaching and fertilising an egg. They work best when used together with a chemical spermicide, as there is always a slight risk of sperm getting past the barrier. Hormonal methods include pills, injections and subcutaneous implants. They alter the female cycle, preventing ovulation and therefore conception. Technically, intrauterine devices (IUDs), such as the 'Copper-T', do not stop conception but prevent a fertilised egg from being implanted in the womb.

Choose and use your method carefully – not all are suitable for everybody, and some are more reliable than others. If artificial methods do not suit you, consider natural family planning. Your doctor or family planning clinic will be able to help.

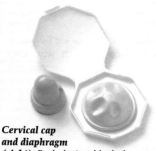

Cervical cap and diaphragm (right) Both devices block the entry of sperm to the uterus. Users need to be fitted by a doctor or nurse and taught insertion and removal. Reliability is good when used with a spermicide and left in place for about eight hours after intercourse.

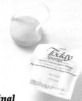

Vaginal sponge A modern version of an ancient idea uses a disc of polyurethane foam impregnated with spermicide. Sponges are disposable but need to be left in for six hours after intercourse. They are not very effective.

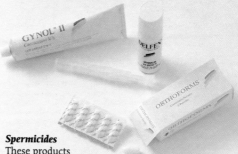

Spermicides These products are available as creams, pessaries, foams or gels. They destroy sperm chemically and most kill the AIDS virus. On their own they are not very effective, but work well with most condoms, diaphragms and caps.

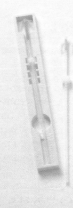

Intrauterine device (IUD) A small plastic and metal device placed in the womb provides extremely reliable contraception. Drawbacks can include heavy periods and an increased risk of infection, so not generally advised for women who have not had children. Fitting must be done by a doctor or nurse.

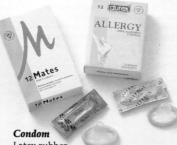

Condom Latex rubber condoms are simple, safe and effective, particularly if used with spermicide. They also offer the best protection against sexually transmitted diseases. Men may find sensation is reduced, and some couples feel condoms interfere with spontaneity.

Female condom One of the newer barrier methods uses a tube of polyurethane plastic held in place by flexible rings to line the vagina. It is bulkier than the male condom but does not require spermicide and can be inserted any time before intercourse. Reliability is as good as for the male condom.

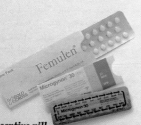

Contraceptive pill Oral contraceptives contain female sex hormones in doses that prevent ovulation. Taken regularly, they provide outstanding protection, but there are long and short-term side effects and users need regular medical checkups. Various types are available to meet individual needs.

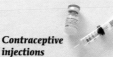

Contraceptive injections Depending on the drug brand (Noristerat or Depo-Provera), injections of synthetic progesterone can be given every 8 or 12 weeks. Like the pill, they prevent ovulation and are highly effective. Particularly suitable for women who cannot remember to take a pill every day.

Implants Soft tubes that slowly release synthetic progesterone are inserted under the skin of the upper arm under local anaesthetic. The hormone makes the womb less likely to accept a fertilised egg and may also stop ovulation. The contraceptive effect lasts five years. The procedure takes ten minutes and no stitches are needed. However, many women suffer side effects such as irregular bleeding, headaches and nausea. Removal can sometimes be difficult.

with a continuous production process that yields about 200 million sperm every time the man ejaculates. Each sperm would have to be dealt with, both to avoid pregnancy and to prevent any remaining damaged sperm from forming an abnormal embryo. This is very different from the role of the female pill, which has only to prevent the release of one egg once a month at a particular point in the woman's hormonal cycle. Another complicating factor is that sperm live for about 70 days inside the testes, so it would take ten weeks for the pill to start working. Thereafter one missed pill would set the whole process back to square one.

An injectable male contraceptive is much more likely. Weekly injections of the male hormone testosterone have been shown in trials to produce reversible male infertility. The brain interprets the high levels of testosterone as evidence that the testes are excessively productive, with the result that it shuts down the production of both testosterone and sperm. A thrice yearly version may be available by the end of the century.

RISKS OF INTRAUTERINE DEVICES

I'm considering having an IUD fitted, but I have heard that they can cause infections. How much of a risk is this? And how often should an IUD be changed?

Women who are fitted with an IUD (intrauterine device) are about 1½ to 2½ times more likely to develop a condition known as pelvic inflammatory disease (PID). This is thought to be due to infectious organisms passing up the thread of the IUD into the Fallopian tubes. Women with an IUD who are under 30, especially those who have had several sexual partners or who have previously had PID, are most at risk. Your doctor will be able to offer individual advice.

If you do decide to go ahead with an IUD, be sure to have any infection treated first, and once the device is in place report any symptoms to your doctor as soon as you notice them. Warning signs of infection include pain during or after intercourse, pain in the lower abdomen, and unusual vaginal discharge, often accompanied by a fever. Infections are easily treated with antibiotics, but if left they can become serious and may even cause infertility.

Doctors advise an annual checkup, and changing an IUD about once every three to five years, depending on the type of device. Very occasionally problems may develop that make earlier replacement necessary.

NATURAL CONTRACEPTION

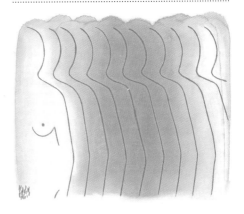

My husband and I like the idea of the rhythm method but I'm worried about its effectiveness. Doesn't it also involve long periods of abstinence?

In theory at least, if you follow it carefully and have a reasonably predictable menstrual cycle, the rhythm method can be about as effective as the IUD or barrier methods such as the condom and diaphragm. In practice, however, it has a higher rate of failure, mainly as a result of not following the procedures strictly enough.

The rhythm method is based on calculating the time of ovulation. This usually occurs 12 to 16 days before the woman's next period. As an egg lives for up to two days and most sperm survive for up to five days in the womb, sex must be avoided (or another form of contraception used) for at least eight days of the cycle – five days before ovulation, the day of ovulation and two days after.

As it is difficult to estimate accurately the exact time of ovulation, it is wise to combine several different techniques (see panel, left). Chemists also sell ovulation predictor kits that can help to improve accuracy. However, some other form of contraception will be needed for the first six months or so, until you have established reliable records. You should also remember that the time of ovulation can vary from month to month. Illness, shock, stress, even going on holiday, can all affect a woman's cycle.

If you decide to use natural family planning, it is essential to be trained in the techniques by a specialist doctor or nurse.

CAUTION Although ovulation is the most fertile period, pregnancy is also possible at other stages of the menstrual cycle. This method is not suitable if an unplanned pregnancy would be a disaster.

Estimating ovulation

Natural family planning depends on predicting ovulation and avoiding sexual intercourse for several days before and after. Various methods are used.

● Calendar method: a six-month record of your periods shows the average length of your menstrual cycle, and the range of variation.
● Temperature method: take your temperature every morning before getting up. A slight rise indicates ovulation has occurred. Remember, illness may have the same effect.
● Mucus method: cervical mucus becomes thinner and wetter at ovulation.
● Symptoms such as lower back pain, breast discomfort or a 'twinge' in the ovary can all be signs of ovulation.

CAUTION All methods must be taught by a trained doctor or natural family planning expert.

MORNING-AFTER MEASURES

What is the morning-after pill? Could I use it as a regular form of contraception?

No. The morning-after pill is a high-dose version of the combined pill (which contains the hormones oestrogen and progesterone). It should be taken to prevent pregnancy only in an emergency, such as if a condom splits. The dosage is too high for regular use.

Although it is known as the morning after pill, two tablets are taken up to 72 hours after intercourse and then another two are taken 12 hours later. These may cause nausea and disrupt periods. In most cases, the morning-after pill should not be taken by anyone who cannot take a normal contraceptive pill.

If you need contraception for infrequent or irregular sex, condoms or the diaphragm are the best methods to use. If you need regular contraception but don't want to take a pill every day, or may not remember to, consider hormone implants or injections.

STERILISATION OPERATIONS

We have three children and don't want any more. Would a vasectomy or sterilisation be a good form of contraception and, if so, which is the better option?

For couples in your position, with established families, surgical sterilisation – whether it be vasectomy for men or tubal sterilisation for women, is considered to be the most effective form of contraception available.

Vasectomy involves cutting and tying both of the vas deferens. It is a minor operation done under local anaesthetic with no hospital stay and no side effects, except for some bruising and pain for a few days afterwards. The only drawback is that contraception is needed until two consecutive negative sperm samples have been submitted. This may take 16 weeks or sometimes longer.

Female sterilisation is usually done by cutting and tying, sealing or plugging the Fallopian tubes. The procedure requires a local or general anaesthetic and usually one or two nights in hospital. A few women have irregular and slightly heavier periods afterwards, but otherwise there are few side effects. Sterilisation can also result from removal of the Fallopian tubes, ovaries or the whole womb – a hysterectomy. These operations are major surgery, however, and are not carried out unless a medical condition demands it.

Both vasectomy and simple female sterilisation are extremely safe procedures, but there are several reasons to opt for vasectomy. The risk of death is zero, compared with 5 in 100 000 for female sterilisation. Vasectomy is also a more reliable operation and if a women does become pregnant after being sterilised she has a higher chance of an ectopic pregnancy, which can be life-threatening. Vasectomy is also less expensive and carries a lower risk of complications.

> ### Emergency contraception
>
> Take action immediately if contraception fails or you have unprotected sex and think you may be at risk of an unwanted pregnancy.
>
> ● Contact your doctor or family planning clinic within 72 hours of unprotected sex. If you cannot get to a doctor or clinic, a hospital Accident and Emergency department may also be able to help you.
> ● You will probably be offered a choice of the morning-after pill, which must be taken within 72 hours of sexual intercourse, or an IUD, which must be fitted within five days.

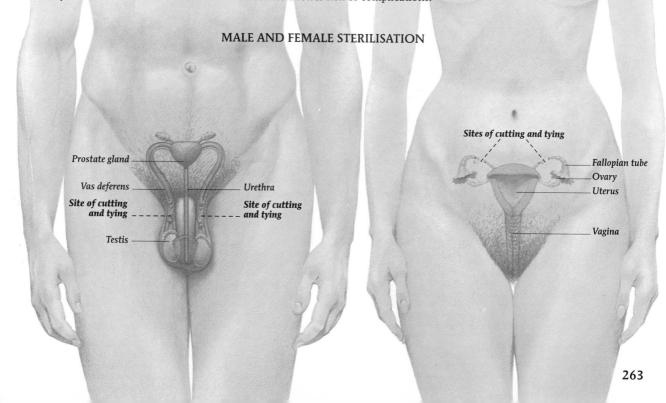

MALE AND FEMALE STERILISATION

Prostate gland

Vas deferens

Site of cutting and tying

Testis

Urethra

Site of cutting and tying

Sites of cutting and tying

Fallopian tube

Ovary

Uterus

Vagina

REVERSING STERILISATION

Can sterilisations and vasectomies be reversed?

Recent developments in microsurgery mean that it is now sometimes possible to reverse a sterilisation operation. However, the surgery is difficult and often unsuccessful. It is easier to reverse a vasectomy than female sterilisation, but even where the man's tubes are reconnected successfully – possible in a third to a half of cases – he may still be left with reduced fertility.

Women who become pregnant after having their tubes surgically reconnected have an increased risk of ectopic pregnancy. It is claimed that the latest type of vasectomy – in which the tubes are blocked by an injected substance – is easier to reverse, but this remains unproven.

Both male and female sterilisation operations should be regarded as permanent and should not be considered by anyone who can imagine circumstances under which they would wish to reverse the decision. The procedure is usually recommended only to older couples who have at least two children, and after extensive discussions with their doctor.

EFFECTS OF A VASECTOMY

I've heard that a vasectomy can affect a man's sex life. Is this true?

No, not in any physical sense. Immediately after the operation the patient may feel sore and have bruised or swollen testicles, which may put him off sex for a few days. Usually he will be back to normal in a week or so. Physically, he can desire, perform and enjoy sex just as before, and the lack of sperm makes no noticeable difference.

A few men who link masculinity with the ability to father children may have a reduced sex drive, but this really is all in the mind. Many more find that freedom from worry about pregnancy enhances their sex drive and enjoyment of intercourse. Only 2 per cent of men claim that their sex life is worse after vasectomy; 70 per cent say it improves; and the rest report no change.

Fertility and conception

Getting fit to conceive

Reducing known health risks before trying to conceive will ensure that your baby has the best possible start in life:

- Don't smoke.
- Drink moderately or not at all.
- Lose weight if necessary.
- Eat a healthy diet, avoiding foods high in fat and sugar.
- Take regular exercise.
- Have plenty of sleep and relaxation.
- Consult employers about potential hazards at work.
- Wear gloves when handling chemicals for the home or garden.
- Have any illnesses or infections treated.
- Consult a doctor about any medication you are taking and any diseases that run in either family.

PREPARING FOR CONCEPTION

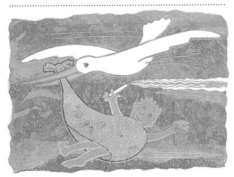

My husband and I want to have a baby. Is there anything we should be doing to get fit before I conceive?

Yes. Experts now recommend that couples start paying special attention to their health about three months before trying to conceive. Being in top condition increases the chances of conception, ensures a healthy pregnancy and reduces risks to the baby in the early weeks before pregnancy is confirmed.

If you smoke, stop. Smoking stunts a baby's growth in the womb, because it reduces the amount of oxygen that is being supplied. The baby is, therefore, likely to be smaller and more vulnerable when it is born. If your husband is a smoker, he should also give up to support you, and to eliminate the risk of passive smoking.

Stop drinking alcohol before trying to conceive – drinking during the first weeks of a baby's life in the womb can reduce its birthweight. Drinking heavily (three to four pints of lager a day) may also reduce your husband's sperm count.

If you have any doubt about your immunity to rubella (German measles), see your doctor who will conduct a simple blood test and, if necessary, give you a vaccination. It is also a good idea to start taking folic acid supplements – one 0.4 g tablet is the daily recommended dose – because it is used to form the baby's cells, and reduces the risk of your baby having spina bifida, and to have a dental check-up to prevent problems in pregnancy when teeth are vulnerable.

Also, avoid uncooked meat, soft cheeses such as Brie and Camembert, raw or lightly cooked eggs and pâté, all of which may harbour listeria or salmonella bacteria, such bacteria can be particularly harmful to an unborn baby. (See also panel, left.)

HELP WITH CONCEPTION

What sort of help is available for couples who have trouble conceiving?

After a year of trying to conceive, a couple's doctor will probably refer them to a hospital fertility clinic. Specialist doctors will give both partners a physical examination to establish their general state of health. They may also suggest changes in diet, such as drinking less alcohol, losing weight or trying relaxation exercises to reduce stress.

Initial tests will check whether the woman is ovulating and whether sperm are getting through the cervical mucus to the womb – two common sources of problems. If sperm are failing to get through, artificial insemination may be offered. If ovulation is sporadic, fertility drugs can be prescribed to stimulate the ovaries. Sometimes these drugs work *too* well, ripening more than one egg at a time and increasing the chances of a multiple birth.

Other common problems include a low sperm count, in which case production can be stimulated by injections of the male hormone testosterone and by keeping the testes cool. Surgery may be necessary for conditions such as fibroids – benign growths in the womb. Blocked Fallopian tubes can also sometimes be corrected, but the success rate is not high – about one in three or four. If these treatments do not succeed or the cause cannot be found, more complicated techniques such as in vitro fertilisation may be considered. Some are available on the NHS, but success rates are not always good.

WHEN TO START A FAMILY

My wife and I are in our late 20s and keep being told that we should start a family soon. Will waiting a few more years really make it more difficult to conceive?

Probably not. Fertility levels do gradually decline with age in both men and women, though this is more of an issue for women because of the absolute limit imposed by the menopause. For women in their 30s becoming pregnant tends to be more a question of time than of anything else. Whereas it may take only two or three months for a woman of 25 to conceive, a woman of 35 may need six months or more. But this may be a result of having intercourse less often as much as of declining fertility.

Fertility is not the only factor to consider, however. Older mothers have to balance the slightly greater risks of Down's syndrome and other complications (see page 269) with, on the positive side, greater maturity, achieving their career aims and, often, greater financial security. The best advice is to wait until you both feel ready. When you do decide that the time is right, you may find it helpful to try natural family planning methods to calculate ovulation – the most fertile period (see panel, page 262).

SELECTING A BABY'S SEX

We have two young daughters and are now trying for our third child. Are there ways of increasing the chances of having a boy?

A baby's sex is determined by its inheritance from the father. About half a man's sperm carry a female, or X, sex chromosome and half a male, or Y, sex chromosome. (The inheritance from the mother is always an X chromosome.) In nature, each time an egg is fertilised there is about the same chance of the baby being a boy (XY) or a girl (XX). Various practices have been supposed to weight the odds in favour of one sex or the other – from eating salt for a boy to douching with lemon juice for a girl. However, all of these remain unproven.

A technically sophisticated, but more controversial, method of selection involves in vitro fertilisation of several eggs and the implanting of an embryo of the desired sex. Alternatively, some fertility clinics claim to be able to separate X and Y-bearing sperm according to their different swimming abilities, though the technique has not been scientifically demonstrated. Neither method has so far shown proven results. Nor is either available on the NHS.

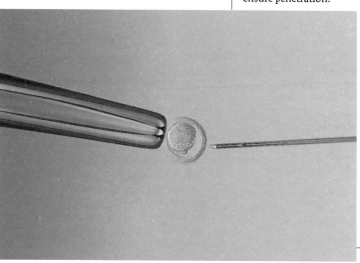

Infertility treatment

Many techniques are used to help couples to conceive. Those listed below are all available on the NHS, although waiting lists for IVF and GIFT can be as long as three years.

Artificial insemination
Semen is injected into the womb at ovulation. If the sperm count is low, donor semen may be used. Success rate: 10 to 25 per cent.

In vitro fertilisation (IVF)
Eggs are fertilised in the laboratory, then placed in the womb. Success rate: 15 per cent.

Gamete intra-Fallopian transfer (GIFT)
Sperm and egg cells are introduced into the Fallopian tube to fertilise naturally. Success rate: 21 per cent.

High-tech conception
In vitro techniques are now so advanced that a single sperm can be injected into an egg to ensure penetration.

REAL LIVES

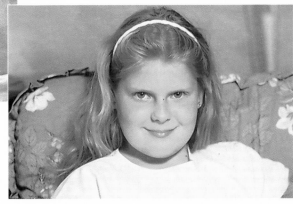

LOUISE BROWN: LIFE BEGINS IN THE LABORATORY

Just before midnight on July 25, 1978, a birth occurred in Oldham General Hospital in Lancashire which made medical history. The world's first baby to be conceived outside the womb – Louise Brown – was delivered healthy and normal to parents who, not long before, had all but given up hope of a child.

Louise's birth was the culmination of 12 years' pioneering research by the British gynaecologist Patrick Steptoe and geneticist Robert Edwards. For nine years Louise's mother had longed for a baby but, because of blocked Fallopian tubes, it seemed she would never conceive. Then Steptoe and Edwards offered her the chance to try their

in vitro – literally 'in glass' – fertilisation technique. They extracted an egg, 'ripened' and fertilised it in the laboratory, then implanted the growing embryo in the womb.

While in vitro fertilisation had been possible since the late 1960s, no successful pregnancy had so far resulted. No one held out much hope that things would be any different in the Browns' case, but as the pregnancy progressed Steptoe and Edwards realised they were on the brink of a revolutionary medical breakthrough.

Since Louise's birth, in vitro fertilisation has become commonplace. However, demand so greatly exceeds supply that couples often have to join a three-year waiting list.

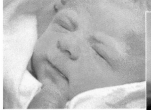

Test tube to teenager *The birth of the first 'test-tube' baby, Louise Brown, brought new hope to thousands of childless couples. Today, there are around 11 000 test-tube children in Britain alone.*

Staying healthy in pregnancy

CALCULATING THE BIRTH DATE

How is a baby's due date determined?

On average, a pregnancy lasts 266 days (38 weeks) from the date of conception. As it is often difficult to be precise about this date, the due date is generally calculated as 40 weeks from the start of the last menstrual period – assumed to be two weeks before ovulation, which is the most likely time for conception. For those women who have irregular cycles, an alternative method is to add seven days to the first day of the last period

and then count backwards three months. Abdominal examinations are also used to judge the stage of pregnancy according to the size of the womb, and ultrasound scans can give an assessment based on the size of the foetus. Ultrasound is less reliable than examination, however, and offers no particular advantage unless there is real uncertainty about the date or about whether the baby is growing normally.

Remember, the due date is only an estimate – few babies arrive exactly on time, though most are within two weeks either side of the calculated due date.

SEX IN PREGNANCY

My wife has just become pregnant and is worried about making love. How safe is sex during pregnancy?

As long as the pregnancy progresses normally and there are no special problems, it should be perfectly safe to continue your sex life as long as you both want to. The baby is well cushioned in the womb and can come to no harm. Even in the late stages of pregnancy, neither intercourse nor the contractions of an orgasm can cause labour to start prematurely, since both the womb and the cervix have to be ready. When a baby is overdue, however, making love is sometimes advised as a way of triggering labour – an effect of the hormone prostoglandin, which is present in semen – but this only works when the birth is imminent anyway.

You may have heard of mothers being advised to abstain from intercourse during the first three months and perhaps the last few weeks of pregnancy. This is usually only where there is a history of miscarriage or symptoms such as bleeding that suggest it may be a risk. Doctors also advise against sex if it becomes painful or uncomfortable at any stage, or if there is any sign of infection.

PUTTING ON WEIGHT

How much weight is it normal to gain during pregnancy? How can I avoid putting on more than is healthy?

Most women gain about 28 lb (13 kg) during pregnancy, although individuals vary greatly and anything between 18 lb and 35 lb (8 kg and 16 kg) is considered normal. The extra weight is created by the foetus, the placenta, the womb, the amniotic fluid, heavier breasts, fluid retention, a larger volume of blood and extra fat, especially on the hips and thighs. Weight gain is also linked to normal weight: in general, heavier women gain more weight than lighter women.

If you are worried about gaining too much weight and you are not yet pregnant, try to get your weight within normal limits (see page 154) before conceiving. If you are pregnant, don't use your condition as an excuse to binge on sweets, cakes and junk foods that are high in calories, but low in nutritional value. You do need to eat a little more, but not much – about 300 kcal extra a day is enough. That's about a single cheese sandwich or ½ pint (285 ml) of semi-skimmed milk and a jacket potato with baked beans.

CAUTION Sudden weight changes in pregnancy or a prolonged period of no weight gain may be cause for concern, and could indicate problems with the baby. If you experience these symptoms, see your doctor or midwife immediately.

WATCHING WHAT YOU EAT

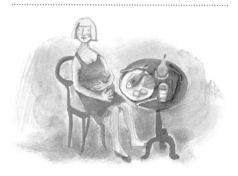

I've never given much thought to my diet but now that I'm pregnant I wonder if I should be more careful about what I eat. Do pregnant women have special needs?

Pregnant women do need to pay attention to what they eat – for the sake of their own health as well as that of their unborn child. The guidelines are not very different from those of a normal healthy diet:

● Eat plenty of wholegrains, fruit and vegetables for vitamins and fibre.
● Have breakfast.
● Avoid junk food, cakes and sweets.
● Choose fresh food rather than processed.
● Use vegetable oils instead of animal fats.
● Drink a pint (570 ml) of milk every day.
● Have at least two servings a day of high-protein foods such as lean meat, eggs, fish, pulses or dairy products.
● Eat food that is high in iron, such as lean red meat, wholemeal bread, dried fruit and leafy green vegetables. Iron is needed to make extra red blood cells to supply the placenta and womb, and the unborn baby.
● Try to drink at least six glasses of water every day.
● Avoid alcohol completely during the first 12 weeks of your pregnancy, and have no more than one or two glasses once or twice a week thereafter.
● Eat foods rich in folic acid, calcium and iron, such as nuts and leafy green vegetables (see chart, pages 46-47).

CAUTION Do not eat liver or liver products during pregnancy. They contain high quantities of vitamin A, which has been linked with miscarriages and birth defects.

Food safety precautions

Most bacteria are harmless, but some – especially those associated with food, such as listeria and salmonella – can be extremely dangerous to an unborn baby. Follow the general advice for food safety on pages 57-59, and in particular:

● Avoid soft cheeses, such as Brie and Camembert, and mould-ripened cheeses, such as Danish blue and Stilton. Both types can carry listeria.
● Avoid raw or lightly cooked eggs because of the risk of salmonella. This includes homemade mayonnaise, ice cream, cheesecake, mousse and hollandaise sauce.
● Don't eat pâté unless pasteurised. There is a risk of listeria.
● Avoid raw or lightly cooked meat because of bacterial and parasitic infections such as toxoplasmosis.

Pelvic floor exercises

Toning up the pelvic muscles can make birth easier, reduce tearing and help to prevent incontinence afterwards.

● Contract the muscles around the vagina as if you were trying to stop urinating in mid-flow.

● Hold for a few seconds, then relax.

● Repeat several times for a few minutes as often as you can. Try to link the exercise with something you do often, such as having a drink.

● Gradually increase the number of squeezes and the length of time you hold them.

TAKING SUPPLEMENTS

Will I need to take vitamin or mineral supplements during pregnancy?

Although a balanced diet will provide you with most of the vitamins and minerals you need, some supplements are generally recommended in pregnancy – in particular, folic acid, calcium and iron. All are needed in much greater quantities during pregnancy and can have serious effects if lacking.

Even if you are only considering becoming pregnant, a daily folic acid supplement (0.4 g) is recommended, and should be kept up until the 12th week. This vitamin plays a vital role in foetal development and helps to reduce the risk of spina bifida.

Calcium supplements are generally recommended to protect bones and teeth – especially important for women who do not eat very many dairy products. In addition, some mothers need iron supplements. However, a woman's blood is naturally more dilute during pregnancy so that, although her blood haemaglobin level may be low, she does not necessarily require extra iron.

Some women have extra requirements. Vegetarians need to take special care to get enough of certain nutrients (see page 30), particularly vitamin B_{12} if they eat little or no food of animal origin. Women who, against all medical advice, continue to smoke during pregnancy are also advised to take vitamin C, as nicotine reduces its absorption. Multivitamin and mineral supplements are recommended for mothers who are very underweight or overweight, on restricted diets, who drink alcohol heavily or who have particular illnesses or pregnancy problems.

In all cases, consult your doctor before resorting to any form of dietary supplement. Not all are suitable for everyone, and some can be dangerous to an unborn baby.

GOOD SKIN CARE

How should I look after my skin during pregnancy? Is there anything I can do to prevent stretch marks?

Many women notice changes in their skin during pregnancy, and it is a good idea to take a bit of extra care. Use plenty of moisturising creams and oils to stop dryness and itching – common problems, particularly in the later months. Wear loose, comfortable clothing, preferably made from soft natural fibres such as cotton, which will allow good air circulation around the body, helping to keep the skin comfortable. Stretch marks are not really preventable, as they depend mainly on hormone production and skin type. Some women never develop them but even those who do generally find that once the pregnancy is over they fade so as to become barely noticeable. The best advice is to avoid putting on excessive weight (see page 267), which could stretch the skin further, eat a healthy diet, and keep your skin well moisturised to prevent dryness, especially on the abdomen, buttocks, thighs and breasts.

Many pregnant women also develop areas of darker pigmentation, often in a line down from the navel. They cannot be prevented but are entirely harmless and usually fade after the birth.

TESTS DURING PREGNANCY

What tests am I likely to have during pregnancy and what will they show?

The first tests will be carried out at your initial antenatal appointment. You will be offered a blood test to check for anaemia, syphillis and rubella, and to identify your blood group. You may be offered a cervical smear test if you are due for one. Throughout your pregnancy your urine will be tested for sugar (a sign of diabetes), protein and for urinary infections. Blood pressure readings will also be used throughout to check for signs of pre-eclampsia, or rising blood pressure, which may stunt the baby's growth if not treated.

From about 12 weeks many midwives and doctors check the baby's heartbeat using a 'sonic aid' instrument that works by ultrasound. If you are concerned about the safety of ultrasound (see facing page) you can choose not to have this test.

At about 16 weeks another blood test, called the Alpha-fetoprotein (AFP) test (also known as a triple test), is offered. An abnormal result is *sometimes* linked to neural tube defects in the baby, such as spina bifida, but the results are not absolutely certain. Some women feel anxious waiting for the results and therefore decide not to have it; others find it reassuring.

From about 14 to 18 weeks most women are offered an ultrasound scan to check the stage of pregnancy. However, as the safety of this test has not been conclusively established, some choose not to have it (see facing page). Women over 35, and those with abnormal triple tests, are also offered an amniocentesis at this stage. Fluid from the womb is drawn off through the abdomen wall to check for Down's syndrome and spina bifida. This test carries a 0.5-1 per cent risk of miscarriage. Chorionic villus sampling (CVS), where a sample is taken from the placenta via the abdomen or vagina, can detect genetic disorders such as Down's syndrome. CVS carries a 1-4 per cent risk of miscarriage.

If you have a special problem, such as Rh-negative blood, chronic anaemia, a family history of neural defects or if you have miscarried before, you may have additional checks such as blood tests and scans.

HOW SAFE ARE SCANS?

My hospital does routine ultrasound scans during pregnancy. What are they for and how safe are they? Can I choose not to have one?

You have the right to refuse any test. The best advice is to discuss whether a scan is necessary with your midwife or doctor.

An ultrasound scan is offered to most pregnant woman at about 14 to 18 weeks. In most cases, the scan is used to confirm the due date and assess the growth of the foetus. Routine scanning has never been proven to offer other benefits to healthy mothers or babies. In fact, it may have disadvantages as scans can be inaccurate. Some experts now recommend that scans be used only in special cases, such as when twins are suspected, if there is bleeding, if the mother smokes or is over 35, if there is any doubt that the baby is alive, or if some other factor means a higher risk of foetal abnormalities.

Although ultrasound scans may often be unnecessary, they are generally considered very safe. Some studies have shown a small link with low birth weight and miscarriage, and there have been suggestions that scanned babies may be more likely to be left-handed, dyslexic or slow to speak. However, all these concerns remain unproven.

OLDER MOTHERS

I am 42 and have just heard that I am pregnant. Will my age have any particular effects on pregnancy and birth?

Yes, there are a number of possible effects that you should be aware of. During pregnancy, older mothers have an increased chance of high blood pressure, which can lead to pre-eclampsia, a serious condition causing fluid retention, headache, nausea, vomiting, abdominal pain and visual disturbances. Mild pre-eclampsia can be treated with drugs, but in more serious cases labour

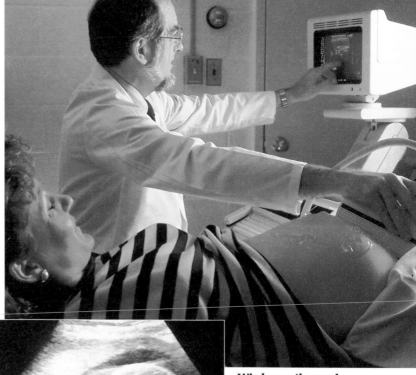

Window on the womb
Ultrasound scans are used in pregnancy to check on foetal development, confirm the due date, identify multiple pregnancies and reveal conditions calling for special treatment. The process is completely painless and uses reflected high-frequency sound waves to build up an image such as that on the left, which shows the baby's head.

may have to be induced or a Caesarean section performed. Older mothers also have a slightly higher rate of miscarriage, and a slightly increased risk of premature birth.

At the birth, an older mother may be more likely to experience complications, and labour may last longer. Interventions such as a forceps delivery or Caesarean section are also more likely.

As far as the child is concerned, the most important risk is the increasing chance of Down's syndrome – 1 in 1 200 for 25-year-old mothers, but almost 1 in 100 at 40. Amniocentesis and other tests to detect such conditions are routinely offered to mothers who are in their mid 30s or older.

On the positive side, older mothers in general are better informed about pregnancy and birth, and tend to cope better with a new baby. One study showed that mothers over 35 adapted better to motherhood, had fewer symptoms and were less troubled by pregnancy than those in their twenties.

GETTING INTO SHAPE TO GIVE BIRTH

Pregnancy places great physical demands on the body, but the fitter you are, the better you will be able to cope. Supple hip joints and groin and buttock muscles make it easier to adopt useful positions, such as squatting during labour and birth; strong leg muscles encourage good circulation which helps to prevent tiredness, cramp and varicose veins; and strong stomach muscles will help with delivery. Being fit will also help you to regain your figure more quickly once the baby is born. Ideally you should try to get in shape before you become pregnant, but it is never too late to take up exercise. Here is a selection of gentle but effective exercises to try.

STRENGTHENING THE BUTTOCKS

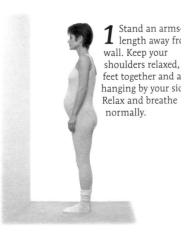

1 Stand an arms-length away from a wall. Keep your shoulders relaxed, your feet together and arms hanging by your sides. Relax and breathe normally.

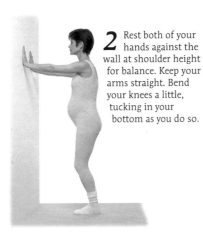

2 Rest both of your hands against the wall at shoulder height for balance. Keep your arms straight. Bend your knees a little, tucking in your bottom as you do so.

3 Using your buttock and thigh muscles, raise your left leg and swing it gently back. Keep the supporting leg bent a little and don't raise your leg too high. Repeat 4 times with each leg.

STRENGTHENING THE LEGS AND LOWER BODY

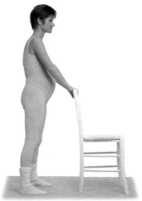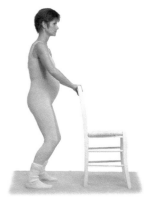

1 Stand with your feet at a comfortable distance apart, and rest your hands on the back of a chair. Use it only for balance.

2 Keep your heels on the ground. Slowly bend your knees, hold for 2 seconds and straighten up slowly. Pause for 2 seconds and repeat 4 times.

LOOSENING THE GROIN AND HIPS

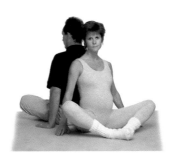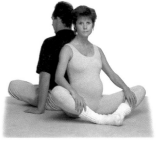

1 Get your partner to help with this exercise, or support yourself against a wall. Sit with the soles of your feet together. Keep your back straight.

2 Resting your hands on the calf muscles, ease your knees down very gently for a count of 6. Never force or strain this movement.

STRENGTHENING STOMACH MUSCLES

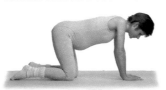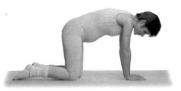

1 Get down on your hands and knees with your knees directly under your hips and your hands beneath your shoulders.

2 Gently contract the buttock and stomach muscles, to arch up your back. Hold for 4 seconds, release, and repeat 4 times.

LEARNING ABOUT BIRTH

What are the benefits of joining an antenatal class? How do I find one and when should I start?

Antenatal classes usually consist of six to eight weekly sessions of one or two hours in the last few months of pregnancy. NHS classes can be found through your midwife, doctor or antenatal clinic. They are free, and most hospitals try to accommodate all first-time mothers. NHS classes are generally quite large and formal, and concentrate on procedures at the particular hospital. Other classes are run by the National Childbirth Trust (NCT). They are smaller and less formal, but charge a small fee. Special attention is paid to self-help and reducing medication and intervention during the birth. Look for your local NCT branch in the telephone directory. Fathers are generally welcome at all classes.

As well as teaching exercises and breathing and relaxation techniques, antenatal classes make sure parents are well-informed about birth. This reduces fear and pain, and enables you to participate more in decisions during labour. Couples who attend classes usually find labour and birth more satisfying, and well-prepared women tend to have shorter labours. Classes are popular, so don't leave it any later than the fourth or fifth month before booking a place.

WORKING DURING PREGNANCY

My daughter wants to go on working as late as possible into her pregnancy. How long is it safe to continue?

It all depends on what your daughter does, her state of health and how well her pregnancy is progressing. Provided her job is not physically demanding, and there are no complications, it should be perfectly safe for her to continue as long as she feels fit and able.

On the other hand, there are certain jobs that pregnant women should avoid. Anything that involves strenuous physical effort, such as heavy lifting, could be dangerous. The same applies to contact with radiation, extremes of cold or heat, and certain toxic chemicals such as lead, carbon monoxide and mercury. Problems such as bleeding or threatened miscarriage may also indicate the need to give up work. If in any doubt, your daughter should consult her doctor.

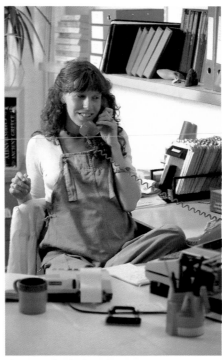

A woman's place... Pregnant women were once advised to take it easy. These days, many prefer the stimulation of a busy workplace.

Problems in pregnancy

NAUSEA AND INDIGESTION

I suffered from morning sickness and indigestion during my first pregnancy. How can I improve things the second time around?

There is no guaranteed cure, but there are many things you can try. Firstly, get plenty of rest and eat small, frequent meals – tiredness and an empty stomach exacerbate the problem. Eat something light – a dry biscuit or piece of toast – before getting up, and have a small snack before going to bed. Some women find vitamin B_6 supplements, foods containing ginger, and camomile, peppermint or spearmint tea helpful. Avoid rich and spicy foods; wear loose clothes, especially at the waist; avoid bending over; and sleep propped up on pillows. Symptoms normally disappear after the third month. Although unpleasant, they do no harm unless you get dehydrated. Seek medical advice if vomiting is severe.

Coping with miscarriage

Losing a pregnancy can be a devastating experience. Along with shock and grief may come a profound sense of disorientation as the couple realise how much planning and energy they were putting into the baby's arrival. Some long for another pregnancy; others are temporarily put off.

Nothing can take away the pain of loss, but talking to others who have been through the experience can often help. To get in touch, contact the Miscarriage Association, Clayton Hospital, Northgate, Wakefield WF1 3JF.

Doctors advise waiting a few months before trying for another pregnancy, to allow female hormone levels to stabilise.

DO'S
— AND —
DON'TS

for preventing varicose veins

Do put support stockings or tights on before you get up in the morning.
Do go for regular walks.
Do circle your ankles when sitting.
Do spend at least 20 minutes a day with your feet above the level of your heart.

Don't stand or sit in the same position for long periods.
Don't cross your legs when sitting.

FIGHTING TIREDNESS

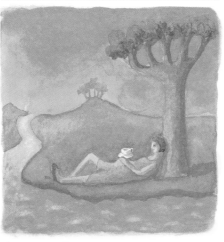

I'm six months pregnant and am starting to feel increasingly tired during the day. Is this normal? How much rest do pregnant women need?

Feeling tired during pregnancy is completely normal. Ideally, you should lie down undisturbed for two hours a day, but if this is not possible, try relaxation exercises for at least ten minutes every day (see pages 190-191). Make sure you have plenty of early nights.

If you have other children, try to arrange for someone else to look after them now and again, and do not hesitate to accept help from anyone who offers.

Tiredness accompanied by symptoms such as dizziness and being out of breath may indicate anaemia. Try eating more iron-rich foods such as red meat and kidney beans and consult your doctor, who may prescribe an iron supplement.

ECTOPIC PREGNANCY

What is an ectopic pregnancy?

An ectopic pregnancy happens when an embryo implants itself and begins to grow outside the womb, usually in one of the Fallopian tubes, which connect the ovaries to the womb. Very rarely, the embryo may implant in the abdominal cavity. As the pregnancy develops, surrounding tissue may be damaged or may rupture, causing severe pain and bleeding.

About 1 in every 200 pregnancies is ectopic, and it is considered a potentially life-threatening condition that requires emergency treatment. Once an ectopic pregnancy is confirmed, an operation is performed to remove the growing embryo. If

the damaged Fallopian tube cannot be repaired, it will also have to be removed. Many doctors advise removing the tube as a matter of course, to prevent another ectopic pregnancy occurring.

There are several possible causes of ectopic pregnancy. Sometimes an egg lodges in the Fallopian tube because of some abnormality in the tube itself, or because of damage to the tube from an infection, such as pelvic inflammatory disease, or from surgery.

It is still possible to have a normal pregnancy with only one Fallopian tube, although the chances of conception are slightly reduced. If an ectopic pregnancy follows a case of pelvic inflammatory disease, both tubes may have been affected. In this case, there is a one in ten chance that the next pregnancy will be ectopic.

FEAR OF MISCARRIAGE

I have had one miscarriage and am now pregnant again. Is there anything I can do to increase my chances of carrying this baby to term?

A single miscarriage does not necessarily affect a subsequent pregnancy. It is not always clear why a miscarriage occurs, nor why some women are more prone to miscarriage than others. Very early miscarriage is, in fact, quite common, affecting at least one in five pregnancies. In many cases the body expels a foetus because there is something wrong – it's nature's safety valve. Only if you have experienced three or more miscarriages is your doctor likely to refer you to a specialist to have the cause investigated.

It is true that a woman who has previously miscarried is slightly more likely to do so again. However, if the pregnancy is progressing normally, there is every chance that it will continue to term. Even so, it is worth taking sensible precautions: don't smoke, eat a well-balanced diet, exercise gently, avoid lifting heavy objects, and consult your doctor about vitamin supplements.

The best advice is to use your own intuition: if something doesn't feel right, don't do it. If you feel happier, avoid sex (but not physical closeness) until the pregnancy is well established and you feel more confident – generally from around the 14th-16th week, when the risk is minimal.

CAUTION Report any bleeding to your doctor and go to bed until it has stopped completely. In most cases it will settle down and the pregnancy will continue normally.

Having a baby

CHOOSING THE RIGHT PLACE

I'm undecided about where to have my baby. What are the pros and cons of hospital and home births?

No one but you can make this highly personal decision. That said, the overwhelming majority of women do choose to have their babies in hospital. Hospitals offer specialist staff and equipment and give mothers a break from home routine and chores, which can be very welcome in the days after birth. Home deliveries, on the other hand, offer the comfort of familiar territory and a sense of being more in control of the process. Don't forget that there is a third option – the so-called 'domino' (domiciliary-in-out) scheme. The midwife helps you through the initial stages of labour at home, then drives you to hospital for the delivery.

Before you make your decision, discuss the issue with your partner and with your doctor, and consider visiting your local hospital to view the maternity facilities. Provided that your pregnancy does progress smoothly, your doctor will probably support whatever decision you make. If you do decide to have a home birth (as is every woman's right if she wishes) and your doctor is not sympathetic, approach another doctor, or write to your local supervisor of midwives (your maternity unit will have the address), who is required to find you a community midwife for a home birth. Alternatively, consider contacting a private midwife through The Independent Midwives' Association, Nightingale Cottage, Shamblehurst Lane, Botley, Southampton SO3 2BY.

RECOGNISING THE START

How will I know labour is beginning? At what stage should I go to hospital?

Labour usually starts with strong, rhythmic contractions. For a first baby this stage can continue for many hours, so doctors generally advise waiting until the contractions are just ten minutes apart before going to hospital. Later births are generally faster, so leave when contractions are 20-30 minutes apart.

Sometimes the first sign that the baby is on the way is a discharge of blood and mucus (a 'show'), or a sudden release of clear amniotic fluid (also called the 'breaking of the waters'). In either case, it is advisable to get to hospital straight away.

DEALING WITH PAIN

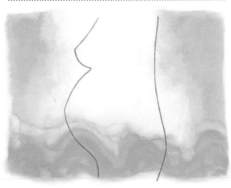

I am worried about how I will cope with the pain of labour. How severe is it and what sort of relief will the hospital offer?

The pain of labour is unlike any other and feels very different from that of illness or injury. All the sensations are restricted to the lower abdomen, lower back and, sometimes, the top of the legs. The pain comes in waves and, at its peak, can be frightening if you do not know what to expect. If you are not already attending antenatal classes, this is one good reason to enrol. As well as psychological preparation, you will learn pain control through breathing and relaxation.

Some women manage with nothing more than natural methods but most choose some form of anaesthetic to help them in the more painful stages. An injection of pethidine, a drug derived from morphine, is usually offered and can be very effective. It lasts for several hours but is likely to make you feel drowsy or slightly drugged. It may also affect the baby, although not seriously.

If you prefer to be more in control of your own pain relief, you may prefer the 'gas-and-air' option – a mixture of nitrous oxide and oxygen that you breathe in as needed from a hand-held rubber mask. It gives a light-headed feeling but does not affect the baby.

Another option is an epidural anaesthetic, which removes all feeling from the waist down but, unlike a general anaesthetic, allows you to stay conscious. It is generally used when a difficult birth is expected, or for Caesarean sections (see pages 274-275).

(see pages 274-275).

Birth choices

Your doctor or midwife can help you to have the sort of birth you want. These are some issues you may wish to discuss.

- Who you would like to be present.
- The equipment and facilities you want and where they are available.
- The chances of needing induction, a Caesarean section or other intervention.
- Pain relief options.
- Freedom to move around.
- Whether you would prefer an episiotomy (cut in the vagina) to natural tearing.
- How to deliver the placenta – naturally or with drugs which make the womb contract.

Hospital checklist

Have your case packed well before the due date. These are the items midwives recommend.

- Sanitary towels.
- Open-fronted nightdress.
- Comfortable day clothes.
- Nursing bra and nursing breastpads.
- Any medicines or vitamin supplements you are taking.
- Glucose tablets for energy during labour.
- Dressing gown.
- Slippers.
- Cotton underwear.
- Towel and washkit.
- Any special foods or drinks, massage oils, remedies or other extras you may want to use.

NATURAL BIRTH

I want a natural birth without drugs or anaesthetics. How can I make sure I have the minimum amount of medication without taking any risks?

Many women feel as you do and most doctors and nurses are sympathetic and qualified to help. You should take the following steps to ensure that the birth of your baby proceeds with minimum medical interference:

● Tell your midwife and doctor that you would prefer to manage without the help of drugs if possible.
● Make sure you can use a birthing pool or have a warm bath to soothe the pain.

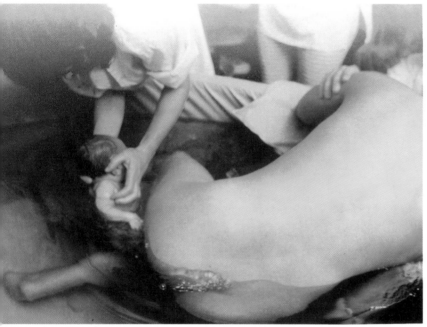

Water baby Giving birth in water is an option available in some hospitals, and pools can also be hired at home. Provided trained staff are on hand to assist, it is considered safe as the umbilical cord is still supplying oxygenated blood. The first breath comes only when the baby is lifted out into the air.

● Be prepared: enrol in antenatal classes, read about the subject and speak to others.
● During labour, try to avoid interventions that increase the need for pain relief, such as induction or continuous foetal heart monitoring. Freedom to move around and change position relieves pain and assists labour. Electronic monitoring of the baby can restrict movement, and you can choose to have it done intermittently, or with an instrument called a Pinard stethoscope, which allows you to move around most of the time.
● Be prepared to change your mind. If you find that you do need pain relief, don't feel that you have let yourself down.
● Investigate methods such as acupuncture and hypnosis (choose a medically qualified

therapist). Ask your midwife about transcutaneous nerve stimulation (TNS or TENS) – a form of pain relief based on small electrical impulses administered from a machine by the mother herself via electrodes placed on the back.

EARLY AND LATE BIRTHS

Why are some babies born prematurely while others are late?

No one really knows. Dramatic hormonal changes occur when labour starts, but it is not understood what triggers them.

Birth does seem to be initiated by the baby rather than changes in the mother's body or anything she may do. Babies born at or before 36 weeks are considered premature and may need special care if their lungs are not fully developed.

Babies born late, or postmature, are less common. Although there is no hard evidence that such babies are in any danger, most doctors will want to induce labour if the baby has not been born by about 42 weeks in case the placenta starts to deteriorate.

CAESAREAN SECTION

I've heard that Caesarean births are becoming more common. When are they really necessary?

At present, about 13 per cent of births in Britain are Caesarean deliveries, a figure some experts believe may be a third to a quarter too high. Like all surgery, Caesarean section carries some risks. In theory, it is

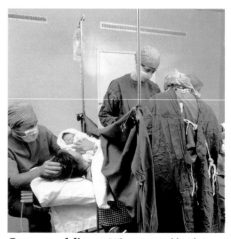

Caesarean delivery When natural birth is dangerous, surgery steps in. Caesarean section takes 30-40 minutes and epidural anaesthesia means mothers can be conscious throughout.

performed only when either mother or baby could otherwise be in danger. Typically, the baby may be too big for natural birth, or lying in the wrong position.

Caesarean rates have indeed been increasing. Partly this is the result of electronic monitoring of the baby's heart, which lets the doctor know instantly if the baby is in distress and needs a prompt delivery. The increasing popularity of epidural anaesthesia has also played a role, since loss of sensation can make normal delivery more difficult. Failed induction can also make a Caesarean necessary, as can a birth that progresses very slowly. Women who have had one Caesarean may need others for subsequent births, but not in all cases.

Mothers who feel unhappy about a proposed Caesarean section should question the medical staff and ask for alternatives, or for a second opinion. In any genuine emergency, it is likely to be obvious whether the operation is essential.

EPIDURAL ANAESTHETIC

I need to have a Caesarean delivery and have been offered an epidural anaesthetic so that I can be conscious when my baby is born. Are there any possible side effects?

An epidural removes all sensation and stops movement from the waist down. It is administered by continuous injection into the area around the spine and is considered a very safe procedure – certainly safer than general anaesthesia for mothers in your position. Usually the only side effects are a slight sensation of grogginess and slowly returning sensation in the legs.

Occasionally, a misplaced needle may cause a long-lasting headache afterwards, and lowered blood pressure makes some mothers feel sick and faint. If severe, drugs may be needed to keep up the baby's blood supply. Very rarely, epidurals fail to work completely, but a larger dose is given for Caesarean section than for ordinary labour, and the operation will not start until anaesthesia is complete. A final dose is given afterwards to prevent postoperative pain.

HOLDING YOUR BABY

Will I be able to hold my baby immediately after the birth?

You should be given your baby straight away, provided its breathing is strong and there are no other problems needing immediate atten-

tion. Even if the baby needs some form of medical treatment it should be given back to you as soon as possible.

If you wish, you can ask to have your baby delivered directly onto your stomach, and if you intend to breastfeed you can put your baby to the breast within seconds of birth.

CHECKING FOR PROBLEMS

Will the doctor be able to tell immediately if there is anything wrong with my baby?

Immediate observation will show up obvious problems such as spina bifida or absent limbs, but these are rare. In the minutes after birth the midwife or doctor will also assess the baby's colour, breathing, heart rate, muscle tone and general responsiveness, and for clues to any other problems. Soon afterwards a doctor will give the baby a thorough examination, checking the spine, heart and lungs, hips, genitals, reflexes, skull, abdominal organs and palate. Blood will also be taken from a tiny heel prick to look for metabolic conditions.

Other disorders – deafness is one – are not detectable at birth. Routine health monitoring and regular checkups are important to ensure early identification and treatment.

VITAMIN K AT BIRTH

My doctor tells me that newborn babies are generally given vitamin K after birth. Why is it needed? Are there any side effects?

Vitamin K is given to babies to prevent bleeding from a rare, but potentially lethal, condition called haemorrhagic disease of the newborn, which is linked with low vitamin K levels and certain liver disorders.

Until recently, vitamin K was generally given by injection shortly after birth, but most hospitals now administer it orally. The supplement is also added to milk formulas for bottle-fed babies. Breastfed babies acquire it naturally, provided they are allowed to feed as long as they wish – it is the richer milk stored at the back of the breast that provides the vitamin.

Some early 1990s research appeared to suggest a possible link between childhood leukaemia and injected vitamin K, but further studies have not supported these findings and paediatricians continue to endorse supplementation. Parents have the right to refuse on behalf of their baby, however, and must give their signed consent before it can be administered by medical staff.

How fathers can help during birth

If you are going to be present, don't feel out of place. You can help your partner in a way that no one else can.

● Stay calm, confident and cheerful. If you feel anxious, don't show it.
● Be sensitive – offer cuddles and reassurance but don't be upset if your partner is aggressive. It's sometimes the only way of releasing tension.
● If, for any reason, your partner is not fully conscious at the moment of birth, be ready to welcome the baby into the world and afterwards describe the moment to her exactly.

What newborn babies can do

Behaviour at birth is dominated by automatic reflex reactions.

● Sucking – an object in the mouth stimulates a feeding response.
● Rooting – the baby turns towards anything that brushes a cheek, searching for a nipple.
● Grasping – stroking hands and feet makes fingers and toes curl up.
● Walking – a baby held upright with a foot on a firm surface will make walking movements.
● Blinking – eyes blink at light, touch and sound.
● Moro reflex – frightened babies fling out their arms and straighten their legs, then draw in their arms. Don't try to elicit the response – you could upset the baby.

Getting back to normal

POSTNATAL DEPRESSION

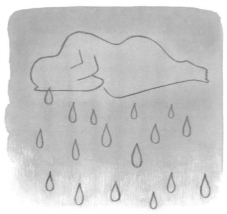

What are the signs of postnatal depression? How common is it?

However much you love the baby, motherhood is never an unmixed joy. If you do feel depressed, console yourself with the thought that you are not alone and that the feeling will pass. Keep a watchful eye on your symptoms, however, and if you ever feel in danger of being overwhelmed or unable to cope, contact your doctor, the Association for Post-Natal Illness, 25 Jerdan Place, London SW6 1BE, or the National Childbirth Trust, listed in the phone book.

Four out of five new mothers experience a temporary letdown and feel weepy and emotional. This can happen any time during the first few weeks after birth. It is a natural reaction to major change, and subsides within a few days. No treatment is needed – apart from kindness and reassurance.

Puerperal psychosis is the most severe form of postnatal depression. It is rare. Symptoms include prolonged, severe sadness, often with irrational fears, extreme fatigue, difficulty in sleeping and feelings of being unable to cope. If sadness persists for more than a couple of weeks, see your doctor.

GETTING BACK INTO SHAPE

What's the best way of getting my figure back after the birth of my baby?

The best way is to breastfeed. Breastfeeding uses between 500 and 1000 Calories a day, so any extra weight often falls away. Also, take up a gentle regime of exercises, such as walking and swimming, to strengthen the muscles weakened during pregnancy and birth. Make sure you eat healthily (see pages 11-15) and get plenty of rest.

It takes several days to lose excess fluid, and several weeks before the womb returns to its normal size. Most women will lose most of their excess weight by about eight weeks after the birth. However, if you put on too much weight during pregnancy it may be difficult to lose, especially around hips and thighs. In this case, a low-fat diet (see pages 34-38) with regular exercise is recommended. If you are breastfeeding, however, check with your doctor, midwife or health visitor before making major dietary changes.

STARTING SEX AGAIN

We've just had our first baby. How long should we wait before having sex?

You will need plenty of time to recover after giving birth to a baby and to adjust to the new demands on your time. Enormous physical and emotional changes are taking place, and your partner ought to be sensitive to this. He too will be feeling the impact of parenthood, and you will both benefit from reassuring cuddles.

Lovemaking can resume as soon as you feel ready. Many women do not feel like sex while they are still bleeding or sore, especially if they have had stitches. If you have had a Caesarean section, you will probably want to wait until you are well on the road to recovery, which may be several weeks.

STRAINED RELATIONSHIPS

Our sex life hasn't been the same since our baby was born. There's nothing physically the matter, so what's gone wrong?

You are not alone. Many couples feel slightly resentful that the baby has changed their daily routine, introduced financial worries, and disrupted their social lives. Fathers often feel excluded because their partners are so involved in caring for the baby. Poor communication, perhaps due to tiredness or lack of time together, can mean that these grievances remain unaired – making intimacy difficult.

Talk about your feelings, your new lifestyle and sex. Try to find uninterrupted time to

---

DO'S
— AND —
DON'TS

for new parents

Do accept help.
Do try to sleep when the baby sleeps.
Do get out of the house every day.
Do ensure that both you and your partner have a daily break from looking after the baby.
Do talk to each other about the changes in your lives.
Do place a limit on visits from neighbours, friends and relatives.

Don't expect to be able to do everything you did before.
Don't feel bad about being stressed – it happens to all parents.
Don't be afraid to admit to mixed feelings – they are common and perfectly natural.
Don't get so tense that you smack, shake, or even shout at the baby. If you feel you can't cope, put the baby in its cot, and leave the room for five minutes.

relax together and regain intimacy. Aim for a wind-down period in the evening, when you have a drink together, and perhaps a bath or massage. When the baby is asleep use some of the time to cuddle up rather than to catch up on chores – but keep a sense of humour about possible interruptions. Also, try to organise regular social time together, by finding a babysitter or asking relatives or friends to help.

GOING BACK TO WORK

I plan to return to work when my baby is six months old. What can I do to ease the transition for both of us?

Organise a childminder in advance, making sure that she shares your views on childcare – for example, on the question of leaving the baby to cry or not. Also, ensure that the carer knows the baby's likes and dislikes, nap times and favourite songs and games. The transition will be smoother if you take things slowly.

● Remain present at first, as the baby gets to know the carer and the surroundings.
● Gradually let the carer take over your routines of dressing, feeding and changing.
● Once your baby seems settled, leave for increasing periods of time (no more than half an hour at first). Your 'goodbye' should be brief, cheerful and confident.
● If childcare is outside your home, always leave a favourite toy or comforter.
● Share a familiar routine with your child at the end of the day, such as the nightly bath, for reassuring renewal of contact.
● If you are still breastfeeding, try adjusting the timing so that you feed the baby before you return to work. It may be necessary to buy or hire an electric pump so you can express milk that the carer can then bottle-feed to the baby.

MATERNITY LEAVE RIGHTS

What are my rights as far as maternity leave is concerned?

All pregnant employees are entitled to at least 14 weeks' maternity leave, regardless of their length of service or hours of work. All employees are also entitled to receive from their employer up to 18 weeks' Statutory Maternity Pay (SMP). The rate of SMP is usually 90 per cent of your salary for the first six weeks and £52.50 per week for the following 12 weeks.

If you have completed a qualifying length of continuous employment (usually two years for full-time staff), you are also entitled to an additional period of maternity 'absence'. This period lasts from the end of your maternity leave until the end of the 28th week after the week you gave birth. However, to ensure these rights, you must give your employer at least 21 days' notice before starting your maternity leave.

CRÈCHE OR CHILDMINDER

Will my baby be better cared for in a crèche or by a childminder in her own home?

At first, a childminder is probably best. The more familiar the environment is to the baby, the better. With a childminder, your baby will have a single carer, and there will probably be fewer children and less noise to upset the baby. However, when the child reaches two or three years of age, a crèche may offer more stimulation, better facilities, such as a playground, and the chance to mix with other children.

As far as quality of care is concerned, most childminders are experienced, often having children of their own. However, a childminder may have other domestic chores and worries, and usually has no back-up. Crèche staff are trained and, as there are several of them, can provide continuous attention.

In all cases, check that your child is happy with the carer. If the child often seems distressed or if you are concerned about the standard of care, make alternative arrangements.

> ### DO'S
> ### ── AND ──
> ### DON'TS
>
> *for choosing a crèche or childminder*
>
> **Do** consider making use of a childminder in a baby's early days.
> **Do** ask for recommendations from local parents.
> **Do** check that a minder is registered with the local authority.
> **Do** ask a childminder to provide references from people such as her GP or health visitor.
> **Do** make sure that the minder's daily routine is one you are happy with.
> **Do** consider putting your child in a crèche by the age of two or three.
>
> **Don't** leave your child with a minder she or he seems unhappy with.
> **Don't** be afraid to make new arrangements if you are dissatisfied with the quality of care your child is getting.

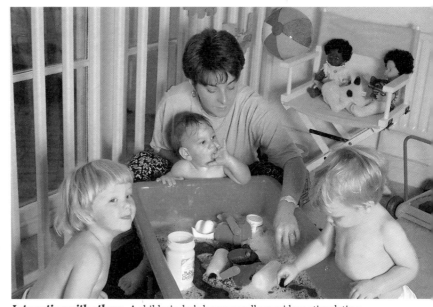

Interacting with others A childminder's home usually provides a stimulating environment. But no matter how many interesting playmates are available, children up to about three years of age still rely on adults to initiate social contact.

The basics of baby care

FACT
— OR —
FALLACY ?

'Bottle-feeding makes babies fat'

Fallacy Only *bad* bottle-feeding makes babies fat. Provided you don't make the formula too strong, don't encourage the baby to drink more than it wants, and don't give sweetened drinks, a bottle-fed baby should be no fatter than a breastfed one.

CONFLICTING ADVICE

Friends and relatives keep giving me conflicting advice about how to look after my baby. How do I know who's right?

Babies have a few basic needs – love, food, warmth and cleaning up. Everything else is detail. Furthermore, the interaction between each mother and her baby is unique, and you are the only person who can be an expert about your child. So listen to others with a sceptical mind, and turn to books only if you're truly stuck or worried. Try that out for a week and see how you get on – you'll be surprised how good a mother's instincts are. Be guided by your baby's responses as to whether you're doing things right – she or he will usually let you know.

Of course, practical advice from books or experienced parents can be helpful. You might, for example, want to ask how to express breast milk or whether you really need a baby walker. You may want to check a book for information, such as signs of illness or allergy. Most books agree on important matters, but the fact that they differ on less basic issues shows that there's no 'right' way to care for a baby.

BENEFITS OF BREASTFEEDING

Which is best – breast or bottle-feeding?

Breast is best. Breast milk is free and readily available. It is nutritionally ideal and complete, at least for babies up to four to six months. Moreover, it contains antibodies that boost immunity, making the baby less likely to get infections (especially gastro-enteritis and respiratory infections) and less susceptible in later life to allergies such as eczema. Breastfed babies are also less liable to develop colic, constipation and obesity.

Ninety-eight per cent of women produce more than enough milk (most could feed twins if necessary). And the supply is self-regulating, as the more the baby sucks the more milk is produced. For convenience sake, breast milk is now often extracted and stored for later use. It can be expressed either by hand or with a manual or battery-operated breast pump, and then kept refrigerated in a sterile bottle for up to 24 hours, or frozen for up to 2 weeks in the freezer of an ordinary refrigerator and thawed. Breastfeeding also helps the womb to shrink, and the mother to get back into shape. If you need help with breastfeeding, contact the La Leche League, BM 3424, London WC1N 3XX.

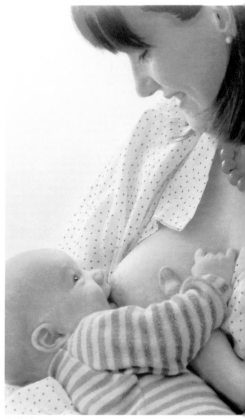

Body language Babies feed in bursts of sucking, with pauses for eye contact – a pattern psychologists think may lay the foundations for turn-taking conversation when speech develops.

BOTH BREAST AND BOTTLE

Can I combine breast and bottle or do I have to opt for one or the other?

You can combine the two methods – any breastfeeding (especially in the first three months) is better than none. However, using a bottle regularly can cause problems with breastfeeding. The baby may start to prefer the bottle, and may stop sucking as vigorously at the breast or even reject it altogether. This is less likely if you use bottles only occasionally, and for a full feed rather than for topping up after breastfeeding.

Bear in mind that if you give bottled for-mula milk, the baby will take less breast milk, and so less will be produced and the supply may dwindle. And since breast milk contains antibodies that protect the baby from infection, a reduced supply means increased risk of illness.

So if you do use bottles for convenience, do try to fill them with expressed breast milk rather than with formula milk.

FEEDING ON DEMAND

When my children were small I fed them on a four-hourly schedule, but my daughter insists on feeding her baby on demand. Which method is best?

Feeding on demand is best: why should a baby be hungry to schedule? With demand feeding, the baby gets ideally regulated nour-ishment, and will put on weight neither too quickly nor too slowly. And since a baby sucks for comfort, to limit its feedings may make it feel that its needs are being ignored.

Demand feeding is probably better for the mother too, if she has the time. She won't have to listen to hungry crying or try to feed a sleepy or uninterested baby. And if she is breastfeeding, demand feeding is more likely to stimulate milk supply.

Most babies soon settle into their own pattern. In the early weeks this may mean short feeds – perhaps every hour or three hours. But, as the baby grows, the interval between feeds will get longer.

Two notes of caution. If a baby seems too demanding, the reason may be poor milk supply, and a supplement may be necessary. And if it seems too undemanding, it may at times need to be woken up for feeding, in order to ensure adequate nourishment.

BREASTFEEDING IN ILLNESS

Is it safe to breastfeed if I am ill?

It depends what's wrong with you. For most minor infections, such as coughs and colds, breastfeeding makes little difference to the baby's chances of falling ill, since mother and baby are in such close contact anyway. For more serious illnesses, breastfeeding may be unwise. Consult your doctor.

If you need medication, breastfeeding might be inadvisable. Some drugs – whether prescription or over-the-counter – can make their way into the breast milk and could affect the baby, so do check with your doctor or pharmacist.

LEAVING A BABY TO CRY

My sister often leaves her baby to cry. It upsets me, but she says it doesn't do any harm. Is she right?

Most probably not. Crying is the main form of communication that babies under one year use. It signals an important need, such as hunger, thirst, discomfort, illness or lone-liness. If left alone, a baby will eventually stop crying – when it falls asleep from exhaustion.

By leaving her baby to cry, your sister risks missing a problem which needs attention. She may also be sowing seeds for future problems. The first year of life is a crucial time for the development of inner security: being left may instil fear or hopelessness in her baby, which may later lead to clingy or attention-seeking behaviour or resignation and withdrawal.

Research suggests that most babies whose mothers respond swiftly and with sensitivity appear more contented, cry less, are health-ier and may enjoy better emotional, intellec-tual and even physical development, with fewer behavioural problems later on.

Calming a tetchy baby

Here are some tips.

- Try feeding the baby.
- Change the nappy.
- Try baby massage, or gently press the soles of its feet for a few minutes.
- If the baby is teething, give it something to chew, or use teething gel.
- If you suspect colic, give the baby its usual medicine, and a gentle cuddle. If it is severe, see your doctor.
- Try rocking or cuddling or stroking the baby, or quietly talking or singing.
- Play with the baby or offer toys.
- Check the baby's temperature, and check for signs of illness (see chart, pages 286-287).

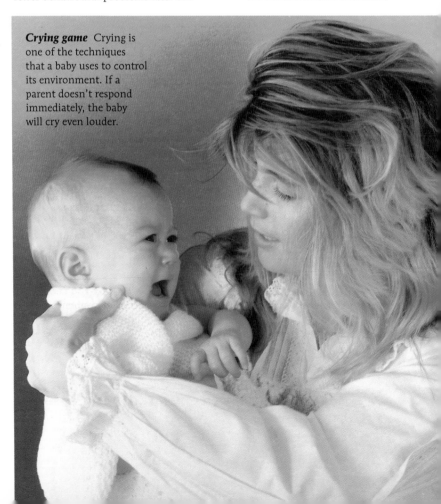

Crying game Crying is one of the techniques that a baby uses to control its environment. If a parent doesn't respond immediately, the baby will cry even louder.

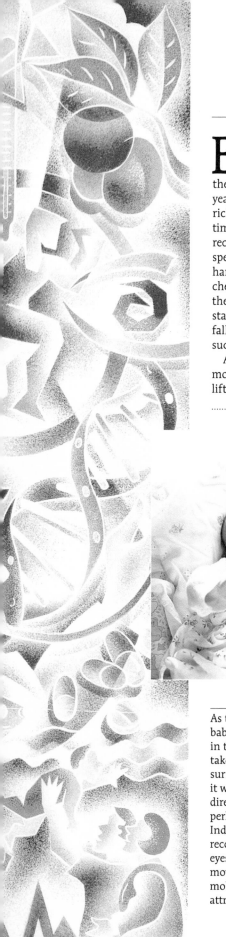

The first year of life

BABIES are born to learn – to learn about people, about language, about the body, about the world around them, about the way things work. The first year of life marks a voyage of discovery far richer and more rapid than at any other time. Some discoveries are subtle – the recognition of faces, the awareness of speech, the coordination of eyes and hands. Others are milestones that parents cherish and remember – the first tooth or the first word, the grim determination to stand upright, the elation when a puzzle falls into place or a new skill is mastered, such as handclapping.

At birth, a baby's skills consist of little more than reflex actions. It cannot even lift its head or see across a room. Yet by the end of the first month, it is already conducting early 'conversations', listening to its parents and responding with gurgles and gestures.

In the months that follow, new accomplishments proliferate as the muscles and nervous system mature. Reflex actions are replaced by voluntary movements, and one new skill serves as a springboard to the next. Once the baby learns to focus properly, for instance, it quickly learns to smile. And sharper hearing leads to a fascination with the human voice – and imitation of it. No matter how random an activity may appear at this stage – flinging out the arms, banging a toy on the ground – it is almost always serving a purpose, and making a contribution to learning.

ONE WEEK

Simple reflex actions characterise the first days of life. Stroke the palm of a baby's hand, and it will grab your finger. Brush its cheek, and it will turn its head in search of a nipple. But it has already made some developmental strides since birth. Although its focusing is limited, it can recognise some colours, for instance, and apparently enjoys looking at human faces. It needs lots of physical contact, and responds well to simple rhythmic movements and sounds.

ONE MONTH

As the first weeks pass, the baby becomes more at home in the world and starts to take an active interest in its surroundings. If spoken to, it will turn its head in the direction of the speaker, and perhaps gurgle in response. Individual faces are now recognisable, and the baby's eyes can follow close-range moving objects. A rotating mobile, for instance, will attract fascinated attention.

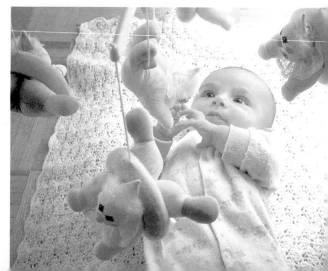

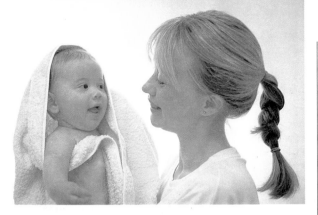

TWO MONTHS

The baby has become a master of smiling. Muscle control is developing fast, and actions are vigorous. The prospect of being picked up prompts enthusiastic kicking and waving.

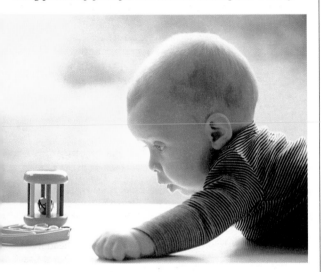

THREE MONTHS

By now muscles are strong enough to lift the head unaided. Objects just out of reach become irresistible and provoke strenuous efforts – not always successful – at grabbing.

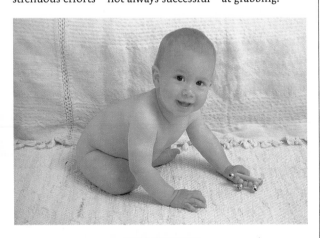

SIX MONTHS

The baby is able to sit up now, with only arms for support. Toys are grasped and handled with ease – and repeatedly thrown aside. Teething gets under way, a major milestone.

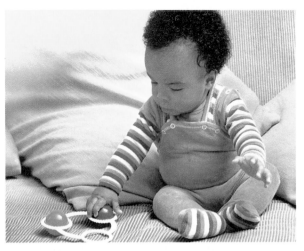

NINE MONTHS

Sitting up and manipulating toys are standard skills, though letting go can present problems. Crawling will start soon, and even standing upright by grasping solid supports. Awareness of strangers is growing, and distrust of them.

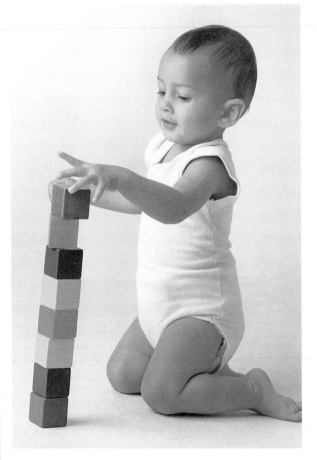

ONE YEAR

Stacking blocks and similar skills are evidence of deft new motor coordination. The baby crawls about rapidly now, and can stand up too, and even walk when supported. First words are just beginning, and a general interest in language.

MASSAGING A BABY

I've heard that massage is good for babies. What is the best way to do it? Is it completely safe?

Baby massage may help to relieve problems such as colic and constipation, and is totally safe as long as you take care. You can massage a baby of any age, but be gentle at first – stroke rather than knead, without applying any pressure. You may want to use books on baby massage or follow your instinct about what the baby likes.

The gentle touch
Massage is a wonderful way to relax a baby, and can be enjoyable for a parent too. It is best begun when the baby is awake but calm – ideally after a bath. If the baby starts to cry while being massaged, pick her up and comfort her as you would normally, and try again later.

Choose a quiet time, and make sure the room is warm enough. Prepare some oil, such as baby or almond oil, by putting the bottle in a basin of warm water. Undress the baby and sit beside her on the floor. Pour a small amount of oil on your hands and massage one area of the body at a time – gently and symmetrically with your palms. Afterwards, wipe off any extra oil before dressing your baby or giving her a warm bath.

A few precautions: never massage immediately after a feed; never push too hard on the stomach; and with very young babies, avoid touching the stomach until the umbilicus has healed.

CIRCUMCISION

Should a baby boy be circumcised? If so, when should the operation be done?

Unless you have religious reasons for favouring circumcision (removing the foreskin) it is best avoided. Most doctors believe that it offers no health benefits in infancy. The foreskin protects the delicate glans (head of the penis) from possible irritation, and may make it more sexually sensitive in later life.

If circumcision is to be done, it should be performed about eight days after birth. It is a simple and quick procedure, though as with any operation it carries a small risk of complications. Occasionally, older boys may need circumcision, if the foreskin becomes infected or is so tight that it hinders urination.

TEETHING TROUBLES

Since she started to cut her teeth, my daughter has been crying and fussing constantly. How can I comfort her? Will it carry on throughout teething?

No, she won't carry on behaving this way. The first few teeth, which appear between four and nine months, can cause these problems, but most babies get used to the sensation of teeth breaking through. Later teeth may simply cause a day or two of fussing, with red cheeks and dribbling.

It may not be teething that's to blame. To find out, massage her gums with a clean finger to reduce inflammation. Although she may initially cry out, if she has teething pain she will appreciate the relief. You could also offer a teething ring, cool liquids, ice lollies or a special teething gel. If nothing helps, the problem may lie elsewhere – perhaps in frustration at trying to master new skills. It is also possible that her behaviour is signalling an illness (see chart, pages 286–287).

Note that teething sometimes triggers nappy rash, a condition which should be treated promptly (see page 288).

WEANING YOUR BABY

*When should I start weaning my baby?
Which foods are best to begin with?*

At four months is the best time. Before four months, all your baby's nutritional needs are met by milk. Giving solids too early may make your baby fat, and places a strain on its immature digestive system. As for weaning too late, milk is no longer enough for an older baby, which needs other sources of vitamins and minerals. A mixed diet should be offered by six months.

The transition from milk to solids should be gradual: too much solid food could make your baby dehydrated, so offer extra fluids, such as cooled boiled water, after a feed. Make sure solid foods are very smooth – puréed or strained – and introduce one food at a time. Stewed fresh fruit or cooked vegetables are a good starting point, but do not add salt or sugar. Avoid foods that are high in fat or starch.

Keep a note of new foods: if your baby suffers from wind or diarrhoea it may be linked to that particular food. In such a case, withhold that food for several weeks before trying again.

PREPARED BABY FOOD

Prepared baby foods are convenient, but how nutritious are they? Do babies also need fresh foods to make sure they get enough vitamins and minerals?

Vitamins and minerals are plentiful in prepared foods, being usually added. Other added ingredients – starch, salt and sugar – are unnecessary and sometimes undesirable.

Most manufacturers now avoid adding salt and sugar when possible. But some baby desserts remain high in sugar, and many meals have a high starch content, so always check labels.

Alternatively, it is easy to make your own prepared foods. Mashed leftovers can be frozen in ice-cube trays or small jars, and thawed and reheated when necessary.

STARTING TOILET TRAINING

I'd like to start toilet training my 16-month-old daughter. How should I go about it? Is she old enough to start?

You can try, but there is little point in doing so unless she is aware of, and can partly control, bladder and bowel movements. This generally starts between 18 and 24 months. Toilet training is best taught in stages, as it involves many skills.

● Encourage your daughter to sit on the potty, clothed or unclothed, and explain its purpose.
● Put her on the potty at exactly the same time every day.
● Encourage her to tell someone when she needs the potty.
● If she uses the potty, offer praise, even if she just sits on it.
● Never force her to sit on the potty for longer than she wishes, or scold her for not using it.
● If at any stage she resists, put the potty away for a few days.
● Teach toilet hygiene at the same time – wiping, flushing and washing hands.

She will probably still need nappies when away from home. And even when dry during the day, she will at first still need a nappy at night. By the age of three or three and a half, she should be fully toilet trained.

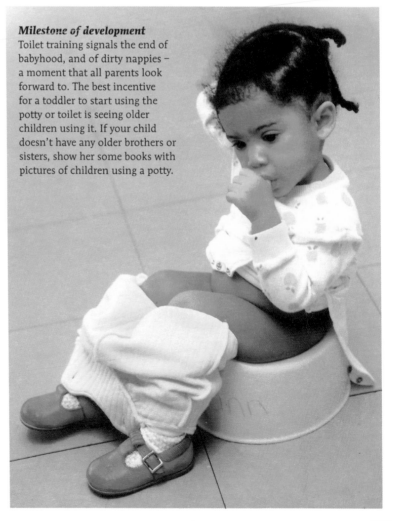

Milestone of development
Toilet training signals the end of babyhood, and of dirty nappies – a moment that all parents look forward to. The best incentive for a toddler to start using the potty or toilet is seeing older children using it. If your child doesn't have any older brothers or sisters, show her some books with pictures of children using a potty.

283

Children and sleep

SLEEPING THROUGH

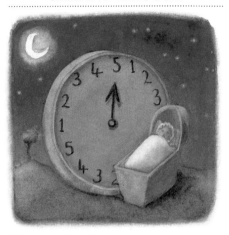

When do babies finally start sleeping through the night? Is there anything parents can do to encourage it?

The average baby manages about five hours' unbroken sleep by three months. However, about one child in three still wakes regularly at age one, and about one in ten does so at age four. It is normal for most young children to have periods of waking, particularly when teething, or grieving, or reaching developmental milestones such as crawling.

There are several ways of encouraging unbroken sleep. First, ensure that the baby's night-time environment and daytime habits encourage sleep. Then, any of three options: take the baby into your bed; break the 'habit' of night waking by leaving the baby to cry for increasing periods before going into the room; go to the baby and soothe it back to sleep. Most parents choose the last route, though it does seem to reward waking, and so risks encouraging it. If you decide to take this approach, keep the baby in or beside the cot, don't turn the light on, and stay quiet – even if you feed the child. Avoid changing nappies unless necessary.

NIGHT-TIME WAKING

My six-month-old baby still wakes up and cries several times during the night. Is there something wrong with him?

Possibly, but it is probably not serious. Babies often experience disturbed nights as they reach milestones, such as learning to sit up

or even using a beaker, or during growing 'spurts'. There may be a simple solution, such as moving your baby's cot or leaving an article of your clothing (unwashed) in the cot. The following are some other possible causes and remedies.

- The same factors involved in daytime crying (see page 279).
- A too rapid transition to weaning.
- Dislike of, or upset from, formula milk or certain foods, such as wheat or eggs.
- A bedroom which is too hot, too cold, too noisy, or too quiet.
- Loneliness or insecurity. Give your baby more attention, cuddling, and reassurance during the day.
- Fear of the dark. Try a nightlight, or take your baby into your bed.
- Lack of fresh air and exercise. Go for a long walk or play outside in the afternoon.
- Eating too much before bed or, conversely, having the last feed too early.
- Too much or not enough sleep during the day.
- Upset or over-excitement at bedtime. Adopt a calming routine, such as bath-feed-song, and stick to it every night.

SHARING YOUR BED

I'd like to take my baby into our bed when she wakes up at night, but my husband says she could suffocate. Is this possible?

No, not unless you are obese, drugged, drunk or otherwise constituting a risk. If you do 'co-sleep', avoid waterbeds or soft mattresses, and make sure that pillows cannot fall on the baby's face. Also, check that the baby is free to move and is not wrapped up.

Co-sleeping has a number of benefits. It calms babies, reduces stress, and stabilises breathing rates and body heat. Parents can notice and respond rapidly to any problems. Co-sleeping is the quickest way to end night crying and resolve sleep problems. It reduces tantrums, and may even help to prevent cot death, which is far less common in societies where co-sleeping is the norm.

However, you are effectively rewarding your baby by taking her into your bed *after* she has woken up, and risk encouraging her to wake up every night. It might be best to let her sleep in your bed from the start of the night. Don't worry about breaking this pattern: she will eventually choose to leave for her bed of her own accord, probably starting with a gradual transition around the age of two.

PREVENTING COT DEATH

What causes cot death and what can I do to protect my baby from it?

Cot death, or SIDS (sudden infant death syndrome), is one of the greatest fears that parents have. It remains something of a mystery, often striking out of the blue, affecting even apparently healthy babies. In some cases undetected heart or breathing problems seem to be involved, but in others even an autopsy cannot identify the cause.

Despite this lack of understanding, doctors have identified numerous factors that increase the risk of SIDS. These include prematurity, low birth-weight, sleeping position and cold weather. Boys are more at risk, as are babies of young, single mothers and mothers who smoke.

The following precautions will help to protect any baby.

● Always lay the baby to sleep on its back or side, never on its stomach.
● Don't overwrap the baby or allow its room to overheat.
● Don't smoke or, if you must, smoke well away from the baby.
● Keep the baby away from people who are ill, especially those with respiratory complaints including even minor coughs and colds.
● Choose an approved baby mattress.
● Breastfeed your baby. Recent research shows that bottle-fed babies have a higher risk of cot death.

BATTLE OVER BEDTIME

Our toddler makes a terrible fuss about going to bed. Would it do any harm to let him stay up until he falls asleep?

It certainly won't do *him* any harm. It's quite possible that he doesn't need very much sleep. Left to themselves, children will take what sleep they need, but not necessarily to the schedule their parents would want.

If you let him stay up, it could become a habit – at least for a while. On the other hand, it could solve the problem: if bedtime fighting is a way of asserting his indepen-

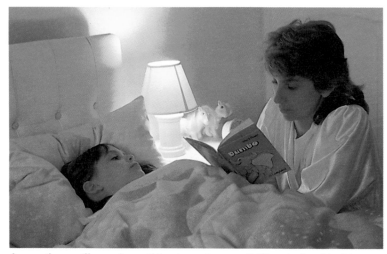

dence, there will now be nothing to make a fuss about. An alternative is to set bedtime half an hour *later* than the time your son wants to go to bed. Make sure he gets up at the same time and doesn't take longer daytime naps. Then gradually bring bedtime forward, by about ten minutes a day, until you get to the time you prefer.

Make sure there is not a hidden reason for his not liking bed, such as fear of the dark. And make bedtime more attractive by establishing a routine that your son likes, such as listening to a story in bed.

BEDWETTING

My five-year-old still wets his bed. Is this a sign that something is wrong?

Not necessarily. All children may occasionally wet the bed up to the age of three or four, and at age five nearly one in ten children still wets the bed. The reason is usually simply that bladder control is slow to develop. Anxiety or occasionally over-excitement may be a contributory factor.

If there is an obvious background to your son's bedwetting, such as a recent move or a new baby in the family, be as loving and reassuring as you can, and pay as little attention to the bedwetting as possible. Buy a waterproof mattress cover and change the sheets without fuss. Never scold or punish your son for wetting the bed. Check that he goes to the toilet just before bedtime, and does not drink too much in the evening. If the bedwetting persists, or if you suspect he has a urinary infection, a nervous system disorder or an emotional problem, see your doctor. He or she might advise you to try an enuresis alarm – a pad placed under the sheet which buzzes when wet.

Telling stories A bedtime book is an ideal way to get children to look forward to sleep, and allows you to enjoy some valuable time together.

DO'S
— AND —
DON'TS

for a quiet night

Do forbid over-exciting television programmes and boisterous play before bed.
Do secure the house so that a child who sleepwalks cannot fall downstairs, get out of windows and doors or otherwise come to harm.

Don't give a child cheese, chocolate or other foods containing sugar or additives in the evening.
Don't try to wake a child who is having a nightmare. Turn the light on and talk calmly. If that doesn't work, just hold or rock the child until he or she calms down again.
Don't try to wake a sleepwalker. Just lead him or her gently back to bed.

IDENTIFYING CHILDHOOD ILLNESSES

Children's illnesses are seldom serious, and most parents soon become expert at judging a child's state of health. Even so, there are times when knowing what to do can be difficult and, in some cases, critical. This chart will help you to identify many of the major childhood illnesses and to take the right action. Always err on the side of caution and seek medical help if in doubt.

EMERGENCIES

These six symptoms indicate a need for urgent action. If you spot any one of them, telephone your doctor immediately or take the child to the nearest hospital accident and emergency department. If no other help is available, call for an ambulance on 999.

1. Unconscious, not fully conscious or unnaturally drowsy.

2. Very pale colouring which persists.

3. Blueness around the lips or face.

4. Serious difficulty in breathing.

5. A fit or convulsion, especially with very high temperature.

6. A rash that looks like bleeding under the skin and does not turn pale when pressed firmly.

SYMPTOMS	POSSIBLE CAUSE	ACTION
Diarrhoea and/or abdominal pain and:		
Listlessness; sunken eyes; very dry mouth; high temperature; rash that looks like bleeding under the skin and does not go pale when pressed firmly; dark urine; infrequent urination; not properly conscious; persistence or worsening of pain.	Possible major illness (meningitis, gastroenteritis with dehydration) or possible appendicitis.	CALL DOCTOR OR GO TO HOSPITAL IMMEDIATELY.
Sore throat; ear pain; aching limbs; headache.	Ear infection, tonsillitis or flu.	Call doctor during surgery hours.
Loss of appetite; nausea; vomiting; cramps; or no other symptoms.	Gastroenteritis without dehydration.	Give fluids, but not milk. Call doctor if no improvement in 6-8 hours or if other symptoms develop.
Fever:		
High temperature but below 39°C (102°F).	Possible major illness (meningitis, appendicitis, chickenpox, rubella, measles) or minor infection (ear, sinus) or minor illness (flu).	Keep the child cool: minimum clothing, lots of fluids. Avoid medication. Call doctor in surgery hours. If temperature rises or other symptoms develop, treat as in next two cases.
Temperature rises suddenly; child distressed or clearly unwell; temperature above 39°C (102°F).	As above.	Give paediatric paracetamol. If the child's temperature has not fallen within half an hour, CALL DOCTOR IMMEDIATELY. Keep the child cool, as above, and sponge with tepid (not cold) water if temperature rises above 40.5°C (105°F), or if child has convulsions or other serious symptoms (see next case).
Temperature persists despite treatment; child has convulsions or other serious symptoms such as vomiting, diarrhoea or signs of dehydration (dark urine, dry mouth).	Major illness, possibly meningitis, appendicitis or gastroenteritis.	CALL DOCTOR IMMEDIATELY. If no doctor available, TAKE CHILD TO HOSPITAL IMMEDIATELY.

CAUTION Never give aspirin to a child under 12, in view of the risk of Reye's syndrome (see page 288).

Fever with runny nose and:		
Not fully conscious; stiff neck; child becomes and stays extremely pale; rash that looks like bleeding under the skin and does not go pale when pressed firmly; dislike of bright light.	Major illness, possibly meningitis or septicaemia.	CALL DOCTOR OR GO TO HOSPITAL IMMEDIATELY.

SYMPTOMS	POSSIBLE CAUSE	ACTION
Fever with runny nose and: (cont)		
Rash of flat, irregularly shaped pink spots.	Measles.	Give fluids. Treat fever (see above). Call doctor during surgery hours.
Rash of tiny pink spots on face, trunk, and limbs; tiny lumps behind ears; not very ill.	Rubella (German measles).	Give fluids. Treat fever (see above). Call doctor during surgery hours. Keep child away from pregnant women.
Rash of blisters in clusters, beginning on trunk.	Chickenpox.	Give fluids. Treat fever (see above). Use calamine lotion on skin. Call doctor during surgery hours.
Swelling under jaw.	Mumps.	Give fluids. Treat fever (see above). Call doctor during surgery hours.
Aching limbs; headache.	Flu.	Give fluids. Treat fever (see above). Call doctor during surgery hours.
Any ear pain.	Ear infection.	Give fluids. Treat fever (see above). Call doctor during surgery hours.
Sore throat; tonsils very red with tiny yellow-white patches.	Tonsillitis.	Give fluids. Treat fever (see above). Call doctor during surgery hours.
Sore throat; sneezing; nasal congestion.	Common cold.	Give fluids. Treat fever (see above).
Rash of itchy blisters with yellow, crusty scabs, spreading gradually outwards from a small area.	Impetigo.	Call doctor during surgery hours. Keep child's towel and flannel away from others.
Abnormal breathing:		
Rapid breathing with high temperature or chest pain; severe paroxysms of coughing, which may cause vomiting or going blue in the face; wheezing; muffled voice; possibly drooling.	Pneumonia, whooping cough or epiglottitis.	CALL DOCTOR OR GO TO HOSPITAL IMMEDIATELY.
Noisy, musical-sounding breathing that is rapid or accompanied by cough; child has been affected in this way previously.	Asthma.	CALL DOCTOR IMMEDIATELY unless wheezing is very mild or the child's difficulty with breathing abates.
Noisy breathing with no other symptoms.	Bronchitis or asthma.	CALL DOCTOR IMMEDIATELY.
Hoarseness; noisy breathing or wheezing with ringing or barking cough; child doesn't look very ill.	Croup.	Keep child in steam-filled room: stay with child. Call doctor if steam brings no relief after half an hour.
Convulsions or jerky movement of limbs and:		
Raised temperature and not fully conscious.	Major illness, possibly meningitis.	Place in recovery position (see page 448). Do not restrain child. CALL DOCTOR OR AMBULANCE IMMEDIATELY.
Unconscious or not fully alert after fit, but no fever.	Epileptic seizure.	CALL DOCTOR IMMEDIATELY. If child has a history of epilepsy, follow the doctor's advice.
Not fully alert; fever; possibly headache.	Major illness, possibly meningitis or encephalitis.	CALL DOCTOR OR GO TO HOSPITAL IMMEDIATELY.
Fever; possibly briefly unconscious.	Fever fit.	Sponge body with lukewarm water; give paediatric paracetamol. If the first attack, CALL DOCTOR IMMEDIATELY. If child has a history of these convulsions, follow the doctor's advice.

Looking after health

CHILDREN'S IMMUNISATION

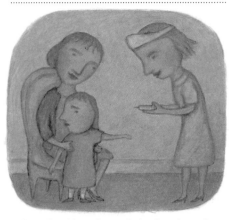

When should I take my baby daughter for her vaccinations?

See your doctor or health visitor, who will give you a booklet for recording your baby's immunisations. Opinions vary slightly about when a child should be immunised, but the following programme is generally recommended:

● A combined injection against diphtheria, tetanus and whooping cough, and an oral vaccine against polio at two months. The second and third doses of these treatments follow at four week intervals.
● An Hib injection (Haemophilus influenzae type b), to protect against meningitis and some breathing problems, at about one year.
● A combined injection against mumps, measles and rubella at about 13 months.
● A combined diphtheria-tetanus injection and an oral polio vaccine at four to five years.

At some time between 10 and 14 years, children are immunised against tuberculosis, and girls receive another rubella vaccination. Between 15 and 18, teenagers have another round of tetanus and polio inoculations.

TROUBLE WITH TONSILS

Our young daughter keeps getting tonsillitis. Should she have her tonsils removed?

Probably not. Tonsillectomy (the surgical removal of tonsils) was once a popular solution to recurrent tonsillitis, but is now recommended only for extreme infection (such as an abscess) or severe obstruction from over-enlarged tonsils. This new restraint is

based on several considerations. First, doctors now know that tonsils actually protect people, especially children, from many infections more serious than tonsillitis. Then, most children who suffer repeatedly from tonsillitis tend to grow out of it in a few years anyway, and conversely, children who have their tonsils removed can still get repeated throat infections. Finally, as with any operation, tonsillectomy carries a small risk of serious side effects.

TREATING HEAD LICE

I've just been told that children at my son's school have head lice. What should I do?

Head lice are common in many schools, and spread easily. Your son may or may not catch them, but short of keeping him away from school, there is nothing you can do to influence events. Head lice do not imply a lack of hygiene: in fact, lice prefer cleaner hair.

If your son is affected, he will probably scratch his scalp constantly, and you may see tiny lice or, more probably, tiny white eggs ('nits') stuck to the base of the hair shafts. You can often detect nits by combing the hair with a fine-toothed comb. If your doctor or health visitor confirms your suspicions, he or she will prescribe treatment – not just for your son but for the whole family. Or you could try one of the special scalp lotions or shampoos available from chemists.

CHILDHOOD RASHES

My baby has a case of nappy rash that will not clear. How should I treat it?

Your baby's nappy rash may have become complicated by a yeast infection or 'thrush'. This turns the skin scaly, and a more fiery red in colour. See your doctor, who will probably prescribe an antifungal cream. As a preventive measure, allow him to go without nappies whenever possible, and use a zinc or castor oil cream at every nappy change.

CAUTION A rash over the whole body, accompanied by a raised temperature or a cough, may be a sign of one of the childhood illnesses (see chart, pages 286-287). If you notice these symptoms, call your doctor immediately.

Growing and learning

THE VALUE OF BABY TALK

Does baby talk serve a useful purpose, or is it better to use proper words even when they can't possibly be understood?

It depends what you mean by baby talk. Most adults, especially mothers, use a particular style of speech when addressing babies: they talk slowly, with a fairly high pitch and an exaggerated 'lilt', in short, simple sentences, leaving clear gaps between words. This helps the baby to understand words and tone of voice, and to keep concentrating.

Baby talk as in 'gee gee' for 'horse' is another matter. It seems to be more for adults' than children's benefit, and is as silly and unproductive as it sounds. The baby can just as easily grasp the real words. And using real words from the start means that the child doesn't have to learn a whole new vocabulary when adults decide he or she is too old for 'baby' words. Even if the youngster mispronounces a long or difficult word, he or she will find it easier to graduate from this version to the correct word than to have to start again with an entirely new word.

LEARNING THROUGH PLAYING

What are the best ways to stimulate a child's intellectual development? Do so-called 'educational' toys and games help?

Games and gadgets help parents: they provide a short cut to amusing and stimulating the child. But, at least until the child reaches school age, you don't really need them. Equal stimulation is provided by exploring everyday objects, places and ideas, and by making things together.

For babies and toddlers, all toys are educational – most learning actually occurs through play. However, *what* they play with is less important than *whom*: advice, attention and encouragement from an adult are the best aids to learning. Give the child maximum freedom to explore the environment, taking care to make your home as safe as possible (see pages 324-328).

After age two or three, a child benefits greatly from playing with other children, though adult company remains enormously stimulating. For older children, toys and games can certainly provide stimulation, but their 'educational' component may be less important than their actual appeal: if a child wants to play tennis, a violin won't be of much interest or benefit.

TEACHING CHILDREN TO READ

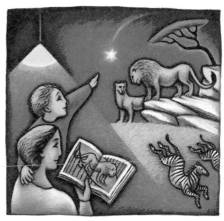

Will it be an advantage to my daughter if she learns to read before starting school? If so, what is the best way to teach reading?

Being able to read before she starts school will not necessarily give your daughter an advantage over other children. In fact, parents are sometimes advised against teaching preschool children to read: the parents' methods will most probably differ from the teacher's, which may cause a clash. However, if your daughter is already beginning to recognise letters and words and asking for details, it would be unwise – and futile – to hold back.

Encourage your daughter by reading to her. Let her see the text, show her when it is time to turn the page and point out words that she may know. Do not adopt a particular school reading scheme: this will only lead to confusion if your teaching methods differ from the teacher's, and boredom if the child is already familiar with the material.

Instead, you might try to make your own books, using simple words about familiar objects and experiences, and with the central character always being your daughter.

The best way of imbuing children with an interest in reading is by your own example. If they see you reading regularly, they will soon realise how useful and pleasurable the written word can be.

DEALING WITH DYSLEXIA

What is dyslexia and what can be done to help children with this problem?

Dyslexia is a particular reading disorder in which letters and words are transposed or reversed. Children with this problem continue to make basic mistakes that others soon grow out of – writing 'p' for 'q' or 'b' for 'd', for example, or reading the word 'tap' as 'pat'. Dyslexia affects only written symbols and in many cases only words – affected children are often able to read numbers and musical notation without problems.

Similar reading disorders can arise from mental handicap, eye trouble and poor or neglected education, therefore a diagnosis of dyslexia is only made when such causes have been eliminated. Dyslexia occurs regardless of intelligence and across socioeconomic backgrounds.

The causes of dyslexia are not well understood but it is thought that disorders of the nervous system may be involved. Inheritance appears to play a part, at least in some cases. It is now thought that dyslexia affects boys and girls equally, but girls experience a different set of symptoms.

Provided dyslexia is recognised early, and treated sympathetically, many of the problems can be overcome. Remedial programmes can teach strategies to improve reading and writing, and parents can help by being supportive and praising all achievements. Further advice is available from the British Dyslexia Association, 98 London Road, Reading, Berkshire RG1 5AU (helpline: 01734 668 271).

LEFT-HANDERS

My three-year-old uses his left hand much more than his right. Will he grow up to be left-handed? Should I encourage him to use his right hand more?

Children in their first year of life generally show little sign of favouring one hand over the other. Between two and three they often switch preferences. Only when they reach three or four is one hand clearly dominant. In the end, about one in ten boys and one in twelve girls grows up to be left-handed.

Encouraging the use of the right hand may have some effect on children under the age of about 18 months. But as for your three-year-old, encouragement will make no difference. He may switch hands or he may not: you must simply wait and see. And don't worry if he does turn out to be left-handed – the drawbacks are minimal.

Children should never be forced to use the right hand. Any such efforts will fail if the child is destined to be left-handed, and pressure can create problems later on, such as stuttering or difficulties in writing.

STAMMERING

My five-year-old son used to speak well, but has recently developed a stammer. My husband thinks that he'll grow out of it, but my mother suggested that we take him to a speech therapist. Is this a good idea?

It depends. Stammering is common in small children learning to speak, seems to run in families, and is more common in boys than girls. It may be triggered by a specific incident, such as a house move or the arrival of a new baby, or by general tension, perhaps through too much discipline. Stammering may also be induced in the presence of certain people who distress the child for some reason or other. Usually this type of stammering disappears as the child settles down, though it may recur with later upsets. Here are some ways in which you could help your son to get through this current bout.

● Be especially loving.
● Create a relaxed home atmosphere.
● Take no notice of the stammering.

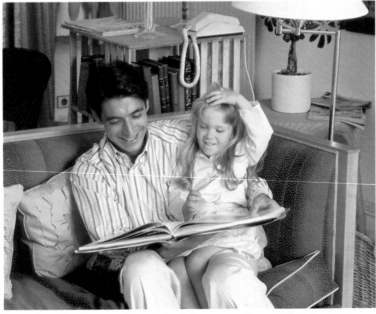

Joys of reading Parents play a vital role in encouraging a child's interest in reading, particularly if there are difficulties such as dyslexia. Keep tempting, attractive books in the house, pay as much attention to entertaining as to conveying information when reading stories, and praise any accomplishments.

- Avoid talking 'at' him.
- Pay full attention when he speaks.
- Don't put him under any pressure.
- Don't get irritated.
- Wait patiently for him to finish what he's saying: don't finish his words for him.

Persistent stammering may be a sign of deeper problems. If there is no improvement after a couple of months, discuss speech therapy with your doctor or health visitor, who may refer you to a specialist.

SEX DIFFERENCES

Should parents try to treat girls and boys in exactly the same way, or are there inborn differences that should be nurtured?

Most people agree that boys and girls have different temperaments and preferred play activities, and these may emerge as early as 18 months. Whether these differences are inborn or due to different treatment is still disputed. There is some evidence for inborn biological differences; for example, male hormones are known to promote aggression. However, there is no doubt that boys and girls are treated differently from birth. Studies have shown that adults, given a baby whose sex they do not know or one dressed as the opposite sex, handle it differently according to the sex they believe it to be.

Moreover, sex differences are reinforced by society – from media images to other children's behaviour. There are counterforces, however. Children who are allowed to play with a range of toys without adult pressure tend to show less sexually stereotyped behaviour. So do children from families where the father plays an active role in their upbringing. Parents are often role-models for their children, so your own attitudes will influence theirs. For maximum even-handedness, provide a range of toys, watch out for stereotyped books and encourage children to consider a range of future roles for themselves.

LEARNING WITH DOWN'S

Our small daughter has Down's syndrome. What does this mean in terms of her learning ability? How can we stimulate her interest and learning skills?

Children with Down's syndrome learn to do most of the things other children do. It is just that their development tends to be delayed. Your daughter will have a certain degree of learning difficulty, but there is no reason why she should not eventually be able to walk and talk, ride a bicycle and read and write. There are a number of measures you can take to stimulate your daughter and give her the best possible start in life.

- Talk to her frequently, read to her, encourage her to play with toys and take her on outings regularly. These activities will help to improve her physical and mental potential and reduce later learning difficulties.
- Arrange speech therapy, if necessary. Children with Down's syndrome often have unclear speech because of muscle weakness.
- Arrange for her to have regular sight and hearing tests, to avoid needless added learning difficulties.
- Accept any special help that may aid her development; for example, 'portage' schemes – special exercises designed to enhance muscle tone. (For further information, contact your local Social Services department.)
- If possible, send your daughter to a mainstream school. Down's children seem to do much better in normal schools than in segregated ones. Many primary and even nursery schools accept Down's children.
- Offer love, support and consideration of her special needs, but don't be over-protective or too lenient. She needs normal childhood experiences and the chance to develop her independence in just the same ways as other children do.
- Lastly, take care not to neglect your other children. Siblings can easily feel isolated and ignored, and your daughter needs their support not their resentment.

For more information and support, contact The Down's Syndrome Association, 155 Mitcham Road, London SW17 9PG.

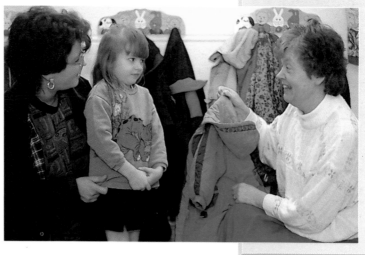

DO'S
— AND —
DON'TS
for your child's first day at school

Do tell your child, in the days before school begins, all about what will be happening there.
Do try to choose a school that will also be attended by your child's best friends.
Do ensure that all items of school clothing are easily recognisable by your child, and clearly labelled with her name.
Do make sure that your child knows exactly where to go at the start and end of the school day, and during breaks.

Don't be surprised if there are a few tears on your child's first day at school. The sheer numbers and noise of other children can be frightening.

Starting school First day at school is often a bewildering experience. Try to organise a visit for your child to meet her teacher beforehand.

Dealing with bad behaviour

NOT SO TERRIBLE TWOS

My two-year-old is impossibly naughty and has to be watched every minute. How can I discipline her in a way she'll understand?

You can't. A two-year-old is not open to rational debate. It is normal for toddlers to be inquisitive and assert their independence. And she *should* be watched or looked after by an adult, because this is just the age when dangers are most present. To increase safety, try to childproof her environment rather than restrict her too much.

She's almost certainly not being deliberately naughty. If she is, that could be a distress signal: she might have a reason to feel anxious, such as family tension or a recent house move, which you should look into. Or it could be a means of attention-seeking, in which case the best way to encourage good behaviour is to pay attention to her, by praising and joining in, when she does things you want, and to ignore or distract her when she does things you don't want. And remember, if you avoid making a big issue out of everything, she's more likely to respect your disapproval on the really important matters.

TEMPER TANTRUMS

Whenever my 20-month-old son doesn't get his own way, he throws a terrible temper tantrum. Is there something wrong?
I really don't know how to handle him.

There is absolutely nothing wrong with your son. Temper tantrums are part of a normal stage of development, and he should grow out of them by the time he reaches three or four.

It's important to realise that a tantrum is actually quite frightening for the child himself – your son really is out of control. The best way of dealing with it depends on the child: it may be best to hold and reassure him, or to ignore him, or to wait quietly by his side until he calms down. Further tips:

● Don't shout and scream – if you do get angry, apologise afterwards.
● Don't try to talk to him during the tantrum.
● Never give in to the demand that prompted it.
● When the tantrum is over, kneel or sit at his level, reassure him and give him a hug. Then carry on with what you were doing.
● Never talk about his tantrums to others in front of him, even if they have a funny side.

TOYS AND AGGRESSION

Do toy guns, bows and arrows and other weapons make children aggressive?

They may do. Children playing with 'aggressive' toys are more verbally and physically hostile towards each other than when playing with toys which require cooperation, sharing and taking turns. Some studies suggest that war toys promote acceptance of brutality and war as normal and inevitable, and that boys who play with such toys are a great deal more aggressive.

However, the toys themselves are less important than a parent's attitudes and the environment in which a child grows up. Emotional neglect or physical brutality plays a far greater role in creating delinquency than letting a child play with water pistols does. But if you do still wish to discourage this form of play, here are some things to encourage.

● Verbal expression of emotions, including anger and frustration.
● Toys or games requiring cooperative play.
● Alternative outlets for high energy and pent-up emotions – any physical activity.
● Creative pursuits such as woodwork.
● Sports and board games which allow competitiveness without violence.

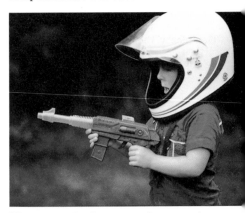

War games Studies suggest that aggressive toys may encourage violence in children, but the really influential factors are parents' attitudes and a child's home environment.

WHEN CHILDREN FIGHT

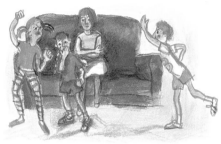

My three children fight all the time, and the two older ones tend to gang up on the smallest boy. How can I make them be nice to each other?

A degree of sibling rivalry is natural, and helps children to learn about tolerance and independence. Sometimes this rivalry gets out of hand, unfortunately, and all you can do then is take a few steps to improve things.

When your children fight, try to stay out of the way. Taking sides or scolding may just make things worse. If they become physically violent or if one child is upset, separate them and refuse to listen to arguments about who was to blame (unless someone was clearly being vicious). Just insist that the fighting stops. If necessary, send them to separate rooms to calm down. As the youngest is being victimised, you could give him a few tips (in private) on standing up for himself.

Encourage your older children to look out for their little brother, but don't force them to or make it a chore. Try to encourage all the children to play together, but don't make them share their toys. Acknowledge their feelings if they are jealous or angry with a brother or sister, and listen to them if they feel they are being treated unfairly.

You can set a good example yourself. Don't 'baby' the smallest child, as the others may then feel jealous. Equally, don't penalise him for being younger, by giving him a smaller ice-cream, say – the older children may imitate your attitude. When they have to be treated in different ways (bedtimes, for example), explain that the same rules did or will apply to everyone at that age.

HYPERACTIVITY

I've always put my six-year-old's boisterous behaviour down to high spirits, but his teacher has started to complain that he is noisy and disruptive in class. Could this be a sign of hyperactivity?

Possibly, but it could just mean that he is bored, unhappy at school, bright for his age or naturally boisterous. True hyperactivity is rare, and affected children are clearly disturbed as well as always being full of energy. For example, they may dislike cuddles, seem miserable, be aggressive, and act in impulsive or reckless ways.

Explanations for the condition vary – from slight brain damage at birth to additives in food or exposure to lead in petrol fumes. No conclusive evidence has been found to prove these theories.

If you feel that your son's behaviour at home is just high spirits, and he seems otherwise happy and well, hyperactivity is unlikely to be the problem. You could check if his diet is involved, by cutting out all unnecessary stimulants (such as caffeinated cola drinks), additives (food colourings and preservatives) and foods that are possibly allergy-provoking (cow's milk, chocolate and tomatoes are common culprits).

Before jumping to conclusions, find out how he is performing at school in other respects. If he is obviously bright and ahead of the class, he may just need more stimulation. Discuss the problem with his teacher.

FACT — OR — FALLACY?

'Spare the rod and spoil the child.'

Fallacy Children who are hit at home are more aggressive than those who are not, and more likely to become bullies and delinquents. Parents who slap or beat a child find that they have to keep on doing so (often with increasing severity), so it's plainly not a tactic that works. And a smack can escalate into serious abuse.

Hitting teaches the child nothing about good behaviour, only about staying out of the way, or timing misdeeds for when the parent cannot see them. The most effective forms of discipline are those that show respect for the child and so promote self-respect and self-discipline. Most children brought up without physical punishment turn into polite, law-abiding, caring adults.

Television and computers

TELEVISION VIOLENCE

How much damage does television violence do? Does it really have a long-term effect?

The effects are very hard to quantify, but experts are certainly becoming concerned. Studies do seem to show that screen violence has a desensitising effect, and the capacity to promote aggressive attitudes and behaviour.

It takes a long time for children to understand the difference between fantasy and reality. While some small children are visibly upset by violence, others seem to copy it: even cartoon films can set them off – biting, hitting, stamping and shouting. Older children may respond to TV violence by becoming rude, hostile and unruly. And there is some evidence that they are more likely to become involved in violence in later life.

Effects of the media on behaviour

If a child has been disturbed by something he or she has heard, seen or read, you might notice one or more of the following signs.

● Difficulty in sleeping, nightmares or fear of the dark.
● Reversion to babyish behaviour such as clinginess or thumb sucking.
● Fear of monsters, witches or fictional characters.
● Increased bullying, fighting or aggression.
● Acting out violent scenes in play.
● Expressing fear for his or her future.
● Unexpected distress over a particular subject.
● Withdrawal, secrecy, hiding objects.
● Rebellious or antisocial attitudes, secrecy, furtiveness or hiding things.

Find out what your child has been watching or reading that has resulted in such negative behaviour. Explain why you feel it would be best to avoid such material in future; for example: 'Hurting people is bad, so I don't want you to watch others doing it.' The child then knows your values even if he or she sees something by accident or outside the home.

Watch television as a family sometimes, if possible. Discuss what you see, especially if the issues raised conflict with your values.

SUITABLE VIEWING

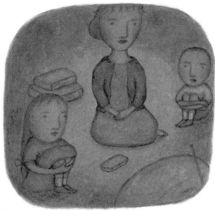

How can I tell which television programmes, videos and computer games are suitable for my children? Could a news bulletin or a crime reconstruction be as damaging as a 'video nasty'?

Unpleasant pictures in any form may disturb children, especially if the images are shown together with frightening music, or as a prolonged, overexciting or highly nerve-racking sequence. Some very small children can even be upset by violent cartoon films, while older ones may be more distressed by graphic news pictures of famine or disaster. Not that such responses are always bad: they indicate sympathy, and can develop a child's social awareness, particularly if parents make a point of discussing the issues involved.

Only you can judge what your children can cope with. Watch their reactions closely and switch off the television if something is causing distress. Don't take a child to a film, or show a video at home, unless you know it contains nothing disturbing.

Computer games are a relatively new area of concern, and you should regulate them in the same way that you would television programmes. Thanks to technological improvements, such games can now use real-life actors and have the potential of being as violent and disturbing as many a 'video nasty'.

In Britain, the computer software industry is not governed by censorship laws, though many large manufacturers have adopted their own voluntary cinema-style ratings. In general, these ratings distinguish between games that are suitable for children and those that are 'adults only'. They may also give a brief description of the situation that each game depicts. For further information and advice, contact The National Council for Educational Technology, 3 Devonshire Street, London WIN 2BA.

Finally, remember that a child's outlook is shaped far more by parents and home than by anything in the media. If you show what you approve of and what you don't, your child is unlikely to be seriously affected, even if he or she is exposed to unpleasant material.

LIMITING TELEVISION

Apart from the negative effects of violent or disturbing programmes, are there any other reasons to limit the amount of television a child watches?

Yes, plenty. Many television programmes do little to stimulate a child's imagination or ability to amuse himself. Watching television is generally a passive, solitary activity that reduces interaction with other family members and friends. Children who watch a lot of television are less likely to read or have hobbies, may not perform as well at school, and sometimes also miss out on play, conversation, sports and other activities.

Encourage your children to be selective about what they watch on television. You may want to limit their viewing to two or three programmes a day, in which case allow them to choose the programmes. Try to watch television with your children so you can discuss what they watch afterwards.

Too much television can be physically harmful too. Children who spend many hours watching tend to get less fresh air and exercise, eat more junk food and are more likely to become obese. Prolonged viewing at close range can also damage eyesight.

EPILEPSY AND COMPUTERS

I have heard that computer games can trigger epileptic fits in some children. How common is this? Are there warning signs?

This is a rare condition, affecting fewer than one child in 4000. Victims tend to be between nine and fifteen, and girls are more affected than boys. Some children show warning signs such as headaches, irritability, lethargy or a general 'odd' sensation before a convulsion, but usually there is no warning.

Any form of flashing light, whether from a television screen, computer game, strobe light or flickering sunlight can trigger an attack. Even geometric patterns have been known to bring on a fit.

CAUTION Never ignore a convulsion in a child (or an adult). Make sure you seek medical help immediately.

Talking about difficult subjects

EXPLAINING SEX

At four, my daughter seems too young for a full discussion of the facts of life, but she has started to ask where babies come from. What sort of explanation should I give?

Give as complete an explanation as she can understand and shows interest in. She is not too young – this is the age when children become curious and you can capitalise on this. If you answer her questions honestly and straightforwardly, you give her the best chance of developing a healthy and matter-of-fact attitude to sex. If you don't answer her questions, she will almost certainly pick up information (probably wrong) elsewhere.

Be guided by your daughter: answer her questions simply and don't be surprised if she loses interest in the details. Use the correct terms for parts of the body, and try to be as cheerful and unembarrassed as you would be explaining anything else. If you find it difficult, or if she is interested in the mechanics, buy a book designed for reading together (make sure you approve of its attitude). It is better to let sex education happen step-by-step along with everyday learning, than to sit down one day for a special session.

SEX EDUCATION AT SCHOOL

When will my children start having sex education at school and what form is it likely to take?

It all depends on the school. In the state-maintained sector, primary schools may offer sex education and secondary schools must do so and must tell parents of the arrangements. All schools must also have a written policy on sex education which parents have a right to see. The teaching is required to encompass moral considerations and family values, and to take account of parents' views. Parents may withdraw children from some or all of the lessons if they wish. In the private sector it is up to the individual school.

Ideally, children should learn the basics of sex and reproduction from their parents, but school sex education can be a valuable addition, especially if parents use the opportunity to discuss the issues again at home. There may be aspects you have missed or which children can talk about more easily among their peers. School discussions are also particularly useful for dispelling playground myths, which teachers may be more aware of than parents.

DANGER FROM STRANGERS

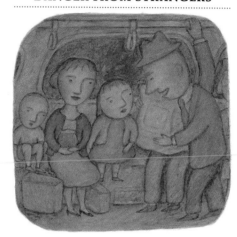

How can I warn my children about horrors such as child abuse without frightening them unnecessarily and making them suspicious of all strangers?

There is no need to scare children unduly, but a healthy suspicion of strangers is, unfortunately, no more than sensible. Instruct your children that unless you specifically give your permission, they must never go anywhere with a stranger or accept presents or treats from people they do not know.

The best way to deal with the subject of sexual abuse is as part of general discussions about bodies and sex. Explain calmly that genitals are private, which is why people keep them clothed in public. Tell children that they have the right to say no to any physical contact that they don't like, even if the person is an authority figure or a relative. Remember that although 98 per cent of abusers are male, boys and girls are equally vulnerable to abuse.

Signs that can indicate sexual abuse include anal injury or pain, vaginal discharge, disturbed or regressive behaviour, disturbed sleep or an unusual awareness of sexual acts. These symptoms can all have other causes, too, so never jump to conclusions. If, after talking patiently and calmly with a child, you suspect abuse, consult a doctor, who will put you in contact with a social worker.

Puberty: how parents can help

Some simple tips can help to smooth this difficult transition.

● Discuss physical changes, sexual relationships and contraception well before puberty.

● Be open and honest, encourage questions, and allay any anxieties.

● Be positive so that you instil confidence not insecurity or fear.

● Reassure teenagers that although they develop at different rates, they'll all be equal in the end.

● Avoid making insensitive or patronising remarks, and don't tease.

● Be gentle with adolescent moodiness and rebellion, and try to remain a source of friendly security.

● Avoid arguing or laying down the law, but set firm limits where necessary.

● Don't be afraid to express your own opinions and needs (for politeness, for example).

EXPLAINING DEATH

My mother has just died. Should we take our six-year-old son to the funeral and how should we explain what has happened?

Take your son if he really wants to go, but otherwise not. If he does choose to go, explain what is likely to happen and have someone there to answer questions and take him home if he becomes upset.

Explain to your son that granny has died and will not be coming back. Unless he has experienced death before – perhaps the death of a pet – he may not understand its permanence. It is a good idea to stress that most people die after a long life. Don't refer to death as 'going to sleep' or you may cause fears about falling asleep.

Children sometimes feel responsible for a relative's death. In such a case, reassure your son that this was not connected with anything he did, said or thought. Don't try to force him to grieve, but do acknowledge his feelings and encourage him to talk about his grandmother and keep photographs or other mementos if he wishes. Try not to overwhelm him with your grief, but admit to being sad or missing your mother.

PREPARING FOR PERIODS

When should I talk to my daughter about periods? How should I prepare her for them?

It is best to explain about menstruation, to both boys and girls, as part of general discussions about sex and reproduction. In any case, make sure your daughter knows about puberty and has any questions about periods answered before the age of nine, as some girls do start this early.

Explain that she will bleed for a few days and will need to wear some kind of protection, and that although her periods may be irregular and infrequent at first, they will gradually settle into a cycle. Show her what sanitary towels and tampons look like and explain how to use them.

Ask your daughter what she already knows so that you can dispel any myths. Never refer to menstruation as 'the curse' or suggest that it might prevent her from playing sport or taking part in other activities. Explain that some women have discomfort, but that there are plenty of remedies, such as simple painkillers. Most importantly, be positive about it yourself and she will be too.

TEENAGE SEX

My 15-year-old daughter has a 'steady' boyfriend and I'm worried they might have sex. How can I convey my feelings to her?

Try talking about *her* feelings rather than yours. She may be confused or worried and a chat could be reassuring for both of you.

If she intends to have sex (or has already done so), the greatest danger is from ignorance – not knowing the facts or where to seek advice. Make sure she understands about contraception and 'safe sex' (see pages 258-260). This won't encourage her to have sex, but will encourage a responsible attitude towards it. Many teenage girls also need reassurance about saying no to sex, so stress that she should wait until she feels ready and that a boyfriend who cares will not put pressure on her. Talk about the relationship between sex and emotions, and discuss the potential pitfalls (physical and emotional) of becoming sexually involved too early.

Remember that while you can tell her your feelings, you cannot stop your daughter having sex – you can only be supportive and try to ensure that she is well informed, confident and able to assert herself. You may also want to remind her that it is illegal to have sex before the age of 16.

A fulfilling family life

EXPLAINING A NEW BABY

I am pregnant with our second child. How should I prepare our two-year-old son?

Even very young children can cope well with change if they have time to get used to the idea and feel involved. Explain the pregnancy and encourage your son to feel the baby move. Make it clear that you love him as much as before. Prepare him for living with a baby, but emphasise things that will stay the same, rather than ones that will change. Introduce any changes, such as moving bedrooms, well before the baby's arrival. Avoid major steps close to the birth – put off starting playschool or toilet training, for example, for a little longer. After the

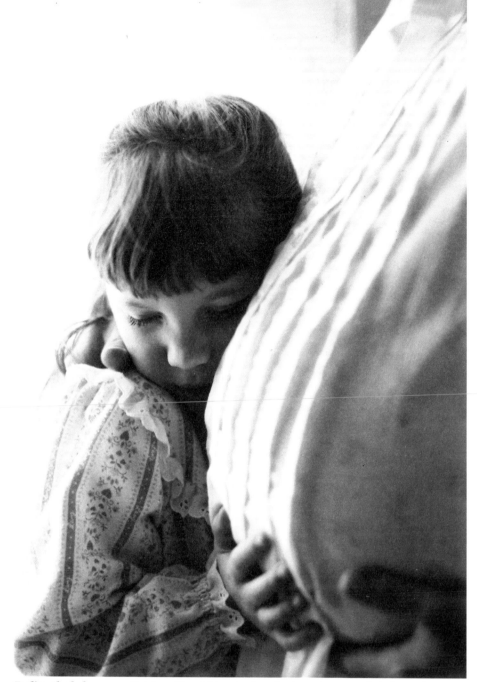

Feeling the baby move Helping older children to share in the excitement of a baby on the way can prevent jealousy later. Make sure to be extra loving and understanding after the baby is born.

birth, give your son plenty of love and attention. Have some small presents ready for him for when visitors arrive with presents for the baby. Encourage everyone to pay as much attention to him as to the baby.

It is possible that your son may regress a little, perhaps wanting a bottle again. Accept this lovingly and don't comment on it. Try to involve him with the baby: let him help with nappy-changing or read to him during feeds. Encourage any signs of wanting to help or hold the baby – just make sure he is sitting on a soft floor.

ONLY CHILDREN

We have a three-year-old daughter and aren't planning to have any more children. How will being an only child affect our little girl? Is there anything we can do to make it easier?

Only children often fare better than popular belief would have it. They tend to get more attention, have high self-esteem, be more secure and are often materially better off. They are usually mature, comfortable with adults, good leaders. Like firstborns, they are generally more intelligent and more likely to get ahead in life than average. However, they can also become isolated, overdependent on approval from authority figures, self-conscious, over-serious and lacking in confidence in mixing with other children. As parents, you can do a great deal to prevent such problems.

● Make sure your daughter has plenty of contact with other children.
● If she is not going to playschool, consider enrolling her.
● Encourage her to take responsibility for herself, to take initiatives and to develop interests that do not involve you.
● Be careful about projecting too many of your hopes and ambitions onto her.
● Let her express her feelings about not having brothers and sisters, but don't make it a major issue.
● Try not to make it always seem like two big people versus one little one. Try to encourage some activities she can share with parents individually.

STAY-AT-HOME STRESS

I gave up work when my second child was born and, although I don't want to go back, I do find it stressful being at home with small children all day. How can I cope better with the situation?

Being at home all day with only young children for company *is* stressful. Full-time work provides a structure, not only to each day, but to weeks and months. When you are at home all day, any kind of framework disappears and everything that happens requires initiative and energy from you. Try to remind yourself of all the changes that have occurred, and don't blame the children.

Getting out of the house and seeing other people is important to maintain your self-esteem and confidence. Join a local mothers-and-toddlers group, or organise a weekly meeting with a group of friends, either with or without children. Make some time to pursue a hobby or interest, and find someone to help with the children regularly – perhaps a weekly childcare swap with another mother. If your children have a daytime nap, use the time to do something you enjoy rather than catching up on chores. If they are older, start a routine 'quiet time for mummy' for half an hour – or more – each day. Get your partner to take over for a while each evening so that you also have an opportunity to relax.

DIVORCE AND CHILDREN

How does divorce affect children?

Most children are unsettled by divorce for at least two years. However, there is no evidence that they are more likely to be delinquent or maladjusted, and with supportive parents they can end up coping very well. Most children long for their parents to get back together, and this desire prolongs the adjustment period.

Initially, young children (up to five or six years) may regress in behaviour, may have nightmares or difficulty sleeping, become weepy and clingy, and are often terrified of being abandoned by the remaining parent. Older children may feel depressed and lonely, have psychosomatic symptoms such as headaches, feel conflicts of loyalty between parents, be more demanding, aggressive or quarrelsome, and tend to drop back on schoolwork. Adolescents vary in their reactions, from sadness to anger to aggression, and may take sides.

Children of all ages tend to blame themselves for the split. As they enter adolescence and adult life, they may worry about making the same mistakes. Their concern is justified – children of divorced parents are less likely to make a stable relationship and more likely to divorce themselves.

SINGLE-PARENT FAMILIES

Do children in single-parent families face special problems?

Yes, but they need not be insurmountable. It is better for a child to be brought up by one happy, loving, supportive parent, than two resentful, neglectful ones. However, life for most single parents is hard – practically, emotionally and financially – and at times this is bound to affect the child.

Apart from material difficulties, single parents generally have less time and energy to spare, and lack support in dealing with conflicts and discipline. Parents on their own may be under more personal pressure, including loneliness, and this sometimes leads to an unhealthy emotional dependence on the child. There may be difficulties with things the child or parent would prefer to be done by the absent parent (telling a daughter about periods, for example). Some single parents cannot help resenting the burden of sole childcare, and children too may feel resentful or guilty about sacrifices made on their behalf.

On the positive side, many single parents try specially hard and develop particularly close, rewarding relationships with their offspring. Children are often quick to acquire a strong sense of responsibility to feel particularly valued as a family member.

MORE TIME TOGETHER

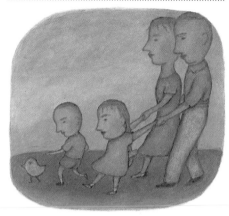

We're all so busy that we seldom seem to have much time together as a family. How can we make the most of the time we have?

Make sure that you set aside some regular time for the whole family, however little, and make it a priority: five minutes a day for a family chat, a weekly outing, or a special mid-week family supper night. Have some time when every member of the family can tell the others what has been happening in their life, and raise any concerns. Encourage open communication on all issues and try to resolve problems early.

Make the most of activities where you can share a chat, such as cooking and gardening. Arrange regular small treats and keep mementos and photographs of special occasions. If you cannot all be together, make social arrangements between individual family members. Try to give each child some individual parental attention every day.

Most of all, when you are together, enjoy one another's company and don't spend the time discussing work or domestic problems.

HOW FAMILIES CHANGE

Are there set patterns and stages in family life or is each family different?

It is not a simple either/or situation. Every family does indeed have its own unique patterns of behaviour and its own stages of development. And yet, many psychologists do believe that there is a certain lifecycle

that most families will go through, although the time spent in each stage varies widely.

Most couples start life together intending to have children within a few years. As time passes, they may come under pressure from relatives as well. When the first child is born a new, highly demanding stage begins, the first as a family rather than a couple. Despite the joy that a baby usually brings, people are often unprepared for all the responsibilities, and many report feeling overwhelmed and exhausted in the early years.

As children grow, parents acquire new responsibilities – to impose authority, make rules and, when school starts, to help youngsters to understand and deal with experiences outside the home. Adolescence brings yet another set of demands as parents have not only to confront their children's independence but very often to face rigorous scrutiny themselves. Despite the difficulties, however, many parents enjoy the teenager stage. Many also report growing closer as couples, a tendency that continues into the stages of children leaving home, retirement and, possibly, grandparenthood.

Although the stage theory is useful for explaining how families change, its weakness is that it really applies only to traditional families. With the varied range of lifestyles in contemporary society, many family arrangements fall beyond its scope.

FAMILY THERAPY

I have heard of families having counselling together. What sort of help is likely to be given and how does a family qualify?

Family counselling is very similar to couple counselling – perhaps noisier. All family members, or various combinations, see the counsellor together to air grievances, discuss the way the family functions and explore interactions between different members.

Counselling can help almost any problem causing disharmony in the family, such as marital conflicts (including affairs), child behaviour problems, a death in the family, separation, divorce and difficulties adjusting to single, shared or step-parenting.

Your doctor may be able to refer you to a counsellor, or you can contact Relate (see page 183) or a counselling organisation such as the British Association for Counselling, 1 Regent's Place, Rugby CV21 2PJ.

A safe place to learn

Families are ideal learning environments for children, but striking the right balance between protection and experimentation is not always easy. Experts offer this advice to parents.

- Encourage natural curiosity.
- Let children do what they can unaided.
- Don't forbid anything without good reason, and explain why.
- Supervise discreetly.
- Emphasise personal responsibility.
- Explain risks but don't exaggerate or overreact to minor mishaps.

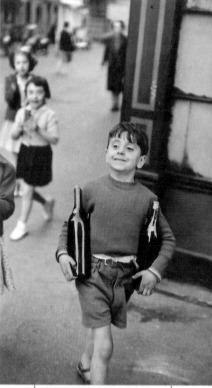

Early exposure Alcohol is a regular part of family life in some cultures. If parents are responsible, children can learn to be, too.

A SAFER HOME AND A SAFER WORLD

*Every breath of air you inhale and every
sip of water you swallow can affect your health.
The way you heat your home, the products you buy for
it and the kind of transport you use affect the environment
as well. By giving proper thought to these matters,
we can all enjoy a safer way of life.*

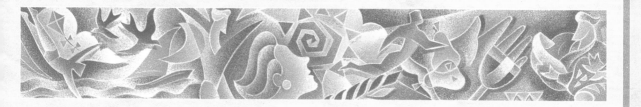

Do you know how to keep yourself safe?

A clean, safe environment can protect your physical and mental health – and a polluted or hazardous one can damage it. A realistic idea of the risks and what you can do about them should be part of everyone's general knowledge. To test your knowledge, tick the right answer for each question and check your score.

1 Where should you fit a smoke detector in a house?

a) On each floor. ☐
b) In the kitchen. ☐
c) At the bottom of the stairs. ☐

2 How long should you air a room after having a new carpet laid?

a) Several days. ☐
b) A few hours. ☐
c) Overnight. ☐

3 Which is more likely to pose a health risk?

a) Water that runs cloudy from the tap. ☐
b) Water that has run through lead piping in an older house. ☐
c) Water with added fluoride. ☐

4 How much are a child's chances of developing asthma affected if one or both parents smoke?

a) Not at all. ☐
b) The risk is slightly increased, but not enough to worry about. ☐
c) The risk is doubled. ☐

5 Which pests are least likely to bring germs into the house?

a) Mice. ☐
b) Cockroaches. ☐
c) Ants. ☐

6 What should you do if you are caught in an electrical storm?

a) Shelter in your car. ☐
b) Stand under a tall tree. ☐
c) Lie down flat on the ground. ☐

7 Which will not reduce pollution from your car?

a) Regular servicing. ☐
b) Letting the engine idle for a couple of minutes if you are stuck in traffic instead of turning the ignition off and on. ☐
c) Fitting radial tyres. ☐

8 Which common plant is poisonous?

a) Amaryllis. ☐
b) African violet. ☐
c) Rubber plant. ☐

9 Which provides the better protection in a motor accident?

a) A seat belt. ☐
b) An air bag. ☐
c) Seat belts and air bags provide equally good protection. ☐

10 What is the best distance for working at a computer screen?

a) 6-14 in (15-36 cm). ☐
b) 14-24 in (36-61 cm). ☐
c) 24-30 in (61-76 cm). ☐

SCORING

Award yourself 1 point for each of these answers: 1(a), 2(a), 3(b), 4(c), 5(c), 6(a), 7(b), 8(a), 9(a) and 10(b). Add up your score.

8-10: You know a lot about what's safe and what's not, and are probably helping to look after the planet, as well as your own health. Even so you may find some surprises in the pages that follow.

7 or less: Learning more about the environment could help you to lead a healthier, safer life. This chapter shows how.

The air we breathe

WHAT IS OZONE?

We are constantly being told to protect the ozone layer, but then I hear that ozone is bad for us. What is ozone, and does it help or harm us?

Ozone is a form of poisonous oxygen created naturally in the atmosphere. It both protects and harms us. Above the Earth a 'layer' of ozone shields us from dangerous ultraviolet radiation. But at ground level too much ozone can harm human and animal health, and can damage plants and trees. Pollution from vehicles, power stations, industry, agriculture and even our homes increases the harmful concentrations of ozone at ground level. Meanwhile the use of chlorofluorocarbons (CFCs) in refrigerators, solvents and propellants damages the ozone layer, making us more vulnerable to skin cancers.

Ozone could turn out to have another influence upon our health: it is one of the 'greenhouse gases' which are thought to play a part in global warming (see page 305).

RISKS FROM THE AIR

I have heard so many scare-stories in the media about air pollution. Is our air really safe to breathe?

Governments throughout Europe are trying to clean the air by tightening controls upon vehicle exhaust fumes, industrial smoke and other pollutants. However, many people in the Western world still breathe a bewildering number of pollutants that are bad for health. Common pollutants include:

● Carbon monoxide – from sources, such as car exhausts, the burning of fossil fuels and tobacco smoke.
● Lead – from leaded petrol and some industrial processes.
● Nitrogen oxides – from power stations, traffic, heating plants, industrial processes and unvented gas appliances.
● Sulphur dioxide – from burning fuel such as coal and oil.
● Particulates – also called 'suspended particulate matter'. They include coal and diesel smoke, fine ash, land dust and sulphates (which come mainly from burning coal and oil).

● Volatile organic compounds – VOCs contain carbon and come from exhaust fumes, synthetic materials (such building materials including chipboard), household and industrial chemicals (such as solvents, wood preservatives and wall insulation), and cigarette smoke.

Research has shown that even low concentrations of these pollutants can irritate the eyes, nose and throat. Exposure to heavily polluted air can cause or aggravate respiratory and cardio-vascular diseases, cause lung damage, cancer and, in some circumstances, even lead to sudden death.

Although you cannot do a great deal to control what you breathe, you can protect yourself to some extent. Avoid walking or cycling near heavy traffic whenever you can find an alternative route or a different time for your journey. If this is impossible, try wearing a face mask that fits snugly. Whichever type you choose, make sure that you change, replace or wash the filter regularly, according to the type of mask and the manufacturer's instructions, otherwise you will breathe in higher concentrations of trapped pollutants. Until you cross a road, keep away from the kerb where exhaust fumes are strongest. Don't do any strenuous exercise in heavily congested areas on still, warm days.

A simple health precaution A cyclist's mask filters traffic exhaust fumes, helping to prevent harmful particles from causing or irritating respiratory complaints.

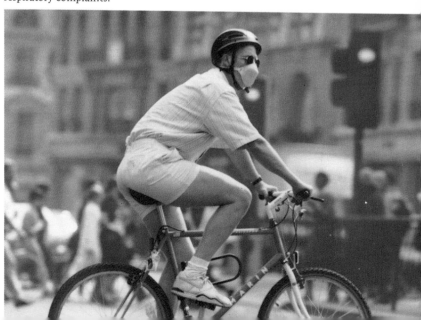

DANGER FROM SMOG

A smoky haze sometimes hangs over my home. What causes this, and is it a danger to health?

This is photochemical 'smog' – a word suggesting the combination of smoke, fumes and fog that you describe. It occurs on still, sunny days when traffic exhaust fumes and other pollutants – from industrial processes and the burning of coal, oil and gas – react with sunlight to create ozone (see page 303). Similar air pollution can also occur on calm, cold days in winter, when pollutants are trapped at ground level by a layer of cold air above. As in summer, the main culprit is vehicle exhaust fumes, but the burning of fossil fuels also plays a part. Even small amounts of smog can cause eye, nose and throat irritation. Asthma sufferers and people with other respiratory ailments, or with a heart or lung condition, can be especially vulnerable. The Department of the Environment provides daily reports about air quality and issues warnings when it expects the quality to be poor. You can listen to a daily recording, free of charge, by calling 0800 55667. Some weather forecasts include a report about air quality.

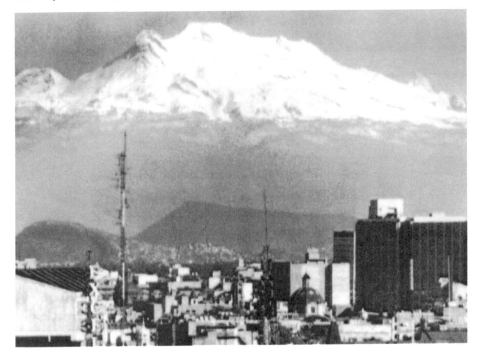

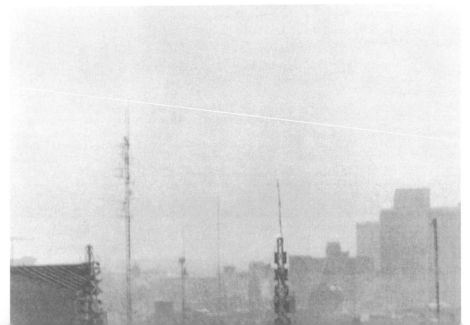

The vanishing city Smog frequently smothers Mexico City, one of the world's most polluted capitals, veiling buildings and mountains and damaging its inhabitants' health. These photographs were taken just three days apart.

GLOBAL WARMING

What is 'the greenhouse effect' and how harmful is it to our wellbeing?

Over the past 200 years an increase in the world's population, industrialisation and other human activities have upset the balance of gases, such as carbon dioxide, nitrous oxide, ozone and methane, in the Earth's atmosphere. These gases act rather like the glass in a greenhouse, allowing the sunlight through and trapping the heat inside. Many scientists fear that an increase in temperature of just a few degrees world-wide could alter regional and seasonal weather patterns, causing crops to fail, droughts, an increase in sea level and the death of some species of animals and plants.

Many governments are trying to reduce atmospheric damage by reducing pollutants, such as vehicle exhaust fumes, that are known to harm humans, animals and plants. Attempts are also being made to reduce the destruction of the world's forests, which produce oxygen and help to 'absorb' carbon dioxide.

DO TREES CLEAN THE AIR?

My daughter thinks that planting more trees in our garden would make our air cleaner. Is this true?

Trees have justifiably been called the Earth's 'lungs'. They produce oxygen, take in carbon dioxide – a major pollutant – and filter harmful particles, such as those from diesel vehicles. Although you would need to plant on a massive scale to make a noticeable improvement in the air quality around your home, every tree makes a small contribution to human health. Trees can also improve our mood and general wellbeing, while feeding and sheltering wildlife.

THE DANGER OF EXHAUST FUMES

What is in petrol exhaust fumes and what harm can they do?

Petrol exhaust fumes include a number of gases and particles that are known or believed to cause health problems. The main ones are:

CARBON MONOXIDE A gas that takes the place of oxygen in your lungs and blood and can be toxic. Even low levels have been known to cause headaches and problems with vision and coordination.

NITROGEN OXIDES Gases that contribute to ozone pollution. They can also cause eye, nose and throat irritation, as well as respiratory problems.

LEAD A metal (see page 320) that can damage the brain and nervous system, and may cause learning problems for children.

HYDROCARBONS Gases from sources such as petrol exhaust fumes that can be poisonous in their own right and also contribute to harmful ground-level ozone (see page 303).

STOPPING DIRTY FACTORIES

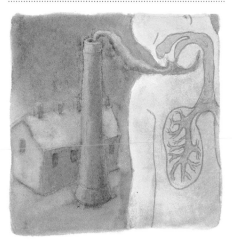

My father has a wheezy chest, which seemed to start when a new factory opened nearby. It produces a lot of smoke, and I wonder whether there could be a link with his poor health?

There could be. Although emissions from power stations and chemical works are regulated and monitored, factory chimneys can send out a variety of compounds and gases, such as sulphur dioxide, that can increase the risk of bronchitis, can make asthmatics more prone to attack and can contribute to a range of lung infections.

Tell the factory about your father's problem and ask what is in the chimney smoke. The information should help your father's doctor to treat his symptoms.

If the factory is uncooperative, or if you need more information, contact the environmental health department at your local council. The environmental health officers (EHOs) will investigate whether the factory is complying with clean air legislation, give you advice about the health implications and, if appropriate, tell you how to make a formal complaint. Advice is also available from your regional office of Her Majesty's Inspectorate of Pollution.

AIRCRAFT EMISSIONS

We live a few miles from a busy airport. Is our health at risk from aircraft exhaust or fuel dumping?

There is no greater risk from air pollution if you live close to an airport than if you live farther away. Aircraft exhaust fumes *are* thought to play a part in global warming because they contain the 'greenhouse' gases carbon dioxide and nitrous oxide. However, the designs for new jet engines have greatly increased fuel efficiency and reduced the amount of fuel released from the aircraft.

In an emergency, aeroplanes occasionally do have to jettison fuel to reduce weight before landing. If fuel dumping becomes necessary, pilots are instructed to try to do so at sufficient height and distance from the airport to cause little or no immediate environmental impact.

Air quality at home

FACT
— OR —
FALLACY?

'Houseplants and cut flowers should be taken out of the bedroom at night.'

Fallacy Although plants release carbon dioxide into the atmosphere at night, a few plants or cut flowers in a bedroom are unlikely to hamper your breathing or cause any other health problem. In large numbers, plants and trees do affect the air we breathe – but generally speaking they are beneficial rather than harmful. In fact, plants and trees are the Earth's main source of oxygen, which they release during daylight hours. They also *absorb* carbon dioxide, one of the greenhouse gases (see page 305), during the day, so helping to ease air pollution.

HOW DUST AFFECTS HEALTH

What is household dust, and how does it affect health?

House-dust can be a health hazard, triggering allergies and aggravating respiratory diseases, such as asthma (see page 350). Dust in the home consists of large quantities of human skin cells, dust mites that live on the skin cells, the mites' droppings, and tiny particles of pollen, minerals, mould and bacterial spores. Household dust can also contain toxic substances from outside, such as lead, asbestos fibres or pesticide residues, which are bad for your health if inhaled in large quantities. To keep dust under control:

● Dust regularly, using a damp cloth, to avoid spreading the dust elsewhere.
● Use a high-efficiency vacuum cleaner that does not blow dust back into the air.

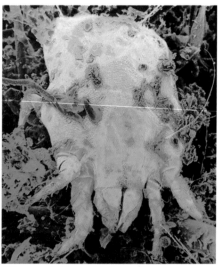

Microscopic hazard A dust mite scavenges among dead skin scales, cat fur and soil.

● Choose blankets and other bed linen that you can wash regularly at temperatures above 58°C (136°F) to kill dust mites and neutralise their droppings.
● Encase your mattresses and pillows in special covers that keep mites and their droppings out.
● Keep rooms well-aired.
● Wash toys regularly, and place them in a freezer overnight to kill the mites.

PASSIVE SMOKING

My husband is a fairly heavy smoker. Are his cigarettes putting the rest of the family at risk?

Yes – unfortunately you and the rest of your family are 'passive smokers', who breathe in your husband's tobacco smoke. While he inhales about 15 per cent of his cigarette smoke, the remaining 85 per cent goes into the atmosphere where you cannot escape breathing it.

You will have to decide on the most effective approach to stop your husband from smoking – you might at least dissuade him from smoking in the same room as you or the children. The following few facts might help your case:

● Babies exposed to cigarettes are more likely to get bronchitis or pneumonia or die from Sudden Infant Death Syndrome.
● Passive smoking doubles children's risk of developing asthma and increases the severity of asthma symptoms.
● Children who are passive smokers are more likely to suffer chronic respiratory disease and cancer as adults.
● Pregnant women exposed to tobacco smoke are more likely to have babies of below-average weight.

KEEPING THE AIR MOIST

The central heating at home seems to make the air dry and my wife often gets a headache. What can we do about this?

Try saving your central heating for very cold weather. Whenever possible use radiant heat sources, such as fan heaters, electric, gas or solid fuel fires. When you have to turn on the central heating, hang humidifying reservoirs from the radiators – as the radiators heat up, the water evaporates, helping the air to stay moist. Keep plenty of plants around the house. If you water them regularly, the evaporation from the leaves and the soil will humidify the air. Another simple remedy is to place shallow bowls of water around the house. You could also consider buying an electric humidifier, but these can be expensive to run and can incubate bacteria if not maintained properly.

A NUISANCE FROM BONFIRES

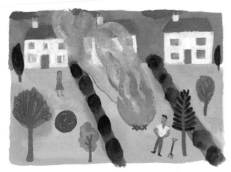

I cannot sit in my garden on some evenings because of smoke from a bonfire in the garden next door. Is there anything I can do about it?

Explain the problem to your neighbours, asking them to avoid still evenings when smoke tends to 'hang around'. If the chat does not solve the problem, contact one of your local council's environmental health officers. They can give advice and check whether the bonfires are a health hazard or a statutory 'nuisance', and determine whether they break pollution regulations or could endanger traffic. Environmental health officers have a range of powers to deal with bonfires and, if necessary, they will take your neighbours to court. You can also obtain information and advice on bonfires and all aspects of air pollution from the National Society for Clean Air and Environmental Protection, 136 North Street, Brighton BN1 1RG. If you have a bonfire yourself, try to avoid weekends and bank holidays when neighbours are more likely to be in their gardens, and don't burn on days when the air quality is already poor.

LIVING NEAR TRAFFIC

We have been house hunting for months and have at last found our ideal family home. It is very close to a busy crossroads and I'm worried about the effect it may have on our health. Should we move there?

It is likely that traffic pollution will be highest near a busy intersection, because cars release more fumes when they stop and start. Traffic pollution is also high when tall buildings trap exhaust fumes along the street.

If you have young children, or are planning a family, you might be wise to consider a house in an area that is less traffic-clogged. The very young, the elderly, and people with a history of heart or lung disease are particularly vulnerable to traffic pollution. In the end, however, only you can weigh the advantages of your dream home against the possible risks from traffic fumes.

BALANCING THE IONS

I've heard that ionisers significantly improve indoor air quality, but I don't want to waste money on a gimmick. Will an ioniser improve my family's health?

There is no clear answer to this question. Many people who use home ionisers say that they are particularly helpful in relieving chest and lung problems. They are also said to help to prevent headaches, migraine, irritable moods, and hay fever. However, many doctors are sceptical that they have any beneficial effect at all.

Ioniser manufacturers say that ionisers work by changing the balance of negative and positive ions (electrically charged particles) in the air. The proportion of positive ions can be increased by electrical fields from television sets, computers and other electrical appliances, by static from synthetic fabrics, by polluted or dry air, and by atmospheric changes before a thunderstorm. It is this increase in positive ions that is blamed for health problems. An ioniser is supposed to charge the air with a high voltage that increases the level of negative ions. However, independent tests in 1992 showed that some ionisers did not produce many ions, nor project them far around a room. Nonetheless, most models cleared tobacco smoke quickly.

DO'S AND DON'TS

for improving the air in your home

Do air rooms frequently: open a window for a while even on cold days.

Do install an extractor fan in the kitchen, and possibly in the bathroom, to take away steam and odours.

Do grow plenty of house plants, especially those which are believed to filter toxic gases, such as formaldehyde from the air. Such plants include spider plants, golden pothos, various types of ficus (fig plants) and chrysanthemums.

Do choose natural fibres, such as cotton, linen and wool, for your clothes and furnishings wherever possible, because synthetic fabrics have been linked to health problems caused by a disturbance in the balance of positive and negative ions.

Do make sure you switch off electrical equipment when it is not in use, to help to maintain the balance of negative and positive ions.

Do put small bowls of water in rooms that do not have any pot plants. This will help to keep the air moist and decrease the positive ions in the atmosphere.

Do have gas appliances professionally checked at least once every year, to prevent any build-up of poisonous carbon monoxide fumes.

Don't overheat your home so that the air becomes dry.

Climate and weather

Fact A sea breeze is certainly refreshing and invigorating, and air quality on the coast is often better than in traffic-clogged cities and industrial areas. Sea and mountain air is rich in negative ions, electrically charged air particles (see page 307). Research suggests that negative ions may have a stimulating, beneficial effect, while too many positive ions may have a depressing effect.

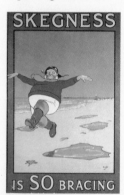

Bouncing with health
Railway companies promoted train services in the 1930s by emphasising the health benefits of the sea.

BEATING WINTER BLUES

I often feel down in the dumps and lethargic in winter. Is this normal, and can I do anything to beat this winter mood?

You are not the only person to feel slightly depressed in the cold, dark days of winter. You may have a mild case of a condition called 'seasonal affective disorder' (SAD). Typical symptoms include sleeping as much as an extra two hours each night, eating extra sweets and starchy foods, losing interest in sex and feeling listless, demotivated and bored. It seems that the problems are triggered by shorter, darker days and vanish during the brighter days of spring. People with severe symptoms are usually treated by daily exposure to a very strong light.

You can help to overcome your winter blues by spending some time each day in bright light. Switch on more lights. If possible, move your desk at work and your dining table at home closer to a window. Get outdoors as often as you can and, if you can afford it, consider taking a short winter holiday somewhere in the sun. Even wearing brightly coloured clothes may help.

SAFETY FROM LIGHTNING

How much danger am I in if there is lightning during a storm?

Two or three people a year are killed in Britain by lightning, but if you remember some simple precautions, you are unlikely to become one of these victims.

If possible, stay indoors during electrical storms. Unplug the television/video recorder and unplug the aerial. Keep away from the windows. Lightning tends to strike the highest points, so if you are outside keep away from tall trees and avoid high ground. If you are caught in the open, you could lie flat on the ground until the storm passes. Don't fly a kite, or ride a bike or horse. If you need to shelter, try to avoid a rocky outcrop where lightning could strike: the back of a deep cave is safe, however.

Metal conducts electricity, so don't stand near metal objects, such as iron fences, lampposts or golf clubs. However, do stay in a car: it is one of the safest places to be. If the vehicle is struck by lightning, the electricity will travel down the sides and be made safe by the car's rubber tyres. If you are swimming when an electrical storm starts, get out of the water as soon as possible.

HEALTH FROM MOUNTAIN AIR

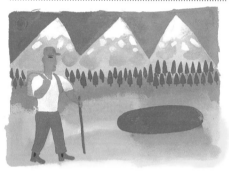

Friends who enjoy hiking say that mountain air can improve your health. Can this really be true?

Clean air and exercise are bound to help you to stay healthy and feel good. If your home is in or near a built-up area, a walk in mountains or even hills will let you breathe air that is much purer than the air you are used to – and you will feel invigorated. The proportion of negative ions (see page 307) in mountain air may also improve your sense of wellbeing. However, if mountain excursions take you over 7000 ft (2100 m) above sea level (for instance in parts of the Alps), you might have trouble breathing easily. At heights over 10000 ft (3000 m) above sea level (for instance the Himalayas in Nepal), you would certainly breathe heavily during exertion, and could be dangerous for anyone suffering from angina.

WINTER COLDS AND FLU

It seems that people catch more colds and flu in winter than in summer. Is this true, and if so, why?

Cases of influenza, other respiratory infections and colds do peak during winter months. These ailments are spread mainly by microscopic droplets of water vapour passed into the air every time we breathe out, and whenever we cough or sneeze. One sneeze propels up to 100000 bacteria into the air at about 200 mph (320 km/h).

People tend to crowd into warm places in cold weather, and often spend more time indoors with the windows closed, so germs are trapped in the air and are more easily passed between people. In summer people usually spend more time outdoors, and windows are thrown open, so the likelihood of contracting colds and flu diminishes.

HEALTH IN DAMP WEATHER

My father's chest complaint seems to be worse during wet weather. Should we try to dry out the air in his home?

Damp housing encourages the growth of mould and the proliferation of mites which can both aggravate chest complaints, so drying out the air in your father's home might well ease his problem: it would be wise to ask his doctor's advice.

You need to find a happy balance between keeping him warm, ventilating his rooms adequately and keeping the air at the right moisture level for his health. Many forms of home heating, such as gas and paraffin, produce a lot of moisture. Airing a room thoroughly in the winter months when heating is in use gets rid of most moisture – even opening a window for a short time each day will help. Your father can also help to fight chest problems by keeping warm, by eating a nutritious diet (see page 11) and by taking some exercise, such as short walks. If your father smokes, he should cut down or, better still, give up all together.

Acid rain

'Acid rain' is a form of pollution caused by acid gases, such as sulphur dioxide and nitrogen oxide, created mainly by traffic, power stations and industry. It can fall as rain, snow, hail, mist and airborne particles. 'Acid rain' can kill trees, plants and wildlife, threatening the whole food chain, and can damage stone buildings.

Clean water to drink

SAFE WATER IN YOUR HOME

Every so often there is a scare about water safety. Just how safe is it to drink water straight from the cold-water tap?

The sources of our drinking water – rivers and natural underground reservoirs – are constantly threatened by pollution from weedkillers, fertilisers and industrial chemicals and metals. However, the water companies in Britain must comply with strict regulations for filtering and disinfecting water before it reaches your home or workplace, so cold tap water direct from the mains is completely safe to drink. It is not advisable to drink water from a hot-water tap. While cold water is piped from the mains, the supply for hot water is stored in a tank in your building and can be polluted by dust, rust, insects or animal droppings.

There are tight legal limits on the amounts of various harmful bacteria, chemicals, metals and other substances that are acceptable in water, and the water companies must test the water regularly and record the results. You have a legal right to inspect the results, but the information is not easy to understand unless you are an expert. If you have any concerns about the safety of your drinking water, you might prefer to contact one of the organisations that can also arrange to have your water supply tested. Speak to your local council's environmental health department or, in England and Wales, contact a customer services committee for water (look in the telephone directory under 'Water'). In Northern Ireland, contact the water executive at the Department of the Environment Information Office.

USING A WATER FILTER

What are the advantages of using a water filter at home?

Tap water from the mains is safe to drink, but many people prefer to remove any minute traces of chemicals, metals and other substances that can legally be left in the water. Whichever filtration system you choose, you must replace the filter according to the manufacturer's instructions, to avoid contaminating the water with harmful bacteria. The three main types of filter are:

● Activated carbon filters (including the cheap jug systems), which are said to remove traces of chlorine (used to purify the water), pesticides and some organic chemicals. They cannot remove fluoride or nitrates. Filters with a carbon block may remove traces of heavy metals, such as lead.
● Distillation units are said to remove most contaminants, but the purified water can taste rather bland.
● Reverse osmosis systems are said to remove virtually all chemicals and minerals, including calcium and magnesium that are good for health.

Plumbed-in filter systems are initially more expensive, but are cheaper in the long run.

FACT —— OR —— FALLACY?

'Bottled waters are purer than tap water.

Fallacy Recent research shows that many bottled waters contain more harmful bacteria than tap water. What is more, 'mineral' water generally contains levels of minerals no higher than tap water, while some 'table' waters are bottled straight from the tap. Bottled waters will not improve your health, so you should drink them only because you prefer the taste.

How water reaches your home

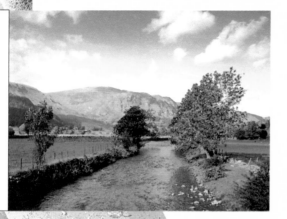

CLEAN water to drink is essential for life and for good health. We take our supplies for granted but the water that comes out of our taps is the end product of some highly sophisticated processes in nearly 1800 water treatment plants throughout Britain.

The plants are managed and maintained by a number of regional water companies, which continually test and monitor their own supplies. Independent tests are also carried out by the Drinking Water Inspectorate and other government bodies to ensure consistent nationwide standards.

1 SCREENING
A filter in the form of a giant sieve removes large floating debris such as leaves and twigs from the river.

Granular activated carbon (GAC) filter
This powerful new design uses a mix of coal, wood and peat that looks like black sand. Urban supplies are often filtered by GAC.

Settlement
Contaminants settle at the bottom of the tank, leaving the water above cleaner and ready to be drawn off for the next stage.

2 STORAGE
After screening, water is stored until needed. Reservoirs are kept as full as possible in case a drought occurs.

Sedimentation
Bands of impurities form in the middle of a funnel-shaped tank when water is pumped in from below. The impurities are siphoned off separately, while the treated water flows over a weir at the top of the tank, and into an outlet pipe.

Fast sand filter
A bed of sand about 3 ft (1 m) thick traps remaining pollutants in water that has been chemically treated.

3 CHEMICAL TREATMENT
Added chemicals help to separate larger pollutants in one of three ways.

a SETTLEMENT

b or SEDIMENTATION

Clean water outlet

c or FLOTATION

Flotation
A water-and-air mixture is bubbled into the tank. The bubbles attract impurities and float to the surface as scum, leaving cleaner water ready to be drawn off below.

Water outlet

Water inlet

Dirt outlet

Air inlet

Water inlet

Clean water outlet

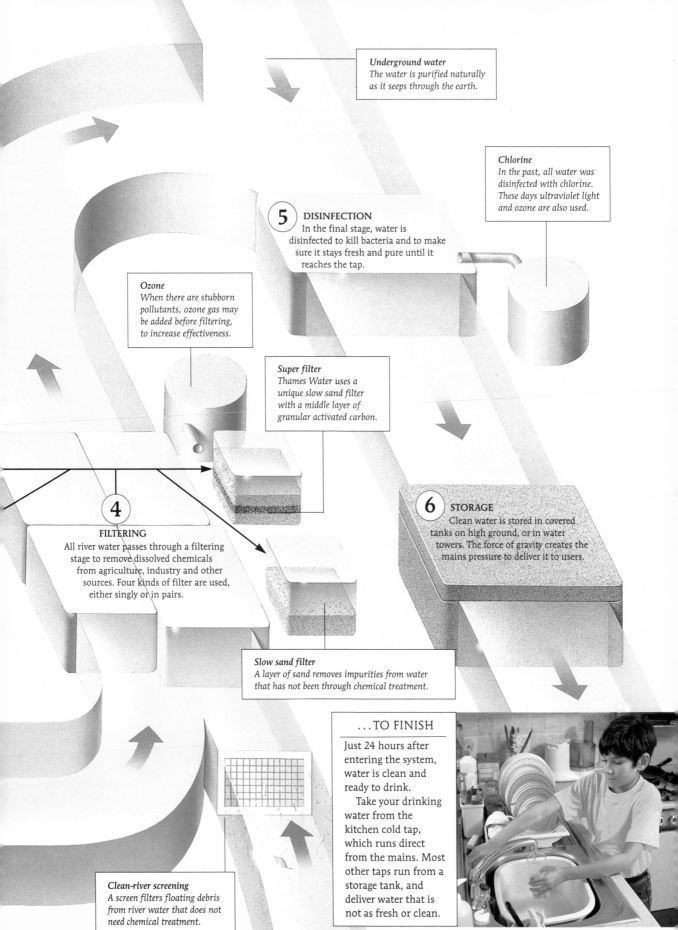

Underground water
The water is purified naturally as it seeps through the earth.

Chlorine
In the past, all water was disinfected with chlorine. These days ultraviolet light and ozone are also used.

5 DISINFECTION
In the final stage, water is disinfected to kill bacteria and to make sure it stays fresh and pure until it reaches the tap.

Ozone
When there are stubborn pollutants, ozone gas may be added before filtering, to increase effectiveness.

Super filter
Thames Water uses a unique slow sand filter with a middle layer of granular activated carbon.

4 FILTERING
All river water passes through a filtering stage to remove dissolved chemicals from agriculture, industry and other sources. Four kinds of filter are used, either singly or in pairs.

6 STORAGE
Clean water is stored in covered tanks on high ground, or in water towers. The force of gravity creates the mains pressure to deliver it to users.

Slow sand filter
A layer of sand removes impurities from water that has not been through chemical treatment.

...TO FINISH
Just 24 hours after entering the system, water is clean and ready to drink.

Take your drinking water from the kitchen cold tap, which runs direct from the mains. Most other taps run from a storage tank, and deliver water that is not as fresh or clean.

Clean-river screening
A screen filters floating debris from river water that does not need chemical treatment.

Protection for teeth Tests show that a small daily intake of fluoride strengthens teeth against dental decay. Fluoride is naturally present in the water in some parts of Britain. In some other parts of the country minute quantities of fluoride are added to the water supply to help combat dental problems.

FLUORIDE – HELP OR HARM?

I assumed that fluoride in water was good for you, but now I hear that it is harmful and can even cause cancer. Is this true?

Fluoride is added to some water supplies and dental products because it has been proved to harden tooth enamel, making teeth more resistant to cavities. However, some children can suffer from 'dental fluorosis' – a rare condition caused by too much fluoride. The combination of drinking fluoridated water and using fluoride toothpaste can severely discolour teeth, making them mottled, or streaked with white horizontal marks. The fluoridation of water has also been blamed for a higher than average number of hip fractures: the theory is that fluoride could make bones denser but less flexible.

Although fluoride has played a major part in improving dental health in Britain, research is being carried out into the effects of fluoride on the immune system, the body's defence system. Several studies have shown that bone cancer can develop in rats fed on a diet high in fluoride. In America, one study has suggested a link between fluoridation and higher rates of a rare form of bone cancer in boys and young men between the ages of 10 and 20 – however the results are still inconclusive.

In the end, the most important thing to remember is that you need enough fluoride to protect your teeth, but not so much that it causes problems. Ask your dentist for advice about exactly how much you need.

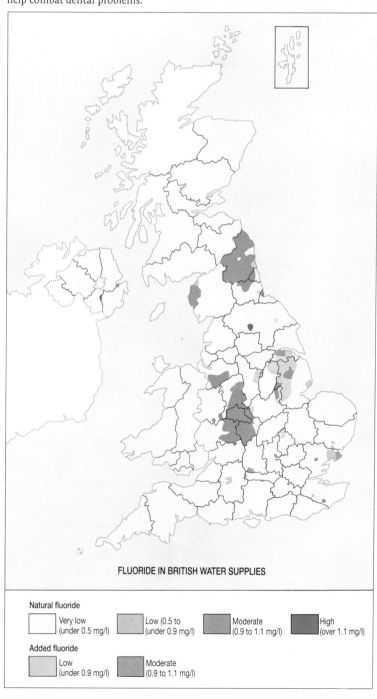

FLUORIDE IN BRITISH WATER SUPPLIES

Natural fluoride

	Very low (under 0.5 mg/l)
	Low (0.5 to under 0.9 mg/l)
	Moderate (0.9 to 1.1 mg/l)
	High (over 1.1 mg/l)

Added fluoride

| | Low (under 0.9 mg/l) |
| | Moderate (0.9 to 1.1 mg/l) |

CLEANING OUR WATER SUPPLY

I've always been told that it is unsafe to drink water from British rivers. What is in the water that could cause harm?

Most British rivers are gradually becoming cleaner, but it is still impossible to tell by eye whether or not water is safe to drink. The water companies filter and disinfect river water to make it safe to drink (see pages 310 and 311). Apart from leaves and other types of debris, rivers contain five main forms of contamination.

- Treated sewage effluent – at strict limits.
- Nutrients – including nitrates, from crop fertilisers, and phosphates (see page 329).
- Pesticides and herbicides – chemicals for killing pests and weeds which can seep through the soil, polluting underground water, or can run off into nearby streams.
- Industrial pollution – poisonous chemicals discharged by factories. Some go directly into rivers in strictly controlled amounts after treatment. Other chemicals may seep through the earth and pollute underground water supplies because of poor storage, handling or disposal arrangements. Among the most dangerous of these pollutants are solvents used in processes such as dry cleaning and the manufacture of computer microchips.

● Waste dumps – poisons, such as heavy metals from domestic batteries (see page 320), can leak into water supplies even ten years after a tip has been closed.

CLOUDY WATER – WHAT TO DO

Why does my tap water sometimes look cloudy or have small particles floating in it, and is it safe to drink when it is like this?

Cloudiness or visible particles in tap water are often caused by work being done to nearby water mains. Normally, your water authority will tell you when work is planned. Occasionally, however, a burst main will stir up a sediment and cloud your supply. If you are concerned, telephone the water authority – find the number under 'Water' in the directory – and ask for advice. Usually, you will be told to run the water until it looks clear or to boil it for several minutes and allow it to stand so that any sediment sinks to the bottom. Pour the water carefully, leaving any sediment behind. If the problem recurs, contact your local council's environmental health department.

WORRIES ABOUT LEAD PIPES

We have just moved into a Victorian house, and I am worried that our water pipes might be lead. How would this affect our health, and what can I do about it?

Lead can cause brain damage to children: it is associated with poor coordination, slow reading and a small vocabulary. Although lead water pipes were once common in older houses, many have now been replaced. However, lead solder is still used to join some copper pipes, creating a potential source of contamination. The risks are slightly higher in soft water areas because soft water dissolves lead more quickly than hard water.

Contact an environmental health officer through your local council, or contact your water authority, to test your supply. In some areas, councils give grants to replace lead pipes. If you do have lead pipes and cannot replace them immediately, take the precaution of running your drinking water for a few minutes every morning before using it. Always take water from the kitchen cold tap for drinking and cooking.

Rivers, pools and the ocean

HEALTH IN PUBLIC POOLS

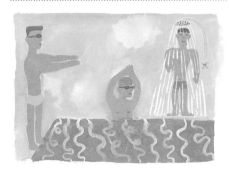

My sons love swimming – but are there any health risks from public pools?

The water in public swimming pools in Britain is continually filtered, disinfected and tested to ensure that it is safe to swim in. It is possible to catch illnesses, such as dysentery, gastrointestinal problems, swimmer's ear (an ear inflammation) and polio from infected water, but your sons are unlikely to be at any risk. Even athlete's foot and verrucas (types of foot infection) are largely controlled by the chlorine used for disinfecting the pool water. Teach your sons to shower after their swim, and to dry their feet thoroughly. A hygienic pool has clean, litter-free changing rooms, and all swimmers are expected to take a shower *before* they go in the water.

SAVING POLLUTED RIVERS

I have recently seen several dead fish floating in a river near our house. Does this mean the river is polluted and, if so, who should I contact?

Dead fish and surface scum are common warning signs that a river could be contaminated. There are many possible sources of the pollution, including industry, sewage works and farms, with contaminated water going straight into the river or running off the land. If you are worried that a river has been polluted, ring the free 24-hour national hotline run by the National Rivers Authority (NRA) on 0800 807060. In its first year of operation (1993-4) the hotline took 30000 calls. Prompt action by members of the public allowed the NRA to trace and stop

DO'S AND DON'TS

for coping with swimming pool chlorine

Do wear goggles to protect your eyes, and a swimming hat to protect your hair against the 'drying' effects of chlorine.

Do rinse your eyes in clean, luke-warm running water after swimming. Tilt your head so that the water runs away from the other eye.

Do shower and wash your hair after swimming.

Don't ignore red or itchy skin blotches. See a doctor if the problem lasts more than a day.

contamination that might otherwise have caused severe damage to rivers, lakes and beaches, and to bring prosecutions against some of the polluters.

DETERGENT DRAINAGE

I am campaigning to clean up a local river. How can I make sure that my washing machine doesn't drain into it?

If you live in a pre-war house, you probably have only one drainage system that leads straight to the sewer, so the problem is unlikely to arise. Most post-war houses, however, have two drainage systems: one takes waste water to the sewer, while the other takes rainwater to a nearby river. If a washing machine outlet pipe empties into the wrong drain, it can pollute the river with dirty water and detergent – an offence which could lead to prosecution. To check your outlet, turn on the kitchen taps to see which drain they empty into. Then run your machine to see where its waste pipe empties. If it runs into the same drain as the tap water, it is going to the sewer. If it runs into a drain that is fed by your rainwater gutters, the water is going untreated to the river. To prevent pollution and prosecution your pipe must be re-routed.

HOW SAFE IS THE SEA ?

We have a traditional seaside holiday every year, and our children love swimming in the sea. How can I find out which beaches are safe for swimming from?

The best way to check whether your favourite beaches are up to standard each year is by contacting the local council's environmental health officer (find the number in the telephone directory for the area), or by buying an annual beach guide, such as *The Reader's Digest Good Beach Guide.*

Beaches used by the public are supposed to reach standards set by the European Community for the cleanliness of water and beaches. There are more than 400 British beaches designated as 'bathing waters'. Most of them achieve the required standards each year and advertise the fact on display boards or by flying a blue 'clean beach' flag. However, some of Britain's beaches are still sometimes polluted by untreated sewage that has been discharged into the ocean and washed back ashore. For the time being such beaches do not have to be closed to the public or display warning signs.

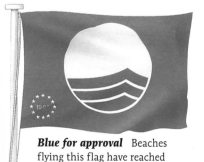

Blue for approval Beaches flying this flag have reached European standards.

CAMPAIGN SAVES WATER

At home in New Zealand microbiologist Lianna Stupples was accustomed to drinking clean water straight from its source. When she moved to Britain in the 1980s Lianna was alarmed to discover from a Government report that weedkillers were getting into some water supplies. As water can be drawn from rivers and underground sources miles away from a tap, the report calculated that 16 million Britons could be drinking quantities of poisonous chemicals that were well above the European Community's legal limit.

Two of the herbicides in the water – atrazine and simazine – were known to cause genetic and birth defects and had been linked to fertility problems in animals. Although the chemicals were on the Government's list of poisons that had safer alternatives, local councils, British Rail, farmers and others were still legally using them throughout the country. Lianna decided that it would be wrong to ignore the situation. She got together with like-minded people and organised volunteers to talk to councils and British Rail about alternative methods of weed control. With the help of the environmental group Friends of the Earth, she produced an education pack, which was sent to all the water companies. This proved to be the turning point.

'The water companies realised that they would not have to spend a lot of money on taking the chemicals out of the water if the weedkillers were not used in the first place – they joined our side and things really started to happen,' said Lianna. British Rail was persuaded to use alternative, biodegradable weedkillers, and dozens of local councils voluntarily banned atrazine and simazine. In May 1992 the Government banned their use, except by farmers under strictly regulated conditions.

'It just shows what local people working together can do to change habits,' says Lianna. 'We showed that prevention is better than the cure – it's better not to pollute than to have to clean up later.'

FALLING FERTILITY

I've read some alarming reports about chemicals that are reducing fish and animal sperm counts. Is there any risk to human fertility?

It is possible that chemical pollution could eventually have an effect on human fertility – but the research is inconclusive. Studies in America and Europe show that the sperm counts of young men today are significantly lower than their fathers' sperm count when they were young, and that cases of cancer of the testicles have significantly increased over the past 50 years. Most research currently focuses upon a number of chemicals that mimic the hormone oestrogen and have been linked with changes in fish and reptile fertility and human fertility problems, such as falling sperm counts, testicular and breast cancer and endometriosis (a gynaecological disorder). Some scientists believe that several chemicals in rivers could be responsible, including pesticides, herbicides, synthetic hormones in the contraceptive pill and other drugs, waste from electronic engineering, paper bleach, some types of plastics (including some used to make babies' drinking bottles), washing powders, cosmetics and detergents. Other theories blame sewage outlets or the increased consumption of dairy products from cows treated with oestrogen to increase their milk yield.

Dealing with noise

THREATS TO HEARING

I live in a very noisy neighbourhood. Could this damage my hearing?

It is highly unlikely that living in a noisy neighbourhood will damage your hearing, only in an occupational setting is irreversible hearing damage likely. However, continual noise can cause other problems – some children have problems in concentrating and experience learning difficulties, while some adults cannot sleep at night and this may cause them health problems.

If you really are worried that the noise levels around your home may be damaging your hearing, contact an environmental health officer (EHO) through your local council. EHOs can give you advice and, in some cases, take legal action to reduce noise. The first indication of a hearing problem is difficulty hearing the consonants in words.

HOW TO COMPLAIN

Noisy neighbours are driving me mad. If there's not a radio blaring, then there is a dog barking, a child yelling, or a car being revved. They refuse to be more considerate, so what more can I do?

Contact your local council's environmental health department and give specific examples of the noise and the dates on which it occurred. If an environmental health officer (EHO) considers the noise is a 'nuisance', there will be an investigation. If necessary, the EHO will issue a 'noise abatement' notice: if the problem continues, the EHO can take your neighbours to court. You are also entitled to complain directly to a magistrate's or sheriff court if you do not wish the local council to be involved or if you are unsatisfied with the EHO's action. Alternatively, you can take civil action – but this could be costly, and it would be sensible to get legal advice first. You can get a free information booklet about noise from the Department of the Environment in London.

REDUCING NOISE AT HOME

Is there anything we can do to make our home quieter throughout the day?

Yes – you can cut out some of the noise from outside and reduce some of the sounds from inside your home.

● If possible, insulate exterior walls.
● Install any form of double-glazing – it will significantly reduce noise from outside.
● Plant hedges or trees between your house and the road.
● Seal any holes that let in noise. These could be cracks or damage around window frames or gaps in the brickwork around pipes or cables.
● If your doors are hollow, replace them with solid doors, making sure that they fit the frames snugly.
● Choose thick carpeting with a good underlay, whenever possible. Fit carpet to steps and staircases.

Everyday noise levels

Noise is measured in decibels (dB), with a special scale (dB(A)) that takes account of the impact upon our ears. The British safety level for noise is 85 dB(A), but prolonged exposure to sound above 80 dB(A) can damage your hearing permanently. The decibel scale rises by multiples, with the loudness of a sound doubling every 3 dB(A).

A whisper measures 30 dB(A), and an ordinary conversation measures 60 dB(A). Sounds such as the ringing of a telephone, 65 dB(A), and traffic noise in a street, 70 dB(A), are just below the safety level. However, a car horn at 100 dB(A), a baby's scream – which can measure up to 100 dB(A) – a pneumatic drill at 120 dB(A) and a jet engine at 135 dB(A) are above it.

● Place book shelves and other heavy furniture against exterior walls.

● Listen to household appliances in operation before you buy them, whenever possible. If you have any choice, select a quiet model.

● If any existing appliances are noisy, have them serviced and oiled.

● Stand appliances, such as dishwashers and washing machines, on rubber or cork mats, and cover the sides with foam pads.

● Sew a thick lining between your curtains and the outer lining, to muffle any noise from outside.

● Choose upholstered furniture and scatter cushions: fabric helps to muffle noise.

● Leave heavy outdoor shoes at the front door and wear footwear with soft soles.

HARM TO UNBORN BABIES

We live near an airport and are expecting our first child in six months' time. A friend says that the noise of the aeroplanes could harm our unborn baby. Is this true?

There is no clear answer to this question. Researchers are investigating reports of a higher rate of birth defects and low birth weight in babies born to women living near large airports. However, until there is firm evidence one way or the other, you might like to insulate your home against noise (see page 315) and to get advice from your local council's environmental health department. You can also get a free booklet from the Department of the Environment, London.

Living with radiation

RADIATION EXPLAINED

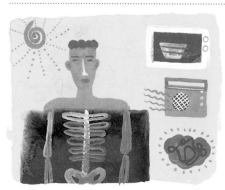

What is radiation and why is it often described as being dangerous?

Radiation is a type of high-speed energy that is all around us. It travels either as electromagnetic waves – such as light and radio waves and radiated heat – or as radioactive particles, which can be found in various substances such as rocks and radon gas.

There are two basic categories of radiation. 'Ionising' radiation (such as X-rays and nuclear radiation) is powerful enough to convert atoms into charged particles called 'ions'. Less powerful radiation, called 'non-ionising' radiation (that includes lasers, microwaves and radio waves) leaves the atom intact but generates heat.

Some radiation is natural. It comes from the Sun, soil, buildings, food and even our own bodies. Radiation is also created by human technology, such as medicine, coal burning, luminous clocks, smoke detectors, nuclear power plants and nuclear weapons.

Whether it occurs naturally or results from human activities, radiation can both help and harm us. We rely on radiant energy from the Sun for the light and heat, but prolonged exposure causes skin burning and eventually cancer. The doses of radiation delivered by X-rays and medical lasers are perfectly safe for most people. In high doses, X-rays and lasers can destroy human tissue and X-rays can cause cancers. They can also be used to *treat* cancer (radiotherapy).

Most of our exposure to radiation is low level 'background' radiation from the Sun. Radiation from human activities, including nuclear fallout from Chernobyl and radioactive waste from power stations, laboratories and hospitals accounts for only 15 per cent of our exposure.

LIFE NEAR A NUCLEAR STATION

Are people who live near a nuclear power station at greater risk from radiation than someone who lives miles away?

Nuclear power stations release low-level radioactivity into the atmosphere, but coal-fired power stations also release natural radioactivity – as fly ash. The National Radiological Protection Board says that the radiation doses to people living near a nuclear power station are extremely low, and are dwarfed by the natural radiation to which we are all exposed. However, some research suggests an increased risk of leukaemia and other cancers in people living near nuclear power plants. For instance, one study shows an increase above the national average in childhood cancers near the nuclear reprocessing plant at Sellafield in Cumbria. Nonetheless, some scientists believe that the 'clusters' could be due to other causes. At present there is no conclusive evidence to prove a link between the cases of leukaemia and the nuclear installations. British Nuclear Fuels is funding a 16-year study of babies' genes in west Cumbria. The researchers hope to discover whether a particular gene, or a combination of genes, makes people more vulnerable to diseases such as cancer, cot death or heart defects.

SAVING THE OZONE LAYER

What is the hole in the ozone layer, and why does it make us more vulnerable to damage from radiation?

A 'layer' of ozone (see page 303) encircles the Earth, protecting us from dangerous levels of ultraviolet radiation from the Sun. In 1984 scientists discovered a 'hole' in the ozone layer above the Antarctic. It is now estimated to be about the size of the United States. The depletion of this protective shield makes us more vulnerable to radiation from sunlight, with an increased risk of developing skin cancers and eye diseases, such as cataracts. Health experts warn against prolonged periods of sun bathing and recommend using a sun screen product (see page 140). Human activities, such as the use of chlorofluorocarbons (CFCs) in refrigerators and as propellants in aerosol cans, are blamed for the ozone hole, so many environmental groups and some manufacturers and governments encourage the phasing out of the use of the suspected chemicals.

RADON AND HEALTH

Friends living on the other side of town recently discovered that their home was contaminated by radon. What are the health risks from radon, and how can I find out whether my home is affected?

Radon is a radioactive gas naturally emitted by all rocks – especially granite – which rises from the ground and collects in buildings. The colourless, odour-free gas accounts for half of all natural radiation on Earth. But it is estimated to cause about 5 per cent of the deaths from lung cancer each year in Britain.

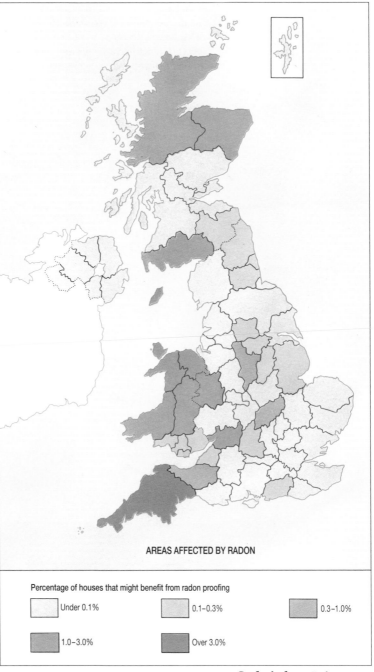

AREAS AFFECTED BY RADON

Percentage of houses that might benefit from radon proofing

Under 0.1%   0.1–0.3%   0.3–1.0%

1.0–3.0%   Over 3.0%

The danger occurs when a large amount of radon becomes trapped in an enclosed space, such as a house.

The problem can affect homes in many parts of the country, but there are particularly high risks in areas where the the rocks are fractured granite, limestone or sandstone. Parts of Cornwall, Devon, Somerset, Derbyshire, Northamptonshire, Wales and northern Scotland have high concentrations of radon, and some districts are designated

Geological gas Radon, formed by the breakdown of uranium in certain rocks, affects homes in various parts of Britain. Protective measures can be taken.

as 'radon affected areas'. New homes have special radon proofing, and local council grants are sometimes available to install protection in older homes. Recommended action usually includes sealing floors, installing exhaust fans in basements and cellars, and making sure that buildings are adequately ventilated. For advice contact your local council's environmental health department, or the Radon Survey at the National Radiological Protection Board (NRPB), Didcot, Oxfordshire, or the Department of the Environment in London. The test for radon involves leaving two small detectors in your home for three months.

COMPUTERS AND PREGNANCY

My first baby is due in five months' time and I am worried that radiation from my computer screen might harm my unborn child. What are the real risks?

People working at visual display units (VDUs) *are* exposed to low levels of radiation and electromagnetic fields, and one American study suggested that there were double the number of miscarriages among women who worked for more than 20 hours a week at computer visual display units. However, the National Radiological Protection Board, which advises the British Government on certain types of radiation, says there is no firm evidence that radiation from computers can damage the unborn child or cause a spontaneous abortion.

Pregnancy can be a stressful time, so you should talk to your doctor and employer about your fears and get advice from your health and safety representative, if you have

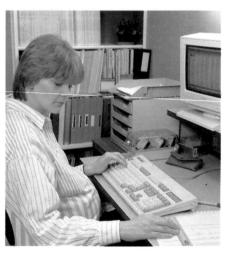

Before birth Many of today's youngsters were 'introduced' to computers early in life.

one, and the Health and Safety Executive: Information Centre, Broad Lane, Sheffield S3 7HQ. Make sure that you sit properly at your computer (see page 144) and that the lighting around your desk is adequate. If working at your VDU becomes uncomfortable, your employer might be able to find you alternative work until after the birth.

MICROWAVE OVENS

I have just bought a microwave oven and my mother is now bombarding me with scare stories. Are microwave ovens safe?

A brand new microwave oven is unlikely to prove a health risk. However, a problem can arise if the door safety lock or the door seals are faulty allowing microwave radiation to escape from the oven.

When you buy a microwave oven, make sure that it has not been damaged in transit. Place it in a part of the kitchen where it is unlikely to be knocked, and follow the manufacturer's instructions carefully for safe use. Clean the door seal regularly using a mild soap solution, not an abrasive. Check the oven regularly to see that the door closes properly: if you suspect a problem, get the oven checked by a qualified engineer who will check for any radiation leak.

DANGER FROM POWER LINES?

How safe is it to live near an electricity pylon or power cables?

It seems that some people who are exposed for long periods to the low-frequency electric and magnetic fields from pylons, power cables and electricity substations could suffer health problems. Possible links have been suggested with a wide range of illnesses, including depression, insomnia, headaches, slow reaction times, disrupted sleep patterns, birth defects, reduced fertility, brain tumours, adult cancers and childhood leukaemia, and a weakened immune system.

According to the National Radiological Protection Board there is as yet no conclusive evidence to prove that electromagnetic fields cause leukaemia or any other type of cancer. If you are concerned about your health, ask your local power company to test the electromagnetic field in your home. This will, however, reveal only the daytime levels, and it is now known that levels often increase significantly at night when cheaprate electricity is being used, either in your own home or in the neighbourhood.

ELECTROMAGNETIC RADIATION

Is it true that radiation from ordinary household appliances could harm me or members of my family?

Any effects from the very low level of electro-magnetic radiation from household electrical appliances, such as hair dryers, toasters, washing machines, refrigerators, freezers and vacuum cleaners, are minimal because the electromagnetic field decreases within a few inches, and the time you spend close to the appliance is usually brief.

Some researchers believe that there may be risks to a foetus if a pregnant woman has frequent and prolonged exposure to low-level electromagnetic fields (for instance from an electric blanket or water bed). However, the National Radiological Protection Board states that the evidence provided so far is weak and inconclusive.

Using electricity safely

ENSURING YOUR WIRING IS SAFE

We have recently bought several new household appliances. How can we make sure that our wiring is safe?

About 40 people a year die in Britain as a result of electrical accidents and many more are injured, so you are right to be concerned. It is fairly easy to spot some of the signs that suggest that your wiring or items of electrical equipment may need attention:

● A trip switch cuts out or a fuse blows.
● Lights are intermittent or flicker.
● A flex is worn, frayed or blackened.
● A plug or socket is blackened.
● You have sockets with round pins or lights with woven flex covers rather than insulating plastic – these show that the wiring is old and should be replaced.

If you are using socket adapters, because you have so much electrical equipment, or using extension cables, because sockets are in the 'wrong' place, have extra sockets installed: this could prevent a fire and remove the risk of tripping over the extension cable.

So much of your home's wiring is hidden, that your safest course of action would be to have the whole house checked by a qualified electrician from your local electricity company or an independent company. Some checks can be made using a socket tester for the circuits, but these can be expensive and will not necessarily help you to pinpoint any fault. You will still need the help of an expert.

For your own safety and that of your family, tackle only the jobs you feel competent to do properly. If you have any doubt leave them alone and consult a qualified electrician. Never attempt any work on microwave ovens, television sets, or any other electrical item that states it should be repaired only by a qualified person. Jobs such as replacing an element in an electric kettle, renewing the flex on an iron, fitting a new seal to a washing machine door, refrigerator or freezer door, and fitting a new drive belt to a washing machine or tumble dryer can usually be tackled safely using only a basic tool kit. But such repairs should only be attempted by a competent handiperson.

GARDEN POWER TOOLS

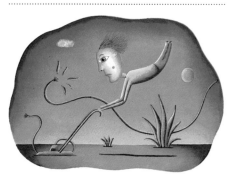

As our garden is very small, we feel that an electric mower is more appropriate than a petrol one, but are electric mowers safe to use on wet grass?

Garden tools and equipment can be used in damp conditions, but never use them in the rain. Electric mowers *are* safe but, as with any electrical appliance, you must use and maintain them with care. Buy a residual current device (circuit breaker) and plug it into the mains socket before plugging in the mower. Remember that the mower blades continue rotating for a while after the power has been switched off: keep your clothes, hands and feet well clear. Work methodically, making sure that the cable is always behind the mower, to avoid cutting through the flex and electrocuting yourself.

Living with metals

AVOIDING LEAD POISONING

Why is lead considered a threat to children's health and how can I protect my own children?

The levels of lead emissions from factories, smelting plants and vehicle exhausts are controlled by law. Nonetheless, environmentalists are still concerned about the amounts present in air, water and soil. When large quantities enter the bloodstream, lead can damage the kidneys, brain and nervous system. Lower doses can impair the physical and mental development of children, and lead has also been linked with hyperactivity and poor hand/eye coordination.

Children can inhale lead while walking or playing near busy roads. Lead in drinking water, mainly because of old lead piping, is another risk. Also, small children sometimes swallow flakes of old paint containing lead. To protect your children:

● Replace any lead piping in older houses (see page 313).
● Teach young children not to eat soil, which can contain lead dust. Get them to wash their hands after playing outside.
● Remove any old, flaking gloss paintwork around the house with a chemical stripper and repaint with a modern lead-free paint. The most likely danger areas for lead-based paints are pipes and other metalwork painted with gloss paint.
● Encourage children to play as far away from main roads as possible.
● Don't let children put toys in their mouths. Some old toys are made from lead or are decorated with lead paint.

DEALING WITH OLD BATTERIES

I rely on batteries for a number of household gadgets, but I've heard that they can contaminate the soil around rubbish tips. How can I avoid causing pollution?

You are right – domestic batteries do contain quantities of mercury, lead and cadmium that have in the past polluted soil and water, and have been blamed for illnesses including cancer and kidney disease. But you will be glad to know that battery manufacturers are trying hard to reduce the amounts used.

About 90 per cent of household batteries are now free from mercury. In 1994 legislation was passed to reduce environmental damage from batteries, and from January 1996 all batteries on sale in the European Union must be labelled with their heavy metal content. The Department of Trade is looking into ways that old batteries could be separated and recycled.

Many local authorities provide collection points for old car batteries: nearly 90 per cent of a car battery can be recycled.

COPPER THERAPY

I've heard that wearing a copper bracelet can cure arthritis. Is this true?

No, but plenty of sufferers say that copper *relieves* the pain of arthritis and rheumatism, and people have been wearing copper for relief since ancient times. One theory is that traces of copper penetrate the skin, helping to replenish a low level of essential copper in the body. However, there is no scientific proof that copper really works.

In an Australian study in the 1970s three out of four volunteers said that they gained relief from arthritis by wearing copper, but an American study in 1991 concluded that copper was useless. What *is* certain is that you will come to no harm by wearing a copper bracelet – and it might even help.

NICKEL AND SKIN PROBLEMS

I love fashion jewellery, but every time I wear inexpensive earrings my ears become sore and inflamed. Is this normal?

Dermatologists believe that between 10 and 20 per cent of Western women are allergic to inexpensive metals. The main culprit is nickel, a hard-wearing alloy used in jewellery and other items, that can cause skin irritation. It should not be worn immediately after ears are pierced. Gold and silver may also prompt an allergic reaction, although usually only when they are mixed with other metals. Stainless steel seems to be the least risky metal. Try wearing earrings with stainless steel clips and posts, or those marked as hypoallergenic (unlikely to cause allergies). See your doctor if any inflammation is very painful or lasts several days.

ALUMINIUM POTS AND PANS

A while ago there was a scare about the possible link between aluminium saucepans and Alzheimer's disease. What is the current view?

At one time some scientists did believe that aluminium from the purification of drinking water, cooking utensils and a variety of other sources could cause this form of dementia. The theory was based upon animal research and the presence of traces of aluminium in the brains of some Alzheimer's patients. However, more recent studies show that aluminium is unlikely to be to blame for the human disease. The most current advice is that using aluminium pots and pans does not increase the risk of getting Alzheimer's disease.

Nonetheless, some health and medical experts still advise against cooking acidic foods, such as apples and tomatoes, in uncoated aluminium pans. They are concerned that the acid can leach aluminium into the food, and may cause brain damage.

Home heating and insulation

USING GAS SAFELY

My sister says that I shouldn't use my gas fire with the window shut. Is she right?

No, but there must be enough ventilation for the gas fire to burn safely. Without adequate ventilation, your fire will produce carbon monoxide, a colourless, odourless poisonous gas that can make you feel sick, dizzy or sleepy, and may even lead to disablement or death if high enough concentrations build up.

When a gas fire is installed, appropriate ventilation must be fitted by an engineer registered with CORGI (the Council of Registered Gas Installers), the organisation that oversees gas qualifications and standards. This could be a chimney, flue, air brick, or an extractor fan – the form of ventilation depends upon the type and make of fire. If you have any queries about ventilation, get advice from your regional Gas Consumers Council office (see your local telephone directory, or the back of your gas bill).

Check that your fire burns with a blue flame. If the flame is yellow or orange, there is insufficient air, and you should stop using it and contact an engineer registered with CORGI. Get your fire serviced every year – this is a legal requirement for landlords – and let some fresh air into your rooms each day to keep the atmosphere fresh and to prevent building up harmful fumes.

BURNING SOLID FUEL

We have two open fires and a wood-burning stove in our house. Could they pose any health hazard?

Whenever they burn, wood, coal and coke give off carbon monoxide – a gas that can cause heart and respiratory diseases, and can even kill. However, you can avoid health problems by ventilating rooms well and by having the chimneys swept regularly to ensure that the smoke escapes up the chimney, not into your home. Closed stoves that burn solid fuel are generally considered safer than open fires because less smoke can waft into your rooms.

INSULATING FOR WARMTH

I'm very susceptible to cold, but I cannot afford to keep my central heating on all the time. Would insulating my home make a significant difference, and if so what is the best way to do it?

Effective insulation could make an important contribution to your comfort and a valuable saving on your heating bills.

Check whether there are any draughts from ill-fitting windows or doors, or from skirting boards and letterboxes. You can buy special metal, foam or plastic strips for insulating windows, doors and letterboxes from DIY stores. Alternatively, you could make

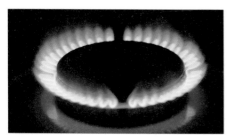

Ring of fire A gas hob produces a bright blue flame when it is burning safely.

fabric draught excluders for the bottoms of doors, or even stuff paper around loose window frames. Heavy curtains, or light-weight curtains with thermal linings, also improve heat retention in the room and reduce the draughts that can make people feel especially chilly. Double glazing provides excellent insulation, but can be expensive. As a cost-saving alternative, secure plastic sheeting to windows with double-sided tape or magnetic strips.

The most significant heat loss from your home is probably through the roof if it has not been insulated. Some local councils give grants towards the cost of insulating lofts, and you should call them for information. The Energy Action Grants Agency also gives advice: ring free of charge on 0800 181667.

INSULATION AND POLLUTION

I have heard that an over-insulated house can be a health hazard. Is this true?

If you seal your home tightly and do not let in any fresh air, you could be breathing higher concentrations of air pollutants, such as carbon monoxide and household dust that can harm your health. No one wants a draughty home – but you do need to venti-late rooms, to keep the air fresh and to pre-vent the build up of harmful particles and fumes. Open a window for a short time every day, or install a fan to draw in air from outside. Keep major cleaning or redecorating projects to times of the year when the weather is mild enough to open the windows to clear the air.

INSULATING WITH GLASS FIBRE

We have decided to insulate our loft with glass fibre. Is it safe to do this ourselves?

Glass fibre and mineral wool are safe to use if you take some simple safety precautions to prevent them from spreading around your home and irritating your skin and throat.

● Follow the manufacturer's instructions.
● Use a face mask designed for mineral fibres – it should be marked BS 6016.
● Wear rubber gloves and overalls with long sleeves.
● Tuck your sleeves into the gloves and your trousers into your socks.
● Keep the hatch closed whenever you are working with glass fibre or mineral wool.
● Open the bags or rolls of insulation only when you are in the loft.

● Put waste and any off-cuts into plastic bags and seal them before taking them out for disposal.
● Use a new dust mask each time you work with glass fibre or mineral wool. Wash all protective clothing before wearing it again.

THE RISK FROM ASBESTOS

The insulation around the hot-water pipes in my loft contains asbestos. Should I have it removed?

If the asbestos seems to be in good condi-tion, leave it alone. Asbestos is most danger-ous when it is being broken up, because it releases minute fibres that can lodge deep in the lungs, causing respiratory problems or lung cancer.

If the asbestos is damaged or crumbly, or could be disturbed during building work, get expert advice before deciding whether or not to have it removed.

CAUTION Never attempt to remove asbestos yourself. Ensure that the contractors work safely (see panel, left), and do not try to sweep, dust or vacuum up after them.

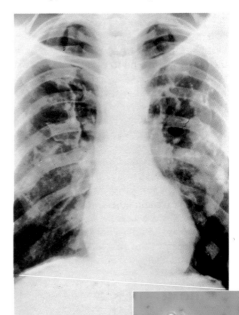

Fibre damage Air sacs in the lungs stiffen, causing breathing problems after microscopic filaments of asbestos (right) are inhaled. The damage looks like white patches (above).

Making a safe, healthy home

CITY VERSUS THE COUNTRY

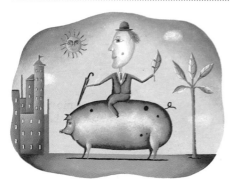

Would we have a healthier life if we moved from our home in the city to the country?

It depends. Life in and around a city can be stimulating and exhilarating, but crowds, traffic jams, noise and dirt can take a toll on your physical and mental wellbeing. For many years there has been a trend for families to leave British cities for country areas, but a lot of people are disappointed by their expectation of 'the good life' and go back to a city within a few years. When you move to the country, you tend to escape air pollution and traffic noise, and usually encounter less aggressive behaviour and crime. However, there are drawbacks that can damage your health and even make your life a misery.

Many newcomers to the country become isolated, finding it difficult to make friends among local people, and spend many hours travelling to social and cultural activities, schools and shops. Some districts do not even offer the peace and quiet anticipated. Before you make any decision to move, get to know a country area during different times of the year: winter could be bleak and journeys long and difficult.

HOMES ON TOXIC LAND

Every so often there is a scare about housing estates discovered to be on toxic land. What safeguards exist?

Local councils keep lists of land that has been contaminated by previous activities, such as smelting, mining, gas works, chemical processing and landfill rubbish dumps, but the lists do not necessarily cover every patch of contaminated land. Before it can approve any new buildings, a council must check that there will not be any health risks from the proposed use of the land. The council has the power to insist that land is made safe before any construction begins.

Occasionally, however, land is found to be contaminated around *old* homes. You would need legal advice to discover whether you had any claim for compensation against a previous owner or the original development company, if it still exists. Generally speaking, however, it is a case of 'buyer beware'. Your solicitor's prepurchase 'search' should include checks on previous use of the land. This may become easier when the Department of the Environment publishes new guidance on researching former use of land.

If you are concerned about the safety of the land around your house, or around a house you would like to buy, check the list of contaminated land at your local council offices. You may have to pay a fee. It is helpful to talk to local people, especially older residents, about the history of the area. You can also get advice from the environmental group Friends of the Earth: 26-28 Underwood Street, London N1 7JQ.

HEALTH HAZARDS FROM DAMP

During winter, our house gets damp patches on the walls. Are they bad for our health, and how can we prevent them?

The patches are not a health hazard in themselves, but damp housing encourages the growth of mould and mites and can increase the risk of respiratory illness, such as asthma. Condensation often causes damp patches: it usually occurs during cold weather, appearing on cold surfaces including windows, areas behind wardrobes and north-facing walls. To reduce the amount of condensation in your home:

● Use lids on saucepans.
● Dry clothes outside or use a tumble dryer with an outside vent.
● Avoid, whenever possible, extensive use of fuels, such as paraffin, that produce a lot of moisture as they burn.
● Ventilate rooms – especially kitchens and bathrooms – to remove moisture.
● Insulate the loft and consider cavity insulation for the walls.

DO'S AND DON'TS

for furniture and furnishings

Do try to buy and use chairs that give your back adequate support.
Do use chairs that are the correct height for tables. This is especially important if you spend long periods reading, writing or using a computer at a table.
Do try to buy furniture that has fire-resistant or fire-retardant materials. Look for the safety label (see page 324). Watch out for upholstered furniture that conforms with the British safety standard BS 5852.

Don't choose chipboard and plywood for all your furniture if you have other options. These materials contain formaldehyde, a chemical which gives off fumes. These can irritate your eyes, nose and throat, and stonger concentrations can cause nausea, headaches, fatigue and even breathing difficulties. These problems usually subside reasonably quickly however.

DO'S AND DON'TS

for using naked flames

Do keep clothes away from open fires and gas flames, taking extra care if you are wearing long sleeves or loose clothes.

Do keep lighters and matches out of children's reach. If possible, store them in a locked cupboard.

Do dispose of matches and cigarettes carefully in ashtrays, not in wastepaper bins where they could set light to paper and other flammable rubbish.

Do fit childproof fireguards. Ideally, they should be attached to the wall and cover the entire fireplace.

Don't dry clothes or tea towels near a gas cooker or open fire, where they could easily catch light.

Don't leave an open fire unattended unless it is protected by a fireguard.

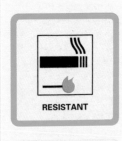

RESISTANT

Filling material(s) and covering fabric(s) meet the requirements for resistance to cigarette and match ignition in the 1988 safety regulations

CARELESSNESS CAUSES FIRE

Resists fire Look for this safety label when choosing furniture and furnishing fabrics.

SAFETY IN THE BATHROOM

A guest slipped and fell in our shower when he was staying with us. Are there any precautions I could take to prevent any other accident in the bathroom?

Use a non-slip mat on the floor of the shower and in the bath. Mop up spills and splashes immediately to reduce the risk of slipping on the bathroom floor. Consider fixing grab handles to the wall if your bath or shower does not already have any. This is especially important if elderly or infirm people are using the bathroom. It is also worth checking that rugs and bathmats have non-slip backings – these are usually rubber.

Ask everyone who uses the bathroom to keep it free from glass containers: remember that some cosmetics and medicine bottles are glass. If your medicine cabinet is in the bathroom, consider moving it to another part of your home. You might also wish to ban china or shell soap dishes from the bathroom, because they could shatter, causing injury. To prevent electric shocks, make sure that your bathroom light has a pull cord rather than a switch. Don't ever allow anyone to use portable electrical appliances, such as hair dryers and heaters, in the bathroom. The only exception is an electric shaver plugged into a special safety socket.

MAKING STAIRS SAFE

We are moving from a bungalow to a two-storey house. How can we make sure that the stairs are safe?

Staircases *are* potentially dangerous, but you can avoid accidents by following some simple safety precautions:

● Make sure that stairs are well lit, with light switches at the top and bottom.
● Fix handrails to both sides of the stairs, wherever possible.
● Teach toddlers to crawl or to walk on all fours backwards down the stairs until they are confident walkers.
● Keep the steps and the areas at the top and bottom of the stairs free from tripping hazards, such as toys and shoes.
● Replace glass doors at the bottom of stairs.
● Fit safety gates at the top and bottom of staircases if you have small children.
● Consider replacing open ladder-type treads with a traditional staircase (with risers and treads) to prevent things from falling through the gaps.

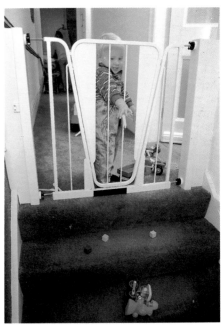

Essential safety barrier This toddler can throw his toys downstairs in safety, because he is protected from falling by a stair gate.

● Watch out for frayed or loose pieces of carpet. Secure or replace any worn areas immediately.
● Remove any horizontal banisters and landing rails that children could use as 'ladders', to prevent falls.
● Check the distance between banisters to ensure that toddlers can trap their heads between the uprights.

FIRE PROTECTION AT HOME

How can I protect my home from fire?

There are many simple precautions to reduce the risk of fire in your home:

● Install smoke detectors on each floor.
● Keep a fire extinguisher or fire blanket in the kitchen.
● Shut internal doors before you go to bed, to delay the spread of any fire that does break out.
● Check visible wiring and sockets regularly and call in expert help if you see any signs of damage (see page 313). Have any round-pin sockets and plugs replaced, because they are very old and likely to be dangerous.
● Have secondhand gas or electric heaters and cookers checked by a qualified engineer before use. Get a registered engineer to fit gas appliances (see page 321).
● Never smoke in bed.

- Get chimneys swept regularly, to prevent smoke from filling rooms.
- Never leave a child alone in a room with a fire, hob or oven that is on, or that the child could turn on.
- Keep paraffin heaters away from doors and other busy areas where they could be knocked over.
- Turn off paraffin heaters before filling them and never move them when they are switched on.
- Try not to store paraffin and other flammable liquids inside your home.

CHOOSING COLOURS

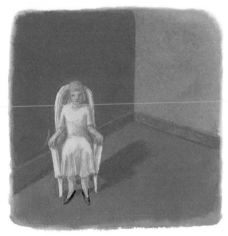

Is it true that you can be influenced by the colours you choose for your walls?

It is well known that colour has an influence on mood – we even talk of 'feeling blue' or 'seeing red', and one form of alternative therapy uses coloured lights and paints to treat patients. Mood and wellbeing can also be affected by the lighting levels and the combination of colours and textures around you. However, researchers generally accept the following guidelines for decoration.

- Pink – usually warm and welcoming. Some deeper shades can be stimulating.
- Red – can be warm, but it may also be confrontational, causing tension and other changes, such as an increased pulse rate, a rise in blood pressure, an increase in muscle tension and increased brain activity, all of which can be measured electrically.
- Orange – warm and stimulating, but can be overpowering as a strong colour. Apricot and peach tones can be comfortable and relaxing to live with.
- Yellow – can brighten a room, and can make you feel peaceful and optimistic.

- Green – pale green is considered restful and is often used for rooms where people spend a lot of time. Bright green is cheerful and stimulating.
- Blue – pale blue is calming and can increase the sense of space, but in some rooms, particularly north facing ones, pale blue can feel cold and bleak. Dark blue can give a sense of solidity and security when used on floors, but it can be oppressive on large areas of walls or on ceilings.
- Purple and lavender – can be calming in pale tones, but strong purple can disturb your focusing ability.
- Brown – beige through to chestnut are the most frequently used colours in homes. Most shades are warm and calming, although some browns can be depressing and bleak.
- Black – on large areas black can be oppressive. On smaller areas, or as grey, it can be cool and peaceful.
- White – often makes rooms seem larger, lighter and cleaner, but large expanses of pure white can seem cold and clinical, and may cause eyestrain. White softened with a hint of another colour is popular for walls.

SAFE COOKING WITH GAS

Which safety aspects should I check when buying a gas cooker?

Gas cookers are safe when they are installed, used and maintained according to the manufacturer's instructions.

By law, all new cookers sold in Britain must meet strict safety standards. Look for the Kitemark label and the British Standard, BS 5386. If you have children, you might like to buy an oven with a 'cool-wall' that prevents oven doors from becoming hot on the outside. Some gas hobs have a safety lid that cuts off the gas supply as soon as the lid is even partially closed. If you are buying a used gas cooker, be sure to select a reputable dealer. Have a secondhand cooker checked by an engineer who is registered with CORGI (the Council of Registered Gas Installers). Make sure that a stability bracket is fitted to any free-standing model to prevent it from being tipped over.

Read the manufacturer's instructions carefully before using the cooker, and have the oven serviced every two years.

CAUTION It is illegal and dangerous to install, repair or service your gas cooker yourself. The work must be carried out by a CORGI-registered engineer.

DO'S AND DON'TS
for dealing with a fire

Do close doors and windows to reduce the air flow.
Do help everyone to leave the building promptly and safely.
Do dial 999 for the fire brigade if you cannot tackle the fire safely.
Do stay outside until a fire officer says it is safe to go back inside.

Don't tackle a fire unless you can do so without risk to yourself.
Don't set off a fire extinguisher unless you are certain it is the right sort for the job – don't use water (red extinguisher) on electrical fires.
Don't open a door if it feels warm to the touch.
Don't shout or run – you could trip, or make others panic.

Keeping children out of danger

SAFE CLIMBING FRAMES

We are thinking about buying a climbing frame for our three-year-old daughter, but are they safe for her age group?

Climbing frames *are* safe if you observe a number of simple guidelines – and they can be well worth the investment. For this age group a ready-assembled climbing frame, with sturdy bars and platforms, is the best choice. The structure should not have any gaps that are between 4 in and 9 in (10 cm and 23 cm) above a drop. This is to prevent a child's head from becoming trapped between two horizontal bars.

Stand the frame over something soft, such as grass or carpet, and make sure it cannot tip over. If you buy a self-assembly kit, follow the manufacturer's instructions carefully. Never let your child climb on a frame unless he or she is supervised by an adult.

PLANT HAZARDS FOR CHILDREN

Some plants, trees and fungi commonly found in British gardens, homes or the countryside can cause health problems if touched or swallowed – and some, such as the death cap mushroom, can be lethal if eaten.

Although there are few deaths in Britain from poisonous plants, children's natural curiosity makes them particularly vulnerable to rashes, abdominal pain and sickness from playing with hazardous plants. Scores of plants can cause unpleasant or even dangerous symptoms. Those illustrated are just a few that children are likely to encounter as they grow up.

It is important to teach children from an early age not to touch or eat any leaves, stems, flowers, berries, seeds, bark, bulbs, roots or fungi. If, however, a child does become ill and you suspect that a plant is to blame, call your doctor immediately, or go to a hospital accident and emergency department. If you know which plant your child has touched or eaten, make sure that you take a cutting with you to help the medical staff to give the correct treatment. You may give the child a small drink of milk or water to ease any stomach irritation, however, do not under any circumstances attempt to induce vomiting.

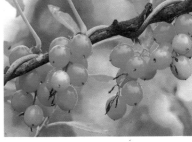

Black bryony This hedge climber has poisonous red berries that last from July until October or even later.

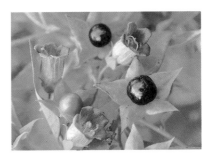

Deadly nightshade All parts of this plant are highly poisonous. Its black berries ripen in August.

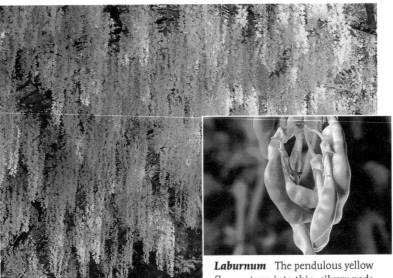

Laburnum The pendulous yellow flowers turn into thin, silvery pods with small dark poisonous seeds.

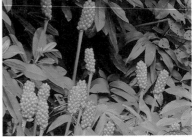

Cuckoopint The red berries are harmful if swallowed and may irritate the skin and eyes on contact.

SELECTING SAFE TOYS

I have read several stories about children who were injured by toys. How can I make sure my children's toys are safe?

The Child Accident Prevention Trust recommends buying from a reputable supplier to ensure that any safety labels are genuine. The Kitemark symbol, awarded by the British Standards Institute, shows that toys have been independently tested and conform to British safety requirements.

● Read the instructions and any safety warnings on the packaging.

● Teach children how to play safely.
● Keep toys intended for older children away from younger ones.
● Avoid toys with small parts for the under fives. Watch out for anything that could be swallowed and cause choking, such as eyes, bells, buttons or snap-together beads. Give any suspect parts a tug before giving the toy to the child.
● Remove any pins or packaging materials that could be swallowed or are sharp.
● Play with the child and toy for the first half hour to detect any problems. This is especially important with secondhand toys.
● Ensure that riding toys, including rocking horses, cannot tip over when in use.

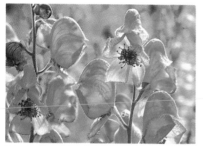

Monkshood Don't confuse this tall, purple wild plant with horseradish – all parts of this plant are highly poisonous.

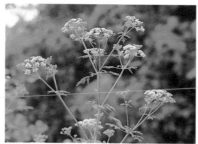

Hemlock Eating any part of this tall, umbrella-like plant could kill you. It grows in open woods and damp places.

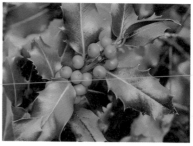

Holly The red berries of this evergreen which appear from October to February may cause a stomach upset if swallowed.

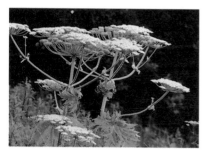

Hogweed Children make peashooters from the stems of this roadside plant, but skin contact can cause a severe rash.

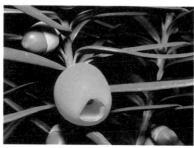

Yew October sees the poisonous berries ripening on this churchyard tree. The bark and leaves are also toxic.

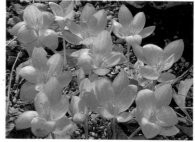

Autumn crocus All parts of this pretty plant are poisonous. Herbalists use small amounts of the poison to treat gout.

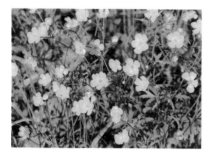

Buttercup Most varieties of this common yellow plant irritate the skin in varying degrees.

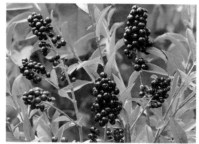

Privet Watch out for this common hedge plant, because the berries and leaves may be poisonous if swallowed.

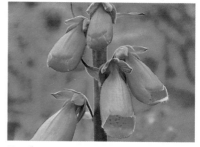

Foxglove Tiny quantities of the poison from this wild and cultivated plant are used in drugs to treat heart conditions.

● Don't use hinged toy boxes if you can find an alternative: they can trap children's fingers or fall on their heads.
● Keep toys tidy – accidents often happen when children or adults trip over toys.
● Give children safety equipment for cycling (see page 339) and skate boarding.

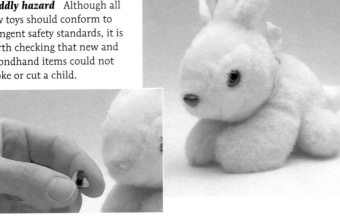

Cuddly hazard Although all new toys should conform to stringent safety standards, it is worth checking that new and secondhand items could not choke or cut a child.

DO'S
— AND —
DON'TS
for child safety

Do keep sharp objects (such as knives), matches, lighters, medicines, cleaning and gardening chemicals, poisonous substances and small objects that could easily be swallowed out of sight and reach.
Do fit safety catches to all windows so that they cannot be opened more than 4 in (10 cm).
Do supervise young children at bath time.

Don't let children play with plastic bags – they could suffocate.
Don't let children play with curtain cords or tie-backs. They could strangle themselves.

CHILDPROOFING THE HOME

What measures can I take, without spending a fortune, to make my home as safe as possible for children?

It is important to remember that there is no substitute for adult supervision, but making the house physically safer will make parents' lives easier. Begin by getting down on the floor for a child's eye view of the world. Remove anything that a child could pull over or put in its mouth: hazards include breakable ornaments on low shelves or tables, and poisonous cleaning materials in accessible cupboards. All homes are different so any hazards will vary, but the suggestions in the panel (left) will make most homes safer.

CHILDREN AND ELECTRICITY

Our baby daughter is learning to crawl. How can I ensure that she doesn't come to any harm from electrical equipment?

The first and simplest precaution is to plug safety covers into all electrical sockets that are not in immediate use. Make sure that sockets are kept switched off until they are needed. Check that any electrical heaters are either wall-mounted, out of her reach, or wired securely into a wall fitting. Also make sure that there are no trailing flexes that she could pull, trip over or chew with possibly disastrous results.

Before too long your daughter will pull herself up to a standing position on anything she can grip. This could be the flex of a table lamp, iron, hair dryer, food mixer, or electric kettle. If possible, keep these items out of her reach. You might have to put them away until she is in bed.

When your daughter learns to toddle, she will also climb on chairs. This will put some electrical appliances kept on work surfaces within her grasp. Consider buying a playpen so that if you do have to leave the room for a moment, you will at least know that she is in a hazard-free area. Even if she has a few tears of frustration, they are a small price to pay for her safety.

KEEPING POISON OUT OF REACH

We keep our house as clean as possible to minimise the risk of germs, but we have heard that many cleaning products could hurt our child or his friends. What can we do to prevent this from happening?

You are right to be concerned. Every year in Britain, some 35 000 children under five years of age are accidentally poisoned in their home.

One of the greatest problems is that many people find it convenient to store cleaning chemicals under the kitchen sink – where children can also reach them easily. Ideally, all cleaning chemicals should be kept in a locked wall cupboard. If this is not possible, fit a child lock to an under-sink cupboard. Consider reducing your stock of cleaning products by trying some alternative methods and materials (see panel, opposite).

Whenever there is a choice, buy cleaning materials with child-resistant tops. Always replace the cap immediately after taking out the amount you need for the job in hand. Stay alert while you work. The Child Accident Prevention Trust says many accidents happen when an adult is distracted in the middle of a job and leaves the chemical unsupervised for a moment.

Never pour cleaning materials into other containers. They may not be strong enough to store the chemical safely, and it is all too easy for an adult or a child to mistake bleach poured into an old lemonade bottle, or white spirit left in an old mug after cleaning a dirty paint brush.

Home and garden chemicals

CARE WITH CLEANING

Every so often you hear about accidents involving household cleaning products. What safety precautions should I take?

All cleaning products need to be used with care. Always read and follow any instructions on the pack, and do not expose yourself to unnecessary contact – by using a spray in a confined space, for example. Even products that are not actually hazardous can cause discomfort or irritation if you get them in your eyes or on your skin. Never mix chemicals: you could cause an explosion or create toxic fumes.

Oven cleaners and drain cleaners are among the most hazardous household products, and can seriously burn your skin and eyes. Use alternatives (see panel, right) if possible. If you have to use any toxic or corrosive substances (see page 337), wear heavy-duty rubber gloves or other recommended protection. Keep the room well ventilated and try not to inhale directly above the cleaner. If you ever splash a chemical product in your eyes or on your skin, rinse the affected area under luke-warm running water for several minutes, and get medical attention immediately if a burning sensation persists.

'GREEN' FOR THE WASH?

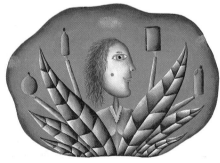

I'm confused by the ingredients in laundry liquids and powders. What are they all for? Does it make any difference to health and the environment to buy 'green' products?

The long names of ingredients in laundry products can make it hard to know exactly what you are buying. All these products have some impact on the environment, but those with so-called biodegradable ingredients – which break down quickly in the environment – generally cause fewer problems. Most laundry products are detergents with various other added ingredients, some of which can cause allergies and other health problems. Green products contain many of the same ingredients as others but not usually phosphates, optical brighteners or perfume. This list of ingredients may help you to choose between the various brands.

● Detergents – chemicals for removing dirt. They break down quickly but large quantities can kill wildlife. Some green laundry products use soap made from vegetable oils instead of detergents, which are usually petroleum-based. Some detergents known as surfactants have been blamed for fertility abnormalities (see page 315).

● Phosphates – water softeners. They are not harmful in themselves, but do encourage the growth of algae that can lead to skin and other health problems if they get into the food chain. High concentrations of algae deprive rivers of oxygen ('eutrophication'), killing waterlife.

● Enzymes – biological chemicals that break down other substances. Those used in washing powders are known as proteases, since they act on proteins, helping to remove blood, sweat and food stains. Washing products with enzymes are labelled 'biological'. Some people find they cause skin or respiratory irritation, and prefer to use non-biological types.

● Fragrances – blamed for some allergies.

● Optical brighteners – also called 'fluorescers'. They have no actual cleaning power but make washed clothes look a brighter white. They are sometimes blamed for skin rashes and a stabiliser called ethylene-diamine-tetra-acetate (EDTA), added to some brighteners, is suspected of forming toxic substances in waste water.

● Polycarboxylates – petroleum-based, nonbiodegradable substances recently introduced as an alternative to phosphates. It is too early to judge environmental effects.

● Silicates – water softeners used mainly to replace phosphates. They may encourage the growth of algae, leading to eutrophication.

● Bleach – the whitening agent sodium percarbonate is thought to be harmless, but sodium perborate can damage plant life by leaving the element boron in water.

Alternatives to household products

There are many tried and tested ways to keep your home sparkling clean and fresh without needing to use any of the harsh chemicals that can cause injuries and have been blamed for harming the environment.

● Try cleaning and disinfecting toilets, sinks and basins with a teaspoon of borax (a natural crystalline powder) dissolved in a pint of hot water. Pour the mixture down the lavatory, or use it to wipe around sinks and basins.

● For glass, tiles and mirrors, mix an equal quantity of white distilled vinegar with water, pour into a spray bottle, spray and buff with a lint-free cloth.

● Try an old-fashioned plunger to unblock drains. If that does not work, pour a handful of table salt and a handful of baking soda down the plug hole followed by a pint (570 ml) of boiling water. Leave overnight. Run the taps for a few minutes in the morning.

● Keep wood clean by rubbing a little cold black tea on it and polishing with a duster. Make a polish with olive oil and vinegar: mix one part vinegar to three parts oil.

● Freshen the air with drops of 'essential oils' (concentrated fragrance) in radiator humidifiers, with bowls of pot pourri or by burning rosemary twigs.

ALTERNATIVE WEEDKILLERS

I'm worried about using weedkillers on the lawn where our children play. Can we eradicate weeds without using chemicals?

You are right to be cautious. Some garden weedkillers are poisonous and babies and small children are notorious for putting their fingers, earth, grass, toys and anything else they play with in their mouths. Fortunately, there are other ways to control weeds.

Try planting weed-resistant grass seed, and don't cut the lawn shorter than 3 in (7.5 cm): the roots will become stronger and the grass will cut out the light that many weeds need to flourish. Weeds that are not near shrubs or flowers can be killed by pouring boiling salted water over them. Or you could try to make the time to pull the weeds out by hand. If you are lucky, you may even be able to persuade the children to help you by turning it into a game with a prize for the one who collects the most weeds. If that does not work and weeding by hand consumes too much time and hurts your back, why not just leave the weeds. Daisies and speedwell can look pretty on a lawn. When your children are older, you can reconsider using a chemical weedkiller. In the mean time, if you do resort to chemical control, follow the safety precautions below.

AVOIDING GARDEN HAZARDS

I don't like using chemicals in the garden, but occasionally there seems to be no alternative. How can I make sure they don't affect my family's health or harm any plants or other wildlife by accident?

The golden rules are to read the instructions on any garden chemicals with great care, and to follow them in every respect.

For your own safety, protect your hands with rubber gloves or gardening gloves whenever you handle any poisons. As a precaution, always wear goggles or sunglasses when spraying herbicides or pesticides, to shield your eyes from stray drops.

Try not to inhale directly over open containers. Avoid spraying on windy days, when it is much harder to control the direction of the spray and you are more likely to inhale droplets or get them on your skin or in your eyes. Wind also increases the risk of spraying plants you do not intend to treat. If possible, spray insecticides in the evening to avoid killing bees and other desirable garden insects. If you have a pond or stream, take care to prevent chemicals running or blowing into the water, where they could kill fish or other aquatic life.

Keep children and pets indoors when you use chemicals and try to keep children off treated grass for a few days, or until rain disperses the residue. Teach young ones not to suck their fingers or put things in their mouths, and to wash their hands when they come indoors.

Some chemicals have to be diluted before use. Mix only as much as you can use immediately. Never leave containers of chemicals unsupervised if you have children.

If you cannot use a toxic product straight from its original container, try to use a bucket, spray or other container kept especially for the purpose and labelled with a skull and crossbones symbol. Never transfer a poison to a food or drink container – an accident could be fatal. Store all chemicals out of reach of children.

CRAFTS AND HOBBIES

I do a lot of craft-work and model-making at home, and have been told that some of the materials I use could be dangerous. What sort of precautions should I take?

You are right to take care. Many crafts and hobbies make use of poisonous or flammable materials: some oil paints contain small amounts of lead or cadmium, while some of the solvents used in painting and printing give off toxic fumes. Pottery clay can contain silica or asbestos, and working with some photographic chemicals can be risky too.

Accidents can happen in seconds, but you can reduce the risks substantially by following some basic rules.

● Try to work away from normal living areas, ensuring that the room or workshop is well ventilated.
● Choose the least toxic materials you can find. Try water-based paints rather than oils. To avoid inhaling powdered paints and dyes, use ready-mixed products dyes and glazes whenever possible.
● Read instructions before use, and follow them carefully.
● Store materials away from children's reach, ideally under lock and key.
● Never leave poisonous liquids in old drinks bottles, cups or mugs – you could mistake the contents.
● Store flammable materials or liquids away from naked flames and heaters, to avoid setting fire to them.

- Do not smoke in the work area.
- Install a smoke detector and keep a fire extinguisher near your work area.
- Wear suitable protective clothing, such as goggles, dust mask, ear-plugs or gloves.
- Clear up any mess as you go, and clean the work area carefully when you have finished. Use a damp cloth to avoid spreading dust.
- Fit a residual current device (RCD) on any power tools or electrical equipment, and regularly check all wiring and sockets for damage (see page 319).
- Never leave any materials or equipment unattended, and always unplug tools and put materials out of reach when you finish working. If there are children about, you should ideally put everything out of harm's way even when you go to the toilet.

Problems with insects and animals

GETTING RID OF FLIES

Every summer we are troubled by flies and wasps in the kitchen. What can we do to get rid of them?

Flies and wasps can both spread disease, so you do need to deal with the problem. Your first line of defence is to avoid attracting flying insects into your kitchen.

- Empty your kitchen bin regularly into a well-sealed outside bin.
- Use rubbish bins with tightly fitting lids. Given the chance, flies will breed on any food waste they can find.
- Wipe up spilled liquids and sweep away crumbs and any other food debris as soon as you notice it.
- Put food away in the refrigerator or cupboard as soon as it is no longer needed.
- Keep food in covered containers: replace lids on jars immediately and cover any food that is cooling with a protective mesh cover, clean towel or piece of foil.
- Do not leave ripe fruit in open bowls: it will attract wasps and flies.
- Keep pets out of the kitchen: if possible, find somewhere else for them to eat and sleep. If they do have to eat there, remove any uneaten food promptly.
- Wash dirty dishes as soon as possible.

It might also help to fit a fine mesh insect screen over any windows opened regularly in summer. Other protective measures include using an old-fashioned fly swatter, hanging up a sticky flypaper or installing an electric insect repelling device that releases vapour from a tablet. If you prefer, try traditional repellents, such as placing bowls of citrus peel, dried mint leaves, lavender, cedarwood or cloves in the kitchen. If you use a fly spray, read the instructions, and take care to avoid contaminating food. Some sprays can harm pets or aggravate respiratory problems.

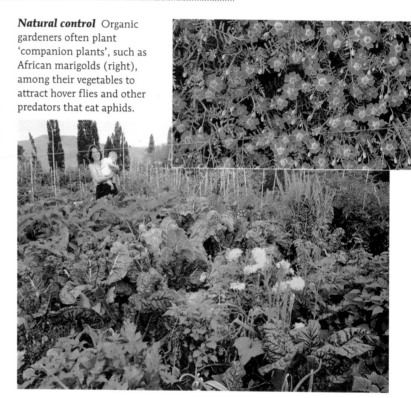

Natural control Organic gardeners often plant 'companion plants', such as African marigolds (right), among their vegetables to attract hover flies and other predators that eat aphids.

CONTROLLING GARDEN PESTS

Our garden is plagued by insects but we don't want to use chemical deterrents. What are the alternatives?

Chemical insecticides are highly effective, but you are wise to be cautious about using them. In many cases, the long-term effects on people and the environment are still unknown. In their place, you could consider plant-based pesticides, such as derris and pyrethrum, that are popular with organic gardeners. Alternatively, you can make an aphid spray by filling a bucket with nettles and water, covering it and stirring the mixture every couple of days for a fortnight. The nettle water will also nourish your plants. You can keep down greenfly on roses by spraying cool washing-up water over them.

Some plants naturally repel certain pests: try planting garlic near roses, or marigolds near tomatoes. Nasturtiums, rosemary and petunias also have a reputation for driving pests away, and interspersing plant species can make it difficult for some insects to recognise their favourite meal. On the other hand, if you prefer to plant groups or rows of the same flower or vegetable, cover seedlings with a tent of fine netting or cheesecloth until they are larger and more able to withstand attacks.

Slugs and snails are a common problem too, especially after a period of wet weather. Try filling saucers with beer and placing them in the ground with the rims level with the earth. Molluscs are attracted to the beer, fall in and drown. Otherwise, try collecting them by hand at night with a torch.

ANT INVASIONS

My house seems to be infested with ants. Even the tiniest scrap of food attracts a column of them. Are they a health hazard, and how can I get rid of them?

Ants are unlikely to spread diseases but they can give you a nasty bite. Your best course of action is to keep your home clear of food debris: if you have small children who are still messy eaters, clear up thoroughly after every meal. Keep food in sealed containers and block up any holes in the brickwork or around windows. There are many effective commercial ant killers available, but most of them are also poisonous to humans: use them with great care, following the manufacturer's instructions. Alternatively, you may prefer to try traditional methods, such as crushed mint leaves or a mixture of dried mint, chilli powder and borax.

DEALING WITH COCKROACHES

I was appalled to see a cockroach scuttle under the fridge at my son's flat. Does this mean that he and his student flatmates should improve their hygiene?

Better hygiene would certainly help to prevent another infestation, but first of all your son should contact his local council's environmental health department. They will offer advice and apply insecticides.

Cockroaches usually get into buildings through cracks and crevices in brickwork. Old buildings with damaged brickwork, leaky pipes, damp cellars and inaccessible drains are particularly vulnerable, and your son might need his landlord's help to improve the building.

In the mean time, find a diplomatic way to tell your son about the health hazards from cockroaches: they can carry many germs, including those that cause typhoid and food poisoning. Encourage your son and his friends to clear away food and to wash up soon after a meal. Advise them to keep food in sealed containers and to wipe out cupboards and sweep regularly under kitchen equipment, such as refrigerators.

CHILD AT RISK FROM PETS?

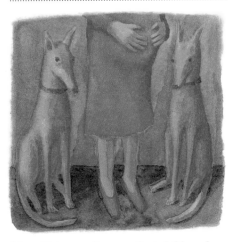

My wife is expecting our first child, and I'm worried that our much-loved dogs could become jealous of the baby. Is this likely?

Dogs have occasionally become jealous and attacked babies, but many pets seem to welcome a newcomer, so don't worry until you have seen how the dogs respond. Give them plenty of affection but, as a sensible precaution, never leave them alone with the baby. Say 'no' firmly if they growl at your new son or daughter. Teach your child from an early age to treat all animals gently, to make animals comfortable, and especially not to pull their tails or ears. Make sure the child never puts its face too near to a dog's face. At such close quarters children are especially vulnerable if the dog becomes aggressive, and even a friendly animal can pass on germs or parasites when it licks. Warn against approaching any dog while it is eating: even the best-natured dog can become aggressively protective of its food. Cats may also need watching – they have been known to sit on sleeping babies and suffocate them.

A MOUSE IN THE HOUSE

We always thought our home was hygienic, but we've recently spotted a mouse in our kitchen. Where have we gone wrong?

Don't feel so guilty. Mice are often attracted by scraps of food, but they are also great opportunists and will squeeze through gaps of less than a quarter of an inch (6mm) to find shelter and nesting sites. Even if your home is spotless, it could be vulnerable to unwanted visitors when doors are left open or when brickwork, windows or pipes are damaged. If you maintain your high standards of hygiene and block up any holes or crevices in the walls, you are unlikely to be troubled by mice again. However, you must get rid of the mouse already in your kitchen, because it could carry disease. Your local council's environmental health department will give you free advice, and may even lay traps or rodent bait free of charge.

INFECTED BY PARASITIC WORMS

My little boy has been complaining of an itchy bottom, and a friend suggested he might have worms. Is this likely and, if so, how could he have picked up something so disgusting?

Children are frequently infected by roundworms or threadworms, but they rarely come to much harm. Teach your son not to put his fingers or toys in his mouth and to wash his hands after playing outside.

Roundworms – *toxicara canis* from dogs and *toxicara catis* from cats – and threadworms are parasites that release their microscopic eggs in the faeces of a host animal.

Roundworm eggs usually incubate in the soil. They are picked up by humans, particularly by children who play in parks or gardens used by dogs or cats, and hatch in the intestines. The worms leave the body when the infected person defecates. If your son has an unexplained persistent fever, a skin rash or respiratory problem after playing outside, you should take him to the doctor, who may prescribe medication. Quite often, however, roundworm infection remains unrecognised because there are not necessarily any clear symptoms: the problem usually clears up without treatment.

Threadworms are more usually spread from person to person – often between members of a family – and may cause rectal or vaginal itching. They can sometimes be seen in the faeces or around the anus where they look like small threads of white cotton. Usually the problem is cured by drugs. All members of the family should be treated at the same time, even if they have no symptoms.

AVOIDING TOXOPLASMOSIS

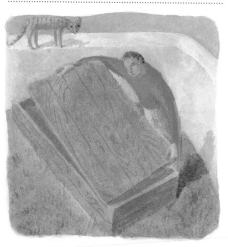

Local cats have started using my daughter's sandpit as a toilet and I'm worried about the risk of toxoplasmosis. Just how dangerous is this disease?

In children and most adults the disease is not a serious cause for alarm, and it can be treated with antibiotics. Toxoplasmosis may not produce any symptoms. When it does, it may seem like flu – with a sore throat, headache, swollen glands and general weakness. For pregnant women and people with AIDS, however, the disease can be very dangerous. If infection occurs during pregnancy, doctors may prescribe antibiotics to try to prevent harm to the foetus.

Toxoplasmosis is caused by a parasite in the faeces of infected cats, and can be caught from garden soil, sandpits, undercooked or raw meat and unpasteurised milk. To prevent infection, always cover the sandpit when it is not in use, and replace the sand regularly. Teach your daughter not to put her fingers or toys in her mouth and to wash her hands after playing in the sandpit or garden. In addition, The World Health Organisation recommends that pregnant women:

● Avoid handling cat litter trays. If this is unavoidable, do wear rubber gloves to protect yourself against contamination.
● Wash your hands after touching cats.
● Wear gloves when gardening.
● Avoid undercooked and raw meat, unwashed fruit and vegetables and unpasteurised milk and milk products.

Dangerous dogs

Pet dogs can provide companionship, but all breeds are potential biters and should be watched when children are around. Under the Dangerous Dogs Act, dogs that are thought to be especially risky, such as Pit Bull type breeds and Japanese Tosas, must be muzzled in public places.

Staying well at work

SICK BUILDING SYNDROME

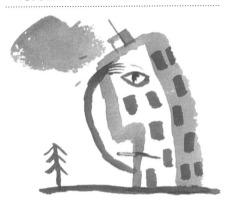

One of my colleagues is convinced that we work in a 'sick' building. What might this mean for our health?

A building is described as 'sick' when the air is contaminated and causes problems such as headaches, nausea, nasal congestion, eyestrain, tiredness, allergies and stress. Many 'sick' buildings are so tightly sealed that insufficient fresh air gets in and air conditioning systems continually circulate bacteria and pollutants, including insulating materials, formaldehyde from pressed wood furniture, glues, synthetic materials, tobacco smoke and fire-retarding chemicals. Other factors, including artificial lighting, room temperatures that are too high or low, and a dry atmosphere, have also been blamed.

If you and your colleagues are concerned about your health, talk to your employer. Explain any symptoms and when they occur. You could also get advice from the Health and Safety Executive and from the health representative at work, if you have one. In most cases, an expert has to be brought in to identify the source of the problem. Remedies usually involve improving the ventilation or removing any contaminants.

RISK FROM PHOTOCOPIERS

My son, who uses a photocopier all day, has recently developed a rash on his hands. Is the equipment to blame?

Photocopiers are not hazardous to people who use them occasionally, but those who work with them all day and have to change the toner can suffer from skin problems and headaches. Your son's employers are responsible for training him to use the equipment correctly and providing any necessary protective clothing. If your son's skin is sensitive, he should get medical advice, wear rubber gloves when he fills the toner reservoir, and wipe up any spilled toner before he removes the gloves.

Some people get headaches from looking at the light when the copier is operating, or from inhaling small amounts of ozone, a poisonous form of oxygen, given off by most photocopiers. These problems can usually be prevented by closing the photocopier's document cover when the machine is operating and by ventilating the photocopying area well, to disperse ozone. Many photocopiers have a special filter to break down ozone but this works well only when it is changed regularly. If your son's machine does not have a filter, he could ask to have one fitted. If the area around the photocopier is stuffy, he could ask for the machine to be moved nearer a window, or ask for a fan to be installed.

ENOUGH LIGHT ON THE SUBJECT

I seem to finish every day at work with a headache. Could the lighting be to blame?

It could be – you can get a headache from working in poor or flickering light – but your problem could also be caused by eyestrain from sitting too close to your work, working at a badly positioned computer screen (see opposite), being under stress (see page 186), drinking too much coffee (see page 50) or working in a 'sick' building (see left). Alternatively, you might need to have your eyes tested for spectacles (see page 126).

Lighting levels are not specified by law, but everyone needs enough light – ideally natural light – to do their job safely and without visual fatigue.

If you have a problem, talk with your company's personnel officers or health advisers, if you have them. Guidelines published by The Health and Safety Executive could help you and your employer to identify and eliminate any lighting problems.

In some factories, where rotating machinery is used, special safety lights need to be installed. Offices can sometimes avoid problems by opting for high frequency fluorescent lights with an imperceptible flicker.

COMPUTER SCREEN SAFETY

I sit at a computer terminal every day and am worried that my work could damage my eyesight. Is my employer obliged to pay for an eye test and, if necessary, to provide me with glasses? What else should I do to protect my eyes?

All employees whose jobs involve regular work at a computer screen, or visual display unit (VDU), can request an eye and eyesight test if they are concerned that their work may be affecting their health. The test must be carried out by a 'suitably qualified' person – in practice, usually an optician. You are entitled to further tests at regular intervals after the first test – these could be frequent if you are having visual problems that could reasonably be considered to arise from working at a VDU. Your employer is also obliged to pay for any corrective spectacles you need for VDU work. However, any spectacles, must be used solely for screen work, and your employer need pay only for the lenses and a basic frame.

You can help to avoid eyestrain by adjusting your distance from the screen and your working position. The Health and Safety Executive recommends that screens should normally be viewed at between 20 in and 24 in (about 50 cm to 60 cm). Position the screen so that daylight or reflections do not fall on it: ideally sit at right-angles to a window. Adjust the brightness of the screen so that you can see the characters clearly without squinting or straining. If you are touch typing from a document, use a document stand placed alongside the screen so you do not have to keep turning your head.

If possible, try to avoid spending the entire working day at your screen. Regulations require employers to plan breaks or changes away from the screen. The Health and Safety Executive suggests that short frequent breaks are better than longer infrequent ones – it is better to rest your eyes *before* you feel tired than to rest to recover. Stretch, blink and change your focal length during your time away from the computer – making a telephone call or organising some paperwork could provide the short break you need. Try the de-stressing exercises on page 193.

To avoid straining your upper body, adjust your chair height so that your elbows are bent at roughly right angles and your wrists remain almost straight. Avoid resting your wrists on the desk or typing with your wrists steeply curved and your hands raised in the 'cobra' position. Adjust your keyboard angle to find a comfortable height and, if possible, use a modern split keyboard to help to avoid any wrist or arm strain.

Keep your feet flat on the floor or on a footrest. Adjust the back rest of your chair to support your lower back and keep your shoulders straight. If necessary, use a lumbar support or cushion to move your weight slightly forward and improve your comfort.

PROTECTING YOUR EARS

I work in a very noisy factory where we have to shout to make ourselves heard. What can I do to protect my hearing?

You'll be glad to know that noise levels and the length of time you are exposed to noise at work are controlled by law, and employers are obliged to protect your hearing. Speak to your supervisor or safety representative, if you have one, to check if your employer has had a noise assessment carried out.

Find out, too, what action has been taken to reduce noise levels where possible, to minimise the time you are subjected to noise above 85 dB(A) – see page 315 – and to provide ear protectors for periods when you cannot avoid high noise levels. Always wear any protective equipment provided, making sure that it works correctly. If you have hearing difficulties, see your GP or, if there is one, the company doctor.

Your welfare at work

Employers have a legal duty to look after you while you are at work. They must ensure, so far as is reasonably practicable, that you will not come to harm because of the way you have to work, or the way the workplace is organised and equipped. Employers are obliged to train you to work safely, to warn you of any hazards (such as dangerous chemicals), to provide any necessary protective clothing and to circulate safety information. But welfare at work involves everyone, not just your employer. You have legal responsibility to watch out for yourself and others affected by your work – whether colleagues, customers or members of the public.

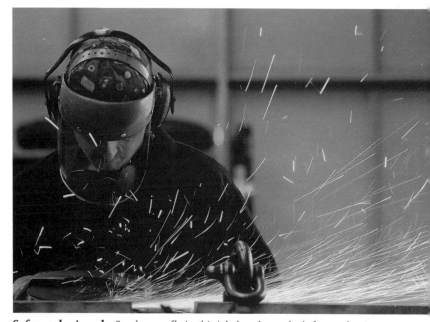

Safeguards at work Sparks may fly in this job, but the worker's face and eyes are protected by a visor, while ear defenders shield his hearing and gloves keep his hands safe. Factory workers are not the only ones to need protective kit – catering, cleaning and medical staff also have to take special precautions.

AIRBORNE ILLNESS

What is legionnaires' disease? How much of a risk is it in modern air conditioning?

Provided they are well maintained, very little – even though air conditioning systems are one of the main culprits for spreading this pneumonia-like disease.

Legionnaires' disease was first identified in 1976 when 29 people died after becoming ill at an American Legion convention in Philadelphia – hence the name. The bacteria – *Legionella pneumophilia* – thrive in warm undisturbed water in rain tanks, air conditioning systems and shower heads. Even though so many people died in America, the death rate has not been repeated in subsequent outbreaks.

British health and safety experts now recommend that hotels and other institutions should keep the temperature of main water tanks and air conditioning systems above or below the main reproduction range – 20°C (68°F) to 60°C (140°F). So far, this appears to be keeping the problem under control.

REPETITIVE STRAIN INJURY

Are computer keyboard users the only ones at risk of injury from repetitive work, and is there any way to avoid problems?

The health problems that are sometimes called 'repetitive strain injury' or upper limb disorders are often associated with keyboard work, but injuries from frequent and forceful finger, hand or arm movements can occur in occupations as diverse as assembly line work, food preparation, packing, dressmaking, construction, decorating, farming and laboratory work. A number of otherwise healthy people have had to take time off work or even give up a job because of pain or, in the worst cases, actual disablement.

Some such injuries, such as tenosynovitis (inflamed tendons) are well understood by doctors. Other work-related injuries have less obvious symptoms and have caused controversy. However, the Health and Safety Executive (HSE) accepts that hand and arm disorders can be caused, or made worse, by work tasks. Other activities, such as sports or housework, are sometimes also to blame.

Preventing problems
Don't ignore persistent aches and pains but get medical help and have a word with your employer as soon as you notice any problem. The HSE can provide information to help staff and employers to assess and deal with risks at work – and your employer is legally obliged to look after your health and safety at work. Common solutions include adjusting the way you sit or move while working, redesigning your work area to avoid awkward movements, improving equipment, rotating jobs, or even changing the way you carry out your work (see also page 335).

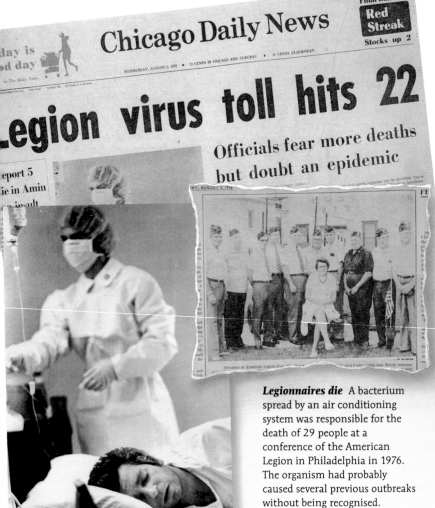

Chicago Daily News

Final markets
Red Streak
Stocks up 2

WEDNESDAY, AUGUST 4, 1976 · 15 CENTS IN CHICAGO AND SUBURBS · 25 CENTS ELSEWHERE

Legion virus toll hits 22

Officials fear more deaths but doubt an epidemic

Legionnaires die A bacterium spread by an air conditioning system was responsible for the death of 29 people at a conference of the American Legion in Philadelphia in 1976. The organism had probably caused several previous outbreaks without being recognised.

ADJUSTING TO NIGHT SHIFTS

I often feel tired and irritable after working night shifts. Why is this, and what will it do to my health? Is there anything I can do to adjust more easily from sleeping at night to sleeping during the day?

You are not alone. Many people feel tired or suffer digestive upsets when they have to stay awake during normal sleeping hours. Although travellers who fly into different time zones usually recover from their jet lag within a few days, shiftworkers find the stress of continual adjustment much harder, especially if they work for just a night or two before returning to daytime shifts. A study showed that shiftworkers can get up to four hours less sleep during the day after a night at work than they would normally manage at night. So it is small wonder that you feel tired and irritable. If you go short of sleep for long, you could have trouble concentrating, be unable to work safely, develop headaches, back pain or even mild hallucinations.

Setting the body clock

Research shows that shiftworkers can avoid problems by finding ways to adjust the 'body clock' or 'body rhythm' – the complex range of natural factors, including your temperature, hormone levels, alertness and powers of concentration. Although scientists do not fully understand how the body clock works, it seems that we are naturally attuned to being active during daylight and sleepy at night. We are at our lowest ebb just before dawn – known as the 'zombie zone' in the United States and 'the hour of the wolf' in the Netherlands – the time when most shiftworkers' accidents and mistakes happen.

By exposing shiftworkers to carefully timed bursts of bright light at night, American researchers have shown that the body clock can be cheated into moving forwards or backward, depending on the timing of the light, so that workers are more alert at night and more sleepy between shifts. Shift staff help to maintain the illusion of night during daylight hours by wearing dark glasses on their way home from work and having heavy bedroom curtains that block out all daylight. Another study, conducted with a group of nurses, showed that they too adapted more easily to night shifts if their bedrooms were totally darkened during daylight hours and their working areas were brightly lit.

Solutions to try

Speak with your employer. It may be possible to improve the lighting in your workplace and to modify your work times. Research shows that the best shift pattern moves from early, to late, to night shifts – so allowing you to adapt more easily and avoid too great a 'sleep debt'. Don't attempt to fight your body's natural rhythms with large doses of stimulants, such as coffee. You will not sleep well later on. At home, consider practising relaxation techniques before going to bed (see pages 190-193), and wear ear-plugs. If problems persist get your doctor's advice.

RISK TO THE FAMILY ?

I want to have a baby but I'm worried about toxic chemicals used where I work. Could they harm an unborn child?

Research suggests that prolonged exposure to high concentrations of certain chemicals, and to some other materials, could harm a growing foetus or affect a worker's children and other members of a family.

The suspect chemicals include ethylene oxide, used to sterilise surgical instruments; vinyl chloride, used in the manufacture of plastics; and arsenic and its compounds, widely used in industrial processes. Other materials that have been blamed for family health problems include asbestos, lead, nickel and manganese.

What the law says

By law – regardless of whether or not you are pregnant – your employer must keep full information about all hazardous materials used at work. He or she must also do everything reasonable to remove or reduce health risks, train you to work safely and to avoid health problems, and provide you with the appropriate protective equipment, such as aprons, overalls, gloves, goggles and masks.

If you are pregnant, have given birth within the last six months or are breastfeeding, your employer is legally obliged to make sure that the kind of work you do and your working conditions will not put your health or your baby's health at risk. If any risks still exist, your employer should alter your working conditions or hours of work. If this is not possible or would not avoid the risk, you must be offered a suitable alternative job with comparative terms and conditions. To get full benefit from the legal protection of your health and safety you must notify your employer in writing of your condition.

Protecting yourself

If you *do* work with high-risk chemicals or materials, make sure that protective equipment is cleaned and maintained at your workplace, or by a special contractor. Never take work overalls or any other items home to wash with the family's clothes: you could carry harmful particles (such as asbestos) or chemical traces with you.

If you are self employed, it is your responsibility to check the risks and the precautions required in your work. You can get advice and information, as can employers, from the Health and Safety Executive's Information Centre: Broad Lane, Sheffield S3 7HQ.

Hazard symbols

Employers must display hazard signs wherever workers need to take special precautions.

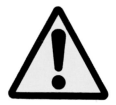

Warning Watch out for hazards in this area.

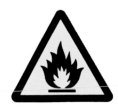

Flammable This will catch fire easily.

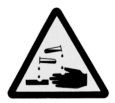

Corrosive Skin contact is highly dangerous.

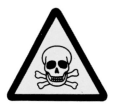

Toxic Do not touch without protective gear.

Harmful
May cause limited health risk if inhaled or ingested or if it penetrates the skin.

Irritant
May cause inflammation and irritation on immediate or repeated or prolonged contact with the skin or if inhaled.

Watch out Health problems could occur.

OCCUPATIONAL HAZARDS

I believe that my breathing problems started at work. What rights do I have to protection at work and to any compensation from my employer?

Many people work with substances, called respiratory sensitisers, that can cause allergies and lead to respiratory diseases, such as asthma. The Government says you could be at risk if you work with isocyanates (found in spray paints and used in the production of plastic foam), laboratory animals, dust from wood, flour or grains, some glues and resins and soldering flux. Some people are completely unaffected by respiratory sensitisers. Others notice allergies such as eczema, or breathing problems within six months of starting work. Others still experience problems only after decades of exposure.

Your employer is responsible for protecting you from anything that could be harmful. You must be trained to work safely, and be given suitable protective clothing, including respirators where appropriate. It is up to you to follow safety instructions carefully.

If you have breathing problems, speak with your employer and your doctor as soon as you notice any symptoms. If you were hurt or became ill because your employer failed to look after your health and safety adequately, you may be able to claim compensation. If the illness or disability means that you are no longer able to work, you will probably be eligible for a pension. For help and information you should contact your trade union, if you are a member, or the Health and Safety Executive (see below).

WORKPLACE INFORMATION

Who can I contact for advice about my welfare at work?

Two organisations share responsibility for enforcing workplace health and safety law: the Health and Safety Executive (HSE) and your local authority's environmental health department. Between them they cover the health, safety and welfare of workers and those affected by work activities (such as shop customers and rail passengers).

The HSE is responsible for factories, building sites, schools, hospitals, farms, railways and local authority and government departments, while local authorities take care of shops, restaurants, offices and hotels.

You can obtain free advice and information from both bodies. Look in your telephone directory for the address of your local environmental health department, or ask at a Citizens Advice Bureau. For general information, get in touch with the HSE Information Centre, Broad Lane, Sheffield S3 7HQ. For specific enquiries, contact your nearest HSE area office (look in the telephone directory). If you are a trade union member, you can get help from your safety representative, if there is one, or from union headquarters.

Getting about safely

SEAT BELTS AND AIR BAGS

I have just bought a new car which is fitted with front air bags. Do I still need to wear a seat belt when driving?

Yes you do. It is a legal requirement for drivers and passengers to wear seat belts, unless they have a medical exemption certificate. Air bags cannot replace seat belts, but they do provide additional protection. In head-on crashes, a front air bag stops your head and upper body from hitting hard parts of the car interior, helping to prevent head and chest injuries. Collisions from the side and rear do *not* inflate front air bags, so your seat belt is still your only protection in such an accident. Seat belts also stop you from being flung through the windscreen in a car crash.

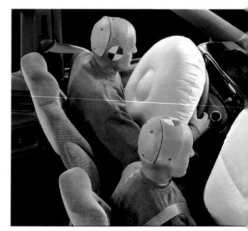

Rapid protection Nitrogen fills air bags within 30 thousandths of a second after impact to cushion against upper body injuries.

PREVENTING CHILD INJURIES

What should I consider when selecting a child safety seat for a car?

You must choose the correct seat for your child's age and weight, but it is equally important to fit the seat correctly.

Seats for babies are rear-facing to prevent head and neck injuries in an accident. Infants that weigh more than 20lb (9kg) can usually sit in forward-facing safety seats – but check the car and safety seat instructions first. If a child under three travels on a *front* passenger seat, the child must, by law, be restrained in a seat suitable for that age. Children over three years of age must also be strapped in: use a toddler seat, booster seat or the car's own seat belts, as appropriate. Check that belts and child seats conform to one of the British or European Standards – these are BS AU202, BS AU185, BS AU186, BS 3254 and ECE 44.

CAUTION Never put babies in a rear-facing safety seat in the front of a car with a passenger air bag. In an accident, the air bag could crush the baby.

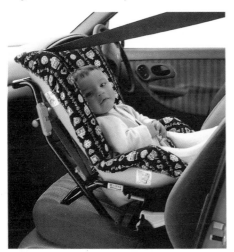

Travelling backwards This rear-facing child seat provides comfort and safety.

SAFETY ON TWO WHEELS

My children are old enough to cycle on minor roads. How can I help them to become safe and responsible road users?

The Royal Society for the Prevention of Accidents advises that children under nine years are too young to cycle safely on roads. However, if you are sure that your children are old enough and mature enough to cope with traffic, then it is time to start some road safety training. The best way to teach is by example. Cycle with your children, pointing out the dangers and showing them how to negotiate difficult junctions. In addition, consider enrolling them on a cycling safety course – often run free of charge by schools, councils, the police and cycling groups. Ask your local police station, council highways department or library for information. It will also help to emphasise these safety issues.

Road sense

Help your children to learn and observe the Highway Code. Teach them to ride at least 3ft (about 1m) from the edge of the road to avoid drains and other uneven surfaces and to allow a narrow safety zone if a vehicle drives too close. They should take care not to get too close to any vehicle and to signal well in advance of any turn. Encourage them to dismount and walk across busy or difficult junctions, particularly when turning right.

Cycle maintenance

Get your children to check their bikes before every trip, looking out for worn brake blocks and tyres, a loose chain or steering, worn or frayed brake or gear cables, or broken lights.

Safe clothing

Make sure your children wear helmets that conform to official safety standards: BS 6863:1989, or ANSI Z 90.4, or SNELL B90, or AS 2063.86. Help them to choose comfortable clothes that will not catch in the wheels or chain. Ensure that they wear a reflective or fluorescent belt so that they can be seen easily by other road users.

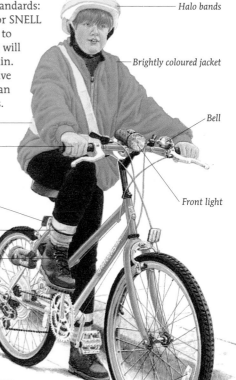

Halo bands

Brightly coloured jacket

Bell

Front light

Reflective/fluorescent belt

Gloves in winter

Rear light

Reflective bands

Laces tucked in

Reflective strip on spokes

Staying visible Brightly coloured clothes, reflective and fluorescent belts, and clear hand signals given in plenty of time all help to make cyclists to be seen by other road users.

AVOIDING ASSAULT

I occasionally feel a little vulnerable when walking alone along a street after dark. Are there any special precautions to take in such a situation?

Although the risk of attack is low in most parts of Britain, it is still wise to take a few precautions. Research suggests that people who appear confident and purposeful are less likely to be attacked than those who seem nervous and uncertain.

Keep to the centre of the pavement and where possible walk facing any oncoming traffic so you can see what is going on. Walk in comfortable shoes that would allow you to run or walk briskly in the unlikely event of feeling threatened. Women who usually wear high-heeled shoes might be wise to carry them with them and change at their destination. Avoid quiet short-cuts or alleys. After dark, try to keep to well-lit roads.

If you are being followed or pestered, walk or run towards lighted buildings, shops, or anywhere that is likely to be busy. Shout or scream if you feel threatened. Although it is illegal to carry a weapon, some people like to carry a personal alarm that can scare off an attacker and help to raise the alarm. Keep yourself fit and, if it would increase your confidence, learn self-defence.

How to make a difference

A rural code

Many people enjoy spending some of their free time in the country, but the number of people involved in leisure activities and their occasional carelessness can put a great deal of pressure upon the countryside and rural environmental services. To avoid harming the countryside, or the livelihood and wellbeing of the people who live there, or the food that is produced, always follow the Countryside Code.

● Leave livestock, crops and machinery alone.
● Take all litter home with you.
● Keep to public paths across farmland.
● Use gates and stiles to cross fences, hedges and farm walls.
● Fasten gates after you.
● Keep dogs under control at all times.
● Guard against all risk of fire.
● Avoid making unnecessary noise.
● Protect water, animals, trees and plants.

BEACH ALERT

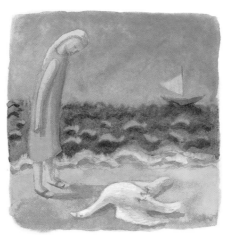

If I see a dead bird or rubbish on a beach, I feel that I ought to do something, but who should I contact?

You can help to protect beaches and marine life in several ways. Collect any bottles, cans or papers you come across and put them in a rubbish bin. If you find medical rubbish, such as a syringe, do not touch it but ring the police or the local environmental health department (listed in the telephone book under the name of the local council). If you see canisters, drums or other containers that could contain chemicals, contact the police or coastguard and warn others in the vicinity, particularly children.

You can also play a part in helping to stop beach and sea pollution. If you see brown foam, brown scum or oil on the sea or on the beach, or if you see dead birds, alert the National Rivers Authority (telephone 0171 820 0101) or tell your local environmental health department: they will try to trace the source of the contamination and stop it.

To help injured and sick animals or birds, contact the local branch of the Royal Society for the Protection of Animals.

Even by reporting *dead* animals, you could help scientists to find out more about pollution and other dangers to wildlife. Report deaths of whales, porpoises and dolphins to the Marine Biological Services Division of the Department of Zoology at the Natural History Museum, London. Contact the Institute of Zoology, Regents Park, London, if you see any dead seals.

REDUCING CAR POLLUTION

Like many other people, I rely on my car to get around. Can I do anything to minimise the pollution that a car inevitably causes?

Yes – every effort towards reducing vehicle exhaust fumes makes a small contribution to reducing pollution levels. Every car-owner can practise these simple measures.

● Save fuel by walking, cycling or using public transport whenever possible.
● Avoid short trips by car – your car burns twice as much fuel within the first few minutes of starting up as it does during normal running on a longer journey.
● Before buying a new car, check whether the vehicle has a high or low fuel consumption. If buying a petrol vehicle,

try to choose one that uses unleaded fuel and has a catalytic converter and a carbon canister (a fitting that reduces pollution). If buying a diesel vehicle, check that it has an oxidation catalyst (that reduces pollution).

● Use unleaded fuel if possible. If you have an old car, check whether it can be converted to run on unleaded fuel.

● Have your car serviced and tuned regularly and make sure the air filter is changed at least every 15 000 miles (24 000 km).

● Keep your tyres at the correct pressure – soft tyres can increase fuel consumption by up to 6 per cent. If possible, choose radial tyres, which improve fuel efficiency by about a mile per gallon (about 1 km per 4.5 litres).

● Drive at a steady, moderate pace whenever possible: stopping, starting, rapid acceleration and high speeds use extra fuel.

● Avoid letting your engine idle for more than a minute. It creates extra fumes and consumes unnecessary fuel.

● Report the registration number of vehicles emitting heavy exhaust fumes to your local environmental health department. Vehicles with smoky diesel engines should be reported to the Department of the Environment or the Department of Transport.

A VOICE IN A MILLION?

My family tries to do its bit for the environment, but are we fooling ourselves that our efforts really make any difference to the world around us?

Simple actions, such as separating and recycling rubbish, riding a bicycle occasionally instead of always getting around by car, and using phosphate-free laundry products will all help. You won't instantly reduce Britain's deep pits of rubbish that take decades to rot, nor immediately affect the Western world's traffic exhaust emissions that are blamed for so many breathing ailments. Nor will you prevent all potentially hazardous waste from reaching the rivers and seas. However, you can rest assured that your efforts do play a small but important part in protecting both the community and the environment.

If you feel you could do even more, why not contact like-minded people in a local, national or even an international conservation group? Local libraries usually have lists of organisations, and many will welcome children as well as adults. You do not have to wave banners or become a full-time campaigner to get involved and make a valuable

contribution. Many people have made a difference to the world around them simply by alerting others to possible threats to human health and the environment.

GETTING DEVELOPMENT RIGHT

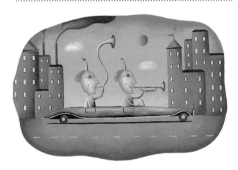

New buildings are going up all round my town. What safeguards exist to protect people and the countryside from new development, and how much say can I have on what is built around me?

There are a number of safeguards to protect people and the environment from oppressive or harmful building development, and local residents can have a big say in what is built. However, the impact you can make on building proposals depends to some extent upon staying alert to what is going on around you and finding out what is planned.

Every planning authority – usually your local council – must produce a 'development plan' setting out policies for use of the land over the next ten to fifteen years. You can make your views known, either as an individual or through local residents', conservation or business organisations, during the obligatory consultation period and public inquiry. Keep an eye on your local newspapers for information about the next development plan. Look at the current plan at your local council's planning office or library.

You can also comment on individual planning applications – for new buildings, changes in the use of land or buildings, or for changes to a preservation order (for a tree, building, district or site of special scientific interest or natural beauty) – and at public inquiries into development plans.

Councils must tell people living or working close to any site affected by a planning application. Local residents' and conservation groups often monitor *all* the applications in their area so they give councils their opinion of plans that could affect the health of the wider community and the environment before it is too late.

Recycling your rubbish

Conservationists estimate that everyone in Britain throws away about a third of a ton of domestic rubbish every year. Yet with just a little effort, most household rubbish can be separated and recycled, saving raw materials and fuel, and helping to prevent pollution from landfill sites and from rubbish incineration.

Many towns in Britain now have collection points for paper and cardboard, glass, metal and plastic. Some places also collect oil, old refrigerators and worn-out batteries.

To help prevent pollution and to protect natural resources:

● Separate and recycle as much of your rubbish as possible. Try to buy food and drinks in glass or aluminium containers that can be recycled.

● Avoid buying items in unnecessary packaging.

● Buy food in bulk – it uses less packaging.

● Reuse polythene bags.

● Make a compost heap from vegetable scraps, if you have a garden. Use the well-rotted material to fertilise the garden and improve the soil.

● Try to find a garage that sends worn car tyres to Britain's tyre-fuelled power station or to be recycled. Buried tyres take decades to rot, can be an eyesore and create a fire risk. Don't be afraid to buy remoulded tyres – they are safe and save valuable resources.

HELP FOR CHRONIC HEALTH PROBLEMS

*Most illnesses are cured sooner or later,
but some keep coming back or simply never abate. To
live better with a chronic condition, you need to understand it,
know the treatments that are available, and find the
best ways to carry on with normal life.*

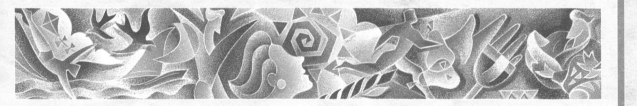

How much do you know about chronic illness?

Chronic illness doesn't mean only arthritis, heart disease and the like – it includes asthma, allergies and dozens of other conditions. Yet even those who live with them often know little about such complaints. Find out how much you know by trying this quiz. Tick the right answers and check your score below.

1 What is a chronic illness?

a) An illness that is serious. ☐
b) An illness that continues for a long time or that keeps coming back. ☐
c) A fatal illness. ☐

2 Which of these chronic health problems is most common?

a) Gout. ☐
b) High blood pressure. ☐
c) Diabetes. ☐

3 What proportion of the British population suffers from hay fever?

a) Over 10 per cent. ☐
b) 2 - 5 per cent. ☐
c) Under 2 per cent. ☐

4 What is the main difference between an allergy and an intolerance?

a) They are essentially the same, but allergies are worse. ☐
b) You can grow out of an intolerance but a true allergy lasts for life. ☐
c) People with allergies have a different kind of antibody in their blood. ☐

5 Which statement about acne is true?

a) Eating chocolate and other oily foods makes it worse. ☐
b) It can be treated with antibiotics. ☐
c) It affects only adolescents. ☐

6 Which of these three statements about asthma is true?

a) It is safe, and even advisable, to take exercise if you have asthma. ☐
b) Country air is better for asthma. ☐
c) Asthmatics should try not to use an inhaler unless they really have to. ☐

7 Which should an ulcer patient avoid?

a) Smoking. ☐
b) Spicy food. ☐
c) Acidic food. ☐

8 Which symptoms would you see in someone with high blood pressure?

a) Redness in the face and irritability. ☐
b) Fatigue and muscle cramps. ☐
c) There are no special symptoms. ☐

9 Which is most important if you have high blood cholesterol?

a) Being careful not to overexert yourself in strenuous activities. ☐
b) Cutting down on cheese, butter and fatty meat. ☐
c) Cutting down on high-cholesterol foods, such as prawns and liver. ☐

10 Which one of these common drugs may prevent a heart attack?

a) Antibiotics. ☐
b) Tranquillisers. ☐
c) Aspirin. ☐

SCORING

Award yourself 1 point for each of these answers: 1(b), 2(b), 3(a), 4(c), 5(b), 6(a), 7(a), 8(c), 9(b) and 10(c). Add up your score.

8-10: You seem to know a great deal about chronic illnesses and how to cope with them.

5-7: Your knowledge is quite good but you may still have more to learn.

4 or less: Perhaps you are fortunate enough never to have been affected by a chronic complaint. Even so, you could find it useful to know a little more.

Living with a long-term illness

THE MEANING OF 'CHRONIC'

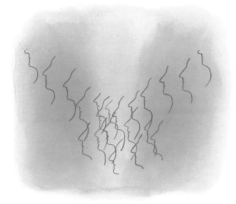

Why are some conditions classified as chronic? Are they always serious?

Doctors use the term 'chronic' to describe any illness or symptom that goes on for a long period of time. Depending on the condition, the duration may vary from months to years to a lifetime. Although many such illnesses are considered incurable, they can very often be well controlled. The symptoms may come and go and there may be periods when the illness goes into remission, sometimes to the extent that there is virtually no evidence of it at all.

Chronic conditions are generally distinguished from acute illnesses, which occur suddenly, last for a short time and produce rapid changes, such as a high temperature or severe pain. In some but not all cases, acute symptoms worsen until they reach a crisis, after which healing occurs steadily until the patient is back to normal.

Infections tend to follow the acute pattern, while chronic disorders more often develop slowly or take the form of occasional flare-ups with long periods of remission in between. Many chronic complaints also fall into the general category of 'degenerative' disorders – conditions that involve damage to the structure or function of body tissues.

Not all chronic conditions are serious, however, or cause permanent damage of any sort. Many people have mild allergies or suffer from migraine headaches from time to time without finding their lives significantly affected. Other patients manage by means of good dietary measures, a generally healthy way of life, or regular medication to control conditions such as diabetes, epilepsy and migraine. Often they manage to remain almost entirely symptom-free and go on to have a normal life expectancy.

CAUSES AND PREVENTION

What causes chronic complaints? Is there any way of preventing them?

Chronic illnesses are very varied and can have many causes. In the vast majority of cases, however, genetic inheritance plays a major role in determining people's vulnerability. This is not to say that everyone who inherits a certain gene or pattern of genes will inevitably develop a condition such as asthma or heart disease, but rather that the *chances* are greater than in the population as a whole. Depending on other factors, such as environment, diet and stress, such diseases may or may not develop in someone who carries the genetic predisposition. Prevention generally depends on identifying people who may be at risk, giving preventive advice on diet, exercise and other health issues, and providing monitoring to pick up any problems before they have a chance to become serious.

TREATING CHRONIC PROBLEMS

If chronic illness can't be cured, what sort of treatments and help can sufferers get?

The important thing to remember about a chronic illness is that it is likely to be a permanent fact of life. This means that the patient has to learn how best to control the symptoms in order to live as full and active a life as possible. Often simply following a healthy way of life, with a good diet, plenty of exercise, adequate rest and stress kept under control, is enough to keep well most of the time. Other people may need drugs to counteract effects such as narrowed blood vessels, a tight chest or an allergic reaction. In some advanced conditions, surgery can help by replacing worn, painful joints or a damaged heart valve.

More than any other factor, attitude determines how well people cope with a chronic illness. Whatever their physical state, those who live life to the full invariably fare better than those who see themselves as invalids.

How common is chronic illness?

As with acute illness, the incidence of chronic illnesses varies greatly and there are no general rules. Some chronic conditions are very rare while others affect a large percentage of the population. Some, such as asthma, are on the increase, possibly because of growing pollution.

Increased life expectancy and better treatments for acute conditions also mean that more people are living long enough to develop slow-acting, long-term complaints. Accurate figures are difficult to establish, but current estimates put the incidence of chronic conditions as follows.

- **Very common (more than 1 in 20)**
  Allergies.
  Asthma.
  High blood pressure.
  Osteoarthritis.

- **Common (1 in 20 to 1 in 100)**
  Chronic bronchitis.
  Diabetes.
  Psoriasis.
  Rheumatoid arthritis.

- **Fairly common (1 in 100 to 1 in 500)**
  Epilepsy.
  Gout.
  Schizophrenia.

- **Uncommon (1 in 500 to 1 in 2000)**
  Ankylosing spondylitis.
  Down's syndrome.
  Multiple sclerosis.
  Parkinson's disease.
  Ulcerative colitis.

Keeping allergies under control

Does diet hold the answer?

One way of diagnosing a food allergy is by means of an exclusion diet. This involves cutting out suspect foods from your diet – either one by one or in groups – and then gradually reintroducing them. The results can be quite decisive, provided the tests are properly set up and conducted under medical supervision. Before beginning, start recording what you eat, and when, and any symptoms that occur.

CAUTION Exclusion diets can be dangerous. Never go on one without consulting your doctor.

DO'S
— AND —
DON'TS

for dealing with allergies

Do try to identify and avoid allergens.
Do stay indoors on dry, windy days and in the mornings in spring and summer when pollen levels are high, if you suffer from hay fever.
Do avoid chemical irritants, such as perfume, household cleaners and chlorinated pool water.
Do dust and vacuum frequently – every day if possible. Vacuum your mattress when you do the bedroom.

Don't clutter your house with ornaments that collect dust.

WHAT ALLERGIES ARE

Every year in summer my husband's eyes start to itch and water and his nose begins to run. The doctor says it's an allergy, but what exactly does that mean and what's causing the problem?

Your husband's watery eyes and runny nose occurring together are classic symptoms of hay fever – one of the commonest allergies there is. Hay fever (sometimes called allergic rhinitis) is usually produced by grass pollen irritating the respiratory tract, so it could be the fresh growth of grasses in summertime that is to blame.

An allergy is an exaggerated response by the body to a foreign substance (or allergen) that enters or comes into contact with it. Allergens can be ingested with food or drink, breathed in with air, injected into the bloodstream by an insect sting, or simply touch the skin. While most people are unaffected by contact, people with allergies react badly because they possess particular allergic antibodies in their blood which go into action to fight such substances, triggering the release of body chemicals such as histamine, that cause allergic symptoms including itching, sneezing, rashes and wheezy breathing. In the case of hay fever, allergic antibodies to

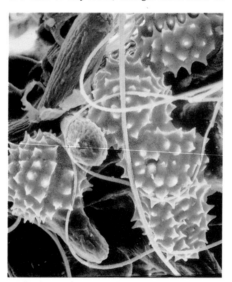

Airborne irritant Pollens are responsible for many allergy and hay fever symptoms in spring and summer. These highly magnified pollen grains come from a goldenrod flower.

grass pollen are constantly circulating in the bloodstream. For people like your husband, the simplest way of preventing attacks is to avoid coming into contact with grass pollen as much as possible. If symptoms do occur, taking antihistamine drugs – available over the counter in chemists – can help to control them. For daytime use, or when driving, ask for a formula that does not cause any drowsiness. If antihistamines prove ineffective, a doctor may prescribe alternative medication such as a steroid nose spray.

No one really knows what makes some people but not others develop allergies in the first place. Inheritance plays some part and exposure early in life to irritating substances, such as house dust or cigarette smoke, may also have an effect. The problem is very common, however, and affects between one in ten and one in three people.

ALLERGY AND INTOLERANCE

My doctor says I have an intolerance to certain foods but not an allergy to them. What's the difference?

These are medical terms used to indicate the mechanism by which the disorder occurs. True food allergy results from the production in the body of abnormal allergic antibodies to particular substances in food. Babies who are allergic to cow's milk, for example, have allergic antibodies to milk circulating in their blood. Every time the antibodies detect cow's milk, they go into action against it, causing allergic symptoms.

By contrast, people who suffer from food intolerance do not have allergic antibodies in their blood. In many cases the exact mechanism of the problem remains a mystery but in others a cause can be identified – babies who cannot tolerate cow's milk, for example, lack an enzyme needed to break down milk sugar. In either case, the child may well grow out of the problem. In older children and in adults both allergies and intolerances tend to remain for life.

Food allergies and food intolerances can produce similar symptoms, although intolerances are generally much less severe in their effects. Reactions including eczema, asthma and rhinitis are typically signs of an allergic condition rather than an intolerance. In practical terms, the real differences between allergies and intolerances are not very great. Avoiding trigger substances is the key to staying well in either case. Problem foods are often the same: dairy products, citrus fruit, eggs, wheat, nuts, cheese, chocolate, fish and strawberries. The symptoms from coffee, red wine and chemical additives may show an intolerance but not an allergy.

FINDING THE CAUSE

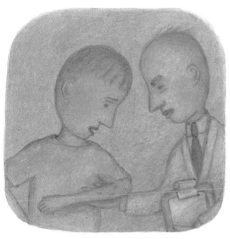

I'm sure I have an allergy of some sort but I can't seem to pinpoint the cause. Is there a test I could have?

You may well have an allergy, but it is also possible that whatever symptoms you are experiencing could have another cause, so it is important to see your doctor for diagnosis.

Once other possibilities have been ruled out, the process of trying to identify allergies

begins. The first step will be self-observation. Your doctor will probably ask about the timing of your symptoms. Are they seasonal, for example, or do they occur all year round? Are they worse in the morning or at night? Places that affect you can also be a giveaway. Do the symptoms occur more at home or at work? Indoors or outside? In town or in the country? In houses where there are pets?

If the results are inconclusive your doctor may suggest laboratory tests. Two kinds are used – skin tests and a blood test known as RAST (radioallergosorbent test) or CAP (a newer version if the RAST test). Both are available on the NHS and although none is foolproof, they can often help to identify the offending substance or substances.

In skin testing, tiny amounts of suspected allergens are pricked into the skin. If you are allergic, your skin will become irritated or develop a weal. The most reliable skin tests are those for pollen, dust, moulds and other airborne allergens. Some food allergens also show up very well – skin tests for fish, shellfish and nut allergies (which can be very violent) are usually extremely reliable. Other food reactions, however, may yield less clearcut results. Skin tests are simple to perform and cause only minimal discomfort. The procedure is considered entirely safe, even for children, and there is no danger of a serious allergic reaction occurring, however violent the allergy itself.

Blood tests cause a little more discomfort, and are more expensive and often less sensitive than skin tests. However, the new CAP procedure is more sensitive than the RAST test and is replacing it in many laboratories.

How drugs help

Allergy sufferers can find relief from several types of medication.

● Antihistamines counter the effects of body chemicals that are responsible for causing allergy symptoms.
● Decongestant tablets or nose-drops relieve nasal and sinus congestion by narrowing blood vessels.
● Bronchodilators are inhaled directly into the air passages and provide immediate relief from respiratory symptoms by widening the bronchial tubes. They can also be used for prevention.
● Steroid nasal sprays and inhalers reduce and prevent respiratory symptoms and are very safe as only tiny amounts of the drug enter the bloodstream. Tablets are also used.
● Sodium cromoglycate eye drops, powder or spray can prevent respiratory symptoms.

Dealing with skin complaints

HAND RASHES

After doing the washing-up, my hands tend to break out in an itchy rash of red blisters. My pharmacist says it's dermatitis, but what does this mean?

Dermatitis is a very general term, used for any type of skin inflammation. Your symptoms probably fall into the category of contact dermatitis – a reaction to something in direct contact with your skin. One obvious possibility would be an allergy to the brand of washing-up liquid you are using, although there is a variety of other irritants that could also be contributing to the problem.

You may find that your symptoms disappear if you are scrupulous about wearing plastic washing-up gloves, preferably with a cotton liner, or if you change to a different detergent. If not, consider other possible irritants – metal jewellery, woollen gloves, hand creams, bath soap and contact with pets affect many people. Occasionally foods such as raw chicken or raw fish cause symptoms.

Good hand care can be a help, too. Wash your hands in lukewarm water, use a mild, unperfumed soap and dry well. Remove any rings and bracelets before doing housework, taking a bath or washing your hands, and don't allow your hands to soak in water. If the problem persists, consult your doctor.

Steroid creams and skin disorders

Steroid creams don't cure eczema but suppress inflammation and relieve symptoms and rashes. However, long-term use can lead to problems such as thinning skin. More potent types can also suppress the adrenal glands if used in prolonged or large doses, particularly on thin skin or raw areas.

To reduce side effects, use the smallest dose of the mildest preparation that gives relief. Follow your doctor's instructions precisely or, if you buy mild hydrocortisone cream over the counter, ask the pharmacist for advice.

Do not apply steroid preparations to the face. Use creams for moist or weepy skin and ointment for dry skin.

Foods that can cause skin trouble

Many people with skin trouble find that avoiding certain foods relieves their symptoms. These are some common problem foods.

- Dairy products.
- Wheat.
- Shellfish.
- Chicken.
- Eggs.
- Citrus fruit.
- Strawberries.
- Mushrooms.
- Foods with additives.
- Nuts.
- Tomatoes.
- Chocolate.

FIGHTING ACNE

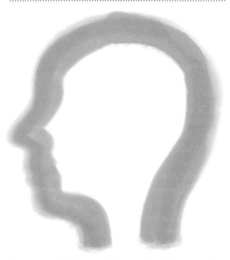

I've been fighting a 25-year battle against acne. Absolutely nothing seems to work. Am I destined to be an old lady with spots, or is there a miracle cure?

Acne is an embarrassment that cannot be cured, but can be controlled. It occurs when there is a blockage of the sebaceous glands that prevents the oily substance sebum from reaching the surface of the skin. This creates infection and inflammation. In some cases it produces no more than the mild unsightliness of blackheads or tiny pimples. In other cases, pockets of pus develop or even painful cysts. Although acne almost always begins at puberty, it can persist well into adulthood and your situation is by no means unusual.

The causes of acne are still something of a mystery. Higher levels of certain sex hormones at puberty are probably responsible, at least in part, but there is also some evidence of a genetic connection. Certain drugs can trigger or aggravate the problem, particularly corticosteroids and androgens, which increase oil production in the skin. Cosmetics with oily bases can also exacerbate the problem. Contrary to popular belief, there is no evidence that eating chocolate and other oily foods causes acne.

Treating acne

To keep acne under control, avoid squeezing or picking spots – you could end up scarring your skin. Stop the build-up of bacteria by washing with medicated soap and warm water. If you use over-the-counter lotions, follow the instructions exactly. Exposure to sunshine or sunlamp rays may also help, but take care to avoid sunburn and to protect your eyes (see page 139). A healthy diet with plenty of fresh fruit and vegetables is generally good for the skin. See your doctor if the condition persists. He or she may prescribe antibiotic creams or a vitamin A gel or lotion known as tretinoin, which can have good results. Oral antibiotics are sometimes also given, but a fairly lengthy course of about three months or more is needed. Women may also be offered a hormone treatment known as Dianette. In severe cases, treatment with the vitamin A preparation isotretinoin may be suggested, but this needs to be administered in hospital.

PREVENTING PSORIASIS

My son suffers from psoriasis from time to time. Is he likely to ever grow out of it? Why does it occur and is there anything we can do to prevent outbreaks?

Your son's problem is unlikely simply to go away, but it can be treated and controlled. What causes psoriasis is not known for sure, though there is a tendency for it to run in families and there are some indications that hormones may play some part. The problem arises during the natural process of skin renewal. For some reason, more new skin is produced than is needed to replace the skin being shed from the body. The new growth accumulates under old skin and produces thick red scaly patches, or plaques.

Relieving symptoms

There is no guaranteed way of preventing further outbreaks, but it will be helpful if you encourage your son to take care of his skin and, in particular, to avoid minor injuries such as burns and scratches. Exposure to natural sunlight or to ultraviolet light from a sunlamp can also help if the problem is mild. Be careful to avoid sunburn and follow the safety precautions on page 139.

For relief when outbreaks occur, try using emollients such as petroleum jelly to alleviate the itching and dryness. Shampoos, gels and creams containing coal tar are very effective at removing dead skin – don't be put off by the medicinal smell or messiness of using them. Your doctor will be able to prescribe dithranol in the form of a cream or ointment – also messy, but effective in slowing down new skin production. This medication has to be used very carefully as it can burn healthy skin, and must never be applied to the face, groin or armpit.

Prescribed steroid creams are simpler to use and very good at reducing inflammation, but they can make the skin thinner, so use them carefully and sparingly. Alternatively, try vitamin D creams and ointments. Many people find them effective and they are both odourless and non-staining.

CONTROLLING ECZEMA

I've had eczema for several years and, although it has periods of getting better, it never completely disappears. Why is this? And what is the best way to keep the condition under control?

Your experience is not unusual. Some cases of eczema, especially those that start in childhood, do eventually disappear. Others, like yours, may go on for years. Part of the problem with treating eczema lies in the difficulty of identifying the cause. Some eczema is caused by allergies – usually to foods, chemicals, fibres or other irritants in contact with the skin – which can be notoriously difficult to identify. In many cases a tendency to eczema appears to be inherited, but there are often other aggravating factors involved, ranging from exposure to cold air and wind to emotional stress.

Because so many elements affect eczema, there is no simple cure suitable for everyone. Even so, eczema can usually be well controlled. GPs will prescribe steroid creams, which need to be used with care but are highly effective. Over-the-counter remedies can also help – try calamine lotion to soothe irritation, and zinc and coal-tar ointments to get rid of dry, thickened skin. If your condition is mild, petroleum jelly may be all you need to keep the skin soft. If itching is severe, however, you may need to use antihistamine tablets or cream. Oral antihistamines can cause drowsiness, so avoid taking them before driving or on other occasions when you need to be alert.

Finding the cause

Longer-term measures depend on identifying the cause. If you suspect an allergy, ask your doctor about a skin test to check your reactions to a range of likely irritants. You can also experiment for yourself by seeing if eczema improves if you wear soft cotton next to the skin rather than wool, avoid certain soaps, or use bedding made of synthetic materials instead of feather and down or wool. Exclusion diets can often help to identify some food allergies, but these need medical supervision – ask your doctor's advice. Further help and advice can be obtained from the National Eczema Society, 4 Tavistock Place, London WC1H 9RA.

A CURE FROM CHINA?

I've heard that Chinese herbal treatments sometimes have more success at treating skin ailments than orthodox Western medicine. Where can I find out about them? Are there any risks?

Chinese herbal practitioners do prescribe a range of treatments for skin problems such as eczema, psoriasis and acne, and there is some evidence that they can be effective.

In traditional Chinese medicine, practitioners view each case as unique, so treatments are prescribed only after consultation and there are no over-the-counter remedies. Normally, a prescription is given for a herbal concoction, which you brew for yourself as a tea and drink at regular intervals. The mixture may be adapted as treatment progresses. Most of the herbs used are imported and are available only from Chinese herbalists, who cannot legally sell them without a prescription from a recognised practitioner.

For further information, you can contact the London School of Acupuncture and Traditional Chinese Medicine, 60 Bunhill Row, London EC1Y 8JS. To obtain the names and addresses of qualified practitioners of traditional Chinese medicine, contact the Register of Chinese Herbal Medicine, PO Box 400, Wembley, Middlesex HA9 9NZ.

CAUTION There have been some reported cases of liver damage and other health problems resulting from Chinese herbal cures, and there is no way of checking on exactly what they contain. Approach all such treatments with caution and always consult your doctor before being tempted to experiment with any. Never stop your ordinary treatment suddenly.

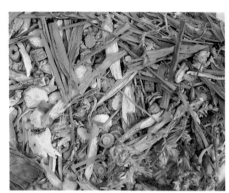

Plants with a purpose Chinese herbal remedies have had some success in treating obstinate skin conditions. Patients infuse a tea from an individually prescribed mixture.

Helping a child with eczema

Childhood eczema can be very distressing, but simple measures can relieve many symptoms.

- Reduce inflammation with prescribed steroid creams. Use sparingly to prevent side effects.
- Don't bath the child too often; this could dry out the skin.
- Use an emollient or emulsifier such as aqueous cream (available over the counter from a chemist) for cleaning and moistening the skin.
- Try over-the-counter bath products such as Oilatum (made from oatmeal) and Bath E45 to relieve itching.
- Ask your doctor about using antihistamines to suppress itching during the night.
- Keep your child's nails clean and short to prevent skin damage from scratching.
- Try cotton gloves or pyjamas with built-in mittens to stop scratching during the night.
- Use plain water without soap for bathing and washing.

Asthma and chest complaints

WHY ASTHMA HAPPENS

My chest has become very wheezy and sometimes I find it difficult to breathe. Could I be developing asthma?

Very possibly – but you will need a proper medical diagnosis to find out, so see your doctor. Your symptoms could also have other causes that need treatment.

Children with asthma Most young asthmatics can learn to control their condition well with just a simple inhaler, but for higher doses of drugs a nubuliser may be needed (below). The machine pumps air or oxygen through a solution of the drug.

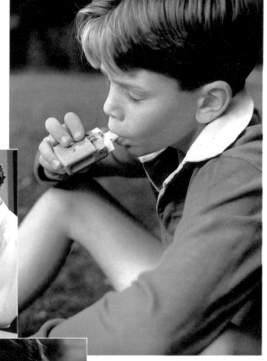

The right technique Asthma inhalers (above and left) need coordinated breathing, which can take practice to get right.

Safer medication A plastic chamber (right) known as a spacer can be placed between mouth and inhaler to make taking asthma drugs easier and safer. With a spacer, patients can breathe naturally and will experience fewer side effects.

Breathing difficulty and wheezing noises are two of the first signs of asthma – noticeably on the increase in Britain. Asthma now affects about one in twenty of all Britons and many more children than adults – estimates range from one in ten to one in seven.

If asthma is responsible for your symptoms, you have probably also experienced occasional tightening of the chest and you may have noticed that you are coughing a lot. These are signs that the airways are constricted, hampering normal breathing. The airway linings are naturally sensitive, and much more so in the case of asthmatics. When substances such as smoke or pollen are breathed in they cause irritation and inflammation, and the passages constrict. This makes it difficult to breathe in, and even harder to breathe out as the airways are naturally narrowed when expelling air. The result is wheezy, laboured breathing.

If you do have asthma, you have probably noticed your symptoms worsening in certain situations – for example, when the environment is dusty or polluted. Pollen, cigarette smoke, certain drugs, most notably aspirin, and even changes in hormone levels or the weather may also be triggers. About half of all asthmatics find attacks are brought on by allergic reactions to such substances.

Before assuming that you have asthma, however, see your doctor. He will help you to pinpoint the cause of the problem and if necessary prescribe medication to ease your breathing. Whatever is wrong, some sort of treatment will be able to help.

PREVENTING ATTACKS

Asthma attacks are becoming a way of life for my children. Surely there is some way of preventing the problem, or at least reducing the frequency?

There are so many ways an asthma attack can be set off that prevention can be difficult. Nevertheless, there is still plenty you can do. Reducing house dust levels is probably the single most effective step, and helps in nearly all cases since dust mites and their droppings are a major cause of asthma. Of course, you cannot hope to eliminate every microscopic particle of dust from your children's surroundings, but by getting rid of some of it you will be cutting down the risk.

Clean all children's bedrooms thoroughly every day, or teach them to, and vacuum the whole house as often as possible.

Pillows and mattresses are both notorious traps for dust and dust mites. Replace any feather pillows you have with foam rubber, change feather duvets for synthetic ones, and vacuum the mattress whenever you do the floor, preferably every day. Also consider buying anti-allergy mattress covers, pillow slips and sheets, which can provide a barrier to dust and mites. Alternatively, cover your children's mattresses with plastic sheets.

Unfortunately, even cuddly toys can be a danger to asthmatic children. And so can pets. This can be a difficult dilemma for parents. Remember, even if a pet does have to be sent to a new home, discarded animal hair and microscopic skin particles will still be left behind throughout the house. After the animal has gone, you will need to clean each room thoroughly from top to bottom.

It is also important to ensure that your children are using their medication properly. If they need to take regular doses, try turning the routine into a game or giving small rewards from time to time.

AIR POLLUTION

I keep hearing that there may be a link between traffic pollution and asthma. Just how much of a risk do exhaust gases pose to asthmatics?

Air that is polluted by car exhaust fumes is not good for anyone's health – asthmatic or not. Asthmatics have an additional reason to be concerned, however, since car fumes can certainly provoke attacks. It is thought that the problem is caused by tiny particles in exhaust emissions which are highly irritating to the extra-sensitive lung linings of asthmatics. The problem tends to be worse in winter when people use their cars more and cold air constricts the airways, making breathing more difficult anyway.

Parents of asthmatic children should be particularly concerned. Recent trends have shown an increase in asthma attacks among children which is said to correspond to an increase in car exhaust pollution, with those living near busy roads most affected.

Scientists have also shown that pollution may undermine a healthy baby's defences, leaving the lungs more vulnerable to irritation from pollen, animals, dust mites and other allergens and possibly increasing the chances of developing asthma. A move to the countryside is not necessarily a solution

either. Traffic fumes travel far and wide and in farming areas there are crop sprays and a high concentration of different pollens to contend with.

The best advice for people with asthma, as for everyone else, is to avoid heavily polluted areas as much as possible, particularly for children's play and sporting activities. Wearing a mask (see page 303) in a busy street may help, as will staying indoors when pollution levels are high. Close windows and air vents when driving in congested areas.

TROUBLE IN SUMMER

Why does my asthma get worse in the summer? What can I do about it?

Summer is a high risk season because of the vast array of pollens wafting around in the air at this time. Air pressure is also often high and winds light, trapping pollution at ground level. The mixture of pollen and pollution is thought to be particularly dangerous for asthmatics.

You can protect yourself to some extent by staying indoors and keeping windows and doors shut. Avoid country outings if flowering crops and trees make things worse, and keep your grass short so that it doesn't flower and release pollen. Watch for pollen and pollution levels every day in the press and on radio and television, and try to avoid going out when they are high.

If you have to go out, consider a preventive dose of medication first.

RELIEF FROM ASTHMA

How do asthma drugs work and how safe are they? Is there any other way to treat an attack?

Drugs are the only medically recognised way to relieve asthmatic symptoms, and they can be very effective, even life-saving. Use them as soon as symptoms appear, to control the attack in the early stages.

Children's asthma and asthma attacks brought on by exercise and allergy can generally be treated with non-steroid drugs called beta-agonists, the commonest being salbutamol and terbutaline. They occasionally cause side effects such as hand tremor, nervous tension and rapid heart beat, but the risks can be reduced by using the correct inhaler technique and taking the exact dosage prescribed. Non-steroids help to relax the muscles of the air passages, opening them up and easing breathing. They do not relieve

DO'S AND DON'TS

for living with asthma

Do try to lead as normal a life as possible.
Do keep a record of your attacks so that you can identify likely triggers.
Do avoid emotional and physical stress as much as possible.
Do carry your medication with you.
Do keep healthy with exercise and a good diet.
Do wrap a scarf around your face in winter to avoid taking in cold air.

Don't ignore symptoms.
Don't be afraid of your treatment. Discuss any fears about drug side effects with your doctor.
Don't behave like an invalid, or treat an asthmatic child (or adult) like one.
Don't smoke or expose other asthmatics to cigarette smoke.

DO'S AND DON'TS

for inhaling steroid drugs

Do use a plastic spacer when inhaling steroids.
Do rinse your mouth out after using an inhaler.

Don't ignore side effects such as weight gain or digestive upsets. A change of medication may be needed.
Don't cut down on medication suddenly.

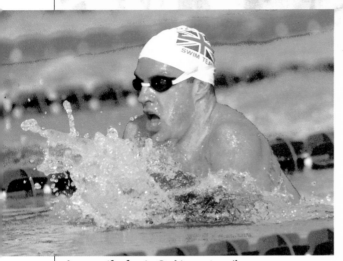

ADRIAN MOORHOUSE: ATHLETE WHO TRIUMPHED OVER ASTHMA

Among the best On his way to a silver medal in the 100 m breaststroke in the 1991 European Championships, British swimmer Adrian Moorhouse proves that asthma is no bar to sporting achievement.

Sporting prowess, you might think, is dependent on perfect health. Not so. Several leading figures in the sports world suffer from some forms of chronic illness – diabetes, breathing disorders, and so on. Their condition represents a hurdle rather than a barrier, and in some cases it may even serve as an inspiration to greater striving.

Take Britain's Adrian Moorhouse, one of the world's top breaststroke swimmers in recent years – multiple gold medallist at both the Commonwealth Games and the European Championships, Olympic gold medallist at Seoul in 1988, breaker of world records... and an asthmatic since the age of five. His achievements in the swimming pool and in the record books provide a heartening lesson to anyone trying to come to terms with a chronic condition.

For Adrian, an asthmatic attack may be triggered by cat fur, or feathers, or even air pollution. In his high-pressure life he has to take constant precautions – to avoid feather beds in hotels, for instance. One factor not so easily avoided is polluted air. It is perhaps no coincidence that one of his most disappointing races, a below-par performance in the 100 m breaststroke final during the 1984 Olympic Games, took place in Los Angeles, a city notorious for air pollution.

As an asthmatic, Adrian has also had to avoid pushing beyond certain physical limits during training. If he does over-exert himself, he risks becoming run down and more susceptible to chest infections such as colds or flu, which might then aggravate or be aggravated by his asthma.

In some ways, however, asthma has made a positive contribution to Adrian's swimming career. It was on his doctor's advice that Adrian took up swimming seriously in the first place, as a means of easing and strengthening his breathing. And conventional attitudes towards asthma, discouraging to say the least, made him only more determined to excel, 'to find a way around it' and to confound the doomsayers.

Adrian is living proof that asthma is no disqualification to success or pleasure in sport. 'I think it's important for people with asthma to find out for themselves what they are capable of,' he says, 'and not to be put down by people telling them what they can and can't do. You can work out your own limits and push yourself as far as you want to go.' That goes as much for a few lengths in your local pool or a round of golf, of course, as for Olympic breaststroke.

inflammation, however, so the most severe attacks may not respond completely.

Steroid drugs are used to prevent symptoms of asthma by reducing inflammation and mucus secretion in the airways and by reducing the effect of the triggers. They work only if they are taken every day, irrespective of whether symptoms occur or not.

Steroids are usually inhaled directly into the lungs, where the problem starts. They reach the airways rapidly and small doses are generally effective and rarely produce side effects, although hoarseness and oral thrush infection are possible. Risks are reduced by washing out the mouth after inhaling and by using a prescribed plastic 'spacer' between the inhaler and the mouth. Steroid tablets

may also be prescribed for severe cases for a short time. Large doses over a long period carry more risks than inhaled steroids and can thin the bones and cause osteoporosis.

There are also some asthmatics who claim to have found relief from non-drug therapies, but so far their value has not been medically proven. Acupuncture, for example, is said to relieve wheezing and protect against exercise-induced asthma attacks. Hypnosis and other relaxation techniques, such as yoga, may help by relieving stress.

Such treatments are considered safe, provided they are not used as substitutes for orthodox medicine. Ask your doctor before attempting them, and do not be tempted to abandon your prescribed medication.

SPOTTING SYMPTOMS

I've had a few coughs that went on for weeks or even months. A friend says this may be a sign of chronic bronchitis. Is it possible she's right?

She could be. A mucus-producing cough that persists or keeps coming back is often diagnosed as chronic bronchitis. But coughing can also indicate other conditions, such as asthma, so you will need to see your doctor for a proper diagnosis. The mucus of chronic bronchitis is usually white or grey and the sufferer may wheeze persistently for a long period. In acute bronchitis, by contrast, the condition occurs suddenly, the mucus is green or yellow, and the problem usually disappears within two weeks.

Chronic bronchitis is brought on by the bronchial tubes becoming inflamed and irritated by something you breathe in, often cigarette smoke. Pollution; cold, damp weather; obesity; and recurrent chest infections can also play a part. The most common sign is coughing and mucus, but in some cases the airways are narrowed and blocked as well, making breathing difficult.

TREATING BRONCHITIS

What can you do to help yourself if you have chronic bronchitis? Is there any way of preventing it from flaring up from time to time?

The first and most important thing is not to smoke. Avoid smoky atmospheres and ask your friends, family and colleagues not to smoke in your presence. If necessary, speak to your employer about creating a smoke-free area for you to work in. Other forms of air pollution can also affect your chest, so try to avoid industrial areas and congested routes, or consider wearing a filter mask outdoors (see page 303). In some cases you may also need bronchodilator drugs to relax and open the airways, ease breathing and encourage mucus expulsion. Any prescribed medication should be used exactly as directed.

It is also very important to avoid respiratory infections such as colds and flu. Keep your distance from anyone with symptoms, however minor, and build up your resistance with a nutritious diet and regular exercise. Don't let yourself become exhausted or put yourself under high levels of stress, both of which can make you run-down and susceptible to infection. You may also wish to consider a winter antiflu jab as a preventative

measure. In winter, try to keep heating levels about the same in every room of the house, so that you are not constantly moving from warm to cold and back again. Remember, however, that a very high level of heating can easily dry out the air and make chest mucus thicker and harder to expel. When you go out in cold weather, wrap a scarf around your mouth and nose.

A technique known as postural drainage may also help to expel mucus. Lie with your head below the level of your chest – either raise the foot of your bed a few inches or hang your head over one end. As mucus drains by force of gravity into the windpipe, it can be coughed up.

'COLD' AND EMPHYSEMA

I have been told that I have chronic obstructive lung disease, or COLD. What does this really mean and what sort of treatment and self-help is worth trying?

Your condition is caused by a combination of two separate but similar lung disorders – chronic bronchitis and emphysema.

Although they are separate illnesses, they quite frequently occur together, and both are associated with cigarette smoking. In most cases COLD, also known as COAD (chronic obstructive airway disease), first appears as chronic bronchitis, which causes congestion in the lungs and air passages.

If chronic bronchitis becomes worse or if the patient experiences recurrent respiratory infections, emphysema (and COLD) may develop. Emphysema damages tiny air sacs in the lungs (alveoli) which become permanently inflated, making the lungs distended and inelastic. Breathing becomes difficult,

DO'S
— AND —
DON'TS

for controlling chronic bronchitis

Do keep your distance from anyone who has a respiratory infection, even a mild cold or a winter cough.

Do eat a healthy diet.

Do take regular exercise of some sort.

Do get plenty of rest.

Do avoid stress.

Do avoid damp rooms and buildings.

Do try to avoid exposure to sudden temperature changes.

Do consider a humidifier if the air in your home is very dry.

Do wrap a scarf around your mouth and nose if breathing in cold air affects you badly.

Don't smoke.

Don't spend time in smoky places.

Don't overheat your home to the point where it dries up the moisture in the air.

Don't let yourself get cold or shivery.

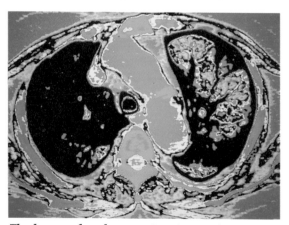

The damage of emphysema On a CT scan the lungs show up in cross-section as two black areas. Coloured patches within the right lung indicate emphysema.

particularly breathing out, placing an extra strain on the heart. Treatment for COLD and emphysema is very similar to that for chronic bronchitis (see page 353). It usually involves prescription bronchodilator drugs to open the airways and help breathing. Antibiotics may be given to treat or prevent respiratory infections, which can be serious if you are already struggling for breath. Seek medical advice immediately you notice any sign of possible infection, such as mucus changing colour. Some patients may also need oxygen from time to time. If necessary, your doctor will help to organise any home equipment you may need.

Helping yourself
If you are or have been a smoker, giving up entirely is now essential. A good posture can also help by making breathing more efficient. Try to sit and walk as upright as possible, with shoulders back and spine straight. Don't try so hard that it becomes uncomfortable or feels unnatural, however, and try to stay relaxed. Muscular or nervous tension can inhibit breathing, so practise relaxation and breathing techniques (see pages 190-192). As with chronic bronchitis, always use medication as prescribed and lead a generally healthy life, eating well and taking as much exercise as you are able.

Coping with digestive trouble

Who gets ulcers?

● Smokers are twice as likely to get ulcers as non-smokers. Smoking also slows healing and increases the likelihood of recurrent problems.
● Regular users of aspirin and other non-steroidal anti-inflammatory drugs are at risk, as these drugs irritate the stomach lining and reduce protective mucus.
● People whose close relatives have ulcers are three times more likely to develop the problem.

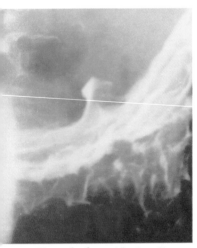

Stomach ulcer A barium X-ray can diagnose an ulcer – which shows up here as the small white mushroom shape in the centre.

CAUSES OF PEPTIC ULCERS

I've been told I have a peptic ulcer but I don't really know much about the condition. What are ulcers and why do they occur?

Peptic ulcers are painful eroded areas in the lining of the upper digestive tract. Depending on where they form, they are described as gastric (in the stomach), duodenal (in the upper part of the small intestine, or duodenum) or oesophageal (in the food pipe). The word 'peptic' is derived from 'pepsin', the name of an enzyme secreted by the stomach lining. Together with hydrochloric acid, pepsin helps to break down food once it enters the stomach.

Normally, the digestive tract lining is protected from contact with the corrosive digestive juices by a layer of mucus. Sometimes, however, the balance between protective mucus and acidic juices is upset and the lining of the stomach or digestive tract is damaged, forming an ulcer. Many factors can play a part in the process, including excess acid production by the stomach or, more commonly, inadequate mucus production. Other factors are often involved as well, including smoking. Alcohol can also irritate the stomach lining and weaken the mucus layer, leaving it vulnerable to damage by even normal amounts of gastric juices. Aspirin, ibuprofen and similar drugs can also reduce the amount of mucus produced, especially when taken regularly.

Recent developments in ulcer research also point increasingly to bacterial infection as a major factor in certain types of ulcer.

The bacterium *Helicobacter pylori* is often found associated with stomach and duodenal ulcers, and appears to attack the stomach lining. Many ulcer patients who have so far failed to respond to conventional types of treatment are now being given antibiotics to treat bacterial infection, often with dramatically successful results.

RELIEF FROM ULCERS

Is a bland diet essential if you have an ulcer? What other forms of treatment are there?

Milk puddings, steamed fish and other bland foods were once generally recommended to ulcer patients. These days, however, medical thinking about food and ulcers has changed completely. Doctors no longer prescribe a universal diet for ulcer sufferers, but are much more inclined to encourage each patient to work out a personal eating programme. Few foods cause problems for all ulcer cases and about the only general dietary advice is to avoid large quantities of tea, coffee and alcohol. Most people soon learn their limits by trial and error.

Otherwise, few ulcer patients need a special diet. Milk can relieve ulcer pain very effectively, but is less widely recommended than before because instead of neutralising stomach acid as was thought it now appears that milk may actually stimulate acid secretion. Likewise, the traditional advice about avoiding spicy and acidic food is no longer given as there is little evidence that they do aggravate ulcers. Smoking is best avoided, and aspirin and similar drugs can cause problems too. Other drugs can be highly effective, however. Antacids and newer drugs known as H$_2$ blockers have the effect of reducing acidity, relieving pain and promoting healing. Antibiotics may also be given to combat *Helicobacter pylori* infection.

LIVING WITH A HERNIA

What is a hiatus hernia and what can patients do to control their symptoms?

A hiatus hernia (gastro-oesophageal reflux disease, to give it its technical name) occurs when part of the stomach protrudes through the diaphragm at the weak point where the oesophagus passes through the abdominal cavity. Unlike some other hernias, nothing is visible externally, and often there are no symptoms at all. When symptoms do occur, they are very similar to indigestion or heartburn – the cause being stomach acid flowing up into the oesophagus.

Obesity is thought to play a role in causing hiatus hernias, so patients are advised to get their weight down if necessary. To relieve symptoms, they should also avoid smoking, eating very large meals and, if possible, lying down or bending after eating. Some people also find it helpful to sleep with their head propped up on pillows, or to take antacids.

Doctors can advise on other types of treatment. If symptoms are severe, a drug such as omeprazole may be prescribed. If nothing else works, surgery may be suggested but it is not always a permanent solution.

COELIAC CHILDREN

Our nine-month-old son has coeliac disease. So far, feeding him a special diet hasn't been difficult, but how can we keep it up as he grows older?

People with coeliac disease have a digestive system that reacts badly to gluten – a type of protein in grains such as wheat, barley, rye and oats, and in products made with them. Such foods are relatively easily avoided in the early days, but once children start going to birthday parties, visiting friends and eventually attending school, things can get more difficult and it helps to be prepared.

One of the most important factors will be not letting your son feel deprived or left out. Once he is old enough to share in family meals, start using gluten-free flour in cooking, so that he eats the same as the rest of the family. Keep gluten-free bread in the house for him and if others have biscuits

and cakes make sure there are also treats available for him. In time, you will need to explain your son's condition to him, and to friends, other parents and schoolteachers.

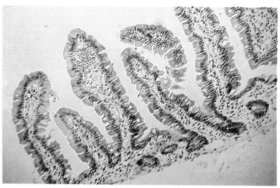

Normal gut The mucous membrane of a normal, healthy intestine is heavily convoluted to provide a large surface area for efficient absorption of nutrients.

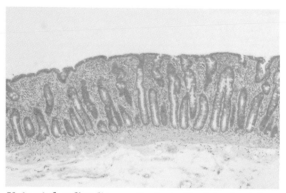

Untreated coeliac disease Contact with gluten has left the intestinal mucous membrane flat and unable to digest food properly. A gluten-free diet will reverse the damage.

Don't go on about it, however – the less fuss the better. Accept invitations to parties and meals, and take gluten-free food along for your son. When other children come to your home, provide gluten-free food for everyone.

TREATING CROHN'S DISEASE

My brother has just been told he has Crohn's disease. What is this condition and how can it be treated?

In Crohn's disease the ileum, or the lower part of the small bowel, becomes inflamed and less able to absorb nutrients from food. If left untreated, sufferers experience severe stomach pain and chronic diarrhoea.

Although there is no cure for Crohn's disease, anti-inflammatory drugs such as corticosteroids can effectively control and even sometimes prevent symptoms. A drug called

Living with a stoma

Coming to terms with a colostomy or ileostomy operation can take time for patients and families, but help is available.

● Hospital staff are highly trained to assist with physical problems, and can provide short-term emotional support and encouragement.
● Counselling is also available. Ask your doctor or seek information from hospital staff.
● For support, advice and contact with other stoma patients, contact the British Colostomy Association, 15 Station Road, Reading, Berkshire RG1 1LG.

DO'S
— AND —
DON'TS

for controlling irritable bowel syndrome

Do keep fit and active, and take plenty of exercise.
Do include lots of fibre in your daily diet.
Do consult your doctor about prescription drugs to reduce overactivity of the bowel muscle.
Do consider drug therapy if anxiety or depression is a problem.
Do keep a record of what you eat and drink to identify problem foods.
Do follow your doctor's advice on diet.

Don't ignore signs of stress – do something about them (see pages 190–195).

azathioprine can help to prevent recurrent attacks and antibiotics are sometimes also given to fight infections.

All these medications can have unpleasant side effects, such as nausea, headaches, dizziness, acne, anaemia and weight gain. Your brother will need to work closely with his doctor to monitor drug reactions so that adjustments can be made if necessary.

ULCERATIVE COLITIS

My sister is suffering from ulcerative colitis. What is this illness and what is her outlook for the future?

Ulcerative colitis develops when the large intestine becomes chronically inflamed and ulcerated, causing bouts of bloody diarrhoea and abdominal cramping. The cause is not understood and while some patients recover completely after the first attack, many find that symptoms persist, going through better and worse patches from time to time.

Even if your sister's illness is of the sort that persists, the outlook is good – provided she looks after herself, gets plenty of bedrest during bad attacks, and uses drugs such as corticosteroids if prescribed.

Fewer than a quarter of the people with ulcerative colitis ever have symptoms severe enough to require hospital treatment. However, if the disease cannot be controlled with medication or if complications develop, surgical removal of the colon may be needed. Sometimes the upper intestine can be joined to the rectum to allow normal evacuation. In other cases the entire colon and rectum are removed and an ileostomy performed.

Both types of surgery can bring about a dramatic improvement in health, although patients will inevitably require time and support to adjust to the effects. Modern techniques mean that an artificial reservoir can often be created internally, so that relatively normal bowel action can continue.

IRRITABLE BOWEL SYNDROME

The so-called irritable bowel syndrome seems to be in the news so often. What is it and is it related to inflammatory bowel disease?

Irritable bowel syndrome (IBS) is a chronic condition in which certain parts of the bowel contract too quickly, and others too slowly, causing a 'spastic' movement that accounts for the condition's other names – spastic colon and spastic colitis. Symptoms include constipation alternating with diarrhoea, and abdominal cramps and bloating. Because the condition involves disturbances of the muscle rather than inflammation or tissue damage, irritable bowel syndrome is considered a far less serious condition than inflammatory bowel disease, a general term for those complaints involving intestinal inflammation such as Crohn's disease and ulcerative colitis. Despite the similar names, there is no link between the two conditions.

The causes of irritable bowel syndrome are not clear, although stress and other psychological factors are thought to play a role. Treatment may include medication to reduce intestinal spasm or to relieve diarrhoea and, for some patients, a high-fibre diet. There is no single cure for the disease. Most patients have to use trial-and-error experiments to find what works best for them.

AFTER A COLOSTOMY

My husband needs to have a colostomy operation and is very apprehensive about the future. How will it affect his life?

Your husband's worries are entirely understandable, but you can reassure him about the future and explain that he will be able to lead a completely normal life.

The operation itself involves creating an opening, or stoma, in the abdomen through which body wastes can be eliminated into a special pouch, or appliance.

Like anyone coming to terms with a major change, your husband will need time to get used to living with a colostomy. His first fear may be about protecting the stoma, but it is tough and resilient and the normal rough and tumble of everyday life will not damage it. The idea of using a colostomy pouch can cause a great deal of apprehension, but it soon becomes routine and patients receive excellent help from medical staff.

Many stoma patients worry about diet, but there is no need to do anything special except to ensure a good intake of fibre to help digestion and elimination. To prevent problems with wind, any increase in high-fibre foods should be done gradually.

A colostomy need not have any effect on sex or intimacy. When problems arise, it is usually because of attitudes and emotions, rather than physical difficulties. If you can be positive and show plenty of love and support you will make things much easier for your husband. It will take time to get used to things, but don't anticipate problems – life often returns to normal surprisingly easily.

Help for incontinence

WHO GETS INCONTINENCE?

What causes incontinence and how is it treated? Is it inevitable as you get older?

The inability to control discharge of either urine or, less commonly, faeces from the body can have several causes, but simple ageing is not a sufficient explanation. The problem does become more common with age, but it is by no means inevitable.

Urinary incontinence
There are several types of urinary incontinence. So-called urge incontinence occurs when the need to pass urine is so powerful that it cannot be controlled long enough to reach a lavatory. The problem is generally ascribed to an overactive bladder. Treatment involves training to control the bladder, and with drugs to reduce bladder activity.

Stress incontinence occurs when coughing, sneezing, laughing or moving puts pressure on the bladder, causing a leak. Weak pelvic floor muscles are thought to be to blame. Pelvic floor exercises, as done in pregnancy, may help (see page 270).

Another form of urinary incontinence – overflow incontinence – occurs when the bladder cannot be entirely emptied because of an obstruction such as an enlarged prostrate. When the bladder fills up, urine can overflow. Treatment is usually by surgery.

Faecal incontinence
The problem is usually the result of diarrhoea or excessive use of laxative pills. If the leakage is very watery, impacted faeces could be causing a blockage – see a doctor for treatment. Faecal incontinence in toilet-trained children can be a sign of fear or insecurity. Consult your doctor for advice.

AID AND ASSISTANCE

What sort of assistance is available when incontinence cannot be cured?

Most chemists stock a wide variety of aids, such as pads and pants for women, and bags and dribble pouches for men. Doctors can also prescribe some aids on the NHS.

People with incontinence can also ask to have a district nurse visit them at home to discuss the problem and to help with bladder training or pelvic floor exercises. If necessary, patients can be referred to specialist continence advisors to have their condition assessed, and to receive help and advice on managing it. Occupational therapists can also help by teaching better ways of coping with everyday activities that cause problems.

The Continence Foundation operates a helpline on 0191 213 0050. Further help and advice can be obtained from the Association for Continence Advice, The Basement, 2 Doughty Street, London WC1N 2PU.

DO'S AND DON'TS
for living with incontinence

Do ask your doctor what help is available from your local authority. There may be a laundry service, for example.
Do ask your local social services office about financial assistance if you need home alterations or fittings.
Do ask a doctor or nurse about aids.
Do reduce your caffeine intake if it exacerbates the problem.
Do persist with treatment and aids.

Don't be ashamed or embarrassed to mention the problem.
Don't drink less fluid.
Don't think that nothing can be done.
Don't try to do too much yourself when you really need expert help.

Liver and kidney complaints

WHAT IS CIRRHOSIS?

What is cirrhosis and is it always caused by heavy drinking?

Cirrhosis is a form of chronic liver damage. It is often, but not always, caused by alcohol abuse, especially when combined with poor nutrition. It also sometimes develops as a complication of hepatitis and, although not contagious like viral hepatitis, it is considered more serious and causes more deaths. Cirrhosis can also be caused by other diseases of the liver, as well as by congestive heart failure, cystic fibrosis, some inherited disorders and, in rather less common cases, by prolonged exposure to high doses of certain drugs or particularly toxic chemicals.

Over time, cirrhosis damages normal liver cells, replacing them with scar tissue. Eventually the liver can no longer perform its vital roles of metabolising fats and proteins, regulating blood sugar, storing nutrients and filtering wastes from the blood. The legs may swell up as fluid collects, and jaundice may develop, giving a yellowish tinge. Confusion and coma occur in the late stages.

Where drinking is the cause, the progress of cirrhosis can be slowed by avoiding alcohol. In other cases, treating the underlying causes may help. In a few cases, a liver transplant offers the only possibility of a cure.

TYPES OF HEPATITIS

Why are some types of hepatitis considered so serious, while others are not? Are they all contracted in the same way?

Hepatitis is not a single, simple illness but a condition that can have several causes. The word itself means only inflammation of the liver, which can arise from numerous different illnesses.

Most cases of hepatitis are caused by a viral infection, either by one of several so-called hepatitis viruses or as a complication of another viral condition, such as glandular fever. Hepatitis can also result from alcohol or drug abuse, or exposure to toxic chemicals such as dry-cleaning fluids. Some medical drugs can inflame the liver, too, and similar effects are sometimes associated with disorders of the immune system, such as rheumatoid arthritis.

Depending on its type and severity, hepatitis can clear up quite rapidly or continue for months or years. In some cases recovery is complete, in others the patient gets better but remains an infectious carrier, and in yet others there is a risk of permanent scarring (cirrhosis), cancer or even death. The condition is considered chronic if it lasts for six months or more.

Five separate hepatitis viruses have been identified, known as hepatitis A, B, C, D and E. Hepatitis A is spread by faecal contamination, usually through food, water, utensils or bodily contact. This is common in developing countries but by no means unknown in the West. Hepatitis E is similar. In both cases, patients usually make a good and complete recovery relatively quickly.

The B, C and D viruses are potentially much more dangerous. They are not passed on in human waste, but in similar ways to HIV – by unprotected sexual intercourse, shared hypodermic needles, tattooing and, in the past, by blood transfusions (although screening has now largely removed this risk). While hepatitis A and E have an incubation period of about two to seven weeks, B, C and D can take much longer – up to six months in the case of hepatitis B. The risk of permanent liver damage or death is also greater. In addition, the B, C and D viruses can remain in the blood for years, causing chronic illness and a continuing risk to others.

Hepatitis sometimes has no symptoms. When they do occur, they typically include fatigue, mild fever, loss of appetite, nausea, aching joints and dark urine. Most patients recover with bedrest, good nutrition and abstinence from alcohol, drugs and other agents that strain the liver. If severe liver damage occurs, however, a transplant may offer the only hope of recovery.

SLOWING KIDNEY FAILURE

Is there any way of slowing down or halting kidney failure once it has started? Can a change of diet do any good?

To some extent it depends on the cause of the problem. Where kidney failure is the result of a condition such as diabetes or high blood pressure, diet can certainly help by controlling the underlying condition (along with measures such as medication and exercise).

Although there is still a lot to be learned about any more direct link between diet and kidney disease, there is some evidence that a reduction in protein intake is beneficial for certain patients, as large amounts of protein can overload the kidneys and most people in the West eat more than they require. However, some kidney patients actually appear to improve on a diet that is rich in protein, so personal advice from a dietician or doctor is necessary in each case.

The only general advice for all kidney patients is to keep up a good intake of starchy carbohydrates and to limit salt consumption – salt encourages fluid retention, so working against the kidneys. If you are tempted to try any drastic dietary changes, always ask your doctor's advice first.

KIDNEY TRANSPLANTS

How successful are kidney transplants? Is the outlook better than simply continuing with dialysis?

The outlook for a kidney transplant patient is very good, especially if the donated organ comes from a relative. But even where this is not the case, the success rate is very good.

Although it is possible for a patient with chronic kidney failure to lead a relatively normal life with dialysis, the recommended treatment is usually a transplant. Despite the benefits, however, it is important to remember that this is a serious operation and that complications are possible.

Although drugs can usually prevent rejection, it remains a possibility in any transplant operation. The drugs themselves can cause problems too. They work by suppressing responses in the immune system, and so leave patients more vulnerable to infection. There can also be other side effects, such as nausea. By comparison with a life of regular dialysis, however, which can mean spending long hours in hospital several times a week, most patients would gladly opt for a transplant. The major problem they face is the shortage of donor organs currently available.

Helping others
There are about 5000 people waiting for kidney transplants in Britain, including babies just a few days old. You can help them by carrying a donor card (right) and registering as a donor on the national database – see page 251.

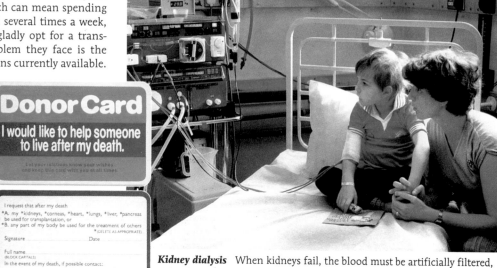

Kidney dialysis When kidneys fail, the blood must be artificially filtered, either by machine, as here (haemodialysis), or by making use of a membrane in the patient's own abdominal cavity (peritoneal dialysis).

A better life for diabetics

UNDERSTANDING THE PROBLEM

What is diabetes and why do diabetics have to avoid sugar?

Diabetes – properly diabetes mellitus – is a condition that arises when the pancreas fails to produce enough or any of the hormone insulin, or becomes resistant to it. The result is that blood sugar cannot be properly used by the body. Instead of being absorbed by the muscles and tissues for use as fuel, it accumulates in the bloodstream and is excreted in the urine. Testing for sugar in the urine is one way of detecting diabetes.

Diabetics do not have to avoid sugar completely, but they do have to keep close watch on their intake. The kidneys are not designed to handle large amounts of sugar and if too much builds up in the blood, they may not be able to get rid of it fast enough. The result can be excessively high blood sugar levels. Many diabetics find they can control their condition simply by watching what they eat and staying generally healthy. Others have to inject insulin or take tablets to keep their blood sugar level relatively stable.

There are several causes of diabetes. In many cases, there is an inherited tendency towards the disease but this alone need not bring it on – it is thought that another precipitating factor is usually involved as well, such as a viral infection affecting the pancreas. Some races are more at risk of developing diabetes than others, and obesity, lack of exercise and ageing all increase the risks. It can also develop as a side effect of certain medical drugs and as a complication in some illnesses. Pregnancy sometimes precipitates temporary diabetes in the mother.

ADULT DIABETES

It came as a shock to hear that a long-standing friend now has 'type II' diabetes. What is this illness?

Type II diabetes (also known as maturity-onset or non-insulin dependent diabetes) is the less severe, but more common, form of diabetes. It tends to develop gradually over the years, often without symptoms, and can remain undiscovered for a long time. Most people who develop it are in their 40s or older when the diagnosis is made.

In type II diabetes, the pancreas continues to produce some insulin, but the amount is either insufficient or for some reason the body fails to use it properly. Blood sugar levels rise, but not dramatically high. Some patients need to inject insulin but most are quite able to control their sugar level with a combination of diet, exercise, weight loss and, if necessary, oral medication.

Staying well with diabetes

Most cases of diabetes can be very well controlled by following these simple guidelines.

- Watch your weight.
- Keep blood sugar levels steady with well planned and evenly spaced meals.
- Take regular exercise.
- Use medication if it has been prescribed.
- Report any new symptoms or changes in your condition to your doctor as soon as you notice them.
- Don't misinterpret feeling well. It simply means that your control regime is working properly – not that you can afford to relax it.
- For further advice contact the British Diabetes Association, 10 Queen Anne Street, London W1M 0BD. They can also provide contact with other diabetics, self-help groups and specialist counsellors.

DO'S
— AND —
DON'TS

for diabetic diets

Do watch calorie intake.
Do keep your weight under control.
Do limit sugar, fat and alcohol consumption.
Do eat plenty of fruit, vegetables and grains.
Do involve all the family in planning meals.

Don't skip meals.
Don't eat between meals.
Don't feel you must buy expensive slimming or diabetic foods. A normal healthy diet, low in fat and sugar, is better, easier and cheaper.

ILLNESS IN CHILDHOOD

How common is childhood diabetes? And why do youngsters with the illness need to give themselves insulin injections?

Childhood diabetes – also known as 'type I', insulin-dependent or juvenile-onset diabetes – is only about one-tenth as common as the type II, adult-onset form of the illness. However, it still affects many people – currently about 60 000 children in Britain alone.

Artificial insulin is needed to make up for the lack of the hormone being produced by the pancreas. Unlike type II patients, who usually manufacture some insulin, type I diabetics generally produce none at all, or very little, often as the result of damage due to a viral infection. The type I illness tends to develop rapidly and as it does the body loses its ability to absorb energy from sugars and starches in the diet, leading to weight loss. Without regular and careful use of insulin, blood sugar levels can rise and fall to dangerous levels. In extreme cases, this can cause coma and death. Patients need to be scrupulous about taking their medication and have to go through life carefully balancing insulin and blood sugar levels.

Complications are possible in later life – mainly affecting vision and circulation – but with a carefully controlled diet and good medical treatment the risks can be greatly reduced. Not smoking is another key factor in preventing problems.

LOW BLOOD SUGAR

What is low blood sugar and why are diabetics at risk from it?

Within certain limits, some fluctuation in blood glucose levels is normal, even for non-diabetics. If blood sugar falls below a certain level, however, it is considered abnormal – a condition known as hypoglycaemia. Diabetics who have to inject insulin can be prone to this, since it is not always easy to administer exactly the right amount of insulin for the amount of sugar in their blood. If they give themselves too much insulin, their blood sugar level can fall dangerously low. Not eating enough, skipping meals or taking too much exercise can also all push up the insulin level in the blood causing a sudden decline in blood sugar.

Minor dips can happen from time to time, and are generally harmless, but if the blood sugar remains very low for any extended period serious damage may be done, particularly to the brain. Provided diabetics monitor their blood sugar levels regularly and take steps to correct any imbalance, serious hypoglycaemia can usually be prevented.

Symptoms of hypoglycaemia can include sweating, dizziness, a racing pulse, weakness, confusion, shaking, headache, hunger, tingling sensations, jerky movements, pallor and, in extreme cases, unconsciousness.

The remedy for hypoglycaemia is a quick dose of sugar – sweet tea, chocolate, glucose tablets or even a sugar lump will do. If hypoglycaemia results in loss of consciousness, injections of the hormone glucagon (available on prescription) will boost the sugar level and rouse the victim. As hypoglycaemia is always a risk for insulin-dependent diabetics, they are advised to keep both sugar and glucagon on them, and to make sure family members and colleagues know how to inject glucagon. See also page 459 for first aid.

For any further information, contact your local British Diabetes Association or write to the organisation's headquarters at 10 Queen Anne Street, London W1M 0BD.

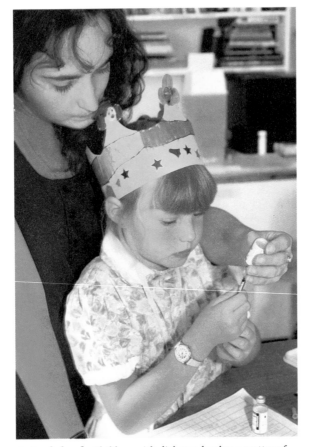

A steady hand Children with diabetes develop a matter-of-fact attitude to injecting themselves with insulin. Parents can find it hard deciding when to help and when to let go.

DIABETES AND PREGNANCY

I have had diabetes since early childhood and would now like to have a baby. Since I have heard that there could be a risk of complications, I am wondering about my chances of a normal pregnancy?

Your chances of a healthy pregnancy have already been greatly increased by considering the issue *before* conceiving. Complications can indeed arise during pregnancy, but provided you always have your diabetes well under control your pregnancy should be normal. Begin now by trying to stabilise your blood sugar concentration as much as you can. Ideally, you should aim to have normal blood sugar levels for at least two months prior to conception. If you have any complications, such as circulation, kidney or eye problems, try to get them well under control before attempting to conceive.

In pregnancy

When you do become pregnant, see your doctor early for referral to an obstetric unit in your area, where expert advice is available. They will also monitor both you and the unborn baby closely during the pregnancy and provide expert help if there is any sign of a developing problem.

During pregnancy you will need to keep your blood sugar levels as stable as possible, both for your own sake and to reduce the risk of illnesses such as jaundice or hypoglycaemia (low blood sugar) in the baby.

Inherited diabetes

You are probably also concerned that your baby may inherit diabetes from you. The disposition towards diabetes does run in families. But the sort of diabetes you have, which develops in childhood, may never manifest itself even if it is passed on to a child. You can help to protect your child and to prevent the illness from developing by encouraging healthy eating and regular exercise, and by keeping an eye on weight during childhood.

HOW EXERCISE HELPS

I've heard that exercise can help diabetics to control their condition – and might even prevent it from developing in some people. Why is it so beneficial?

There is evidence that middle-aged men who exercise regularly and avoid obesity have a lower risk of developing diabetes than those who do not. For those who already have diabetes, exercise is also extremely beneficial. As well as improving health generally, exercise helps with weight loss – a continual struggle for many diabetics. It also increases the body's metabolic rate – the rate at which fuel is burned for energy. This helps to lower blood sugar levels and enhances the body's use of insulin, making drugs and injected medication more effective. The well-known importance of exercise for reducing blood pressure and lowering cholesterol levels is especially relevant to diabetics, who have a higher risk of heart disease.

People with non-insulin-dependent diabetes can, if they have both the condition and any complications under control, be as active as non-diabetics in similar condition. But they do need to get their doctor's agreement before starting any new activity.

Insulin-dependent diabetics have to be more careful, particularly if unfit, as strenuous or lengthy exercise sessions could cause a dangerous drop in blood sugar. The risks can be lessened by eating before exercise, and possibly by reducing their insulin dose. Before starting any exercise programme it is essential for them to consult a doctor about precautions to prevent low blood sugar.

FACT ⸻ OR ⸻ FALLACY?

'Skipping meals can cause hypoglycaemia in healthy people.'

Fact But these are rare cases and the condition is mild, without the serious effects it can have for diabetics.

Slim young women in particular can develop hypoglycaemic symptoms such as faintness, hunger, anxiety, cold sweats, rapid pulse and irritability if they go too long without food or engage in intense physical exercise. They have smaller stores of the muscle fuel glycogen than men – particularly older, fatter men.

The problem can easily be avoided by having regular meals; by eating starchy foods such as bread, potatoes, rice and pasta; and by cutting out very sugary foods and alcohol. If symptoms do appear, eating or drinking something sweet will cure them.

Controlling high blood pressure

UNDERSTANDING THE PROBLEM

What is high blood pressure and why is it considered so dangerous?

High blood pressure (hypertension) is excessive force generated by the heart as it pumps blood through arteries in the body. Some variations in blood pressure are normal and unavoidable, even in people who are in the peak of health. But when blood pressure is persistently and abnormally raised, serious damage can be caused to vital organs including the brain, heart and kidneys.

Hypertension is caused by arteries becoming narrower as their wall muscles thicken, making it more difficult for blood to flow through them. The result is that the heart has to work harder to produce more pressure than is normally needed to keep up a steady

FACT
—— OR ——
FALLACY?

*'Losing your temper
can make your blood
pressure go up.'*

Fact Anger is a powerful emotion which can have dramatic effects on the body as well as the mind. Anger precipitates the release of the hormones adrenaline and noradrenaline, sending up the heart rate, increasing the flow of blood to the muscles, and causing blood pressure to soar immediately. So far, however, it is not known if this short-term response is dangerous to blood-pressure patients.

Longer-term emotional tension is another matter, however. Being continually angry, irritable or unable to relax is definitely not good for your blood pressure, heart or general wellbeing. Psychologists term such people 'type A' personalities and have suggested a possible link with an increased risk of heart attacks (see pages 175-176).

and adequate flow of blood around the body. This extra pressure can eventually damage the artery walls if it is prolonged, possibly speeding up the process of atherosclerosis, in which fatty deposits, or plaques, form on the lining of artery walls. This may cause a further narrowing of the arteries and increase the possibility of blood clotting.

Without treatment there are some serious health risks, including angina, heart attack, stroke and damage to the kidneys. One of the greatest dangers is of high blood pressure going unnoticed and undiagnosed since, contrary to popular belief, it does not necessarily cause any symptoms at all.

To reduce the risks, high blood pressure patients may be advised to reduce the fat and salt in their diets, cut down or give up smoking, drink only in moderation, stay fit with regular exercise, and find ways of relaxing and dealing effectively with stress. In cases of sustained high blood pressure, medication is likely to be needed, probably long term.

Measuring blood pressure

A blood pressure measurement consists of two separate readings. The first is recorded when blood pressure is at its highest, which is as the heart muscle pumps out blood. This is called the systolic pressure. The second, and lower, reading – known as the diastolic pressure – is recorded when the heart relaxes between beats. The readings are usually written in the form of a fraction with the systolic measurement given on the top and the diastolic underneath (120/70, for example).

The normal blood pressure for a healthy young adult is generally considered to be about 110/75. It is common for this to rise slightly with increasing age – at 60 a reading of about 150/90 is normal.

BLOOD PRESSURE DRUGS

How effective are drugs that are given to control high blood pressure?

Medication can be very successful against high blood pressure but it needs to be used carefully and side effects are possible. Report any reactions or new symptoms to your doctor as soon as you notice them – there may be a simple solution. Commonly given drugs include the following.

● Diuretics or 'water pills' expel sodium and fluid from the body and reduce the volume of blood. They are best taken in the day because of increased urination. Side effects may include impotence and gout.

● Beta-blockers may be used with diuretics or on their own, to reduce the amount of blood being pumped by the heart. Side effects include fatigue, cold hands and feet, sleep disturbance and wheezing. Beta blockers are not suitable for people with asthma or breathing trouble.

● ACE inhibitors work by dilating the blood vessels, so reducing the pressure within them. Occasionally, blood pressure can fall too low, cause fainting or lightheadedness.

● Calcium-channel blockers also have the effect of widening the blood vessels. Possible side effects include flushed skin, headaches, swollen ankles, nausea and rashes. Taking the medication with food reduces the risk.

IMPROVING YOUR DIET

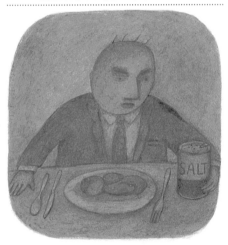

My doctor tells me my blood pressure is too high and that I ought to lose weight – something I've never yet managed to do. Should I go on a diet and, if so, what sort? Are crash diets justified if there is a pressing health reason? And does the kind of food I eat matter, or just the calories?

Certainly go on a diet (see page 153), but keep clear of crash weight-loss programmes. It is almost impossible to get all the nutrients you need from fewer than about 1000-1200 Calories a day – twice as much as some extreme crash diets provide. Sudden changes in eating and weight are not good for the body and dramatic effects seldom last long.

Bear in mind that as you seem to have been overweight for a long time, your regular diet clearly needs to be reconsidered. You may find that by just changing to healthier eating habits (which means more fruit, vegetables and wholegrains, and less sugar and fat) you lose weight quite naturally without dieting. As you suggest, it is not just calories that count, but what you get them from. Try to eat more fibre (see page 20) and to cut down on fat in general and in particular on saturated fat – found mainly in animal and dairy products (page 36). Reducing your salt intake will also help (page 39).

ADOPTING HEALTHY HABITS

Can changing your way of life do away with the need to take drugs for high blood pressure, or decrease the amount of medication you have to take?

It may do, depending on the individual case and the severity of the problem. Certainly, the vast majority of blood pressure patients could benefit from changes such as giving up smoking (or even cutting down), drinking only in moderation, taking more exercise, losing weight, improving their diet, and practising relaxation techniques. If the patient's blood pressure is only slightly above normal

such measures alone may be enough to correct it. But patients who have a sustained diastolic pressure of over 100 are likely to need medication as well, probably for the rest of their life. Drugs are also generally required when high blood pressure is hereditary or when it is associated with diabetes, organ damage or high blood cholesterol.

In a few cases, patients improve so much by adopting healthier habits that they are able to reduce or even give up medication. Usually they are obese people who work hard at losing weight, improving their diet and taking more exercise. It is impossible to predict which patients will do particularly well, however, so it is probably wisest to regard medication as a permanent part of life.

CAUTION However well you are doing, never stop a hypertensive drug suddenly or without medical advice. It could precipitate dangerously raised blood pressure, palpitations or a heart attack.

Heart and circulation trouble

DEFINING HEART DISEASE

Why is heart disease so serious and what causes it? Who is most at risk?

Heart disease (properly, ischaemic heart disease or coronary artery disease) occurs when the supply of blood to the heart is reduced because of narrowing of the coronary arteries. Britain has some of the worst figures in the world for heart disease, which is currently the leading cause of adult deaths.

Almost everyone develops some narrowing of the arteries as time passes, but when it is severe the results can be life-threatening. The process occurs when fatty deposits, or atheroma, build up and harden on artery walls, forming raised patches called plaques – a process known as atherosclerosis or arteriosclerosis. Eventually the artery walls lose elasticity and the plaques start to obstruct the flow of blood. When this happens in the coronary arteries, the heart receives an inadequate supply of blood and is deprived of oxygen and nutrients. This causes the chest pain of angina, especially when the heart is under pressure – during exercise, for example, or when the person feels stressed.

Narrowed arteries also increase the risk of blood clots, not just because a smaller clot will block them but because plaques can

cause cracks in the normally smooth inner surface of the arteries. Where cracks occur, clots may form. If a clot completely blocks a coronary artery, the result is a heart attack.

Many factors, both preventable and not, are involved in heart disease – high blood pressure, high cholesterol, smoking, inactivity, diabetes, heavy drinking, a family history of heart disease, being male and even just growing older can all increase the risks.

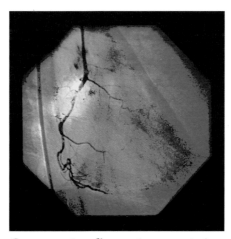

Coronary artery disease A computerised scan shows the heart in red, with the right coronary artery (in black) obstructed by a narrowing in the highlighted yellow area.

Cholesterol testing

A cholesterol test is advisable for anyone affected by risk factors such as smoking, a family history of heart attacks, obesity or high blood pressure.

Doctors do cholesterol testing in the surgery free of charge. Results usually take a week. Pharmacy and home tests give results in minutes, but can be rather less reliable.

Understanding results
● Normal – below 5.2 mmol/l.
● Slightly raised – 5.2–6.5 mmol/l. Cutting down on saturated fat may correct the problem.
● High – 6.5 –7.8 mmol/l. A strict diet is needed and possibly medication if there are other risk factors.
● Very high – over 7.8. Drug therapy is generally recommended.

Reversing heart disease

Research in the United States strongly suggests changing your way of life can not only stop heart disease from progressing but also reverse some of the damage.

In one study, subjects were required to make radical changes in various aspects of the way they lived. They gave up smoking; switched to a diet low in fat with no meat, no poultry and no fish; and had their dietary cholesterol intake drastically reduced.

The diet included fruit and vegetables, pulses such as kidney beans and lentils, and grains and grain products such as pasta. Low-fat milk and yoghurt were permitted. Egg white (high in protein but free of fat) was also allowed, but not egg yolk (high in fat and cholesterol). Tea, coffee and cheese were banned, but alcohol and sugar were allowed in moderation. Salt was denied to those who had high blood pressure.

Subjects were also required to take exercise amounting to half an hour's walk a day, and were taught techniques for mental relaxation and stress control.

At the end of the trial, subjects who had stuck to the programme were found to have significantly improved their condition.

CAUTION Don't embark on any radical programme except under medical supervision.

ANGINA AND HEART ATTACKS

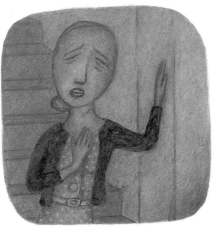

What is the difference between an attack of angina and an actual heart attack?

Angina, or *angina pectoris*, is a severe chest pain, commonly described as a sensation of intense tightening. It occurs in the middle of the chest behind the breastbone from where it may spread out to other parts of the body, mainly the arms, neck and jaw.

Any form of severe stress, either physical or emotional, can trigger an angina attack. Under physical exertion or stress the heart rate can increase, as the body requires an increased supply of blood and oxygen in the blood. If the flow of blood to the heart muscle is insufficient owing to a narrowed coronary artery, the heart muscle is deprived of oxygen and the chest pain of angina is the result. The pain is usually relieved as soon as the patient manages to rest and relax.

Angina is sometimes mistaken for a heart attack, but they are quite distinct conditions. A heart attack happens when a coronary artery becomes blocked by a blood clot, completely cutting off the supply of blood to a part of the heart muscle. The pain is severe and prolonged, and the damage is permanent. In contrast, the shortage of blood that causes angina is temporary and does no lasting damage to the heart muscle. Angina is a warning sign, however, and does sometimes lead to a heart attack.

DRUG TREATMENT

What sort of drugs are available to treat angina? Are there any risks of side-effects?

The classic treatment for angina is glyceryl trinitrate (GTN) and other nitrate drugs, which dilate the blood vessels and increase blood supply to the heart muscle. At the first sign of an attack, the patient slips a GTN tablet under the tongue, or doses himself in the same place with a GTN spray. The drug dissolves instantly, relieving pain in minutes. Nitrates are also given in the form of long-lasting skin-patches which allow continuous absorption as a preventive measure.

Other drugs are also used to counteract angina, including a second group of blood-vessel dilators called calcium-channel blockers. Beta-blockers, such as atenolol, can also be effective. They slow down the heart and reduce its workload. While all of these drugs help to relieve the symptoms of angina, none can cure the underlying condition (coronary artery disease), so they generally need to be taken indefinitely

The side effects of angina drugs are not usually serious. While nitrate medications may cause headaches and faintness, it is usually only at the beginning. Calcium-channel blockers may cause skin flushing, headaches, constipation or swollen ankles. Beta-blockers sometimes increase tiredness and reduce the flow of blood to the limbs, resulting in cold hands and feet.

To prevent angina attacks, always carry your medication with you and always make sure to get your prescription renewed well before your supply ends. Dose yourself just prior to attempting anything energetic, such as taking exercise or climbing a long flight of stairs, and when you feel an attack may be imminent. If you use patches, you may want to apply one before going to bed to prevent an attack during the night.

CHOLESTEROL IN THE DIET

What is the relationship between cholesterol and heart disease? Why are some types of cholesterol considered more harmful than others?

Cholesterol is manufactured in the liver and is one of several fatty compounds that are found in human blood and tissue. The body needs it to build cell membranes, make the protective sheaths around nerve fibres and to produce substances such as vitamin D and certain hormones. Too high a level of cholesterol, however, is linked to the development of fatty deposits, or plaques, on the linings of arteries. Eventually, plaques can build up to such a degree that they begin to obstruct blood flow. Depending on which arteries are affected, the result can be an increased risk of a heart attack or stroke.

Since cholesterol is a fatty substance, it cannot dissolve in water and has to be transported in the bloodstream by special molecules known as lipoproteins. There are two main types of lipoproteins – high density lipoproteins (HDLs) and low density lipoproteins (LDLs). Of the two, only LDLs pose a health risk, since they supply cholesterol to the body tissues and are responsible for depositing it on artery walls. HDLs, on the other hand, are protective, since they transport cholesterol away from body tissues and artery walls, returning it instead to the liver to be reused or excreted. Having either high LDL levels or low HDL levels puts you at greater risk of heart disease. Having high HDL levels, however, protects you.

The best way of reducing harmful cholesterol is to cut down on saturated fats (see page 36) in your diet, such as high-fat dairy products, fatty meat and hard margarines made from hydrogenated oils. Take plenty of exercise – it not only strengthens the heart but reduces overall cholesterol and raises the proportion of beneficial HDL cholesterol. It is also important to control your weight – obesity is linked with raised blood pressure and high blood cholesterol.

CONSIDERING A PACEMAKER

My doctor has suggested that a pacemaker could help my heart condition, but I find the idea alarming. How much would it interfere with normal life?

Pacemakers are used to regulate the heartbeat when it is too slow, too fast or erratic. They work by transmitting small electrical impulses to the heart from a tiny battery generator at just the right rate to keep the heart beating normally.

For people with permanent conditions, a pacemaker is generally installed within the body, usually in the chest, and connected to the heart by means of a thin wire passed through a vein. The batteries last for several years, and replacing them requires only minor surgery.

There are several types of pacemaker available. Depending on your condition, you may be offered either a fixed-rate instrument that beats at a steady rate no matter how active your heart, or a demand pacemaker that discharges impulses only when necessary, as when the heart slows down or skips a beat.

Pacemakers are no longer as sensitive to electronic interference as they once were but it is still necessary to avoid powerful electrical fields such as those found near electricity pylons and generators. Some ultrasonic medical and dental equipment can also affect a pacemaker, so wearers are advised to inform anyone who treats them. Some security systems can also be triggered by a pacemaker, or interfere with it, and it is worth mentioning you have one to staff at airports and other high-security premises.

In all other respects, life with a pacemaker is normal – with the advantage of being able to forget about your condition. Your doctor should be able to advise you further, or you could contact the British Heart Foundation, 14 Fitzhardinge Street, London W1H 4DH.

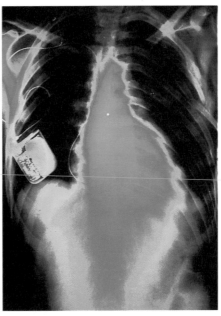

Pacemaker in position Once fitted behind the ribs, even this relatively large pacemaker is barely noticeable to the carrier. Batteries may now last as long as ten to twenty years.

ANGIOPLASTY AND SURGERY

I'm taking drugs for my angina, but they don't seem to be providing the relief I need. What other forms of treatment could I consider at this stage?

There are two treatments that might now be considered to deal with the obstructed arteries causing your problem: a relatively simple procedure known as angioplasty, and the more radical option of bypass surgery.

Angioplasty is suitable only for less serious cases and involves fairly minor surgical intervention to widen narrowed arteries. A thin tube, or catheter, tipped with a small inflatable balloon, is inserted into an affected artery and the balloon inflated where the narrowing occurs. The fatty deposits causing the obstruction are squashed back against the artery wall, opening up the passageway and allowing blood to flow more freely. The operation requires only a local anaesthetic and a day in hospital. Full recovery normally occurs within about a week.

If the blockage is too severe or extensive for angioplasty, your doctor may advise a coronary bypass operation, which effectively creates a new blood pathway to the heart. The procedure involves taking a section of vein from the leg or of the mammary artery from beneath the breastbone and grafting it to form a bypass around the affected part of the coronary artery, to restore a normal flow of blood to the heart. The operation usually requires about seven to ten days in hospital and two or three months for full recovery.

AFTER A HEART ATTACK

Since I had a heart attack I've been feeling rather anxious about the future. What lies in store for me?

A heart attack is a frightening experience, and it is quite normal to feel a little apprehensive about the future. Take comfort from the fact that there is a great deal you can do

to speed your recovery and protect your future health. The most important first step is to adopt the right attitude. Don't think of yourself as an invalid, or let others treat you as one. Your aim is gradually to get back to normal without, of course, putting yourself under undue strain. Friends, family and colleagues can help greatly by offering encouragement and support.

No one knows precisely why heart attacks occur so it is impossible to guarantee that any particular regime will prevent a subsequent attack. Nevertheless, doctors do know that certain factors greatly increase the risks – particularly smoking, high blood pressure and being overweight. If necessary, take steps now to deal with these problems. If your blood cholesterol is high, you may also need to reduce your fat intake, particularly saturated fat (see page 36).

Moderate exercise such as gentle walking and swimming is generally considered safe for recovering heart-attack patients, and you should gradually be able to resume a normal sex life and get back to activities such as driving. You will probably be back at work in a few months, but take it slowly at first and avoid subjecting yourself to stress or strain.

Getting over a stroke

WHY STROKES HAPPEN

What happens when you have a stroke, and what causes the problem?

Most strokes occur when a local blood clot blocks one of the cerebral arteries or when a blood clot that has occurred in the heart is pumped out to lodge in a blood vessel of the brain. In other cases the problem is the result of a burst blood vessel haemorrhaging into the brain. Without an adequate supply of oxygen and glucose – transported in the blood – brain tissue dies.

In general, damage to the right side of the brain can cause paralysis on the left side of the body, impaired spatial perception and loss of memory. Damage to the left hemisphere of the brain is more likely to result in paralysis of the right side of the body, speech impairment and difficulty in understanding and remembering words.

Not all strokes cause such serious damage. A 'mini-stroke' or TIA (transient ischaemic attack) has all the hallmarks of a full-blown stroke, but the effects are temporary and

subside completely within 24 hours, leaving no trace. Some patients are not even aware of what has happened, but recognising and treating a TIA is essential – it can be a warning of more serious trouble ahead.

Strokes are usually associated with other underlying health problems, including narrowing of the arteries, heart disease or high blood pressure. Diabetes increases the risk too, as do weakened cerebral blood vessels, which can cause bleeding into the brain.

PREVENTING FUTURE PROBLEMS

A while ago my husband suffered a 'mini-stroke' and our doctor warned us that he could have another one. How great is the risk and is there anything we can do to prevent this happening?

About one in three people who have had a mini-stroke (or transient ischaemic attack – TIA) go on to have another mini-stroke or a full stroke within five years. The risk is highest in the first year and declines steadily after that. You and your husband can take heart from the fact that proper treatment and care can significantly reduce the risks.

The most important treatable risk factor for stroke is high blood pressure, or hypertension. If your husband's blood pressure is at all raised, it is vital to take steps now to lower it, including keeping weight down, not smoking, cutting down on fatty foods, drinking alcohol only in moderation, taking regular exercise, practising relaxation methods and, of course, taking any prescribed drugs.

Many stroke patients are also treated with aspirin, which has been shown to reduce the risk of further attacks. Patients whose problems arise from severe narrowing of one of the major arteries to the brain may be offered surgery to rebore the artery. Those with blood clots from the heart are now routinely treated with anticoagulants.

For further information and help, contact The Stroke Association, CHSA House, Whitecross Street, London EC1Y 8JJ.

LOOKING AHEAD

A week after having a stroke, a friend still has a speech impediment and partial paralysis in one arm. What are his chances of eventually making a full recovery?

It is very difficult to say at this early stage. There are some people who recover full physical and mental functioning during the first few months following a stroke. Others take longer but, with hard work and the help and support of therapists and family members, eventually make a virtually complete recovery. But many people do suffer continuing effects of one sort or another.

Your friend's most dramatic improvements will probably occur within the first six months. In almost a half of all cases the patients recover enough to return to their normal, independent life in the first year.

Your friend has already started out on the path to his recovery and is almost certainly receiving physiotherapy to prevent problems associated with immobility, such as muscle weakness and respiratory complaints. Later on, as his needs become clearer, an individual rehabilitation programme will be drawn up for him. Depending on the progress he makes and the difficulties he experiences, it may include physiotherapy to improve balance or spatial perception, or to retrain muscles; speech therapy for language difficulties; and occupational therapy to relearn basic skills such as washing, dressing and eating.

Depression sometimes follows a stroke – not surprisingly. Provided it is recognised, it can be overcome with proper treatment. As a friend, you can help, too, by staying positive and giving encouragement at every step on the way to recovery, however small.

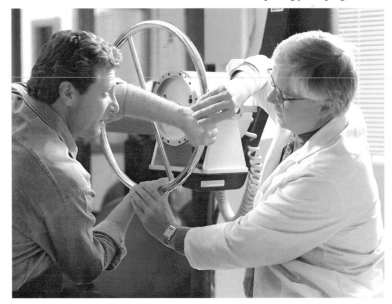

Road to recovery Getting over a stroke takes courage, commitment and persistence. With the help of expert therapists, patients can make surprisingly fast progress.

Help for nervous system disorders

CAUSES OF EPILEPSY

Our young daughter, who is just 13, has been diagnosed as epileptic. What causes her seizures and is it usual to develop the problem at this age?

Epilepsy is a physical condition brought on by sudden, brief disturbances in the way the brain operates. Epilepsy seizures occur when normal electrical signals in the brain misfire. In most cases they happen spontaneously but, in a small minority of patients, external factors such as flickering or flashing lights can trigger attacks. Most seizures, of whatever sort, are of short dur-ation – from just a second to a minute or two.

There are two main types of seizure: generalised, affecting the whole brain, and partial, affecting a much smaller area. In a generalised seizure, the person loses consciousness and in severe attacks (known as 'grand mal') may go into convulsions. In a partial seizure, by contrast, there may be no more than a fleeting moment or two of confusion or disorientation. A partial seizure, however, can sometimes develop into or trigger a generalised one. Children sometimes experience a type of generalised seizure known as an 'absence' seizure in which they momentarily lose consciousness. To others it may appear as if the child is simply daydreaming or as if attention has suddenly wandered.

Epilepsy can develop at any age but most cases are diagnosed in childhood or early adolescence, so your daughter is quite typical. In many cases there is no identifiable cause, although occasionally it can be connected with other conditions, ranging from head injury and brain disorder to drug use, poisoning or certain illnesses.

CAUTION Never leave an epileptic alone during any type of seizure. Treat seizures as described on pages 458-459.

PREVENTING SEIZURES

What sort of help is available to control epilepsy? Do anti-epileptic drugs have any dangerous side effects?

The outlook for the treatment of epilepsy is very good. With the right kind of medication, about seven out of ten people suffering from the illness never experience another attack, and even among those who continue to have seizures, most will have fewer than ten throughout their life.

A variety of drugs is used to control different types of epilepsy. Like all medicines, they can produce unwanted side effects – in this case generally double vision, sleepiness or unsteadiness – but these can usually be well controlled by careful dosage. In rare cases, epilepsy may be treated by surgery if drugs prove unsuccessful or if only one specific part of the brain is affected.

If you are taking medication for epilepsy, it is important to report any side effects to the prescribing doctor as soon as you notice them. Women who are considering becoming pregnant also need to discuss the matter with their doctor, as there is a risk of birth defects with some anti-epileptic drugs.

If a person with epilepsy remains seizure-free for an extended period, his or her doctor may eventually consider discontinuing drug therapy. But this is a decision that needs to be carefully weighed, and epileptics should never be tempted to stop taking prescribed medication suddenly or without first seeking

medical advice. Abrupt withdrawal has in some cases been known to cause seizures and other health problems.

Epileptics may also find it helpful to contact the British Epilepsy Association, Anstey House, 40 Hanover Square, Leeds LS3 1BE.

SUFFERING FROM MIGRAINE

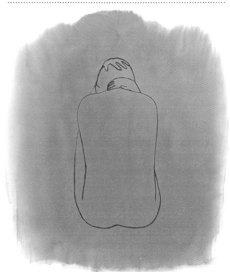

What happens in a migraine attack? Why do they occur and what sets them off?

Migraine often begins with subtle changes in mood or behaviour – often unaccountable feelings of elation or depression, or of ravenous hunger or a craving for sweet foods such as chocolate.

Within a few hours, sometimes even the next day, the main attack starts. In classical migraine, the person experiences an 'aura' effect, in which he or she sees flashing lights and strange patterns in front of the eyes. This usually lasts from about 20 minutes to about an hour, and then fades to be followed by a severe headache. However, most people with migraine simply experience a headache without any preceding aura stage – this is known as common migraine.

The pain of migraine is not like a normal headache. It is intense, disabling and throbbing – the result of dilated blood vessels. Sometimes there is nausea or blurred vision. Migraine can affect any part of the head but typically occurs on one side only. Duration varies from several hours to several days.

What causes migraines is still a mystery. Attacks are thought to begin with the blood vessels in the brain suddenly becoming constricted (this may be the cause of the aura when it occurs), and then dilating. A wide variety of factors can trigger attacks, ranging from stress, anxiety and fatigue to bright or flashing lights, noise and heat or cold.

Hormones also appear to play some role. Women are more affected than men, and migraine often starts at puberty. The contraceptive pill exacerbates migraine in some women, and changing hormone levels at different times of the menstrual cycle can bring it on. Attacks often cease during pregnancy or after menopause.

TREATING MIGRAINE

What can I do to help prevent attacks of migraine? Are drugs the only answer?

There are many approaches to dealing with migraine, and drugs are just one of them. The best method, of course, is prevention. Start keeping a diary and recording every attack you have from now on, and the circumstances in which it occurs, including what you were doing, how you were feeling, what you had eaten and so on. You may well find that this is enough to show up some trigger factors that you can avoid. But be cautious about assuming a food connection – it is not unusual to crave food (particularly chocolate and sweets) just before an attack. The migraine may follow the food, but that does not mean it was caused by it.

·Looking after yourself generally can go a long way to preventing migraine. Stress is well known for provoking attacks, so make a special effort to get enough sleep, to take regular exercise, and to practise relaxation techniques such as described on pages 190-193. Experts believe food acts as a trigger only in a small minority of cases. When it does, the commonest problems seem to be with alcohol (especially red wine), chocolate, cheese, citrus fruit, nuts and drinks containing caffeine such as coffee, tea, cola and cocoa.

Drugs cannot totally prevent migraine but they are useful for dealing with attacks in the initial stages. Mild migraines can sometimes be averted by taking aspirin or paracetamol in the early stages, together with a hot, sweet beverage or a fizzy drink. If this is not effective tell your doctor, who may prescribe an anti-nauseant to help the absorption of the painkillers. Take the medication as soon as possible and use more rapidly absorbed types, such as soluble aspirin. Then lie down and rest in a darkened room.

Specific drugs for migraine such as ergotamine and sumatriptan are also available on prescription. These are more likely to produce side effects, however, such as nausea and diarrhoea in the case of ergotamine, and

pain and weakness in the case of sumatriptan. They work by constricting the dilated blood vessels in the brain and are not suitable for anyone suffering from angina (the result of already narrowed arteries). Sufferers can be taught to administer sumatriptan themselves by injection, so that medication reaches the bloodstream immediately the attack begins.

Other drugs, such as pizotifen or the beta-blocker propranolol, may be prescribed to avert more frequent attacks of migraine, but they too can produce side effects.

Some people have also been helped by biofeedback techniques (see page 193). With the aid of monitoring machines, patients can learn to control migraine through bodily responses such as muscle tension and temperature. By learning to raise hand temperature, for example, it is sometimes possible to direct the flow of blood away from the head, relieving pressure on swollen arteries.

MULTIPLE SCLEROSIS

Multiple sclerosis seems such an unpredictable illness. What is it and how does it affect the human body?

Multiple sclerosis (MS) is a disease of the central nervous system in which inflammation damages or destroys myelin, the protective covering around nerve fibres. The nerves become unable to function properly, causing symptoms such as paralysis, tremors and loss of muscle control.

Although the underlying cause of MS is unknown, the main suspects are a slow-developing virus, an autoimmune reaction, or a combination of the two. The disease occurs more often in colder regions than it does in the tropics and is twice as common in women as in men. It primarily strikes young adults, with the first attack typically occurring between the ages of 20 and 30. Onset is rare in children and in older adults. Genetic factors also play a role, since relatives of people with MS have a higher than average risk of developing the disease.

The typical symptoms of MS are sudden, slightly painful loss of vision in one eye; double vision; tingling, numbness or weakness on one side of the body; clumsiness in a limb; and difficulty in walking. After the first attack, symptoms often disappear completely until months or even years later it is followed by a second bout. The pattern of relapses and remissions can continue for many years, after which the symptoms may gradually start to become more disabling.

**DO'S
— AND —
DON'TS**

for controlling migraine

Do keep a record of attacks, noting when and what you eat and drink, how much under stress you feel and any other possible triggers.

Do keep as fit as possible. Regular exercise will also help you to relax more easily.

Do eat regularly. Low blood sugar can set off migraine attacks.

Do learn to cope with stress (pages 190-195).

Do rest in a dark, quiet place if you feel an attack coming on, and take preventative medication.

Do discuss medication or treatment regularly with your doctor.

Don't drive when you have an attack.

Don't prolong attacks by trying to ignore them.

LIVING BETTER WITH MS

What sort of treatment is available for people with multiple sclerosis? Are there any ways to prolong a remission?

Although there is as yet no cure for multiple sclerosis, much can be done to help people who have the disorder to remain active, independent and productive.

Treatment with corticosteroid drugs can sometimes shorten an attack of MS. Other medication can also be prescribed to alleviate more specific symptoms, such as spasm, tremors, shaking and urinary problems.

Physiotherapy is often used to strengthen and relax muscles and to help patients to regain normal muscle functioning following a severe attack. Some people may also need walking aids such as sticks or elbow crutches to help them to move about.

The prospects of a future treatment for MS are good. A trial of the drug beta interferon has indicated that it might help to slow down the progress of the disease. But the results were not considered conclusive and further trials are taking place.

In the meantime, people who have MS are advised to try to maintain optimum health by eating well, making sure they have regular rest periods, and avoiding overwork, excessive fatigue and stress. Exercise is also helpful, as it keeps nerves and muscles working as effectively as possible. Doctors frequently recommend swimming to MS patients, since it provides excellent all-round exercise while supporting the weight of the body.

People with multiple sclerosis and their families can obtain further assistance and information by contacting the Multiple Sclerosis Society of Great Britain and Northern Ireland, 25 Effie Road, London SW6 1EE.

A CURE FOR CHRONIC FATIGUE?

I'm 30 years old with a successful career and a lively social life, but now I've been struck down by ME. What is this illness and how will it affect me in the future?

There is considerable debate in medical circles about the disorder known as ME (myalgic encephalomyelitis), also called chronic fatigue syndrome or post-viral fatigue syndrome. So far, no objective way of diagnosing the illness has been found, nor any simple cause identified, such as a particular virus or bacterium. There is evidence, however, that the disorder may be connected with poor functioning of the body's immune system, damage to tiny structures known as mitochondria in the muscles, and other physical problems. There is also an accumulating body of evidence to support the view that a persisting or reactivated viral infection may be the root cause of many cases.

Many people with ME symptoms also find themselves diagnosed as having a psychiatric disorder (depression in particular is associated with very similar symptoms) and some doctors believe that ME may be a physical manifestation of a more fundamental psychological condition. This view is no longer widely held, however, as it cannot account for accompanying physical abnormalities.

Dealing with symptoms

Despite all the confusion, ME patients do exhibit a clear pattern of symptoms, including mental and physical fatigue, reduced tolerance for exercise, and muscular aches and pains. In addition to fatigue, some patients also experience troublesome mental symptoms, such as memory loss and an inability to concentrate, which can become disabling. Some ME patients also suffer from sleep disturbances, enlarged glands, recurrent sore throats, alcohol intolerance, and unusual unsteadiness and clumsiness.

To keep these to a minimum, try to maintain a healthy way of life, avoiding stress, overtiredness, alcohol and anything else that makes symptoms worse or causes physical or mental strain. Eat well and get plenty of rest.

Treatment and outlook

Your doctor may also be able to prescribe a low dose of a drug such as amitriptyline to relieve pain and improve sleep. About one-third of ME patients suffer from depression at some stage (rather than simply feeling 'low' or frustrated) and then treatment with antidepressant medication may be helpful, although it must be used with care as a few patients (about one-quarter) find it actually makes them feel worse in some respects.

Despite its reputation, ME need not be a life sentence. With good care, most patients do get better, many quite quickly.

SELF-HELP TO BEAT FATIGUE

If medicine can't offer a cure for ME, what can I do for myself?

Self-help can be very effective against this condition and you have already given yourself a head start by recognising the need to take responsibility for your own recovery. As you say, medicine does not have a simple cure for the illness (or even a generally accepted definition of it), but this is not to say that nothing is known about it, or how it should be treated.

Begin by accepting the need to make some adjustments to your life. In the early stages of ME, in particular, it is important to make plenty of time for rest, even if this means curtailing some of the things you want to do. Try to fix your sights on long-term recovery at a slow, steady pace, and don't expect instant miracles. However, do try to adopt a positive, confident approach – many people recover to lead normal or near normal lives.

Balancing rest and activity

Provided you take care in the early stages, you will probably find that you can gradually start to resume some of your former activities. It is only natural to be excited when you notice the first signs of progress, but don't be tempted to do too much too soon, or you could suffer a relapse. Try to find and maintain the right balance of rest and activity at every stage along the way. Once you feel well enough to resume some form of physical activity, start with gentle walking or perhaps swimming in a heated indoor pool. Do not attempt anything so energetic as squash or jogging until you have been in good health for some time. And even then, it is as well to discuss it with your doctor first.

Watching your diet

Take special care with food and drink, too. Watch out for signs of allergic reactions and avoid any suspect foods. Eat plenty of fruit and vegetables, and wholegrain foods such as wholemeal bread and brown rice. Keep all processed food, sugar, salt and foods with additives to the minimum. Avoid alcohol or drink only moderately and watch for any bad reactions – some patients report intolerance.

Getting care and support

Good medical care is also important. In particular, have regular dental check-ups so that oral or gum infections can be treated early. Immunisation is said by some to cause setbacks, so you may wish to avoid it unless vital. Discuss the matter with your doctor and if you do have to be immunised choose a time when you feel well. If you are travelling abroad, get immunised well in advance.

Help and counselling are available from the ME Association, Stanhope House, High Street, Stanford-le-Hope, Essex SS17 0HA and from the National ME Support Centre, Disablement Services Centre, Harold Wood Hospital, Romford, Essex RM3 9AR.

DEALING WITH PAIN

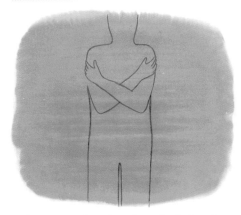

What causes chronic pain and what sort of help can sufferers get?

Chronic pain can have many causes – or none, at least none that medical science can discover. People with painful long-term conditions such as arthritis make up a large percentage of pain patients, as do people with nerve damage. But in other cases pain arises in the absence of any identifiable physical condition at all.

Treatment depends very much on the individual circumstances of each patient. As well as treating underlying causes involving disease or injury, doctors can also prescribe many sorts of pain relief, including drugs that range from aspirin and paracetamol to more powerful sedatives such as morphine. Antidepressants including amitriptyline, or anticonvulsants such as carbamazepine are widely used for nerve-damage pain.

Psychological methods can also be used, including relaxation training, cognitive therapy, hypnosis, biofeedback and meditation. In addition to these, planned exercise programmes are widely prescribed for chronic pain patients. Exercise is known to increase the production of endorphins – transmitter substances that improve mood and function as the body's natural pain relievers.

Alternative treatments such as acupuncture and a therapy known as transcutaneous electrical nerve stumulation (TNS or TENS), have also helped. No one knows how they work, but it has been suggested that they too may stimulate the production of endorphins in the central nervous system. In any case, they appear to be particularly effective in dealing with pain from muscle spasm and tension. Pain patients can also benefit from joining a self-help group – for information and advice contact Pain Concern UK, PO Box 318, Canterbury CT4 5DP.

WHAT PAIN CLINICS DO

I've heard that specialist pain clinics can help people who suffer from recurrent pain. What sort of treatment do they offer and how do I find out more about them?

Most hospitals have an attached pain relief clinic that advises about the dispensing of analgesic drugs, and helps patients to make the best use of medication. Most clinics also

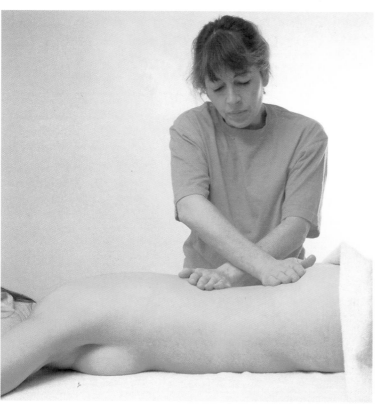

offer nerve block anaesthetic injections to help to locate the site of pain and occasionally to treat it. In addition, hospital clinics provide patients with information and a better understanding of their condition and of what can be done to improve it. Referral is generally either by the patient's own GP or by a hospital specialist.

There are also more than two dozen very highly specialised pain management units in Britain, offering help to patients with complicated or intractable problems. Treatment is generally on an outpatient basis, although St Thomas's Hospital in London can offer NHS inpatient treatment when necessary.

Patients are generally referred to a pain management unit only once they have experienced pain for a long period and nothing else has been able to help. The units operate in a rather different way from hospital pain relief clinics. Their purpose is not to cure pain, but to change the way patients perceive and respond to it. Both mental and physical aspects are dealt with in programmes that use a wide variety of techniques including exercise, breathing and relaxation, as well as mental training to overcome fear of pain.

The goal of treatment is to restore fitness, confidence and independence, and to enable patients to lead a fuller and more active life. So far, all the evidence suggests that pain management clinics are remarkably successful at increasing patients' activity level and reducing dependence on drugs.

Healing touch Some pain clinics can refer patients for treatments such as massage. Since the ultimate aim is independence and self-help, patients may be encouraged to bring a relative or friend along to learn the technique.

Coping with arthritis

DEFINING THE PROBLEM

Why are arthritis and rheumatism always grouped together? Surely they are two quite different illnesses?

These are general terms belonging to the vocabulary of rheumatic illness, but used quite imprecisely in everyday language. Technically, *arthritis* should be used to mean 'inflammation of the joint' and *rheumatism* to mean 'affected by the body's vital fluids' (including the lubricating fluid in joints). In Britain it is probably least confusing to speak

only about arthritis when referring to joint pains and problems, and to dispense with the term rheumatism altogether. There are four main arthritic complaints.

Osteoarthritis
The old-fashioned terms for this illness – degenerative bone disease and wear-and-tear disease – are now considered misleading. Although the condition is often related to changes that come about with age, it can affect younger people too and by no means all older people have disabling symptoms. Osteoarthritis develops when a joint starts

to remould itself in response to disease or damage. It is an extremely complex response and can cause severe, disabling pain. The most commonly affected joints are the fingers, hips, knees and spine – all parts of the body that come under repeated stress, that are at risk of injury, or that carry a significant amount of weight. It is not unusual for only one or two joints to be affected without other parts of the body showing any symptoms at all.

Rheumatoid arthritis

The disorder can start in one joint or in several, with inflammation and swelling of the membranes surrounding the joint, the tubes tendons move in and the fluid-filled sacs (bursae) that allow muscles and ligaments to move smoothly over each other. Later, cartilage and bone may be affected, and inflammation may spread to other joints. Although rheumatoid arthritis is potentially one of the most severely crippling joint disorders, many cases never become severe. Over time, however, and particularly if proper treatment is not received, joint deformity is possible.

Ankylosing spondylitis

In the most common form of this illness, the vertebral joints of the lower back become inflamed and the bones fuse together. Most patients are men between the ages of 20 and 40. Treatment involves vigorous exercise and physiotherapy to prevent the permanently stiffened 'poker back' that used to be associated with the disease.

Gout

Excess uric acid collects as crystals in a joint (often the big toe or another foot or hand joint) producing sudden inflammation and intense pain. Uric acid is normally filtered out of the bloodstream by the kidneys and excreted in the urine, and why some people accumulate very high levels is not known. Men are more at risk than women, however, and heredity probably plays a role.

TREATING OSTEOARTHRITIS

What is the outlook for people with osteoarthritis? How much can drugs help, and what else can patients do to improve their quality of life?

All bones and joints do suffer some natural deterioration with ageing, and the effects are clearly more noticeable and troublesome for people who have arthritic complaints. Even so, there is a great deal that can be done to

treat the symptoms of osteoarthritis and to slow down the development of the disease.

Drugs can help, at least in relieving symptoms. Analgesics are used to relieve pain, and non-steroidal anti-inflammatory drugs can help by reducing joint inflammation and the associated swelling and stiffness. But drug therapy alone is not enough. Patients need to feel in control of their condition.

Firstly, patients should understand their own case as well as possible, so that they can take proper action to avoid further damage. An overweight patient with osteoarthritis in a weight-bearing joint such as a hip or a knee, for example, could clearly benefit from simply losing weight.

Exercise and activity are extremely important to maintain joint mobility and preserve

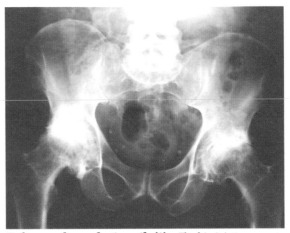

Before ... advanced osteoarthritis The hip joints support the whole weight of the body and experience constant impact – a strain that can take its toll in osteoarthritis. This X-ray shows characteristic damage to both hips.

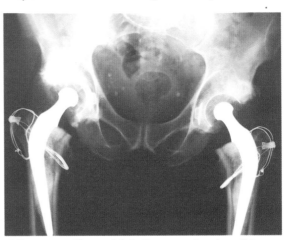

After ... smooth new joints Two operations later (hip joints are replaced one at a time), the patient is mobile and active again. The new joints, made of plastic and metal, should give about ten years of trouble-free service.

muscle tone. Exercise has also been shown to have pain-reducing properties, and it can lift mood too. Patients need to be careful not to strain their joints, however, and to choose the right exercise. Consult a doctor before starting any new activity, and never push yourself beyond what feels comfortable.

Physiotherapy can also be helpful. Therapists teach exercises, relaxation and the use of pain-relief equipment to maintain joint mobility and to strengthen muscles around the affected joints. Exercising in warm water (hydrotherapy) is effective as well, whether done in a heated swimming pool or simply in a warm bath at home.

In serious cases surgical replacement of the damaged joint with an artificial one may be the only answer. Operations such as hip replacements are now routine and highly successful, although waiting times on the NHS can be lengthy.

RHEUMATOID ARTHRITIS

How can I keep my rheumatoid arthritis under control?

Most people with rheumatoid arthritis can lead productive lives, with a level of activity close to normal. These measures may help.

Self-help
Try applying warm compresses or cold packs to sore joints. If appropriate, ask your doctor or physiotherapist about using hand or wrist splints at night to prevent joint deformity.

Rest
Make sure you get plenty of relaxation, rest and sleep, and don't become overtired, particularly during flare-ups. Consider building rest periods into your daily routine.

Exercise
Staying active is vital, for both physical and mental wellbeing. Try swimming and gentle stretching in a heated pool, as well as professional physiotherapy. Take it gently at first and avoid anything that causes pain. You will soon learn through trial and error when to push yourself and when to take it easy.

Drugs and surgery
There are different views about drug therapy for rheumatoid arthritis. Some specialists give drugs known as DMARDs (disease modifying anti-rheumatic drugs) very early after diagnosis on the theory that they will 'disrupt' the progress of the disease, together with steroids to suppress painful inflammation. Other doctors are more conservative, preferring to use ordinary painkillers and NSAIDs (non-steroidal anti-inflammatory drugs) at first, and only to try DMARDs and steroids – which carry a greater risk of side effects – if inflammation becomes severe. Whatever drugs are given, always take them as prescribed and report any side effects or loss of effectiveness.

As with osteoarthritis, joint replacement surgery can be extremely effective for people with long-term, disabling symptoms. Ask your doctor's advice.

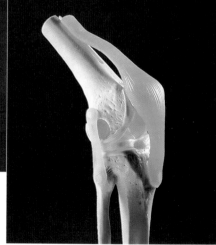

As good as new Manmade joints such as this plastic knee (complete with artificial tendons and cartilage) provide almost instant relief and new mobility.

Knee trouble Attacks of rheumatoid arthritis can come and go for years, affecting one joint or many, often symmetrically. This false-colour X-ray shows damage to the bones of the knee – a clear candidate for joint replacement surgery.

STAYING INDEPENDENT

All sorts of ingenious aids and adaptations have been developed in order to help people with arthritis and other disabling conditions to lead full, active and independent lives. Some aids, such as chair lifts and wheelchair ramps, have to be specially installed in the home; others are small, simple tools such as knives and forks designed for easy use.

Local authorities can provide such aids or give grants towards buying them. Voluntary organisations concerned with particular disabilities can also offer advice and sometimes financial or practical assistance.

If you need further information, contact your own doctor or speak to an occupational therapist at your local social services office. Advice and catalogues are available from the Disabled Living Foundation, 380-384 Harrow Road, London W9 2HU. Aids can be viewed at Disabled Living Centres in many towns.

Upstairs the easy way   Many people find it difficult to negotiate stairs as they grow older. But there is no need to live on one level if you don't want to. Modern chair lifts are compact, convenient and reliable.

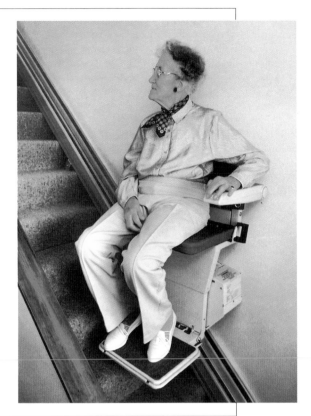

Coming to terms with cancer

REMISSION AND RECOVERY

What does it mean when cancer is in remission? Is it the same as a cure?

Certain cancers and long-term illnesses go through periods in which they develop and others in which symptoms start to improve or disappear altogether. This is called going into remission. Being in remission does not mean that a disease has been completely cured, but it does mean that the first step towards recovery has been taken. When all signs and symptoms of disease disappear, a complete remission is said to have occurred – but even this is not the same as a cure. For a disease to be considered cured, doctors require complete remission to last for a substantial period of time – with cancer, generally for five years.

When remissions occur, medical treatment shifts focus slightly from combating the disease to extending periods of improvement while continuing careful monitoring to detect any returning symptoms. The outlook for cancer is improving all the time. With today's treatments, many more cancer patients than ever before will be alive and well five years after their original diagnosis. About half can expect to live out the full, normal human lifespan – and this figure does not include cases of the easily cured basal cell and squamous skin cancers, which rarely lead to loss of life. Even when cancer does not go into remission, patients may live with it for a very long time – for ten years or more in some cases.

MAKING A CHOICE

How do doctors and patients decide among all the different cancer treatments? Which have the best success rates?

Surviving cancer involves four steps: diagnosis, treatment, rehabilitation and follow-up. When cancer is diagnosed, patients receive help through all four stages from a dedicated

Helping yourself to fight cancer

Overcoming cancer is not just a job for professionals. Patients need to take control too.

● Keep all medical appointments and follow medical advice scrupulously.
● Make sure you have a good, nutritious diet, and increase the proportion of protein and fat to give yourself extra energy. Drink soups, milkshakes, or milk instead of water, tea or coffee.
● Fatigue is a normal part of the disease and its treatment. You might need a nap in the afternoon or a few extra hours of sleep at night.
● Take exercise to stay fit and prevent stiffness, sores, constipation, breathing problems and other conditions related to inactivity. Your doctor can help you to draw up an exercise plan or, if you prefer, just take a walk every day.
● Continue your normal sex life. Physical intimacy is therapeutic and almost always possible. If in doubt, or if there are problems such as pain, ask your doctor for help.
● Talk openly to close family and friends about what you are going through and how you feel about it – isolation makes things worse.
● Fight with your mind as well as your body. Try imagining the cells of your immune system vanquishing cancer cells. Relaxation, breathing and meditation can help – see pages 190-192.

team of specialists, usually led by an oncologist (tumour specialist) to whom the patient is referred by a family doctor.

Members of the cancer team conduct various tests, interpret the results and advise on options such as surgery and chemotherapy. Ultimately, however, all decisions about treatment rest with the patient, who needs to feel confident and knowledgeable about the situation. Doctors are trained to help, advise and support, and welcome it when patients ask questions and take an active part in decision-making.

Three main types of cancer treatment are used, either singly or in combination.

Surgery

Minor surgery alone completely cures 90 per cent of certain types of skin cancer. Surgery can also be an effective treatment for cancer of the breast, lung, bowel, uterus and testicle, particularly if the disease has not spread beyond the original site.

Chemotherapy

Modern chemotherapy has greatly increased the chance of surviving certain cancers, in particular breast cancer and some types of leukaemia (which once used to be almost always fatal but now sometimes needs no other treatment than drugs).

Chemotherapy is also frequently used in treating Hodgkin's disease and for tumours of the testicle and bone marrow.

Radiotherapy

Radiation treatment is sometimes the first option for cancer treatment, particularly in certain skin cancers. But not all cancers are sensitive to radiation and the deeper down the problem is, the harder it is to treat in this way – and the more difficult it is to prevent damage occurring to healthy tissue. Where it is appropriate, however, cure rates can be outstanding – as high as 90 per cent when used in conjunction with surgery for some skin cancers.

SIDE EFFECTS OF TREATMENT

Why do cancer treatments seem to have such harsh and unpleasant side effects? Can anything be done to ease them?

There is some good news for cancer patients – the latest treatments are not only better at combating the illness, but are also safer and less debilitating to patients. Although no two cancer treatments are exactly the same, most patients face some combination of

surgery, radiotherapy and chemotherapy – an onslaught that can be hard on the body. Agents powerful enough to wipe out cancer cells can also damage or even destroy normal cells, causing side effects such as hair loss, nausea, fatigue or infection. But although unpleasant at the time, most problems are only temporary.

Recent improvements in chemotherapy have produced drugs that are able to selectively attack malignant cells only, significantly reducing side effects. Although some improvements have also been made in radiotherapy patients can still experience unpleasant side effects. The severity depends largely on the patient's initial state of health. Tiredness and nausea are the most common problems and both can be eased by medication. Depression is another frequent side effect, and many radiotherapy centres now employ counsellors who are specially trained to offer psychological support during treatment.

Pain control has been improved as well. Some pain is alleviated by cancer treatment itself but pain-relieving drugs are often given – aspirin, ibuprofen, paracetamol, codeine, or even morphine, may all be used.

TALKING ABOUT CANCER

I am finding it very difficult to talk about having cancer, especially to my family. How can I stop this illness from damaging my relationships with those I am closest to?

You are not alone – many cancer patients find it hard to talk about their illness, but it is very important all the same. Remember that although you are the one with the disease, your partner, children, parents and friends are all intimately affected. They are also your main emotional support and you need to have their help and understanding.

Try to be as honest as you can with your family, and don't cover up feelings of uncertainty, doubt or fear. Talking through negative emotions is one of the most effective ways of disarming them.

Couples who don't talk risk misinterpreting each other's feelings and experiencing a sense of rejection that can in its way be as damaging as the illness itself. Cancer can not be transferred by touching, kissing or making love, so there is no reason to avoid physical contact. Appearance and feelings about the body can be affected, however, and it is important for patients and their partners to talk about this.

Telling children about cancer can be especially difficult. Do it as openly and honestly as you can. Very young ones may need to be told in stages so that they gradually come to understand over a period of time.

Friends also need you to talk to them, particularly so that they know what they can do to help. Many people find that focusing on practical issues makes it easier for them to start talking about difficult subjects, and even to cope with deeper emotions.

Your doctor can help too or refer you to a counsellor. Support and advice is also available from the British Association of Cancer United Patients (BACUP), 121-123 Charterhouse Street, London EC1M 6AA.

Attitude makes a difference

SEEING YOURSELF AS WELL

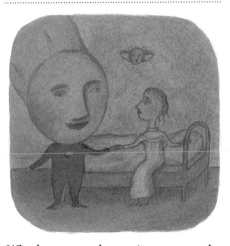

Why do some people seem to cope so much better than others with the same illness? Is attitude important?

Attitude is vitally important, especially for anyone coming to terms with a chronic illness. Any long-term complaint inevitably affects a patient's way of life to some extent, whether because of physical symptoms and restricted activities, or simply by imposing the need to remember regular medication. The important thing, and where attitude can help most, is in not allowing it to become the dominant aspect of life.

In our society, being sick is recognised as a role that sets people slightly apart from normal society and has its own standards of behaviour. Sick people are not expected to work in the same way as those who are well, or to take part in social activities. They are expected, however, to take steps to get well and to seek medical help if necessary. They are often treated rather differently by others, who are generally more prepared to offer help and assistance, but who will also more readily give advice and even instructions to the sick person in a way they would not to someone well. This is known as adopting the 'sick role' and while it is often appropriate for people with acute, short-term illnesses, it can be a dangerous trap for those contending with a more long-term condition. Adopting a sick role as a way of life means giving up a great deal of freedom and independence and sometimes even restricting possibilities such as marriage or a career. To prevent this, a strong, positive attitude is vital. The steps outlined in the panel on the right show some ways of applying it in day-to-day life.

WINNING THE WAR AGAINST CHRONIC ILLNESS

In recent years, new or better treatments such as cataract surgery and joint replacement, have transformed the life of many people with chronic diseases. New immunisations against infectious diseases now prevent death and disability. Along with general health measures – improved diet, housing, and sanitation; screening; stop-smoking campaigns – and higher living standards across the Western world, such advances mean that we are living longer, healthier lives than our forebears.

In the years that lie ahead, the greatest advances in medicine are expected to be made in molecular genetics. Susceptibility to disease depends largely upon how our genetic make-up interacts with the environment we are living in. Scientists are currently busy with an ambitious worldwide project – the human genome project – to map every human gene and its functions. Already such information is being used to diagnose and predict illness, and soon it may be possible to correct abnormal genes – eliminating illnesses such as inherited diabetes and high blood pressure. And if a way can be found to alter the genes that control cell division, the great hope of cancer cure – at least for certain types – may one day be realised.

The right approach

● Don't define yourself by your problem. You can be a diabetic in the surgery, but try not to be at the golf club.

● Find a sympathetic relative, friend or doctor to talk to about your illness, and avoid letting it dominate other conversations.

● Accept real restrictions and look for ways around them. Instead of being upset that you cannot do gymnastics with arthritis, try yoga.

● Help yourself when you can and ask for help when you cannot – don't be a martyr.

● Don't look for special concessions or sympathy.

● Don't suppress negative emotions or feel guilty about them. Talk about your frustrations or vent them through exercise, or try positive thinking or relaxation techniques.

● Ensure you are not in any way contributing to your illness – by eating the wrong foods, for example, or refusing to offload stress if you have high blood pressure.

● Find a doctor you like and trust, and cooperate fully with the treatment.

● Look after your general state of health.

● Enjoy life and maintain all your interests and activities.

MAKING THE MOST OF MIDDLE AGE

*Change is a part of life at any stage - and
the middle years are no exception. Children become
teenagers, and then young adults with lives of their own.
Parents are also growing older, and may need more help than
before. At the same time, careers reach a peak, and the
demands of work pile up faster than ever. Health needs
attention too - good habits learned now lay the
foundation for a fit and active future.*

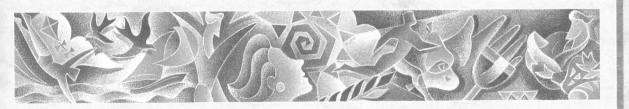

What do you know about middle age?

Attitudes to middle age are changing fast. As people live longer, healthier, wealthier lives, the midpoint of life is getting later, and there are more years left ahead after it is reached. Test your knowledge of middle age with the following quiz. Tick the correct answer for each question, and check your score below.

1 What is the average midpoint of life?

a) 35 for women and 32 for men.
b) 39 for women and 36 for men.
c) About 40 for both sexes.

2 Given the choice, which of these would more middle-aged people opt for?

a) More money.
b) Restored youthful appearance.
c) Advancement at work.

3 Which is the best way to prevent wrinkles in middle age?

a) Avoid smoking and sunbathing.
b) Use a good antiwrinkle skin cream.
c) There is nothing you can do – wrinkles are a natural and unavoidable part of the ageing process.

4 Which of these statements is true?

a) It is natural and healthy to put on weight as you get older.
b) Exercise gets less effective at toning the body as you age.
c) Putting on weight at the hips is healthier than at the stomach.

5 Which of these measures is most effective at counteracting osteoporosis (loss of bone mass)?

a) Taking a calcium supplement.
b) Dieting regularly to stay slim.
c) Taking exercise such as walking.

6 How often does a healthy 40-year-old need a blood-pressure check?

a) Every year.
b) Every three to five years.
c) People without symptoms don't need regular blood-pressure tests.

7 Which of these counts against having hormone replacement therapy?

a) A family history of breast cancer.
b) Menopausal hot flushes.
c) Smoking.

8 What is the average age at which women begin menopause?

a) 45.
b) 50.
c) 55.

9 At what age are people most likely to go through a divorce?

a) Mid to late 30s.
b) 40s.
c) Mid to late 60s.

10 Which statement about heart attacks is true?

a) The risks are about equal for men and women of all ages.
b) Men are always more at risk than women of the same age.
c) Until menopause women are less at risk; then the risks even out.

SCORING

Award yourself 1 point for each of these answers: 1(b), 2(a), 3(a), 4(c), 5(c), 6(b), 7(a), 8(b), 9(a) and 10(c). Add up your score.

8-10: You are clearly well informed and up-to-date about the prime of life.

5-7: Your general knowledge is good but there might be some areas you could know more about.

4 or less: This chapter could hold some surprises. Read on for more information about middle age.

A new stage of life

REACHING MATURITY

What counts as 'middle age' these days – and how long can I expect to live after I have reached it?

The definition of 'middle age' is becoming less clear cut as increasing life expectancy, better health and changing attitudes push back the start of middle age and increase its length. The average midpoint of life is now about 36 for men and 39 for women, but most people do not start to consider themselves middle aged until they enter their 40s. The upper limit of middle age is also receding as more and more people continue working and enjoying good health well past traditional retirement age.

Over the last century, the average life span has increased by about 70 per cent, mainly through a reduction in infant deaths. Life expectancy for the middle aged has also increased – by 40 to 60 per cent.

Improved fitness and social changes have also altered ideas of middle age. The average age of a woman giving birth is now 28 and rising, as more and more women are choosing to establish a career before having children. The result is that increasingly couples in their 30s and 40s have young families.

Midlife is also when career and financial success tend to peak. Ambitions and expectations for later years have expanded, and many people carry on active professional, social and personal lives well into their 60s and beyond.

Changing social attitudes mean that these extended middle years are increasingly seen and lived as the prime of life rather than the start of old age – there has probably never been a better time to be middle aged.

STILL FEELING YOUNG

I'm approaching my 40th birthday but I feel just as fit and energetic as I did at 20. Am I deceiving myself?

Not at all. The physical consequences of ageing make little practical difference to most people until well into their 50s or even older. Apart from the menopause, 'middle age' today is more of a psychological than a physical challenge. Events such as significant birthdays, the appearance of wrinkles

and grey hairs, and noticing the adult status and success of much younger people, often prompt a certain amount of life-assessment.

Such a period of 'stocktaking' can be positive, provided you do not panic, and it often opens the door to a new phase of maturity, with added confidence and creativity and greater awareness of personal achievements, needs and limits.

Middle life often has other compensations too – material comfort, financial security, increased influence and status.

FACING TRANSITION

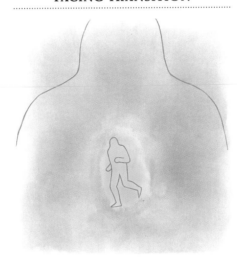

I'm dreading the thought of growing older. Am I heading towards a midlife crisis?

Middle life means facing the downhill slope for the first time – counting the years left rather than the years gone. Once the tasks of early adulthood – finding work, setting up home independently, starting and rearing a family – are accomplished, people begin to assess their progress.

Depending on individual personality and mental state, they may ask 'Where next?', or 'Was it worth it?' or 'What's the point?'. Other events common in this period, such as looking after elderly parents, or facing their death, can add to the sense of being an older generation, the next to die.

By the time they reach their late 50s, many people claim to have undergone a 'midlife crisis'. Some people react by becoming depressed or obsessively concerned with health, appearance or fitness. A few others

---

Living longer

At the end of the last century, the middle of life occurred, on average, at about 22. These days, it arrives some 15½ years later. Women have shown a greater increase, probably as a result of fewer deaths in childbirth.

Years remaining at different ages

1891

	Men	Women
Birth	42	46
40	Figures unavailable	
50	18	19
60	12	13

1988

	Men	Women
Birth	72	77
40	34	39
50	25	30
60	17	21

Power and influence

Middle-aged people now make up about one-third of Britain's population. They already have above-average incomes, greater capital wealth and more spending power than any other age group. The 'baby boom' generation that hits middle age in the 1990s will swell their ranks, and there will be fewer young people to follow them, as the effects of a declining birth rate become apparent. The reduction by a million in the number of potential employees in the 16 to 24 age group over the next decade will inevitably improve opportunities for older people. They will become the first generation to enjoy inherited wealth on a wide scale – acquiring from their parents who were the first generation to make home ownership in Britain the norm.

panic, but crisis indicators such as suicide attempts, heavy drinking and divorce are no more common at this stage of life than at any other.

Most people come to terms with increasing maturity, and a pause for assessment can encourage you to make the most of life. While you may have to abandon some dreams – it is probably too late to become a world-class gymnast or an astronaut – there are few absolute limitations on your capacities in middle age, and there are balancing benefits such as enhanced confidence and

wisdom. Creativity often peaks in midlife, changes direction or emerges for the first time, and many people, especially women, find new enthusiasm for pursuing personal goals after years devoted to others.

Experts recommend these tips for coping in the acute phase.

● Allow yourself to mourn for what is truly gone – lost youth, fertility, some ambitions. Then refocus on positive things.
● Take stock of what you have achieved.
● Remember, middle age is a luxury of

REAL LIVES

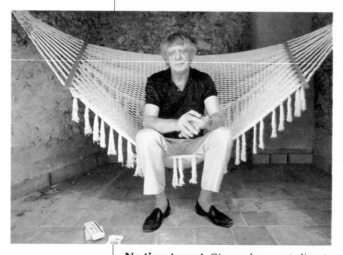

ANTHONY BURGESS: FINDING A VOCATION AT 40

The approach of middle age often nudges people to reassess their lives. Occasionally the result is a 'midlife crisis'. But for some people, midlife brings a new lease of creative energy, or the confidence to strike out in a new direction. Many novelists discover their calling only in their 40s: George Eliot and Catherine Cookson are just two distinguished examples. They can draw on greater experience now than they could in their youth, and perhaps greater powers of concentration too. For Anthony Burgess, one of the most celebrated of English writers at the time of his death in 1993, author of A Clockwork Orange *(1962) and* Earthly

Powers *(1980), there was an extra factor behind his late start – a midlife anxiety of the most intense kind.*

In 1959, at the age of 42, working in Borneo as a teacher in the Colonial Service, Burgess fell ill. He was diagnosed as having an inoperable brain tumour and was given a year to live. He returned to England determined to spend his last months hard at work to provide for his wife's future.

Burgess was a man of many talents, a linguist and a composer as well as a teacher, but the trade he thought most promising was that of novelist, having published a modestly successful trio of novels during the previous four years. He now set to work with a will, turning out four new novels during his 'final' year of life – only to learn, on being re-examined by British doctors, that no trace of the tumour could be found. His energetic and efficient working regime persisted, however. During the next 34 years he wrote a further 50 books or more, not just dazzling novels but learned non-fiction works as well – on language, cultural history and literature. Add to that the occasional screenplay and an enormous number of reviews and articles for British, French and Italian newspapers and magazines, and you begin to get some idea of the astonishing abundance of his literary output.

Throughout his early and late middle age, Burgess's youthful flair, determination and imaginativeness remained at full pitch. Life can indeed begin at 40 or thereabouts, his career suggests, and flourishes after that for as long as you will it to.

No time to rest *Given only a year to live at the age of 42, Burgess worked feverishly to provide for his wife after he had gone. In the event, he lived another 35 years.*

civilisation. In the past, and still in some countries, few survive to have midlife problems. Try to look on this as a transition, not a crisis.

● Try to channel your worries into something productive, such as getting yourself fit.

● Avoid panic behaviour – it may be a good idea to take up water skiing or to go on holiday in the Himalayas, but think very carefully before selling up everything to go and live on a Greek island or making any other irreversible changes.

● Find at least one thing you really want to do for yourself – and that won't undermine your health, marriage, job, family or financial security – and do it.

WOMEN'S EXPERIENCE

Women seem to fear getting older much more than men. Do they really have a worse time in middle age?

Yes, in some ways, at least in the West. As well as facing the menopause and loss of fertility, women often find that social attitudes and circumstances make middle age harder, and women are more likely than men to report feeling disturbed.

Firstly, women are still judged more on physical attributes, and popular perceptions of attractiveness are less kind to women as they age. The custom for men to partner younger women is a major disadvantage for older women.

Secondly, marriage and parenthood are still much greater sources of self-definition and social appraisal for women, so the end of active motherhood poses a greater challenge. Those who have stopped work to care for children may be left relatively financially dependent and with less to fall back on in middle age.

If divorced, they are much more likely to fall into poverty than a divorced man is. For women who are childless, even if by choice, middle age heralds the point of no return in their own eyes and those of others.

Older women are also less likely to have the midlife compensations of money, power and status. But even those who do achieve such compensations may find that they reap fewer rewards from them – for while success increases the social and sexual attractiveness of men it can, even today, be seen as intimidating in women.

Older women generally have less influence in public life, are less visible, are portrayed more negatively in the media, and are rarely given as much respect as is shown to middle-aged men.

Lastly, a woman's future expectations may seem bleaker: most women can expect to spend their last years alone, since husbands are generally older and die younger. There are nearly four times as many elderly women as elderly men living alone.

Because of the importance that culture increasingly places on attractiveness – both sexual and social – women at middle age face much starker losses than men. And little is offered to replace such losses. In other, more 'traditional' societies, by contrast, older women are respected for their wisdom and experience and play an increasing role in advice and decision-making, both in the family and in the community.

What matters most in midlife?

A 1991 Gallup poll investigated the preoccupations of middle age. The results are in order of priority.

Major concerns
● Health.
● Putting on weight (mainly women).
● Loss of sex drive (mainly men).
● Feeling less sexually attractive.
● Hair loss (mainly men).

Top stresses
● Children reaching adolescence.
● Bereavement.
● Children leaving home (mainly women).

Main desires
● More money.
● Greater fitness.
● Change of home.
● Change of job (mainly men).
● Change in appearance (mainly women).
● To have a child, or another child.
● Promotion at work.

Staying in shape

KEEPING BODY TONE

I'm not overweight, but I do feel flabbier than I used to. Is this an inevitable part of growing older?

No – but as time passes it can become much more difficult to keep trim. After the mid-twenties, lean body mass gradually declines with loss of tissue from bones, muscles and vital organs, and lower body water content. Without weight loss, most of this is replaced by fat, which is quite healthy within normal limits (without fat, elderly people can look scrawny and dehydrated). Excess fat, however, turns all too easily to flab. Body metabolism slows down too, so people need less food to maintain the same weight. As well as eating less, it is important to stay active. Exercise helps weight control, slows down muscle and bone loss, and keeps muscles toned. And the more exercise you take, the more improvement you will feel. You also need to watch your posture. Increased fat and reduced mobility encourage 'middle-aged stoop', with rounded shoulders and protruding abdomen. Women are more vulnerable because they start with a thicker fat layer, and can suffer from weakened abdominal muscles as a result of pregnancy. After menopause they tend to lay down fat around the abdomen, rather than on the hips (see panel opposite). The end result is that since many middle-aged people eat more and exercise less, they are at risk of becoming overweight and flabby.

WATCHING YOUR WEIGHT

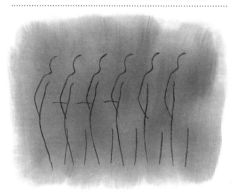

How can I tell if I am in danger of developing middle-age spread and what is the best routine for fighting it?

Firstly, keep a careful but not obsessive check on what you weigh. If you start out within normal limits (see page 154) weigh yourself no more than once a fortnight, if overweight not more than once a week.

Next, check your fat level – the rule that if you can 'pinch more than an inch' on the abdomen you are too fat, is a useful guide. Then think about your risk – if you have a hefty build or your family tends to run to fat in middle age, you need to watch your diet more closely than if you are a beanpole from a family of beanpoles.

Eating well

Whether you need to lose weight or not, the best way to control it in the long term is to establish good, basic eating habits.

Base your diet on filling, starchy foods such as wholemeal bread, potatoes, pasta and wholegrain cereals, and include plenty of fresh fruit and vegetables. If you buy meat, avoid fatty cuts.

Grill, steam or bake your food rather than fry it. When eating at restaurants, try to avoid creamy sauces, dishes that are rich in cream and sugary desserts, and drink alcohol in moderation.

Examine your eating habits to see if they need changing. You may be picking at fattening snacks during the day or having heavy business lunches and still eating a full meal at home in the evening. Some people also find it helpful to keep a food diary for a week

or so, recording everything that they eat, when they eat, and how hungry they feel at the time. This makes it possible to see where the extra calories are coming from, and helps with planning realistic alternatives.

Considering a diet

If you are flabby or overweight, you may want to begin a gradual weight-reducing diet (see page 153) and aim to lose no more than 2 lb (around 1 kg) per week.

Trying too hard to lose weight could be dangerous. Excessive sudden dieting can lead to nutritional deficiencies; and being underweight may increase the risk of developing osteoporosis (weakening of the bones) in later life. Do not, on any account, be tempted by radical, or 'starvation', dieting. You won't have the energy to keep up a rigorous daily routine and, when the dieting stops, you could end up putting on more weight than you were trying to lose.

Staying active

Next, assess your activity level, and how it has changed. Try to take regular exercise, especially if your day-to-day life is fairly sedentary. If the active sports of your youth, such as football, running or squash, seem too demanding, consider alternatives such as walking, swimming or cycling, to keep up your activity level.

Posture and tone

Lastly, keep up both flexibility and posture for a trimmer and fitter appearance irrespective of your weight.

You can help to tone up your muscles by observing a couple of simple rules: never slump over your work while sitting at a desk and always try to sit upright while at the same time pulling in your stomach muscles. Stretching exercises or yoga are excellent to maintain muscle tone and flexibility, and to help to build awareness of posture.

THE VALUE OF EXERCISE

I exercised regularly for many years in my 20s and 30s. Would it be advisable for me to start slowing down now that I've reached middle age?

Not at all. People who develop a regular exercise routine as young adults will benefit greatly from maintaining and developing it as they go through life.

Regular exercise helps to strengthen the heart and circulatory system, reducing the long-term risk of a stroke or heart attack,

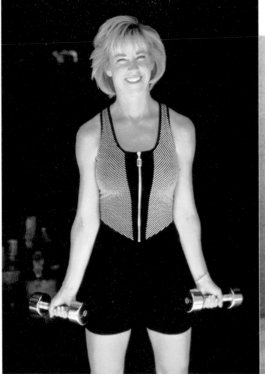

Toning up Activity rather than age is what matters when it comes to keeping a lean, shapely body and good muscle tone – as tennis champion Chris Evert (above) and actress Raquel Welch (right) demonstrate. The rewards last well into later life too.

and is also thought to be responsible for holding back the development of such diseases as arthritis and diabetes.

Exercise also helps to lower blood cholesterol and counters the common mid and later life problems of weight gain, muscle stiffness and reduced flexibility. Although peak performance capacity does diminish with age, proper conditioning can improve the tone of your muscles at all stages of life. Exercising can take many forms, too – see pages 69-72 for advice on choosing.

APPLES AND PEARS – HOW DO YOU SHAPE UP?

Obesity is well known to increase the risk of certain illnesses, but recent research shows that it is not just how much fat you have or what you weigh but where the weight is that matters.

Scientists and doctors now know that having most of your fat distributed on the upper half of your body is a health hazard, irrespective of how much you actually weigh.

So-called apple-shaped people, with relatively thick necks, arms and waists, are much more at risk of heart disease, diabetes and high blood pressure than pear-shaped people with bigger hips and thighs. For women there are added risks from breast cancer, period problems and infertility.

To find out whether you are an apple or a pear, you need to calculate your waist-to-hip ratio. Measure your waist and hips at the widest point, then divide the waist measurement by the hip measurement.

If the resulting ratio is more than 0.8 for a woman or 1.0 for a man, you count as an apple. For example, a man whose waist measures 42 in (106 cm) and whose hips measure 38 in (96 cm) will have a ratio of 1.1 (42 divided by 38), which is a sign of a typical but dangerous 'beer belly' or 'spare tyre'. By contrast, a woman with a waist of 28 in (71 cm) and hips of 39 in (99 cm) has a ratio of 0.7 (28 divided by 39). This is the pear shape – traditionally despised but actually a sign of better health.

GETTING STARTED

I want to start some sort of exercise but I'm worried that, at 47, I may have left it too late. What should I do?

It certainly is not too late to begin a programme of exercises or to take up activities that will provide you with valuable physical exercise and have a lasting effect.

One in four middle-aged people rate getting fitter as the factor which would most boost their confidence, and starting exercise even when elderly can increase strength by nearly 200 per cent.

Brisk walking for at least 20 minutes three times a week is ideal for beginners, and cycling and swimming both help to tone up ageing muscles. Less strenuous games such as golf and bowls are particularly beneficial in helping to keep joints and muscles supple, and many people also enjoy the social side of such activities.

CAUTION If you are thinking of embarking on a programme of exercises or taking up one of the more strenuous pastimes, start gradually and don't overdo it at first. If you have high blood pressure, or heart, chest or back problems, always check with your doctor before starting so that you don't over-strain yourself.

Good looks to last

DO'S —— AND —— DON'TS

for using make-up in middle age

Do keep make up subtle. Strong colours can be ageing.

Do use a camouflage cream on broken capillaries, age spots or other blemishes. A light smear of matt green eye shadow applied first counteracts red blotches.

Do dust your lips with face powder before applying a final layer of lipstick to prevent it running into creases.

Do try doing without foundation and face powder, or try a colourless silicone-containing cream instead for a more youthful sheen.

Don't use creamy eyeshadows if they run into creases. Try powder types instead.

CARING FOR YOUR SKIN

I've always been complimented on my youthful appearance. Is there any way of preventing wrinkles from developing as I reach middle age?

Most people develop fine facial lines in their mid to late 30s, and coarser face and neck wrinkles by their late 40s. Fine wrinkles are due largely to the skin thinning and losing natural oils and elasticity. As a result, excess loose, dry skin settles into familiar patterns such as crow's feet and frown and laughter lines. Coarser wrinkles develop from fine lines in the skin which, over the years, draws away from underlying muscle.

While the unavoidable effects of ageing are responsible for some wrinkling, exposure to the sun causes far more damage – some doctors estimate as much as 90 per cent. This is why face and hands suffer far more than the trunk. Soap, water and smoking accelerate wrinkling too.

The best way to slow down the development of wrinkles is good skin care, ideally from puberty. Once they have appeared, it is even more important to be careful to prevent further damage.

● Never sunbathe. Protect exposed areas from exposure to sun and wind by using sunscreens and moisturisers, and wearing a hat or gloves.
● Don't smoke.
● Choose a gentle soap without chemical additives such as perfumes or antiseptics.
● Wash your face and hands with lukewarm rather than hot water.
● Try to prevent the air in your house from drying out. Hang humidifying reservoirs from central heating radiators in winter.
● Use a moisturiser after washing your face, especially in the mornings and before going outside. Include your neck in the treatment. A moisturiser does not add moisture but seals in what is already there, so apply it while the skin is slightly damp. Cheap brands are as effective as expensive ones.

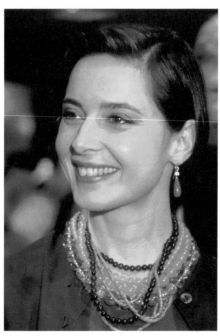

Role model In her early 40s Isabella Rossellini had a modelling contract cancelled on grounds of age. After she spoke out, it was reinstated.

● Use rubber gloves for household chores and apply hand cream after washing.
● Try using face masks or facial scrubs (soapy mixtures containing an abrasive). They remove the dead outer layer of cells, making skin appear temporarily fresher.

'ANTIAGEING' FACE CREAMS

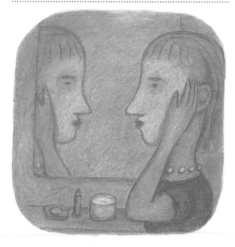

So many cosmetics claim to have rejuvenating properties. They seem incredibly expensive – but do any of them actually work?

Not really. Despite the scientific-sounding claims that are made to promote creams and lotions, there is no over-the-counter cosmetic that can remove wrinkles or reverse or prevent any other signs of ageing. Wrinkles and creases are the result of many factors – including exposure to the sun, hereditary skin type and smoking – none of which can be counteracted by cosmetics.

Most so-called antiageing creams, according to medical experts, are merely sophisticated emollients: substances that plump up the skin by encouraging water retention. Other creams called exfoliating agents contain chemicals that promote the shedding of dead cells on the surface of the skin, exposing new younger-looking skin beneath. You can get the same effect by using a granular cleanser or buffing sponge once or twice a week. Rub gently and stop if the treatment irritates your skin. Avoid such treatments altogether if you have sensitive skin.

British law allows manufacturers to make claims such as 'antiageing complex for the face', so it is up to buyers to be on their guard. In the United States legislation is stricter, and the very same product may be described simply as promoting 'smoothness, radiance and firmness'.

SPOTS ON THE HANDS

My wife has developed small brown spots on the backs of her hands. Is there any cause for concern?

None at all. Liver spots, or age spots, are small, flat, light brown patches like oversize freckles that often appear in clusters on the hands in middle age. Despite the name, they have nothing to do with the liver. Some doctors believe they result from years of over-exposure to the sun, but this is not known for certain.

Most people soon get used to the spots and forget all about them, but if your wife is concerned about the look of her hands she could consider disguising them with cover-up creams or make-up. Applying a sunscreen may help to prevent new spots developing.

Some older people also develop another kind of age spot – tiny, cherry-red spots that appear singly, usually on the trunk. These are called Campbell de Morgan spots, and are also harmless.

TAKING CARE OF OLDER HAIR

As well as going grey in places, my hair seems to be getting thinner and more brittle. How can I keep it looking good in middle age?

Hair growth slows down in middle age while the rate of loss remains the same, so eventually more hairs are lost than replaced. In women, hair usually thins out evenly but men are more likely to develop balding at the temples and crown. Individual shafts get thinner, too, making hair look wispy and fine. Older hair also becomes more fragile and more vulnerable to damage by chemical treatments such as colours and perms.

Greying (really loss of natural pigment) is genetically determined and begins in the mid-30s to mid-40s for most people. It shows more in darker hair, but blonde hair is more likely to end up completely grey.

Treat your hair gently and try these tips to keep it in top condition.

● If possible, avoid brushing or combing your hair when wet, and let it dry naturally.
● Try scalp massage to increase blood flow and promote hair growth.
● Use a mild shampoo suitable for your hair type. Apply conditioner sparingly – it can make hair go limp.
● If your hair is dry, try an oil treatment once a fortnight. Gently heat a little olive oil

Professional beauty treatments

Several specialist techniques are available for those keen to keep their looks. If you are tempted, remember that results are not guaranteed, and treatment can be costly.

● Extensive removal of surface skin – done by skin peeling (dermabrasion), mechanical methods or applying enzymes. It is said to boost skin cell rejuvenation and requires the supervision of a dermatologist as excessive treatment can cause scarring.
● Retinoic acid – a derivative of vitamin A originally used to treat acne. It can partially reverse age changes, especially fine wrinkling due to sun damage. Retinoic acid can be given only under medical supervision, and must be used for two months or more before there is a noticeable improvement. Skin irritation sometimes also occurs.
● Subcutaneous injections of collagen, silicone or fat – used to puff out skin creases. Treatment is usually given by a cosmetic surgeon. Collagen (from animal tissue) needs topping up about once a year, and may cause an allergic reaction. Silicone and fat (taken from the buttocks by liposuction) last longer.
● Cosmetic surgery – the only cure for deeper lines and wrinkles. See page 388 if you are tempted to try.

until it feels pleasantly warm. Rub it into your scalp, cover with a warm towel for 20 minutes, then shampoo and rinse out well.

● If you want to colour your hair, choose a product designed to cover up grey hair. If you notice damage such as split ends or your hair becomes dry, brittle or dull, seek advice from your hairdresser.

● Have your hair professionally cut and styled, and do not be tempted to try permanent tints and waves at home. Wait at least six weeks between treatments.

● Avoid tints that are darker than your natural colour, as the effect can be ageing. Remember that eyebrows and lashes can be coloured too.

● Hormone replacement therapy (see page 394) can sometimes help to reduce hair loss in women, although this is not a sufficient reason for undertaking treatment.

CAUTION Poor hair condition can be a sign of illness, stress, inadequate diet or anaemia. See your doctor if any sudden changes occur.

HELP FOR BALDNESS

I don't want to end up bald like all the other men in my family. What are my options now that I've noticed my hair starting to recede?

Male pattern hair loss is almost entirely due to inheritance, and most men end up in the same position as their father. About one in three notice some hair loss in their 30s and by 50 half have bald areas, either a receding hairline or a monk's crown on top. 'Cures' for baldness have been touted since antiquity, but nothing guarantees success in all cases. Currently available options include:

● Minoxidil: a drug that was originally used for high blood pressure. It has the side effect of increasing hair growth, and is marketed as 'Regaine' for baldness. It does help, but it is expensive. Regrowth takes time, is often patchy, and requires continuous treatment.

● Grafting: plugs of head or body skin containing hair follicles are transplanted to bald patches. Treatment is lengthy and expensive but can produce good results.

● Scalp reduction: a sort of surgical 'scalp lift' that works by removing a wedge of hairless skin and drawing up hairy areas to cover it. It works best on small bald spots.

● False hair: strands of artificial hair are interwoven with existing hair to disguise thinning or small bald patches.

COSMETIC SURGERY

I am thinking about cosmetic surgery. How effective is it? Are there any risks?

Surgery can correct some features of ageing and make you look younger, but it cannot make you 20 again. Anyone who expects it to change their way of life, revive a marriage or relieve depression is doing it for the wrong reasons and is likely to be disappointed. Good candidates, by contrast, have specific, simple goals – 'I just want to get rid of the bags under my eyes' or 'I'm fed up with the shape of my nose'. These are realistic aims that may well be possible to achieve. Before going any further, it may help to try to identify the exact physical effects you want to achieve. If you find it difficult to be precise, it could be a sign not to proceed, or not until you are more certain.

Cosmetic surgery is becoming increasingly popular, with an estimated 70 000 operations a year in Britain. People are also seeking help earlier – at one London clinic, the average age of face-lift patients fell from 65 to 47 between 1986 and 1991.

Provided you choose a reputable surgeon and hospital, cosmetic surgery is no more dangerous than other operations – but also no less dangerous. All such procedures carry risks of infection and scarring, and a tiny but real chance of serious complications. The most common procedures include:

● Liposuction – removal of excess fat from beneath the skin, especially on the chin, abdomen, thighs, buttocks and upper arms. It is considered suitable for small fat deposits, but not for general weight reduction. Possible drawbacks include an uneven effect and loose skin.

● Blepharoplasty – taking a tuck in the upper or lower eyelid to correct sags, bags and wrinkles.

● Full face-lift – pulling loose facial skin up and back towards the ears to smooth out wrinkles and sags.

● Half face-lift – taking a tuck in loose skin of the jaw and chin.

● Breast-lift – tightens sagging breasts.

● Abdominoplasty – removes loose abdominal skin, especially after childbirth or severe weight loss.

Cosmetic surgery is not generally available on the NHS, unless a condition is actually disfiguring. If you do decide to go ahead, follow the advice in the panel, left, and ask your doctor's opinion. He may also be able to recommend an experienced surgeon.

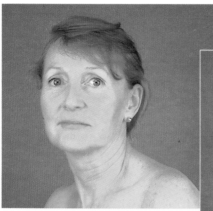

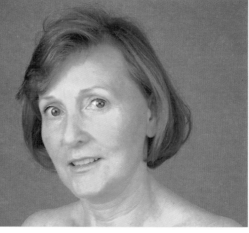

Three months later A successful face-lift (below) has smoothed out lines and wrinkles, giving the youthful appearance she desired.

A certain age... A look familiar to many middle-aged people led Stephanie Williams (above) to try cosmetic surgery. She chronicled the experience in her book, *Diary of a Facelift* (1993).

LOOKING AHEAD

Is there anything I can do now to keep my looks in the future?

As well as good skin and hair care, plenty of exercise and rest, and a healthy diet, you can cultivate habits and attitudes in middle age that will keep you looking healthy and vital well beyond.

● Practise some form of regular relaxation (see pages 190-195) – no one ages well if they feel tense and under pressure.
● Stay happy – people will rate you as more attractive whatever your age.
● Choose clothes carefully. Classic designs that are well cut and unfussy never date.
● Maintain good posture – as well as making you look younger and fitter, it enhances confidence and mood.

Looking after your health

HEART ATTACK RISKS

So many middle-aged men seem to have heart attacks that I have become quite worried. How much of a risk is this and can I do anything to reduce it?

You are right to be concerned. One man in twelve will die of a heart attack before he retires and heart attacks are five times more common among middle-aged men than among women, at least before menopause. Thereafter, risks increase with age for both sexes becoming, in old age, the commonest cause of death.

Some people are much more in danger than others. A huge range of factors can be involved, including a family history of heart disease, high blood pressure, high blood cholesterol levels and obesity. You are also more at risk if you are diabetic, smoke, lead an inactive life, suffer from stress or show aggressive 'type A' behaviour (see pages 175-176).

Drinking very heavily, living in a soft-water area, snoring and a condition known as sleep apnoea (moments when breathing stops during sleep – see page 158) all further increase heart attack risks. However, some simple measures can give protection:

● Have your blood pressure checked regularly. If necessary, take steps to reduce it (see pages 362-363).
● Lose weight if you need to.
● Adopt a healthy diet, low in saturated fat.
● Seek medical advice if you are obese.
● Drink unfiltered tap water if you live in a hard-water area. Filters remove calcium that protects the heart.
● Don't smoke.
● Take regular exercise.
● Practise relaxation every day.
● Avoid heavy drinking.
● Half an aspirin every other day after 50 may reduce the risk of a heart attack – ask your doctor for advice.

FACT
—— OR ——
FALLACY?

'Men are more likely than women to get heart disease.'

Fact (up to a certain age). Men between 35 and 44 are six times more likely to die from heart disease. Women under 40 are believed to be protected by the hormone oestrogen, which may prevent fatty deposits building up in arteries. After the menopause, oestrogen production drops and a woman's risk becomes as great as a man's.

HELP FOR VARICOSE VEINS

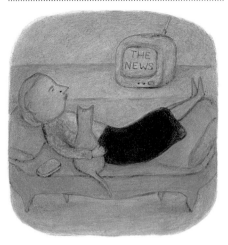

The varicose veins on my legs are becoming more and more unsightly, and more painful. What has caused them and what can I do about them?

Around one person in five suffers from varicose veins. They occur when valves in the leg veins fail to function properly, preventing blood from flowing smoothly up towards the heart. Instead, the force of gravity pushes blood downwards, building up pressure in the veins and causing swelling and pain.

The tendency to develop varicose veins can be hereditary, and the problem is exacerbated by many factors, including hormonal changes during pregnancy which dilate the veins. The primary cause, however, is our upright posture, which places great pressure on the leg valves. The longer you spend on your feet, the more pressure the valves come under and the more likely they are to fail or weaken. This is why varicose veins become more common with age, and among people who spend many hours standing, such as hairdressers and shop assistants.

You can prevent the swelling from worsening, and sometimes even reduce it, by staying on the move. Walking about rather than standing or sitting for long periods, and flex your calf muscles to improve circulation. Whenever possible, try to sit with your feet propped up above waist level. Try to lie down with legs raised above the level of your heart for 20 minutes in the evening. You may also find elastic stockings helpful to support and ease swollen veins. Avoid hot baths, however, and prevent constipation by eating lots of fibre and taking plenty of liquid with it.

If these self-help techniques do not solve the problem, see your doctor, who may then decide to refer you for surgical treatment.

This is usually a minor procedure involving injecting a sclerosing (hardening) agent into affected veins to divert blood through other paths. The leg remains bandaged for up to six weeks, during which time the patient has to take a daily 3 mile (5 km) walk.

If veins are too badly varicosed for injection treatment, or if they recur despite treatment, you may be offered an operation to remove them altogether.

PREVENTING OSTEOPOROSIS

What exactly is osteoporosis and why are middle-aged women particularly affected?

Osteoporosis literally means porous bones. From the 30s onwards bones become less dense, losing about 0.3 per cent of their mass every year as the supporting structure is gradually eroded and calcium leaches out. After the menopause, the loss accelerates in women, sometimes to as much as 2-3 per

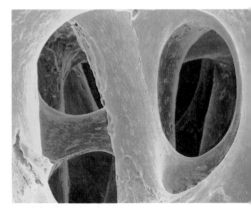

Healthy bone In young adulthood, bones reach their peak mass and calcium density, forming a strong, supple framework.

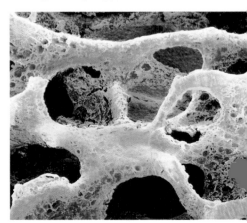

The ravages of osteoporosis Calcium loss leaves bones porous and weak. Prevention is vital as treatment cannot reverse the damage.

cent a year. By the time she is 70, a woman may have only half the bone mass she had at 30. As the losses mount up, bones become weak, fragile and brittle. Eventually, a little height is lost as the spine squashes down slightly. In extreme cases, the upper vertebrae may even become wedged into a dowager's hump. The risk of bones breaking even under minor pressure is also dramatically increased, especially in the wrists, legs and vertebrae of the spine. Up to one in four elderly women at some stage sustain a fracture, often impairing mobility and sometimes causing fatal complications.

The risk of severe osteoporosis is increased by factors such as a family history of the illness, early menopause, poor diet, smoking, alcohol and lack of exercise. You can help to prevent it, or to reduce further bone loss once the process has begun, by taking regular weight-bearing exercise such as walking, and avoiding extreme dieting, smoking and excessive alcohol consumption.

Exposure to daylight will promote production of vitamin D, which is important for calcium absorption. A calcium-rich diet is also important (see page 48), but although calcium supplements are sometimes recommended, there is little evidence that they help. The sooner you adopt preventive measures the better – ideally begin in your 20s to build up maximum bone mass before losses begin. Hormone replacement therapy (HRT) (see page 394) both prevents and reduces osteoporosis, as oestrogen helps to prevent calcium loss.

HYSTERECTOMY ANXIETY

My doctor tells me I need a hysterectomy. I know it's a fairly common operation, but I can't help feeling anxious. Are my fears justified?

It depends on what you are worried about and why you need the operation. In some cases, such as cancer, there is clearly no argument about its usefulness. Most hysterectomies, however, are done to ease menstrual problems, such as heavy bleeding or pain, and such cases are more debatable.

Although a hysterectomy is regarded as a safe operation there are always risks, and side effects are common. Convalescence can last for anything from eight to twelve weeks, and although some women feel better in days others find it is six to nine months, or even a year, before they feel fully recovered. Some women also report psychological difficulties or problems in achieving an orgasm.

If the ovaries are also removed – generally only for a sound medical reason – the operation will precipitate an immediate menopause. Even in operations where only the uterus is removed, menopausal hormone changes generally begin within a few years, whatever the patient's age.

If your problem is menstrual, you might want to consider other options, bearing in mind that when the menopause comes the problem will end naturally. In any case, do discuss the issue further with your doctor – women who feel that they have made their own decision are much less likely to experience problems adjusting afterwards. Ask whether a full hysterectomy is really necessary. New techniques mean that just the womb lining can be removed rather than the whole womb, and often this is all that is necessary. This procedure has fewer complications, needs a shorter hospital stay and recovery period and reduces the psychological effects. Increasingly, doctors are offering this as an alternative, and it is estimated to be suitable in as many as half of the cases where hysterectomy would once have been the standard treatment.

If other options are not advised, ask about the aftereffects you are likely to experience, whether the operation will be carried out through an abdominal incision or through the vagina (which is safer, leaves no scar and makes for a easier recovery, but is not always possible), and whether the surgeon intends to remove the ovaries – if he does, discuss options such as hormone replace therapy (HRT) to avoid early menopause.

After sorting out these issues, make sure you are as fit as possible for the operation, to reduce complications and speed recovery. If you are overweight, try to lose the excess fat. If anaemia is a possibility (heavy periods can be a cause) eat plenty of iron-rich foods. Take exercise to tone your muscles. And if you smoke, stop – at least try to give up for a week (longer if possible) before surgery to minimise the effects of the anaesthetic on your respiratory system.

The operation itself takes between 40 minutes and an hour and you will be encouraged to get up as soon as possible and to move your feet and legs while still in bed to prevent blood clots developing. Stitches are usually removed on the fourth or fifth day and it is normal to go home within a week.

If you are still worried, contact the Hysterectomy Support Network, 3 Lynne Close, Green Street Green, Orpington, Kent BR6 6BS. They can put you in touch with others who have had the operation.

> ### Are you getting the care you need?
>
> A large part of staying healthy is identifying symptoms before they become serious. The following screening schedule is designed to do that.
>
> ● Blood pressure – annual check every three to five years after 40, and more often if it is high.
> ● Eye tests, including glaucoma – every two years, or more often if a relative is affected.
> ● Dental check-ups – every six months.
> ● For men: Monthly testicle self-examination (see pages 162-163). Some doctors advise an annual PSA (prostate serum antigen) blood test for prostate trouble, although it is not always available on the NHS.
> ● For women: Monthly breast self-examination (see pages 163-164); cervical smear test every one to five years; breast examination and mammogram every two or three years from the age of 50 to 64.

Midlife fertility and menopause

CONTRACEPTION IN MIDLIFE

Are some types of contraception more suitable than others for women who have reached middle age?

Most methods are just as safe and effective in middle age as earlier in life, but there are some differences worth bearing in mind.

● Contraceptive pills that contain oestrogen can increase the risk of heart attack and stroke. For women over 40, particularly if they smoke, doctors generally recommend changing to a progesterone-only minipill.

● Intrauterine devices (IUDs) can trigger or exacerbate the heavy menstrual flow some women experience preceding menopause.

● Condoms, diaphragms and other barrier methods may need extra lubrication – as menopause approaches, the vagina sometimes becomes drier.

CAUTION Do not assume you are no longer fertile once menopause starts. Although the chance of a pregnancy is much less, it is not safe to stop using contraception until at least a year after your last period. Wait two years if you are under 50. If in doubt, check with your doctor.

FACING THE END OF FERTILITY

I am in my 40s and although I have two children and have never before thought about having any more, I do feel a little sad at the thought that my fertility will come to an end one day. Is this normal?

Perfectly normal. All major changes in life, even positive ones, provoke contemplation on what has been and what is to come. The end of something which has been precious and important to you is bound to be a little sad, and even women who are certain they want no more children can be slightly wistful or nostalgic.

Your sadness is probably also connected with more general feelings about getting older. If it is very specifically related to fertility, it may still not be too late to think of another baby. If, on reflection, you decide that this is really what you want, discuss the matter with your doctor. Otherwise, allow yourself to grieve for what is inevitable but remember, that this is a stage that will pass.

In the 17th century, three out of four women died before reaching menopause; now only one in twenty does. And however you feel about menopause, it is certainly better than not getting there. Humans are also the only species to have a menopause, which suggests that limiting the childbearing years is an advantage.

STARTING THE CHANGE OF LIFE

I'm nearly 50 and have noticed that my periods are not as regular as they used to be. Is this the start of menopause and, if so, what further signs and changes should I expect now?

Your irregular periods are indeed a typical sign of the changing hormone levels that precede menopause, or the 'change of life'. Menopause usually occurs between 45 and 55, with 50 being the average age.

As menopause approaches, the ovaries slowly become less active. The production of oestrogen and the monthly release of eggs becomes erratic. Periods may get heavier or lighter and cycles shorter or longer. You may miss a period or two, then begin menstruating regularly again for a time. Or you may simply have a final period and then stop menstruating for ever.

Menopause is not considered complete until you have stopped menstruating altogether and your body has fully adjusted to the reduction in hormone levels. This adjustment can take as long as five years after the final menstrual period. Along with changes in the menstrual pattern, some women experience many other menopause symptoms. Others notice almost nothing.

Falling oestrogen levels are generally at the root of any physical symptoms such as hot flushes, night sweats and vaginal dryness. Some women also experience urinary problems (itchy skin, particularly in the genital region), and sometimes increased facial or body hair. Declining oestrogen also accelerates the rate at which bone mass is lost – osteoporosis – and increases the risk of heart disease. Other effects commonly attributed to menopause may have more to do with psychological and social factors than with any physical changes. Western women frequently report symptoms such as depression, anxiety, insomnia, fatigue and irritability, but these are rare in cultures where women acquire new status with age. Remember that every woman's experience of menopause is individual, and try not to approach this stage of life with too many negative preconceptions. Although treatment is available if symptoms arise, by no means all women need medical help. Many report a new surge of energy after menopause, and a heightened sense of wellbeing.

FIGHTING HOT FLUSHES

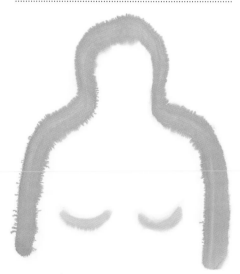

For me, the worst aspect of menopause has been the embarrassment of unpredictable hot flushes. What is the cause of this problem and is there anything that can prevent it?

There is no easy solution to the problem of hot flushes – among the most common and most disturbing symptoms of menopause, and estimated by some doctors to account for more than half of all menopause-related consultations by patients.

The mechanism that causes hot flushes is not fully understood, but it is thought that fluctuating oestrogen levels may be responsible for sudden rushes of blood to the skin. As with many symptoms of menopause, hot flushes affect women in different ways.

Some are fortunate enough never to experience them; others find that they occur only at night. For most, intermittent hot flushes continue for three to five years.

By far the most effective medical treatment for hot flushes is hormone replacement therapy (HRT), which replenishes lost oestrogen (see page 394).

If you cannot have HRT, or do not wish to, an alternative drug called clonidine can give relief. In either case, you need to seek advice from your doctor as these treatments are available only on prescription. You can also help yourself in several ways:

- Wear natural fibres next to the skin.
- Wear loose-fitting clothing and dress in layers you can shed easily.
- Sit near to doors and windows in public places such as restaurants.
- Try sipping a cold drink or splashing tepid water on your face during an attack.
- Tea, coffee, alcohol, stress and sudden temperature changes can all make hot flushes worse – avoid them if possible.
- Some women report improvements when they take vitamin C and E supplements, or use homeopathic or herbal remedies.

SEX AFTER MENOPAUSE

My husband and I are feeling somewhat apprehensive. Will menopause affect our sex life?

Forget your fears. Surveys suggest that for at least 80 per cent of women, sexual responsiveness either increases or stays the same during and after menopause. Indeed, many couples find their sex life revives at this time, when they need no longer be so concerned about pregnancy or contraception, and often have more time together.

Sexual problems do, however, sometimes arise: in particular, reduced vaginal lubrication, changes in libido and worries about appearance and ageing. Midlife crises and relationship problems can also affect a couple's sex life. Many of these problems are temporary and they often disappear once the difficult transition stage is over.

Couples who can discuss their feelings honestly are most likely to enhance their sex life and to resolve any problems that do occur. A little extra effort and mutual attention may also be well rewarded.

- Keep up day-to-day intimacy.
- Don't let standards slip – it is hard to feel sensual to someone wearing bedsocks. Considerate men shave at night.
- Make sure you are fully aroused before penetration, and use a lubricating cream if necessary. Oestrogen creams and hormone replacement therapy can also help – ask your doctor.
- Focus on quality rather than quantity of sex, and be prepared to take more time.
- Consider other ways to improve your sex life (see page 255).

CONSIDERING HRT

What is actually involved in hormone replacement and how should I weigh up the pros and cons?

Hormone replacement therapy (HRT) works by topping up the body's oestrogen levels, which decline naturally at menopause as the ovaries slow down. The results can be dramatic, putting an end to or greatly reducing unpleasant menopause symptoms such as hot flushes, night sweats, skin irritation and vaginal dryness. It also reputedly makes skin and hair look younger.

While psychological symptoms experienced at the time of menopause may well have other causes than just falling oestrogen levels, there is no doubt that many women do obtain an emotional boost on HRT. Some even report increased libido.

For many women, HRT markedly improves the experience of menopause. As with all medication, however, some people are troubled by side effects – principally the return of monthly bleeding. While many women are happy to put up with this, others feel they are losing out on one of the prime advantages of menopause.

HRT is generally considered as extremely safe. An increased risk of womb cancer was found with some early types of treatment based only on oestrogen, but is now avoided by combining oestrogen with a second hormone, progesterone. Women who have had a hysterectomy, however, will still be prescribed oestrogen-only HRT, since they have no risk of contracting cancer of the womb.

Some studies also suggest that there may be a small increased risk of breast cancer with HRT, especially among women with a strong family history of the disease. Against this, HRT halves the risks of strokes, heart disease and fractures in later life, and overall mortality may be reduced considerably.

HRT can be administered in many different ways – tablets, pessaries, skin patches and implants are all available – and almost all women can find some form that is suitable in their case. Treatment may be given during menopause, in the years approaching it, or at any stage when the ovaries need to be removed on medical grounds. The benefits cease when treatment is stopped, so HRT should be seen as a long-term measure; some would say a permanent one.

Although HRT has many strong advocates among the medical profession, there are also opponents, and each woman must decide for herself. Before opting for treatment, discuss the issues fully with your doctor. Information is also available from The Amarant Trust, Grant House, 56-60 St John Street, London EC1M 4DT.

WEIGHING UP THE PROS AND CONS OF HORMONE REPLACEMENT

For a rough idea of whether or not hormone relacement therapy may be indicated in your case, tick any symptoms below that apply to you. Then add up the pluses and minuses to obtain an overall score. The foot of the page tells you how to interpret your score.

Hot flushes - severe.	+3	Family or personal history of breast cancer.	−2
- moderate.	+2		
- mild or none.	0	Family history of osteoporosis.	+3
Night sweats.	+2	Loss of height.	+3
Vaginal dryness or irritation.*	+1	Brittle bones or fractures.	+3
Lack of lubrication during sex.*	+1	Sedentary way of life.*	+2
Soreness or discomfort on penetration.*	+1	Poor diet, smoking or drinking more than 3 units of alcohol a day.*	+1
Period problems (pain, heavy bleeding).	−2		
Urinary symptoms.*	+1	Family or personal history of heart disease.*	+2
Skin or genital itching.	+1		
Hysterectomy.	+1	Troubling increased facial or body hair *	+1
Early menopause (symptoms before the age of 45).	+2	Thinning hair.	+1
		Fatigue, depression or anxiety about your appearance.*	+1
Ovaries removed before the age of 55.	+3		

If your total score added up to +3 or more, HRT may have significant benefits to offer you. Consider discussing it with your doctor.

* Other treatments are available for these conditions. If all your symptoms are in this category, HRT may not be the best choice.

Keeping relationships happy

ISSUES IN MIDDLE AGE

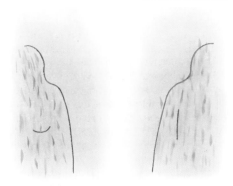

Married friends of mine separated when their children left home. Do marital difficulties increase in middle age?

Not necessarily. Divorce rates peak not when people are in their 40s and 50s – as is often supposed – but among those in their mid to late 30s. However, there are certainly more divorced people among the middle aged, since their number also includes those who divorced earlier on – so at a quick glance it can look as if getting older increases the likelihood of divorce.

Since most couples are aged within five years of each other, they tend to experience middle-age stresses at around the same time, compounding any problems that occur.

Individual concerns often conflict – typically men are wrapped up in work, while women may be more worried about social isolation, menopause or children leaving the home. If one partner goes through a period of personal growth or change, the other may feel threatened. Any crisis reaction, such as having an affair, can be extremely stressful and destabilising.

Boredom with settled patterns of home, social or sexual life becomes a real risk at this stage, too. Sex can suffer if partners are worried about libido or fading attractiveness, or if there are physical problems such as impotence or diminished vaginal lubrication. Sexual incompatibilities often become an issue for the first time in midlife. Women may start to become dissatisfied and men feel threatened or incompetent, especially if they regularly work long hours and find themselves too tired for sex. Simple solutions can often help such problems (see pages 255-256). Most couples survive the difficult patches, and many find they end up even closer than before with more time for each other.

Growth and change can be stimulating rather than threatening, and may bring new interests to share. And even if the frequency of lovemaking declines, couples often report that it becomes more enjoyable and carefree. Many people grow increasingly concerned with personal and spiritual issues, and can be more loving and tender as a result.

RELATIONSHIPS UNDER REVIEW

After 20 years of marriage I am starting to feel dissatisfied and have even found myself thinking of having an affair. Is this a phase or is there something seriously wrong with my marriage?

It depends on the roots of your dissatisfaction. Surveys suggest that up to two-thirds of men and women have an affair at some time during married life. Men are more likely to do so believing that they can 'have their cake and eat it', while women tend to cite real dissatisfaction with their marriage, which may represent more of a threat.

Affairs are more likely in unhappy marriages and those with sexual problems, but when a much younger partner is involved midlife turmoil is a more likely cause. One in five middle-aged men and one in ten middle-aged women admit to contemplating such affairs, but far fewer have them.

If your marriage is really at risk, there will probably also be other signs of trouble, such as boredom, growing apart or sexual difficulties. In middle age all of these can become worse or be felt as less tolerable than before.

When children leave home, hidden problems can be exposed or exacerbated. Women in traditional marriages may start to feel dissatisfied and want more from a relationship, which can place a strain on their partner.

Whether your feelings arise from a personal midlife crisis – which will pass – or from fundamental problems in your marriage it is essential to discuss the matter with your spouse and if necessary, a counsellor – see page 183. Trying to resolve any problems between you, even if it eventually means deciding to go your separate ways, is more productive and far less likely to cause pain or regret than having an affair.

GETTING MARRIED LATE

I'm nearly 40 and thinking of getting married, but I'm worried that I will find it difficult living with someone after many years alone. Is there any way to make the transition easier?

It can be difficult to adapt to togetherness once you are mature, independent and to some extent set in your ways. Even so, the fact that you are aware of possible problems and thinking about the issue gives you a head start in dealing with any difficulties.

The best thing you and your partner can do is to talk about how you imagine life after marriage in as much detail as you can. Try to cover both practical issues and feelings, joint hopes and individual ambitions. Look for possible areas of conflict and consider how to compromise, or at least agree on a strategy for settling arguments. Think about major issues, such as whether you want children and whose career will take priority if there is a choice to be made. Consider your differences, especially on apparently trivial details, such as how tidy you are and how chores will be shared. These tips may also help.

● Find a new place to live which is joint territory, rather than one person moving in with the other.
● Decide what you need in your home together and get rid of anything extra – if you have two toasters, sell one.
● Do things separately but in each other's company whenever possible – do the household bills at the kitchen table while your partner prepares a meal, for example, or read a book while he or she works.
● Have some private space – preferably a room of your own – and an amicable agreement to allow each other time alone.
● Maintain individual interests and friends as well as those you have in common.

KEEPING LOVE ALIVE

We've been blissfully happy together for the past ten years. How can we make sure our marriage stays as good in the future?

Maintaining such a successful relationship depends on good communication, balancing intimacy and independence, and being able to adapt to changes, both in circumstances and within each other. After ten years you have obviously found a successful formula for living together and there is no reason why it should not continue to work for many more years.

However happy you are, it can be wise to check that you are both still blissfully contented. Sometimes one partner (often the man) is unaware of how the other feels, or even of his own personal dissatisfactions brewing under the surface. Never ignore a feeling, however vague, that something is wrong. Talk regularly about your problems, progress, plans and hopes for the future, and try to spot any likely crisis points and discuss in advance how you will cope – especially with major changes such as children leaving home, a wife returning to work or a retirement to be faced. Always remember that a successful relationship thrives on continued thought and effort, and should not be taken for granted because it is so comfortable. And finally, go on enjoying it – determine to grow older vigorously, keep up your interests and enthusiasms and continue to live life to the full, both together and individually.

Family life in middle age

DEALING WITH TEENAGERS

My children are entering their teenage years. How can I prevent the kind of traumas that so many families seem to experience at this stage?

Don't expect serious problems – this can be one of the most enjoyable stages of family life. These tips may help.

● Cultivate mutual respect at home – ban personal remarks about habits, beliefs, appearance, dress sense or choice of friends on either side.
● Make clear, basic rules about safety, respect for other family members and household duties, but otherwise allow teenagers to run their own lives.
● Be sensitive to moodiness and emotional crises, and don't be afraid to admit (and apologise) if you are going through a tense or difficult period yourself.
● Acknowledge, if only to yourself, any jealousy you feel of your children's youth, opportunities or sexuality. Ask yourself if

this could underlie any conflicts and try to deal with your own feelings separately.

● If you hear yourself uttering 'middle-aged' comments about sleeping habits, work, security or settling down, change the subject immediately. Abort any sentence starting 'When I was your age . . .'.

● Try to be open about sex – children need to be able to discuss difficult subjects with you.

RESPONSIBILITIES ALL ROUND

What with three children, a demanding job and elderly parents who depend on me, I feel swamped by responsibilities. How can I cope better?

Your problem is common to many people in the middle stage of life, when responsibilities suddenly tend to accumulate. Somehow, you must find a way of meeting all your commitments while also making time for yourself – and not feeling guilty about it. Remember, if you become so over-stressed that your health suffers, all your dependants will suffer too. If they need you, they need you to be both physically and mentally well.

Start by taking a hard look at your schedule and assessing what, if anything, could be cut out altogether and what might be delegated to others.

Consider what alternative help might be available. Perhaps your parents might qualify for some kind of day care or help from social services, such as meals-on-wheels. Is there a neighbour or a relative who could take over some chores? Can your partner help – by visiting at weekends for example? What about your children? Could they spend more time with their grandparents or go shopping or cook for them occasionally, leaving you time to yourself?

You may also be spending too much time running after your children or fretting about teenage traumas. Perhaps it is time to renegotiate family rules and responsibilities so that others do more to help at home.

If possible, get older children to look after younger ones. Explain to all family members that while you will continue to help and support them where needed, you are going to reclaim a little of your own life too, and ask them to help and support you.

Time off for parents
One way of easing parental pressures is to get older and younger generations more involved with each other. With years of experience behind them and more free time, grandparents can offer a special kind of involvement.

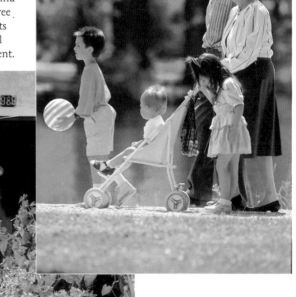

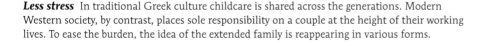

Less stress In traditional Greek culture childcare is shared across the generations. Modern Western society, by contrast, places sole responsibility on a couple at the height of their working lives. To ease the burden, the idea of the extended family is reappearing in various forms.

DO'S
—— AND ——
DON'TS

for dual-career couples with children

Do share chores and childcare – you are likely to stay closer as a couple and as a family.

Do communicate – explain what you want from your partner, and what is expected from your children.

Do spend some time, however little, with each child, and some time together, every day.

Do try to stagger working hours to fit in with childcare arrangements. Consider asking your employer about flexitime or working partly at home.

Do try to wind down on the way home.

Do take a family holiday at least once a year, and short breaks as often as you can.

Don't try to do everything, don't expect perfection and don't feel guilty – either let the dust accumulate or hire domestic help.

Don't bring work problems home or talk obsessively about work when you are at home.

HOW FAMILY LIFE IS CHANGING

The traditional family consisting of a stay-at-home mother, breadwinner father and their two children is rapidly disappearing. Today's 'middle-aged' families – those where the parents are in their 40s and 50s – are among the first to show the full range of effects.

It is now more common for a woman to have her first child in her early 30s than her early 20s. About one in three children is born outside marriage, in most cases to parents who live together. The fastest rate of change, however, is occurring among single professional women in their 30s and 40s who choose to go it alone as parents.

Divorce is also more common than ever and puts an end to one in three British marriages – the highest rate in Europe. Half of all divorced people get married again within five years, in most cases to another divorced person. Second marriages typically occur in middle age, and the age difference between partners may vary greatly. Women are also more likely than ever before to marry men who are younger than they are. Increasingly, remarriage is creating second families a generation younger than existing children. As a result of all the changes, couples may find themselves at midlife with young children, teenagers, adult offspring, or all three. There may be one or two parents, one or two households, and wide age variations between spouses, between children and between parents and children. One or both partners may be divorced or have children from a previous relationship, and they may or may not still remain in regular contact with their ex-spouse and in-laws.

Second families create a complex web of relationships and roles that can be confusing for younger members. Parents need to bear it in mind that children will require time to adjust to step-parents, stepbrothers and stepsisters, stepgrandparents and other new relatives. In time, the arrival of a half-brother or half-sister may need sensitive explanation.

Many of today's middle-aged people have lived through a succession of several different household styles, often starting with a first marriage and children, through separation and divorce, to single-parenthood, to a new step or blended family. They are the ones bearing the brunt of the changes – and the way they meet the challenge may well determine the future of family life itself.

WHEN CHILDREN LEAVE HOME

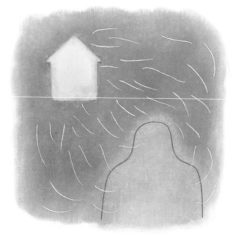

My youngest child is moving out of the house soon, and I feel very happy about it. Is this unusual? Shouldn't I be experiencing the 'empty nest' syndrome?

Not at all. In study after study researchers have found that most of today's parents find the transition to an 'empty nest' a happy time. Indeed, after having teenagers around it can be a great relief. In fact, a far more stressful situation appears to be having an adult child who will not or cannot leave home. Parents who have maintained careers and other outside interests throughout their child-rearing years are likely to have positive feelings about launching their children into the world. Most parents, in any case, experience a deep sense of accomplishment and relief when their parental responsibilities have been fulfilled.

Even so, some parents, especially women who have devoted years of their lives exclusively to raising children, do find the initial months rather strange, and it is sensible to anticipate this and to plan extra activities. Even those couples who report a certain sadness as their children grow up and gain their independence usually find the feelings are offset by their own prospects of increased personal freedom and more time and energy to devote to postponed ambitions.

Once children leave home, even couples who dreaded the change often find renewed intimacy and satisfaction with each other. They usually also form deep, loving friendships with their newly independent offspring of a kind that was not possible before.

BECOMING A GRANDPARENT

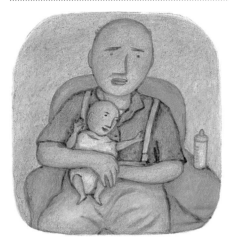

I have recently become a grandparent for the first time. But far from feeling ecstatic, I find I have rather mixed feelings. Is there something wrong?

Don't worry. It is quite common to equate becoming a grandparent with growing older. Even if such feelings are entirely unconscious, the arrival of the first grandchild can understandably provoke mixed emotions.

Like other major transitions, becoming a grandparent can lead to personal stocktaking, which may highlight fears and disappointments in your own life. Inevitably, you will make comparisons between the way you brought up your child and the way your son or daughter treats the new baby. This can lead to friction or rivalry if you allow yourself to feel guilty or critical. It will help to recognise that almost all new parents, whatever their background, want to give their child a better start in life than they feel they had. Don't take this personally – remember, you probably had similar feelings yourself.

Try to look on grandparenthood as an experience that will renew and invigorate your life, not as a symbol of ageing. With current life expectancies, there is every chance you will live to see your grandchildren's children, too. Visit and help as much as you want to and as much as is welcome – remember how stressful a new baby can be. Don't be intrusive but, equally, if you feel taken for granted, be firm about what you are prepared to do – you have already done your share of parenting, after all.

If you detect potential conflicts, try to defuse them. Be honest about your feelings, cautious about offering advice, and avoid comparisons. Make the most of this new stage – grandparents really do have the best

of both worlds, being able to enjoy the baby without the responsibilities of parenthood. Many people find grandparenting even more rewarding than having their own children.

LOSING A PARENT

My wife has become withdrawn since her mother died two months ago. What is the best way to help her?

The death of a mother or father is both a major bereavement and a significant transition in life – one that frequently marks a milestone in middle age. It is quite natural and healthy for the experience to prompt intense reflection on mortality, childhood, relationships with parents and with the bereaved person's own children. Part of your wife's own history has gone, and there may be sorrow about unasked questions and a feeling that it is now too late to make sense of some events of childhood.

Faced with such a loss, people may for the first time contemplate their parent as an individual rather than a mother or father. The future inevitably looks different, too. It can come as a deep shock suddenly to realise that there is no powerful mother or father-figure to come to the rescue and that you are finally on your own in the world.

Give your wife time and space to mourn, cry and contemplate, but be there to comfort and support her in carrying on with normal life at other times. If you have children, this may be their first experience of the death of someone close and you may be able to help by explaining sensitively what has happened (see page 296).

Let your wife talk as much as she wants to about her mother, the past and her feelings now. If she does not broach the subject directly, raise it yourself but don't push her to talk if she would rather not. Avoid general inquiries such as 'What's wrong?' or 'Are you feeling all right?' – to which the answer is obvious. Don't be afraid to offer intimacy or sexual advances. If necessary, reassure her that there is nothing wrong with finding comfort in this way, but don't feel rejected if she is not ready yet.

Finally, accept that your wife will need to talk about her parent, and her feelings, for some time to come, and that she will need you to listen and to give support. Death should never become a taboo subject – it is too much for one person to cope with alone. Nor should anyone who has been bereaved be expected to 'get over it' after a certain amount of time.

(see page 296).

DO'S AND DON'TS

for good grandparenting

Do offer constructive, practical help – learn how to change disposable nappies, for example, or offer to do the shopping or to babysit occasionally.

Do recognise that your son or daughter is the parent now – your role is quite different.

Do stick to the practices and rules your children have set.

Do ask the parents if you are unsure about anything – don't assume you know best.

Don't arrive unannounced or overstay your welcome.

Don't feel you have to babysit or help out every time you are asked.

Don't criticise or continually bring up issues that cause disagreement.

Don't compare your son or daughter's parenting style with your own.

Don't ask leading questions such as, 'Shouldn't he be talking by now?'

Don't allow more television, sweets or other treats than the parents do.

Don't undermine parental authority.

Changes and challenges at work

THE two fundamental ingredients of a happy life, according to the psychiatrist Sigmund Freud, are work and love. Those who work at something they enjoy are most likely to find fulfilment. Few people, however, end up following exactly the career path they planned or getting exactly the job they wanted, and chance opportunities frequently disrupt or enhance even the best-laid career plans.

In midlife many people take a step back, weigh up their achievements, aims and ambitions and, possibly for the first time, give serious thought to what they are doing and why. Midlife reassessments can be painful and occasionally disruptive but, used positively, they can bring huge gains. Use this time to develop a realistic strategy to take you where you want to go, whether that is president of a large corporation or retirement at 50. The unique combination of experience and energy at this stage of life makes it more possible than at any other to fulfil your ambitions.

NEW ROLES AT WORK

No matter how successful your career, there comes a point in midlife when you become aware of being an old hand rather than a rising star. While some people welcome the role of elder, others suffer nostalgia, self-doubt and regret for lost opportunities, leading to jealousy, a need to prove themselves, or competitiveness towards junior staff. In small doses, this can provide a healthy boost to performance, but taken to extremes it can be both exhausting and counter-productive. Don't let this happen to you.

- Remember that older workers have professional advantages such as experience and maturity.
- Don't strive too hard to join younger social circles – you are needed as a mentor, not a drinking or gossip companion.
- Take advantage of youthful enthusiasms – delegating will help you and give others a chance to prove themselves.
- Think of age as adding to your role, not diminishing it – you are now the generation with expertise and experience to pass on.
- Accept and enjoy any teaching or coaching responsibilities you are offered.

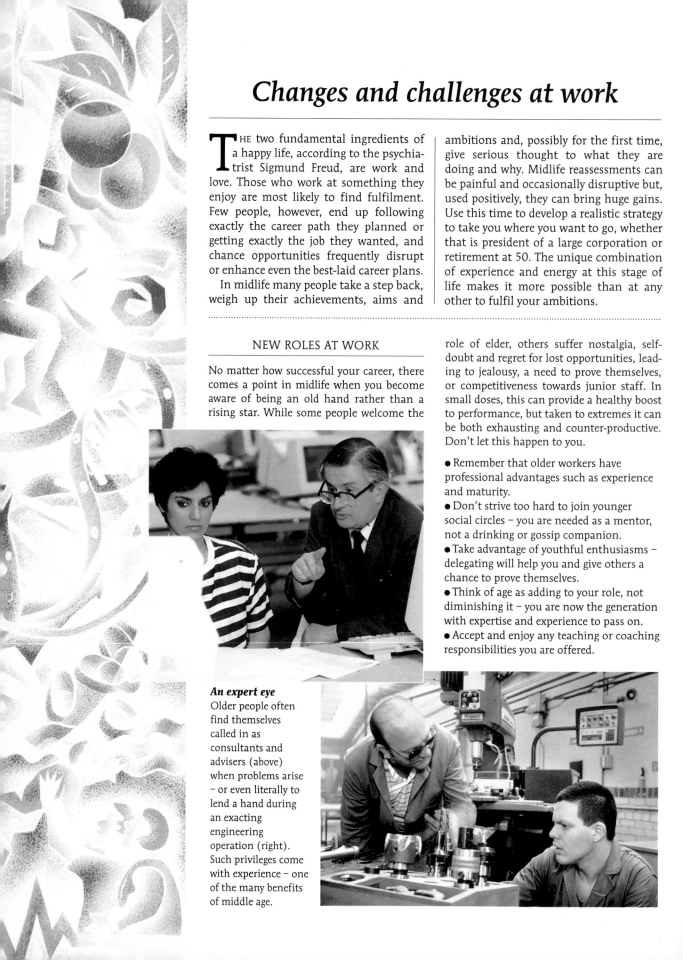

An expert eye
Older people often find themselves called in as consultants and advisers (above) when problems arise – or even literally to lend a hand during an exacting engineering operation (right). Such privileges come with experience – one of the many benefits of middle age.

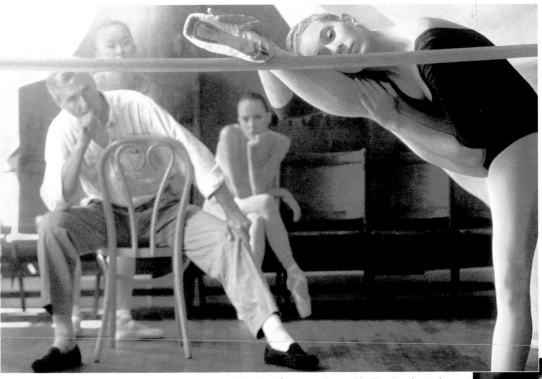

CHANGING TRACK

In some careers, people move steadily up a ladder or slide naturally into new roles as they get older – sportsmen start coaching, for example, and businessmen become company directors. Not everyone makes such a smooth transition, however. If you are thinking about a midlife move, devise a practical, realistic strategy and remember:

● It is easier to find a new job if you are already in work.
● Don't act hastily, and always test the water before committing yourself.
● Don't give up a secure job for a chancy scheme. Be particularly wary of commission-only sales jobs.
● Decide on basic issues. What is your ultimate goal? Do you want to work for someone else or be your own boss? Do you want to work from home? How much money do you require? Do you need income or can you support yourself for a while?
● Find out as much as you can about your planned new career, and ensure you have the necessary experience. Talk to others in the business, or consult a career adviser.
● Investigate the employment market in your chosen field before striking out.
● If you want to start your own business, you need a business plan and financial backing. You also need to know about tax,

Master class In classical ballet the physical demands of performance are punishing, even in youth. Later on, some dancers turn to teaching or choreography instead.

VAT, national insurance, accountancy, health and safety, and employment laws. Further advice and information is available from the Department of Trade and Industry, telephone 0800 500 200.

COPING WITH CAREER PRESSURE

Work pressures tend to peak in midlife and take their toll not only on health but also on family relationships and social life. Many ambitious people eventually rise to slightly above the level where they are most competent, and even high-achievers may feel a threat from younger colleagues and worry about declining status. Those who feel they are not progressing or wonder if they are in the wrong job may become frustrated. These are ways of coping you can develop:

● Don't become anxious about things that have not happened – such as missing out on promotion or facing possible redundancies – but do make contingency plans.
● Make time for your family and do at least one thing each week that you really enjoy.
● Don't resort to self-destructive behaviour, such as heavy drinking or a series of affairs.

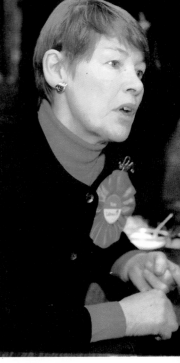

Not acting now In middle age, Glenda Jackson swapped an illustrious career in acting for a life in politics. Her new vocation reflects a general midlife tendency towards wider social and ethical concerns.

- Never take irrevocable steps (resignation, a showdown with the boss) in anger.
- Check your workaholic potential (see panel opposite). Take action if necessary.
- Learn to relax. De-stress yourself at regular intervals with desk exercises or deep breathing (see pages 190-193), or take a walk.
- Learn to recognise stress-provoking situations and take a few minutes to practise relaxation techniques.
- Delegate wherever you can, don't be a slave to the telephone, and learn to make use of your most valuable piece of filing equipment – the wastepaper basket.
- Assess what you really want – to go further up your current ladder, to side step into something more rewarding, to go it alone or to start a gentle climb down that gives you more time for other activities.

KEEPING MENTAL POWERS SHARP

While ageing need not herald a decline in mental abilities, many working people worry that in midlife they will seem out of touch or unable to compete with younger colleagues. Developing a positive attitude towards your abilities at this stage will pay dividends in keeping you mentally alert and active for years to come.

- Refuse to be intimidated by youthful overconfidence or virile displays in more junior colleagues.
- Capitalise on your talents. Studies show

that older professionals are better than younger ones at conserving time and energy and distinguishing between vital and trivial tasks. They are also more likely to be cool in a crisis, accurate, conscientious, tolerant, aware of their own strengths and weaknesses, realistically self-confident and able to learn from mistakes.

- Keep an open mind and actively look for new ways of doing things – older people are often hampered more by caution, rigid habits and fixed patterns of thought than by any physical changes of ageing.
- Don't be frightened by new challenges. Look on them as opportunities to enhance your talents and experience. Ask for help if you need it, and be prepared to learn.
- Don't use your age as an excuse or expect either respect or special concessions solely because of it.
- Don't avoid new technology, or allow it to intimidate you, or make a virtue of your ignorance. Get yourself properly trained and remember that the machines are there to serve you.

UNREALISED AMBITIONS

The stereotype of middle age is one of placid contentment and stability – the time when people are settled in to a marriage, a career, a daily routine. But in reality things can be rather different. Unrealised ambitions and unfulfilled dreams can lead to deep dissatisfaction and the feeling that time is running out. If you are feeling restless but unsure what to do about it, give some consideration to the following questions:

- How far will your current job take you? How long will you have to wait for a promotion? Can your employer ultimately offer the kind of position you want, or would you still be dissatisfied even if you got to the top? If not, would you be any better off somewhere else?
- What are you willing to do to get to where you want? Would you work longer hours, accept more responsibility or travel more?
- Have you got the talent, qualifications and skills to achieve your ambitions? If not, could you acquire them?
- What are your true motives? Are you really striving after a distant goal, or would you be satisfied with some simple changes – different hours, more stimulating tasks, a bigger office or more pay, for example.
- Does anyone know how you feel? You may not get promoted if you are doing a good job and appear perfectly content.

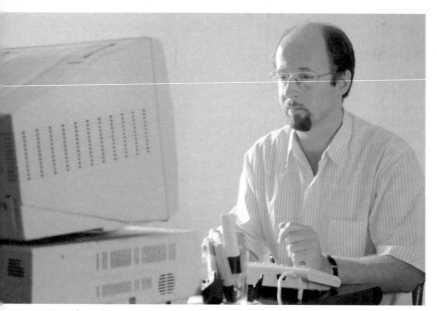

Man and machine Getting to grips with new technology is essential in many modern jobs. Although older people sometimes worry about acquiring new skills, the evidence is that learning becomes, if anything, more efficient and goal-directed.

WOMEN GOING BACK

Midlife brings special rewards for many women. In particular, those who have spent earlier years at home looking after small children can find this a new, liberating time.

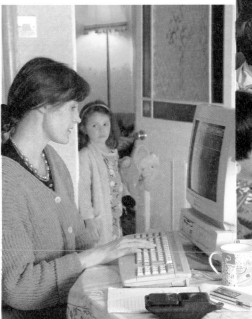

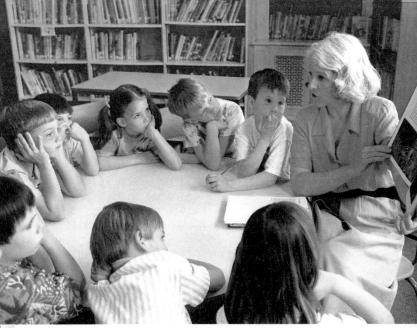

Resuming a career Whether they go out to work or operate from home, mothers make good workers. As well as professional skills, they can capitalise on talents such as planning, stamina, crisis management, teaching and concentration in the face of distraction. If you would like to go back to work but think your skills may be a little rusty, or are not sure where to start, ask your local authority about courses for women returners.

If you want to go back to work after a break, a little preparation before you rejoin the job market can provide a significant advantage.

● If you are not ready for full-time work just yet, go back gradually. Start with an afternoon a week, or mornings only, or consider freelance work at home.
● Maintain or rebuild your contacts. A friendly phone call or a lunch date now and again will keep you in people's minds. Let everyone know you are available for work.
● Keep in touch with new developments in your field. Join the right societies and subscribe to professional journals applicable to your trade.
● Consider retraining to update or add to your skills. Some local authorities run courses specifically designed to help women re-entering the job market.
● Involve your family and get them to help – with chores around the house and with your job-hunting.
● Plan childcare well in advance, draw up reliable back-up arrangements and decide how you will cope with illness, sports days, parent-teacher meetings and other family commitments.
● Put together a good curriculum vitae and practise your interview strategy.

ARE YOU A WORKAHOLIC?

Workaholism has been called the respectable addiction. Its victims are hard-working, motivated, ambitious, dedicated and conscientious – typical successful people. But some are also driven, defensive and unhappy, and the price of success for many is high – a heart attack, a personal crisis, even sudden death in the 40s or 50s. Find out if you – or your partner – could be at risk by answering this questionnaire.

● Do you regularly take work home?
● Do your family complain about seeing too little of you?
● Do you often feel anxious about being late, or become angry when others don't arrive on time?
● Have you ever stayed up all night to get work done?
● Do you often miss important family occasions such as a wedding anniversary, child's birthday or school speech day because of work?
● Do you regularly fail to take all your holiday entitlement?
● Are you constantly rushed or trying to fit more into the time available?
● Do you spend a lot of time getting things exactly right, instead of accepting what is good enough?
● Do you find it difficult to delegate work, or spend a lot of time re-doing or polishing what others have finished?
● Do you often think about work problems away from the office?

If you answered yes to three or more questions, consider seriously whether home and personal life is really getting the proper attention, and think hard about priorities other than work; six or more and you may need help – contact Workaholics Anonymous, c/o 9 Maunsel Street, London 1P 2QL.

Looking to the future

ACTION PLAN FOR HEALTH

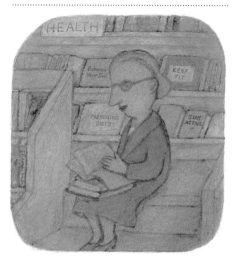

There's so much health advice everywhere these days that I'm left feeling quite confused. What are the most important things to do in middle age so that you stay well in the future?

While good genes and good luck help to determine how kind the ageing process will be to you, there are certain essential rules to follow if you want to maintain your vitality, looks and wellbeing into late middle age and well beyond.

● Stay mentally active. If you stay well-informed, take a lively interest in the world around you, and keep yourself intellectually challenged, your mental agility and capacity for learning will continue to grow.
● Stay physically active. People who are unfit in middle age are three times as likely to die prematurely as those who are even just moderately fit. Exercise also makes you feel more energetic, keeps you supple and looking younger, counteracts osteoporosis and reduces depression.
● Stay involved. Cultivate and maintain friendships, community roles and activities.
● Don't smoke. As well as being disastrous to health, smoking ages the skin dramatically. See pages 156-157 for ways to stop.
● Avoid sunbeds and sunbathing. All ultraviolet rays, natural and artificial, increase wrinkles and skin cancer risks. If you do go out in the sun, be sure to protect yourself (see pages 139-140).

● Eat a balanced diet and try to maintain a healthy weight. A diet rich in fresh fruit, vegetables and wholegrain cereals will keep you well supplied with vitamins, minerals and energy, prevent constipation and other minor ailments, and even help to protect against cancers and some other more serious diseases.
● Keep alcohol intake within safe limits. While a moderate amount may offer slight protection against heart disease, too much puts you at risk of liver disease, high blood pressure and mental failings.
● Avoid medication wherever possible, especially sleeping pills and tranquillisers. All drugs have side effects and these types in particular can cause dependency.
● Don't get upset about growing older. Studies show those who worry more when young are more likely to be ill in old age.

PLANNING FOR RETIREMENT

I will be facing retirement in a few years' time and, to be honest, I have hardly given it a thought. What should I be doing to prepare for it?

Retirement is an important transition in life and one that requires psychological as well as practical adjustment. These are the most important points to consider:

● Make sure your pension provisions are adequate and, if necessary, consider ways of increasing them – you may be able to make additional contributions, for example. Remember also to allow for inflation. People who are more than four months from retirement age can obtain a forecast of their likely state pension by filling in form BR 19 from a Social Security office and posting it to: Retirement Pension Forecast, Benefits Agency, DSS Longbenton, Benton Park Road, Newcastle upon Tyne NE98 1YX.
● Review the provisions you have made for any family members or dependants. If you have not already done so, make a will (see panel opposite) and consider life insurance – the older you get, the more expensive a new policy becomes.
● Assess your likely income in retirement, including occupational, private and state pensions, any state benefits to which you

Early retirement

More and more people are retiring early, either by choice or as a result of restructuring at the place they work. In 1971, two-thirds of people aged 60 to 64 were still working. By 1989, a little over one-third were. Since people are also living longer, the average length of time spent in retirement is increasing in two directions, highlighting the need for good financial planning. Increasingly, people are considering a second career after their first is over. Men who retire at, say, 55, have on average 20 years ahead of them, and women 25 years.

may be entitled, maturing insurance policies, paid work you expect to do, or money from investments. Financial experts say most people live reasonably comfortably on their retirement income, but if you aim to travel extensively, you may need to make extra provision.

● Think about your current level of expenditure and how it will change in retirement. For example, you may save on transport costs with discounted fares and no need to travel to work, but your heating and lighting bills may increase if you are at home all day. Will you be able to afford to keep up the same lifestyle? If not, what are your fixed and unavoidable expenditures, and what luxuries could you give up? Could you cut costs by insulating your loft or driving a more fuel-efficient car?

● Start thinking about what you want to do with your time.

● Try to organise as long an overlap period as possible between work and retirement so that you can adjust to the changes gradually. As retirement approaches, try to reduce your workload and instead start up new activities or spend more time on current leisure interests. If you plan to work from home after retiring, think about organising a work area or office in your house, acquiring any equipment you will need, and letting people know you will be available for employment.

● Consider a pre-retirement course. Some companies run them for staff. Alternatively, contact the Pre-retirement Association, The Nodus Centre, University Campus, Guildford GU2 5RX.

● Prepare yourself emotionally. Think about what you will say when asked what you do, or how you will feel when you are offered a pensioner's discount.

HOW TO GO ABOUT MAKING YOUR WILL

It is never too early to make a will, especially if you have dependants. If you die intestate – without a will – your estate will be distributed among relatives according to a complex legal formula, and may not benefit those you wish. A will also enables you to appoint up to four executors to administer your estate (it is considered wise to have at least two) – usually trusted relatives or friends, sometimes bank officials or solicitors (who will deduct a charge from the estate), or a combination.

If you have children under 18, you should nominate a guardian and make provision for money to be held in trust for them. You can specify any wishes about your funeral and other arrangements, but these are not legally binding. A will can also help with inheritance tax planning – if your estate is worth more than a certain amount, tax is charged at a higher rate unless you take steps to avoid it. Seek advice from a financial planner or from your bank.

To make your will, you first need to draw up a list of everything you own, including money deposited in bank and building society accounts, investments, property, personal possessions and so on, not forgetting any insurance or pension policies that pay out when you die. Then decide who is to benefit from your estate – who is to get specific legacies such as your house, a painting or a car; who is to receive cash gifts; and who is to inherit the rest. You can write your own will on any piece of paper or on a standard form from a post office, or you can employ a bank or a specialist will-writing company. For all but the simplest circumstances, however, it is wise to use a solicitor, who will probably charge in the region of £50.

Whatever type of will you make, you will need two adult witnesses (staff in the solicitor's office, for example) who are not beneficiaries and whose spouses are also not beneficiaries. Executors must be over 18, but can be beneficiaries.

Once drawn up, your will may be kept with your bank or solicitor, or with the Probate Registry who will charge a nominal £1. You can obtain the address of your nearest Registry from the telephone directory or from your local Citizens Advice Bureau. Make sure your executors know where your will is kept and keep a copy at home in a clearly-marked file, together with details of insurance policies and bank accounts.

If you want to change your will, you can add a legal document called a codicil to it or you can revise the whole will, revoking all previous versions. Ask a solicitor to help you. Never mark the will itself – even a paperclip imprint could invalidate it.

You must make a new will if you marry, and it is wise to revise your will if you divorce or if a main beneficiary or executor dies.

Note
The law in Scotland differs slightly. Check with your solicitor.

LIVING WELL IN LATER LIFE

People are living longer, fitter, more independent lives than ever. Advances in medical knowledge offer the hope of a healthier future for all of us. Social attitudes are set to change too, as the numbers of older people - and their expectations - increase.

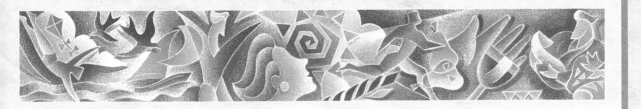

How much do you know about getting older?

There are many misconceptions about old age, even among old people themselves. The following chapter aims to dispel most of them, but before you read on, you might like to try this quiz, and find out how much you already know. Tick the correct answer to each question and check your score below.

1 Do women really live longer than men do?

a) No, the difference is negligible. ☐
b) Yes, by about six years on average. ☐
c) Yes, by about two years on average. ☐

2 What do drivers have to do when they reach the age of 70?

a) Renew their licence. ☐
b) Have an eye test. ☐
c) Take another driving test. ☐

3 How many people in Great Britain are pensioners?

a) One in ten. ☐
b) One in twenty. ☐
c) One in five. ☐

4 What is the full human lifespan estimated to be in the absence of disease or injury?

a) Seventy. ☐
b) Eighty. ☐
c) One hundred and twenty. ☐

5 How does alcohol affect you as you grow older?

a) More strongly – your metabolism slows down and alcohol remains in your system for longer. ☐
b) Less strongly – your body builds up a resistance to alcohol over the years. ☐
c) The same – age bears no relation to alcohol tolerance. ☐

6 Which change do most people need to make to their diet as they get older?

a) Eat fewer calories. ☐
b) Eat more high-energy foods. ☐
c) Eat more protein. ☐

7 At what age does the law say you have to retire?

a) Sixty for women and sixty-five for men. ☐
b) Sixty-five for everyone. ☐
c) There is no legal requirement to retire at any age. ☐

8 At what age do you become too old to undergo heart surgery?

a) Seventy. ☐
b) Age is not a factor. ☐
c) Eighty. ☐

9 How old must you be before your doctor has to offer you an annual check-up?

a) Sixty-five. ☐
b) Seventy-five. ☐
c) Doctors are never obliged to offer annual check-ups. ☐

10 How many people over the age of 65 suffer from glaucoma?

a) One in twenty. ☐
b) One in fifty. ☐
c) One in a hundred. ☐

SCORING

Award yourself 1 point for each of these answers: 1(b), 2(a), 3(c), 4(c), 5(a), 6(a), 7(c), 8(b), 9(b) and 10(a). Add up your score.

8-10: Excellent, if you are not already a senior citizen, you seem to be well prepared to enjoy active and interesting later years.

5-7: You have a reasonable knowledge about the later years, but there is still much you can learn.

4 or less: The pages that follow may help to give you a more accurate view of growing older.

Growing older – staying young

DIFFERENT RATES OF AGEING

I have noticed that some of my friends in their mid to late seventies are still leading healthy, active lives, while others are rapidly succumbing to old age. What causes the difference?

No one is quite sure why people appear to age at different rates, though it is known that genetic factors play a part in determining how long a person will live. Those whose parents have both had long lives are likely to live to a ripe old age themselves. Conversely, susceptibility to a number of diseases – such as heart trouble and some cancers – is also hereditary, though by no means everyone with such a family history will be affected.

People who look after themselves, eating well and staying active in body and mind, greatly increase their chances of a healthy old age, and will not age as fast as those who have a sedentary lifestyle and smoke and drink too much.

Attitude is also a critical factor in determining the state of your health. Recent studies have shown a link between people's own assessment of their health and their mortality. While you cannot will yourself to good health, a positive attitude may mean that you will take better care of yourself.

MENTAL CHANGES

Why have some elderly people I know become less mentally sharp with age, while others seem to remain just as alert and intelligent as ever?

The mind is like the body in that the more it is used, the longer it will continue to be effective. Intellectual power need not decline with age. When older people attend college or university they often outperform their younger fellow-students. One man in his 80s recently completed a postgraduate research degree, commenting that he did it 'to give my wife and me something to talk about'. In the workplace, too, older people are often valued for being more careful, reliable and industrious than younger workers.

True enough, ageing does affect the short-term memory. Older people often seem to forget people's names, or where they put their keys only a moment ago. However, this 'benign forgetfulness' is not usually a symptom of any mental illness. And the long-term memory – retrieving important events from the more distant past – remains acute.

Other noticeable changes include a slowing down of reactions, and increased difficulty in working out problems, learning new skills and grasping abstract ideas.

Mental functioning can also be adversely affected by ill health and anxiety. So it is all the more important to lead an active life – both physically and mentally – in retirement, to enable you to use the wisdom and experience that come only with age.

TOO LATE FOR LOVE?

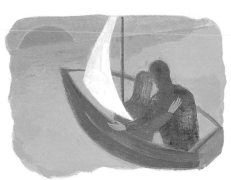

I am 75 years old and am considering marriage to someone of about the same age. However, I am worried about what people might say. Are we too old to get married?

Of course you are not too old to get married. If you love each other and want to spend your lives together, there is no reason at all why you should remain apart. You certainly should not let your chance of happiness be spoilt by anything that others might say. In any case, what most people would probably say is 'Good luck to you', and they will tend to be envious rather than disapproving.

When it comes to sex, don't fall into the trap of believing that this is a pleasure reserved for the young. Many couples enjoy an active sex life well into their 80s. Certainly some conditions such as arthritis and prostate trouble can make things difficult, but with a little imagination – and, if necessary, advice from a doctor – most such obstacles to a happy sex life can be dealt with.

As with any marriage, certain things do need open and honest discussion before you

Pensioner power

The number of elderly people in Britain is on the increase. Of a total population of some 58 million, about 10.5 million have reached pensionable age.

This trend will probably continue. The proportion of pensioners within the general population – about 18 per cent at present – is expected to continue rising, until it levels out at about 24 per cent in the year 2025.

People are not just living longer these days: they are healthier and more active in old age. Fewer than 6 per cent of people over 65 live in 'homes'. Elderly people are also politically and economically more powerful: the over-65s have about a quarter of the country's wealth.

An ageing population raises serious social questions, in particular how the government will continue to pay for medical care for elderly people. At the moment, for every pensioner benefiting from national insurance, there are just under two-and-a-half people contributing to it. By the year 2025, however, there will probably be only about one-and-a-half contributors for every pensioner.

As their numbers increase, older people are organising themselves into pressure groups, to focus attention on their rights and concerns, such as pension levels and the retirement age.

make a final decision – not least, the question of where you will live if you both own a home already. You will also need to discuss your incomes, and perhaps see a solicitor to work out a joint financial arrangement.

STAYING IN SHAPE

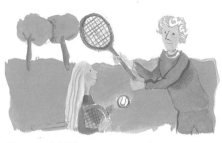

My grandchildren are amazed that their 70-plus grandmother jogs and plays tennis. Is there any reason not to exercise as long as I possibly can?

With any luck, your grandchildren will learn a thing or two from you. Maintaining a sensible exercise programme is one of the best things you can do for your health. Research shows that many conditions associated with advanced age – weakened muscles, brittle bones, creaky joints – are really due more to inactivity than to simple ageing.

Some older people are reluctant to exercise for fear of falling and hurting themselves, or even of provoking a heart attack. These are real dangers, but the risk is even greater for those who avoid exercise. Regular exercise helps you to maintain your agility and balance, and will, in the long term, reduce your chances of suffering a heart attack. People who lead sedentary lives are less fit and agile, and therefore more vulnerable to injury and disease.

An important caution: be sure not to exercise too strenuously, or to start vigorous exercise after a lengthy period of inactivity. Always listen to your body, and take a rest when you feel tired or out of breath.

AGEING IN OTHER CULTURES

I have heard that in China the elderly are held in the highest respect. Is this true?

In Western countries, social status is often linked to the job a person has, so retirement often means a loss of social standing. Less so in many Eastern countries, where people tend to have much closer family links, and where status accordingly often goes hand in hand with old age. In the West, care of the

elderly is considered, at least in part, the responsibility of the state, while in Eastern countries, such as India and Japan, it is regarded as the responsibility of the family. In the People's Republic of China, four out of five old people live with their families, and the state actively encourages children to support their parents and treat them well. After a person has retired from work, he or she still has a role to play as a senior member of the family, and is accordingly held in high esteem.

ATTITUDES TO AGE

Apart from being a bit less steady on my feet and tiring a little more easily I've hardly changed with age in the way I feel or the things I do. So why do people have such negative views of the elderly?

Psychologists and sociologists have been puzzling over this question for some time. The physical and mental changes brought on by time are, in most cases, very slight. A 70-year-old brain has 97 per cent of the cells it had in youth, and 93 per cent of its weight. The heart, lungs and muscles can lose efficiency, but this is more the result of inactivity than of the simple passing of years. A fit 70-year-old may well be in better condition than a fat, sedentary 25-year-old. Some of the most responsible positions in our society are held by older people – many judges, politicians and company directors, for example, are over 65.

Yet despite all the evidence, people persist in attaching negative stereotypes to old age. So widespread and powerful are these stereotypes that old people themselves tend to have them too, at least towards other old people, though they usually make an exception in their own case.

The bad reputation of old age is probably due largely to illnesses that affect the mind, such as dementia, even though fewer than one in ten people ever develop them. Perfectly rational older people – the vast majority – may be treated as if they too cannot remember things, or think clearly. Forgetfulness that no one would comment on in a younger person is all too often put down to age in someone older.

As more people live longer, healthier and wealthier lives – the overwhelming trend in the West – such stereotypes may give way to a more realistic and positive general view of age. In the meantime, it is up to individuals, old and young, to challenge the prevailing prejudice whenever they encounter it.

THE QUEST FOR YOUTH

The basic mechanisms of ageing are not known, so it is not possible to control them. Nevertheless, many attempts have been made to extend human life. For centuries, alchemists struggled, unsuccessfully, to find an *elixir vitae* – elixir of life – to prolong life indefinitely. In China, the Taoists sought the 'pill of immortality'. A variety of plant and animal products – orchids, royal jelly, semen – have been tried, and 20th-century attempts at rejuvenation have included such treatments as monkey testicular grafts, serum therapy, and cellular therapy. While none of these has proved successful, other lines of enquiry are being avidly pursued.

One treatment that has had some degree of success, in rejuvenating women, is hormone replacement therapy (HRT) – often prescribed to relieve the distressing symptoms brought on by menopause (see page 394). The oestrogen used in this form of treatment has other beneficial effects: preventing the sudden acceleration of bone loss that might occur after menopause, offering some protection against heart attacks, and improving the condition of skin and hair. It is possible that, in time to come, men may benefit in similar ways by replacing the testosterone they lose as they get older.

Claims have been made that ginseng, an ancient Eastern remedy extracted from the root of a plant, prolongs life. However, while the extract does have properties that help to combat fatigue and relieve stress, there is no evidence for more dramatic effects.

A nutritional approach to slowing down the ageing process involves increasing the intake of antioxidants, such as beta carotene vitamin E and vitamin C. These are thought to mop up free radicals – molecules responsible for damaging chain reactions and ageing effects in human tissue. Once again, however, there has been no proven success.

Research into the thymus gland – the first gland which deteriorates in adult life – is being carried out in the United States at the George Washington University. A substance called thymosin, derived from the thymus glands of animals, and used experimentally in the treatment of lung cancer, is now being studied as a possible aid to prolonging life.

Scientists are also hoping to identify the genes which control ageing in humans. They have already accomplished this goal in simpler life forms such as worms and fruit flies, and have succeeded in virtually tripling the lifespans of these creatures. Researchers have also managed to extend the lifespan of individual human cells by up to 30 per cent, and hope to produce drugs which will have similar effects on the body as a whole, perhaps within the next 25 years.

Tales of youth The search for eternal youth has long inspired the imagination, giving rise to such tales as H. Rider Haggard's *She*.

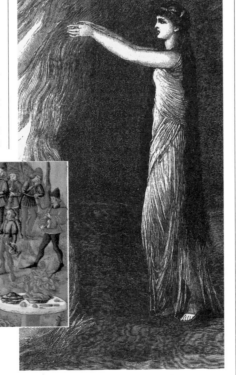

Water therapy For centuries people sought the legendary rejuvenating Fountain of Youth, thought to be in the Bahamas.

EXERCISING TO STAY STRONG AND SUPPLE

No matter how old you are, regular exercise is an important way of keeping fit and healthy. At any age, it strengthens your muscles, keeps your weight down, and helps to prevent heart disease. In your later years, it helps to relieve stiff joints, and to improve balance and blood circulation. The exercises shown below can be practised at home. For them to be really effective, you should do them regularly – every day if possible. Wear something loose and comfortable and make sure that the chair you use is stable and does not have arms. The exercises are very gentle, so there is no need for you to warm up beforehand.

SWIVELLING FOR FLEXIBILITY

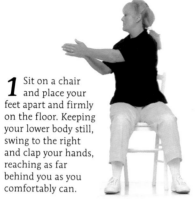

1 Sit on a chair and place your feet apart and firmly on the floor. Keeping your lower body still, swing to the right and clap your hands, reaching as far behind you as you comfortably can.

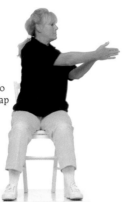

2 Swing round to the left and clap your hands. Make sure that you turn your head to watch your hands. Repeat the exercise four times each way.

STRETCHING FOR MOBILITY

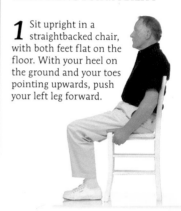

1 Sit upright in a straightbacked chair, with both feet flat on the floor. With your heel on the ground and your toes pointing upwards, push your left leg forward.

SWAYING FOR BALANCE

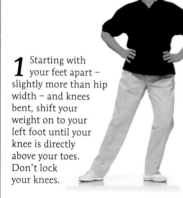

1 Starting with your feet apart – slightly more than hip width – and knees bent, shift your weight on to your left foot until your knee is directly above your toes. Don't lock your knees.

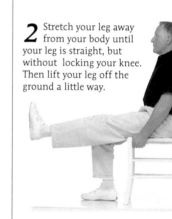

2 Transfer your weight on to your right leg, keeping your body at the same height throughout – don't bob up and down. If necessary, use a chair to help you to keep your balance. Repeat four times.

2 Stretch your leg away from your body until your leg is straight, but without locking your knee. Then lift your leg off the ground a little way.

CLENCHING FOR DEXTERITY

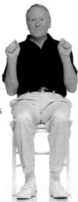

1 Hold up your hands with your fists clenched, so that your knuckles are pointing towards the ceiling.

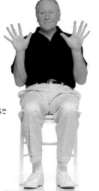

2 Unclench your hands, and spread your fingers wide apart as you do so. Repeat the exercise eight times.

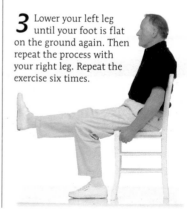

3 Lower your left leg until your foot is flat on the ground again. Then repeat the process with your right leg. Repeat the exercise six times.

Retirement and after

A HEALTHY ATTITUDE

I have worked hard all my life, and was looking forward to retirement as a time of freedom and leisure. But instead I find that I miss my job and am feeling bored and depressed. What can I do about this?

It is perfectly natural to feel at a loose end after retirement – particularly if your job was interesting and satisfying. You are very likely to miss the status and self-esteem that the job gave you, the contacts with other people and organisations, the feeling of being part of a team, and the companionship of your colleagues. No matter how much you may have been looking forward to your retirement, the change from having a recognised and structured occupation to being a totally free agent takes a good deal of adjustment.

Making a success of retirement is mainly a matter of developing a positive attitude, of taking decisions and of keeping active. Resolve to fill your days doing things you particularly enjoy, or things you have always wanted to do but have never had time for before. Many people find voluntary work rewarding, as well as being a good way to make new friends. Charitable organisations are always short of helpers, and you could check with conservation bodies and hospitals as well. Ask at your local Citizens Advice Bureau, public library, or council offices for any information on what voluntary work is available. Taking up a new hobby or sport is another good way of meeting people with similar interests.

If you are interested in learning some new skills, consider joining an adult education class. Courses range from car maintenance, art and cookery to archaeology, classical literature, and philosophy. Find out if there is a branch near you of the University of the Third Age (see page 415). The university has branches all over the United Kingdom. Its courses are designed for the mutual benefit of tutor and student, rather than to provide qualifications. If you want a more serious approach to your studies, many universities are keen to enrol mature students. Write to whichever university you would like to attend, and ask the Registrar about the pre-entry and enrolment requirements. If you would prefer to study at home, the Open University offers a wide range of correspondence courses.

How long should you continue working?

Reaching retirement age does not actually require you to retire. The law allows, but does not oblige, you to stop work at that age. If both you and your employer are happy that you remain in your job, there is no reason why you should not do so. Many people continue working long after the age of 65. The comedian George Burns is booked to perform at the London Palladium when he is 100.

Not that everyone would wish to carry on working beyond, or even up to, the standard retirement age. If you want to retire, you are entitled to, and you might try to arrange early retirement if you can afford it. Family and friends may have ideas for keeping you busy – helping them to start up a new business, for instance – but it is your retirement, so do whatever suits you.

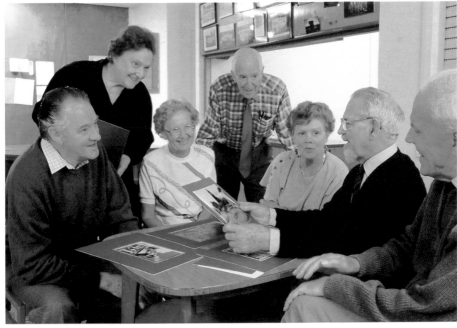

Third Age photography A photographic course at the University of the Third Age offers an opportunity for the students and the course leader to learn from each other. Having completed an assignment, the students and leader meet to discuss one another's work.

EARNING MONEY

I find that I can no longer easily afford some of the things I used to enjoy. Is it still possible to find paid work after retirement?

It is certainly possible to find paid work after you have retired, but it may not be easy. Former employers and clients quickly forget names and faces that are no longer part of their everyday duties. Furthermore, you may have to accept far less pay than before. In fact, if you are interviewed, and really want the job, consider suggesting that you are willing to work for a modest sum. And be ready to answer questions about your last job, your health, and what you have been doing since

Taking time Retirement can give you the chance to exploit the creative skills that you had too little time for during your working life. Here two pensioners perform the delicate task of mending a footstool. Your artistic abilities will never desert you. Picasso was painting when he was in his 80s, and Titian did some of his best work at 90.

New skills It's never too late to learn. One nursing home in London offers pottery classes – teaching patients to make not only pots but also intricate art objects, or even garden gnomes. The standard achieved by the elderly students is high enough for their work to be exhibited once a year, and for some of the goods to be sold.

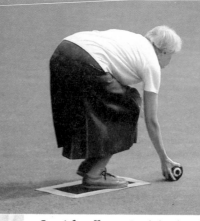

Sport for all ages Bowls has long been a popular sport among elderly people, and is now increasingly popular with younger people as well. Today there are some 750 000 registered players of all ages in Britain – competing with each other up to the highest level.

retiring. Ideally you should have been keeping active, by doing voluntary work, for instance, rather than holidaying at home.

Areas where you may be able to find paid work include:

- Consultancy work, possibly on projects for your former employers.
- Journalism, particularly if you have writing talent or a special field of expertise.
- Teaching, especially supply teaching or coaching. Contact local schools and agencies to find out about vacancies.
- Temporary jobs at supermarkets, chain stores or hotels.

Another option is to set up your own business, perhaps in catering, childminding or gardening. But do be careful. Although it can be exciting and rewarding, it involves considerable financial risk, and calls for an enormous commitment of time and energy.

On with the dance Tea dances are a fun way of meeting people and getting some exercise. Dancing to familiar old tunes is a short cut to recapturing your youth for a while.

RETURNING TO STUDIES

I have been thinking of going back to university to finally complete my degree. I am now over 70. Am I too old?

No, you are certainly not too old to study. As long as you are in good health, there is no reason why you should not return to university, enjoy the experience, and excel in your courses. Furthermore, the mental stimulation you gain from your classes will be complemented by the social benefits of contact with other people on campus.

Some older people do find that it takes longer to absorb new information, and is harder to study in the presence of noise or other distractions than it used to be. So you may need to set aside more time for study, and to find a quiet place.

Research shows that the effects of ageing on one's ability to think and learn are fairly minor. In any case, the greater motivation and experience that older students boast will usually more than compensate for this slight decline in sharpness.

The University of the Third Age

It was the French who originally coined the phrase 'Third Age' (or rather, its French equivalent) to refer to the period of active retirement that comes after the first two ages – youth, and working life – but before the final age of infirmity.

The first University of the Third Age was set up in Toulouse in 1972 to give retired people an opportunity to enrich their lives through study. In 1981 a similar university was set up in Britain, and today has branches all over the United Kingdom. The university does not offer degrees. The lecturers are often themselves pensioners. Subjects range from Classical Greek and Anthropology to Embroidery and Belly Dancing. No previous qualifications are necessary. A small fee is charged for enrolment into each course. If you wish to find out more about the University, ask at your local library for information, or contact the National U3A Office at 1 Stockwell Green, London SW9 9JF.

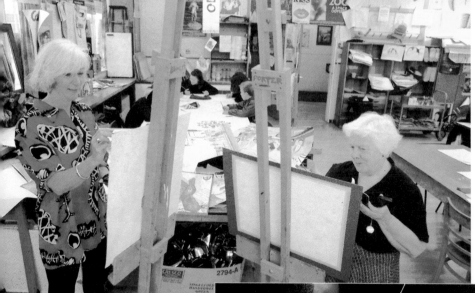

The age for art Contrary to the proverb, you can teach an old dog new tricks. Many people make use of their retirement to acquire educational qualifications that they overlooked when younger – such as A level art.

Archery lesson Being old does not, and should not, mean giving up all forms of physical exercise. Retirement even gives you the opportunity to learn new ones.

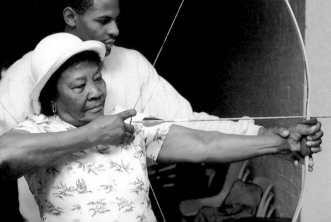

REAL LIVES

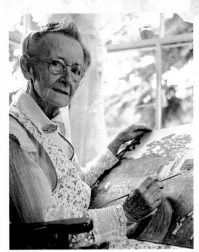

THE FARMER'S WIFE WHO BECAME AN INTERNATIONAL ARTIST

Old master *Anna Moses held her first solo exhibition in 1940 at the age of 80. A critic reviewing the exhibition gave her the name 'Grandma Moses'.*

Grandma Moses was in her 70s when she started painting. Born Anna Mary Robertson in 1860, in the small town of Greenwich, New York State, USA, she left her parents' farm at the age of 12 to become a servant. Some 15 years later, she married Thomas Moses, and they farmed together until his death in 1927.

During her childhood, Anna had drawn pictures and coloured them with berry juice. After her husband died, she started creating embroidery pictures, and it was only when her arthritis got too bad for her to hold a needle that she turned to painting, a pastime that was to turn into a profession and keep her active until shortly before she died.

Her first pictures, in the 1930s, were simply copies of prints and postcards, but she soon started painting scenes of what she called 'old timey' farm life, as she remembered it. Her pictures, painted in the primitive style, were first displayed modestly in a drugstore in Hoosick Falls. Then in 1938 she was 'discovered' by an art collector, and the following year featured in a show at the Museum of Modern Art in New York. Soon her pictures were being exhibited all over the United States. Although she never had an art lesson, she came to be widely heralded as a major modern artist, with paintings such as 'Out for the Christmas Trees' and 'Over the River to Grandma's House'.

Before long, her fame reached Europe, and in 1950 a collection of 50 of her pictures was exhibited in Vienna, Munich, Berne, The Hague and Paris. Two years later, her autobiography, My Life's History, was published. She died in 1961, at the age of 101.

Comfort and safety at home

Bathroom safety

The bathroom can be a particularly dangerous area, as it is easy to slip in the bath or on a wet floor. So it would be advisable to have fitted carpets rather than vinyl or mats underfoot. To prevent slipping in the bath, fit extra handrails and a rubber mat. When taking a bath, be sure to run the cold water first. This will ensure that you are not scalded if you happen to slip. To avoid being scalded in the shower, have a cut-out device or temperature selector installed. And do leave the door unlocked, to make it easier for help to reach you in an emergency.

PREVENTING FALLS

I am not as steady on my feet as I once was. What can I do to reduce the risk of a fall?

Falls are the most common cause of injuries in older people, so do try to 'stumble-proof' your house or flat. Keep the rooms well lit, ensure that electric flexes do not run across the floor or carpets where they could trip you up, and fix rugs down with adhesive corners. Arrange the furniture in your main living area so that you can move easily without bumping into things. Have any electrical sockets repositioned so that you do not have to bend down to reach them. If you are unsteady on your feet, wear shoes that have ridged rubberised soles and non-slip heels to give you a firmer footing.

Steps and stairs

Falls often occur on the staircase or doorsteps, so make sure that the lighting over your stairs is good, and that the stair carpeting is firmly fixed to guard against rucking and the risk of tripping you up. A handrail on the wall opposite the banisters will give you extra support while climbing stairs. If you wear bifocal spectacles, you might find it difficult to judge distance, and should take extra care on the staircase.

Kitchen safety

Slippery floors are a problem in the kitchen, so be sure to wipe up spills immediately. Items that you use on a daily basis should be placed where they are easily accessible, in order to reduce the risk of injuring yourself by straining to reach high shelves or low cupboards. If your grip is poor, a wall-mounted or electric can-opener will make it easier to open tins, and help to avoid injuries.

Bedrooms

Try to make sure that your bed is the right height – when you sit on the edge of the bed, the soles of your feet should touch the floor and you should be able to stand up easily. If you remain sitting on the bed for a short while before standing up, it will help to prevent dizzy spells. Make sure the switch for the bedside lamp is within easy reach for when you wake up in the dark, and keep a torch handy in case of power cuts, or in case you need to move around at night without disturbing your partner.

Take particular care when getting up at night to go to the bathroom. If you are still groggy, the bathroom becomes an even more hazardous area than during normal waking hours (see panel, left).

COMBATTING THE COLD

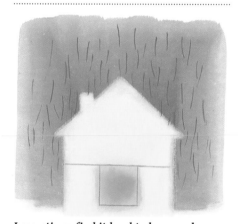

I sometimes find it hard to keep my house warm in winter and I cannot afford to spend a fortune on fuel. What else can I do to keep my home at a comfortable temperature in cold weather?

Living in a cold house is not just uncomfortable but can be perilous, even fatal, to older people, so you are right to be concerned. There is always the risk of hypothermia, a dangerous condition that occurs when body temperature falls below 35°C (95°F).

To prevent hypothermia, you must stay warm and heat at least the rooms where you spend most time. Older people may underheat their homes not only to cut fuel costs but also because they simply do not notice the cold as much as before. If heating bills are a worry, try to keep most of your activities to one well-warmed room, and turn down heating elsewhere. Consider using a chamber pot at night, to avoid taking trips to a chilly bathroom. And be sure not to place your bed against an outside wall.

Since almost half the heat lost from the body escapes through the scalp, it is essential to wear a hat in cold weather, and perhaps a nightcap in bed. Hot food and plenty of hot drinks throughout the day will also help.

BEATING THE WEATHER

As you grow older, your body becomes less adept at adjusting to changes in temperature. In the elderly, continued exposure to cool temperatures – even as mild as 16°C (60°F) – can trigger hypothermia, a dangerous lowering of the body temperature that requires emergency treatment. At the other extreme is heat exhaustion, or heatstroke – life-threatening in its own way. Never ignore symptoms such as fatigue, faintness, dizziness, or nausea during a spell of hot weather.

Cold-weather precautions
● Dress warmly before going out of doors, especially to protect against brisk winds, and always wear a hat.
● If you get soaked in a sudden downpour, change into dry clothes and warm yourself as soon as you can.
● In severe cold, stay at home if possible. If you must travel, don't travel alone.
● Keep the indoor temperature at home at a minimum of 18°C (65°F) – higher when you are ill – and dress warmly.
● Use plenty of covers on your bed, perhaps with a heated underblanket, as your body temperature drops when you are asleep. A woollen night cap is a good idea if your bedroom is cold at night.
● If you take tranquillisers or antidepressants, dress more warmly than you would usually, as they lower your perception of how cold you are. Check with your doctor whether any other medicines that you are taking may cause similar problems.
● Keep physically active, and eat regular, nutritious meals.
● Drink warm liquids such as tea, hot chocolate or soup between meals, but avoid alcohol, as it prevents your body from retaining heat.

Hot-weather precautions
● Take it easy when the temperature rises above 32°C (90°F). Don't try to accomplish too much, or even to do routine tasks as quickly as in milder weather.
● Wear loose-fitting clothes made of cool, porous fabrics, such as cotton or linen.
● Drink plenty of cool liquids – water or fruit juice – throughout the day.
● Stay out of the sun, especially in the afternoon when it is hottest.

Electricity and gas checks

Always have your gas or electricity checked by professionals if you are worried about safety. If the cost is a problem:

● Some electricity boards examine wiring free of charge. Telephone your local office to find out if they will do so.
● British Gas will check gas appliances for free if you are over 60.

Help with heating bills

● Pensioners on Income Support should automatically receive a Cold Weather Payment for each seven-day period in which the local average temperature is freezing or below. The payments are just added on to Income Support.
● According to the code of practice operated by the fuel industries, pensioners cannot have their gas or electricity supplies disconnected between October 1 and March 31, even if they cannot pay their bills.
● Bills can be paid by instalment, or using a pre-payment meter. This will not solve a real money problem, but may help you to budget.
● Local authorities and Age Concern offer grants to help pay for home insulation.
● Further advice on meeting the cost of fuel and other essentials is available from local branches of Age Concern and the Citizens Advice Bureau.

Choosing the right place to live

UNLESS health or financial circumstances dictate otherwise, most of us would prefer to live out the rest of our lives in our own house or flat. Staying in your own home preserves independence, promotes continuity and a sense of belonging, and makes it easier to keep up long-established friendships, activities and social contacts.

Even if it is a struggle to cope at home, do look into the various kinds of support available before committing yourself to a change. A number of organisations have resources – whether financial or in the form of home help – to enable you to keep your own roof over your head: the social services, the NHS, your local authority, and a number of charities. Always think carefully both about what you want now, and what you may need in the future.

If you do decide to move, try to keep the option open of changing your mind. Give your new residence a trial, for a month at least and longer if possible, before finally selling or quitting your old home.

For further information, contact your local Citizens Advice Bureau or branch of Age Concern or Help the Aged.

MOVING IN WITH FAMILY

Living with a grown-up child can work out well, particularly if you like the idea of being part of a family, get on well with everyone in the household, and wish to both give and receive support. Discuss and agree all aspects in advance, including practical and financial details, and consider carefully the issue of your own independence.

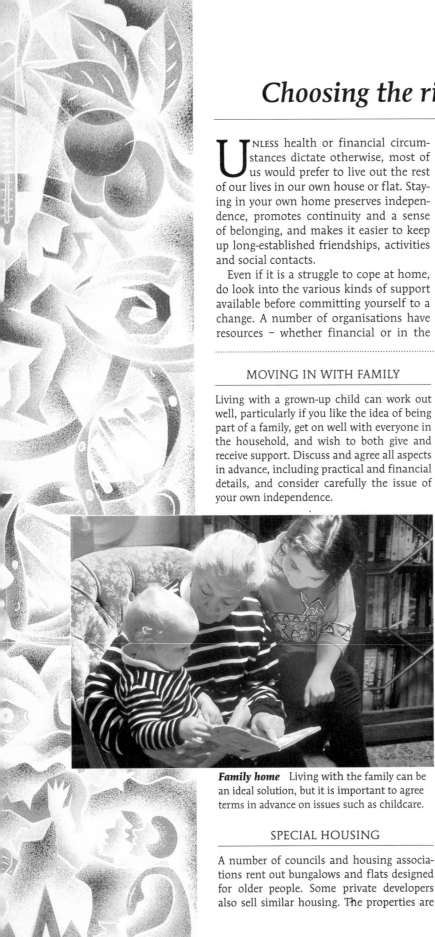

Family home Living with the family can be an ideal solution, but it is important to agree terms in advance on issues such as childcare.

SPECIAL HOUSING

A number of councils and housing associations rent out bungalows and flats designed for older people. Some private developers also sell similar housing. The properties are

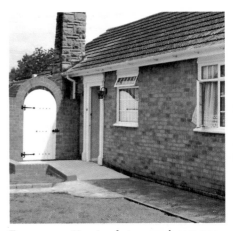

Easy access Housing features such as ramps to doors can make independent living possible for people who would otherwise struggle.

normally situated on level ground close to public services and shops, and often have features such as ramped access, waist-high electrical sockets, walk-in showers and bathroom safety rails. Remember that many of these can be installed in any home, and consider, too, how you would feel about living in a development purely for older people.

SHELTERED HOUSING

People who want the independence of a self-contained bungalow or flat combined with the security of knowing help is always at hand may find sheltered housing the ideal solution. A resident warden supervises the buildings and runs the communal facilities such as a dining room, common room and often a laundry. Each property has an alarm

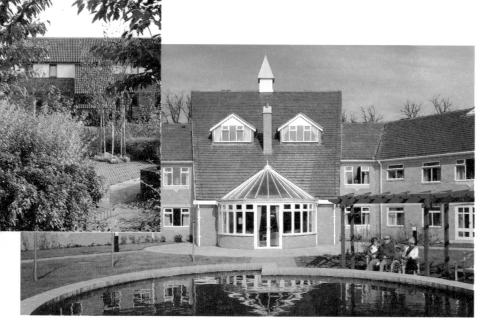

Best of both worlds? Sheltered housing offers a home of your own set in communal gardens and with a warden on call – a combination of privacy and security that appeals to many people.

button and the warden is always on stand-by to answer calls or give assistance.

Some councils and housing associations also offer sheltered housing with additional services such as the provision of meals and visits from care assistants who will help with tasks such as washing, dressing, housework and administering medicines. Such services allow many people who would otherwise be forced to move into a residential home to maintain a more independent way of life.

RESIDENTIAL HOMES

People who have become too frail to live alone but who do not need skilled nursing may consider moving to a residential home. Price, size and quality vary greatly and it is essential to inspect the premises thoroughly before deciding to move in. Talk to the residents as well as the staff, and ask to see the

Communal living Shared lounges and dining rooms mean that moving into a residential home can give a boost to your social life.

rooms, which may be either shared or private. Inspect communal facilities such as lounges and dining rooms and before you commit yourself make sure that you can have a trial period to see if you like it there.

NURSING HOMES

People who require nursing care 24 hours a day may need to consider moving into a nursing home. Most of these are privately run, though they must be registered with the district health authority. Even so, there is still a great deal of variation in quality. Before deciding on a nursing home, arrange a visit to see what it is like. Good homes will also allow you a trial period to make sure you are happy before you decide finally.

Evaluating residential and nursing homes

All homes are inspected twice a year, and it is wise to read the reports as well as visit homes yourself. You can see the reports at the inspection unit of the social services department or ask a social worker to obtain them for you. These are some specific issues to consider.

- How near is the home to family and friends?
- Can your pet come?
- Are there any restrictions on visits?
- Can you go to bed and get up when you like?
- Is it clean? A smell of urine is a bad sign.
- What possessions will you be able to bring?
- Is there a lift?
- Will you have your own room?
- Are there lavatories attached to the rooms?
- Is there an alarm-call system in every room?
- Can you lock valuables away in your room?
- Do you like the people?
- Will you be able to pursue interests such as music or gardening.

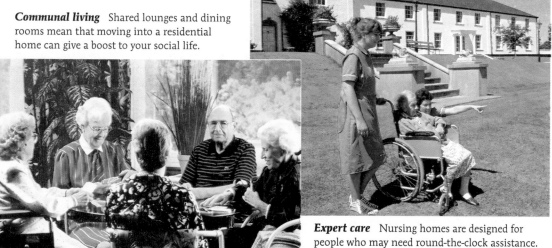

Expert care Nursing homes are designed for people who may need round-the-clock assistance.

Fighting hypothermia

Low body temperature, or hypothermia, can be lethal, so it must be treated as quickly as possible. Symptoms include a pale cold skin, a cool or cold abdomen, a puffy face, muscle stiffness, slurred speech, drowsiness and confusion. If you notice these signs in someone, wrap the sufferer up as warmly as you can, give a hot drink, get him or her to move about, and call the doctor. Do not give alcohol, however, as this will only cause further heat loss. See also page 464.

Alarm button When the button is pushed on a community alarm telephone (below) or pendant (right), a control centre is automatically dialled. Details of the caller will appear on a screen at the control centre. Having spoken to the caller, the officer will send whatever help is needed. Some schemes provide a mobile warden who will respond to any emergency.

GRANTS FOR REPAIRS

My friend's house is badly in need of repair but he cannot afford to pay for it. Can he get any financial assistance, or will he have to move out?

It should not be necessary for your friend to move out of his house. The best way to finance home-improvement work – if personal savings will not cover it – is to get a renovation grant from the local authority. Elderly people who have a relatively low income are usually eligible for such a grant. Your friend will probably have to undergo a means test before his application is fully and finally approved, and he should be prepared for this.

To apply for a grant, he should contact his local council and ask for the renovation grants section. If his home is structurally unstable or in serious disrepair, has inadequate lighting, heating, ventilation or water, or does not have proper facilities for cooking food, then the council must give him a grant. However, he should not start the work before the council has given the go-ahead, otherwise he might find that he will end up paying the bills himself.

There is another source of grants. If your friend is receiving income support, he could try for a grant from the Social Fund. He should contact his local Benefits Agency office for details. Failing that, there may be a local charity that can help with the costs of minor repair work. For further information, he should contact his local library, Age Concern group or Council for Voluntary Service.

COMMUNITY ALARMS

My mother, who is in her 80s, lives alone, and I am worried that she might injure herself one day and not be able to reach the telephone to call for help. What can be done to prevent this from happening?

The worry that an elderly relative may have an accident and be unable to contact anyone for help is a common one. The best solution is a community alarm. It looks and works like an ordinary telephone, but it can also automatically dial a control centre when a button on the phone is pressed. Supplementing the base unit is a pendant – to be worn round the neck at all times – with a push-button on it to activate the phone from up to 75 ft (23 m) away during emergencies. The pendant also contains a small microphone and loudspeaker, enabling the control centre staff to find out what the problem is and to send whatever help is needed.

All the control centres are staffed for 24 hours a day. They are usually run by local authority housing or social services departments, though some are run by commercial organisations. They store each caller's name, address, medical details, contacts – such as the doctor – and friends or relatives who have the key and can let themselves into the house or flat.

Community alarm systems can be bought or rented, the costs varying greatly according to the service on offer. If you want one, contact your local housing or social services department. If they cannot supply you with one, look in the press for advertisements for commercial systems.

Getting out and about

DRIVING AFTER 70

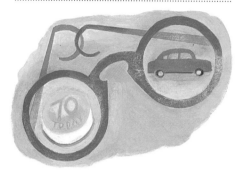

How long is it safe to go on driving? Are there any special tests for older people?

It is safe to go on driving well into your retirement, provided that you are fit and your eyesight and hearing are good. A few weeks before your 70th birthday, the Driver and Vehicle Licensing Agency (DVLA) will notify you that your licence needs to be renewed, and you will have to renew it every three years thereafter. On the application form you must declare any diseases or handicaps that you suffer from.

In fact, drivers of all ages are required by law to notify the DVLA of the onset or worsening of any medical condition that might affect their ability to drive safely – above all, anything affecting the three main requisites of safe driving: good vision, good hearing, quick reaction times. You should write to Drivers Medical Branch, DVLA, Swansea SA99 1TU, describing your medical condition in detail, and giving your driver number or full name and date of birth. The DVLA may then send you a medical questionnaire to complete and ask your permission to get a report from your doctor. They may also ask or require you to be examined by a local medical officer.

BUYING A CAR

I am about to buy a new car. Are there any special factors that older drivers like me should take into consideration when making their decision?

Apart from looking for the features that any driver looks for when buying a car – comfort reliability, performance and economy – you need to bear in mind that if you are like most people you will get a little less agile as the years go by. So power steering, for example, might prove an asset, making parking and U-turns much simpler. Also check how easy it is to open and close the door when seated, and to put on the seatbelt.

Above all, you will need to make sure that you can readily get in and out of the car you-plan to buy. To be certain, check the height and width of the door frame, the height of the seat and the door sill from the ground, and the depth of the floor well.

As guidelines, door-frame height should be about 33 in (84 cm), seat height about 20 in (51 cm), door-sill height 14 in (36 cm), and floor-well depth 4 in (10 cm). Of course, you also need to test the car directly, and to try getting in and out several times, both from road level and from the kerb.

USING A WHEELCHAIR

My sister is becoming more and more dependent on her wheelchair when outdoors, and indoors finds it very difficult to manoeuvre herself about. What can be done to make things easier for her?

If your sister is currently living at home, her family doctor will arrange for a visit from the community occupational therapist and perhaps also the physiotherapist. They will assess her needs and organise suitable home modifications – ramps over small sets of steps, adjustments to the height of the bed and lavatory seat, grab-rails in the bathroom, a stair lift, raised electrical sockets, and so on. In addition, a social worker will call to discuss other support, such as home help or meals-on-wheels, and if necessary to advise on financial assistance.

If your sister is about to be discharged from hospital, the procedure may be slightly different. Her needs should already have been assessed by a doctor, occupational therapist, physiotherapist and social worker, some of whom may now visit her again at home and draw up a list of necessary home modifications. The list is then sent to the social services, who appoint a care manager to work out the costs. If the social services cannot afford the entire package, a compromise will be worked out. If your sister has any difficulties getting assistance, her local branch of Age Concern can help.

DO'S —— AND —— DON'TS
for safer driving

Do exercise to keep your body flexible, so that you can see the road from all angles and manoeuvre the car more easily.

Do have your eyes checked regularly. If you wear glasses, keep your prescription up to date and pick frames that will not interfere with your peripheral vision.

Do have your hearing checked regularly. If you need a hearing aid wear it when you drive.

Do get plenty of sleep before a long trip, and take rest stops as needed along the way.

Don't drive at dusk or daybreak, unless you have to. The light is difficult at these times. **Don't** drive at night if you have any problems with night vision.

Should you drive?

If you are in any doubt at all about whether you should drive, contact the Department of Transport's Mobility Advice and Vehicle Information Service (MAVIS). The address is c/o TRL, Wokingham Road, Crowthorne, Berks RG11 6AU.

The service offers free advice to older drivers about where and how to get their driving ability assessed, and about the range of modifications available to make using a car easier.

STICKS AND FRAMES FOR WALKING

It is not unusual to become slightly slower and more unsteady on your feet as you get older. In many cases exercise can counteract the problem and help to maintain mobility, but some people – those who suffer from arthritis, for instance – may need to use walking aids.

Walking sticks

These are mostly used by people who are weak, or have stiffness or pain, on one side of their body. The stick – usually made of wood, though you can get lightweight aluminium varieties with adjustable lengths – should be long enough to allow the user to walk upright with the elbow slightly bent, and should have a rubber tip, or ferrule, to prevent slipping. Some sticks may have three or four feet for extra stability. The stick should generally be carried on the strong side, so that it moves forward at the same time that the weak foot does.

Walking frames

For those who suffer weakness or pain on both sides of the body, or have severe balance problems, walking frames provide a very stable support. The frames are usually made of a strong, light alloy, and have four rubber-tipped legs to prevent sliding.

Looking your best

DEALING WITH DRY SKIN

As I have got older I have found my skin becoming dry and scaly. Is this a normal part of the ageing process?

A certain degree of wrinkling, drying and loss of elasticity is the natural result of hormonal changes and of wear and tear from sun, wind, cold and other environmental assaults. If you are troubled by dry skin:

- Try to ensure that the heating in your home does not dry out the air too much.
- Keep detergents, bleaches, and other drying substances away from your skin.
- Use only mild soap, or a gentle cleanser. Ask your pharmacist for advice.
- Apply lotion to dry areas immediately after washing, while your skin is still moist.

To help keep your skin supple, apply a cleansing cream and moisturiser night and morning, massaging upwards to counteract any wrinkles or sagging skin. Even men – who tend to have naturally robust skins – can benefit from a moisturiser, particularly since shaving can damage dry skin. Be wary of extravagant claims for expensive products that are supposed to banish your wrinkles overnight. Simply applying sunscreen to the skin when you go out will be more effective, by delaying further wrinkles.

No one knows your skin better than you do. If you think that the dryness and scaliness that you are experiencing is unusually severe, you should consult your doctor. The condition of your skin may be a pointer to health problems. An underactive thyroid, for instance, can cause the skin to look older than it should and to feel thick, dry and cool to the touch. Itchiness that has no obvious cause may simply be the result of your skin's ageing, but it could be a sign of an allergy or illness, such as diabetes, perhaps, or a kidney or liver disorder. If you suspect any such illness, do seek medical advice right away.

CAUTION Never ignore any skin changes associated with moles, lumps, bumps or other growths. See your doctor immediately.

HINTS ABOUT HAIR

I have always been proud of my hair, but as I get older it gets greyer and thinner. How can I best look after my hair?

As you age, your hair becomes more delicate, and starts to thin and lose its colour. If you are worried about your hair being grey, consider tinting it a darker colour. But be careful: you may be sensitive to the chemicals in the dye. Check by trying it out on a small, inconspicuous area first. Also, avoid very dark tints, which can look harsh and obvious. For most older skins, pale tones are more natural and flattering. Silver highlights or streaks can also look attractive, and white hair itself is very striking if cut well. Hair is best worn fairly short, as this gives the facial lines a lift. To keep your hair in good condition, shampoo it regularly, massaging the scalp well to improve the blood supply, and use a conditioner to keep it soft.

If your hair is thinning, consider trying products designed to increase its body and volume – your hairdresser should be able to advise on the most suitable ones. Wigs and hairpieces now look more natural than they used to, so you could consider buying one. Those made of human hair are very expensive, but those made of acrylic, though perhaps not quite so convincing, weigh less, and are cheaper and quite easy to look after.

LOSING HEIGHT

When I measured my height recently I was shocked to find that I am an noticeably shorter than I was in my youth. What happened? Will I lose any more height?

Slight loss of height is a normal part of the ageing process. In midlife, various problems develop: curvature of the spine, compression of the spinal discs, loss of elasticity in the joints, and flattening of the feet. By the age of 70, the body may have shrunk by an inch (2.5 cm) or more. Some people also develop a stoop as a result of bad posture. The best way to combat both the loss of height and the tendency to stoop is by exercising regularly, to strengthen your bones and muscles.

A more substantial reduction in height could mean that you are losing bone mass, a symptom of osteoporosis (see page 437). Although this condition is often regarded as a woman's ailment, men are not immune. As their male hormone levels decline, men between 65 and 70 begin to lose bone mass at the same rate that women do.

Prevention is far better than cure when dealing with osteoporosis. An active lifestyle, a healthy diet containing plenty of calcium,

abstinence from smoking and moderation in consumption of alcohol will all help to keep your bones strong (see page 390). Even if you already suffer from osteoporosis, the same measures are still advisable, to slow the progress of the condition.

CHANGES IN WEIGHT

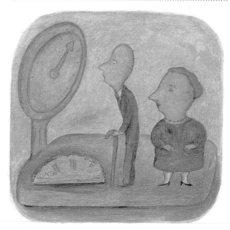

As they got older, my mother got rather fat but my father grew very thin. Why should one put on weight and the other lose it?

As people grow older, their body fat is redistributed. The layer of fat beneath their skin diminishes, and someone who is naturally thin begins to look scrawny. On the other hand, people who are naturally plump – usually women – find that their body fat accumulates in certain places: round the waist and the abdomen, on the thighs, and sometimes under the chin.

A correct diet will help both problems. Someone who is too thin needs to concentrate on receiving sufficient nutrients (see page 11), while someone who is overweight may need to cut down on the amount of food consumed (see page 153).

Choosing colours in later life

White skins tend to lose colour as they age, so keep make-up light and pale – bold colours look unnatural. With paler hair and skin, you will be able to wear lighter colours: pale shades of blue, pink and green or turquoise look very good with grey or white hair.

Darker skins are more resistant to the ravages of age, and colours that suited people in their 20s will still look good in later life. Black skins tend to darken with age, so black women often favour a good foundation cream.

Healthy eating and drinking

TIME FOR A CHANGE?

Should older people continue to eat the same types of meal as before, or should they go on a special diet?

It depends on what sort of meals they have been eating. If they are already following a healthy, balanced diet (see page 11), then there is no need for them to change their

diet, other than to cut down the quantities a little, to compensate for the fall – by up to a fifth – in their metabolic rate. If, however, they have been living on fried foods and foodstuffs high in animal fats and sugar, and drinking large quantities of alcohol, then they would be wise to make changes.

A healthy diet should include plenty of fibre, found in fruit, vegetables, wholemeal bread, pasta, rice and wholegrain cereals.

Fact To maintain a steady weight, a woman over 75 years old will use up 1800 Calories a day, compared with 2100 Calories at 18. The figures for men are 2100 at 75 and 2750 at 18.

This reduction in each case probably has more to do with changes in lifestyle than with the ageing process. People tend to become less active as they grow older. At any age, our calorie requirement is related to the amount of activity undertaken, so slowing down in old age will reduce the amount of food our bodies need. If, for some reason, an elderly person increases his level of physical activity, his daily calorie requirement will go up as well.

In spite of their reduced need for calories, many elderly people continue to eat as much as they always have, and the resultant excess calories are turned into body fat. However, provided the weight gain is not excessive, the additional body fat will do little harm. It may even help insulate against the cold.

On the other hand, because they need fewer calories, and therefore may tend to eat less, elderly people should ensure that their diet is high in nutrient-rich foods, rather than foods full of sugar and fat.

Salt should be used sparingly, as it can lead to high blood pressure; there should be enough salt already in everyday foods for dietary needs. Plenty of liquid – six to eight cups a day – is also important. Alcoholic drinks will not provide that extra liquid, as alcohol has a dehydrating effect. People who feel they must have sugary or fatty foods should eat them only occasionally as a treat.

A BETTER APPETITE

When I was younger, I had a good appetite, but these days I don't seem to enjoy my food as much as I used to. Why is this?

The senses of taste and smell often become a little weaker with age. As they are also very closely linked, a problem with either one can interfere with the other and greatly interfere with your enjoyment of food.

There are several reasons for this gradual loss of taste and smell. The taste buds on the tongue can lose their responsiveness to delicate flavours as you get older, and if you suffer frequently from colds or catarrh your sense of smell will be deadened. Poor dental hygiene can leave an off-putting taste in your mouth that interferes with your taste for food, so make sure that your teeth are kept as clean and healthy as possible, and make regular visits to your dentist.

You can compensate for diminished taste sensations by paying more attention to the texture of your food. Raw or crunchy vegetables might be more interesting to eat than well-cooked ones, as well as being better for you because they retain more of their nutrients. When you are preparing your favourite dishes, experiment with seasonings and garnishes. If you are on a low-salt diet, you could experiment with spices to enhance flavour; and fresh herbs such as basil and garlic are easily available in supermarkets. Even lemon juice can add a delightful new flavour to a recipe.

SOFT FOODS FOR EASY EATING

I have weak teeth and cannot chew very well, but so many soft foods seem bland and boring. How can I vary my diet without causing tooth trouble?

People who have difficulties chewing, for whatever reason, tend to avoid foods with a hard or tough texture. Before you do anything else, however, you should establish whether your problems can be helped by a dentist. If you still need to eat soft foods after being treated by the dentist, there is no reason why your meals should be bland or boring. The following ideas will help you towards a more interesting diet:

● For breakfast have porridge or a soft-textured cereal. Serve it with stewed fruit, or soft fresh fruits such as raspberries, peaches or sliced banana.
● Make a hearty kedgeree by flaking smoked haddock and mixing it with rice and chopped hard-boiled egg.
● Make grated cheese-and-pickle or tuna mayonnaise sandwiches using wholemeal bread. Avoid granary, which may contain hard grains that can damage teeth.
● Follow the Chinese style of slicing meat and vegetables into delicate easy-to-chew strips, and serve these with boiled or fried rice or soft noodles.
● Try the Italian approach. Pasta is very soft and can be served with dozens of different sauces. Risotto is also very easy to make and to eat, whatever the state of your teeth.
● Scoop the flesh from a baked potato, mix with cheese and a little milk, then pile back into the skin and heat till brown on top.
● Cook casseroles and stews until the chunks of meat are so tender they simply fall apart in the mouth.
● Try spicing up tender white fish or chicken with ready-made piquant sauces.
● Enjoy soft-textured vegetables such as creamed spinach, carrots mashed with parsnips, baked aubergine, steamed cauliflower florets or grilled tomatoes.
● For dessert, try soft fruit topped with low-fat yoghurt or fromage frais, or a baked apple or thin pancakes with fruit purée.

SIMPLE COOKING

Since my wife died, I have found it a struggle to feed myself, as she always did all the cooking and shopping. What can I do to make sure I am getting a healthy, balanced diet?

It is quite understandable that you are struggling with your meals, but it is important to avoid falling into the unsatisfactory though common routine of reaching for biscuits and tea throughout the day, and eating little else. Although there are many exceptions, it is often women who buy and cook food for the family, and many newly bereaved husbands have to face the loss of both a lifelong companion and their provider of food. Some widowers have never even shopped for food, let alone shown interest in its preparation or cooking, so the first few forays into the crowded aisles of supermarkets can be somewhat overwhelming.

Your wife probably bought fresh ingredients and made them into seemingly complex dishes. If you lack the culinary expertise to do this, why not try to learn creative cookery – which can be great fun at local classes. Failing that, you may prefer to buy a selection of frozen meals for one, and cook them in the oven or microwave. In addition, work up a list of meals that you enjoy and that are easy to prepare. Some straightforward dishes that you could try are:

● Grilled lean pork chops with fresh or frozen vegetables.
● Lean minced beef cooked in a ready-made sauce and served with spaghetti or potatoes.
● Canned fish (tuna, salmon, pilchards or sardines) with a ready-mixed fresh salad.
● Lean grilled steak served with frozen peas and oven chips.
● A half avocado filled with ready-cooked prawns or drained, canned crabmeat.

The more dishes you can add to your list, the more satisfying and nutritious your new diet will become. With a little practice you will soon be able to invite friends around to your home, confident that you will be able to prepare a meal everyone will enjoy.

Finally, make an effort to get out at least once or twice a week to eat lunch or an evening meal with friends. This will help rekindle the social aspect of eating, which is sadly absent when you dine alone.

VITAMIN SUPPLEMENTS

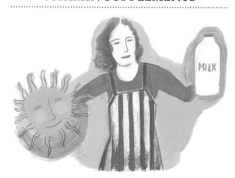

A friend of mine claims that vitamins help to keep her young. Should I take vitamin supplements now that I am over 65?

A vitamin supplement does not turn a poor diet into a good one. If you are healthy, the best way to meet your nutritional requirements is to eat a well-balanced diet. The components of such a diet will deliver

the necessary vitamins and minerals to your body far more efficiently than supplements do. However, because the body's ability to absorb calcium and synthesise vitamin D (which aids calcium absorption) declines with age, many doctors suggest a calcium supplement as a protection against osteoporosis, though there is some doubt as to its effectiveness (see page 48). For most people, drinking a cup of milk a day or sitting in the sun for 10 minutes twice a week meets their vitamin D requirements.

By itself, the ageing process does not necessarily increase your body's need for most nutrients. However, illness, injury, the recuperation process, certain medications, and a poor diet may cause nutritional deficiencies. So older people who do not eat enough suffer chronic health problems, or take prescription drugs regularly may benefit from a multiple vitamin supplement.

HOW MUCH ALCOHOL?

I have always enjoyed an aperitif before dinner, and a glass of wine with it. Is there any reason to give up drinking now?

A little alcohol is usually harmless and relaxing. It stimulates your appetite, increases your feeling of wellbeing, and may even be beneficial to your health. Some studies show that light drinkers live longer than either heavy drinkers or teetotallers. There is therefore no reason for you to give up drinking simply because you are getting older.

Remember, though, that alcohol can react unpleasantly with any drug you may be taking. To be on the safe side, it is always a good idea to ask your doctor or pharmacist whether it is safe to drink while taking a prescription drug – or, indeed, with one you are buying over the counter yourself.

Be aware, too, that drinking affects your physical coordination and reaction times more quickly as you get older, making you more susceptible to car accidents, falls and other injuries. If you have trouble remembering things, alcohol will aggravate the situation. Also, drinking heavily with your meal increases your chances of choking on your food, particularly if you wear dentures.

The recommended limits for safe drinking for older people are:

● Men: about 2 units a day.
● Women: 1 to 2 units a day.

A unit corresponds to half a pint of beer or lager, a small glass of wine, or a single standard pub measure of spirits.

FACT
—— OR ——
FALLACY?

'Alcoholic drinks affect you differently as you grow older.'

Fact As people grow older, their tolerance for alcohol decreases. With age, the metabolism slows down, and the liver filters alcohol from the blood more slowly, causing people to become drunk faster and stay drunk for longer than they did when they were younger.

Furthermore, the way alcohol makes you feel can change as you grow older. Some people start to become hostile and irritable, rather than more relaxed and happy, after a drink or two.

Effortless eating for those on their own

It is all too easy, if you are living on your own, to fall into the habit of not eating properly simply because you cannot be bothered to cook elaborate meals. Here are some easy ways of ensuring a nutritious diet without effort.

● Eat healthy snacks – sandwiches and salads – throughout the day, instead of full meals.
● Prepare dishes such as casseroles that last several days.
● Cook favourite dishes in large quantities, and freeze in portions.
● Take it in turns with a good friend to cook for each other.

Caring for older eyes

Cataract surgery

Cataract surgery involves a relatively simple operation to extract the cloudy lens. It is one of the most successful types of surgery, producing much-improved vision in 95 per cent of cases.

The operation takes about 30 minutes and can be performed under either local or general anaesthetic. After the faulty lens has been extracted, a substitute is needed. The best option is a lens implant, inserted in the eye when the cataract is removed.

Most people suffer nothing more than a few days of mild discomfort after the operation. It takes about a month for the incision to heal.

EYE EXAMINATIONS

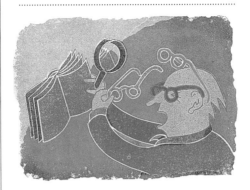

Now that I am over 65, should I have my eyes examined regularly?

A deterioration in eyesight often occurs in old age, so it is important that you have your eyes tested at regular intervals to ensure that they are functioning well, and that you are not suffering from any eye diseases. This is particularly true if you suffer from diabetes or high blood pressure, or have a family history of glaucoma, as these conditions make you more susceptible to eye disease. Regular eye tests will increase the chance of detecting an eye disease early – when there is a greater chance of effective treatment. Furthermore, people who wear glasses tend to change prescription more often as they get older. This is because the lens in the eye gets harder, making it more difficult for the muscles surrounding it to bend it and bring the images of near objects into focus.

The first signs of some disorders, such as diabetes or high blood pressure, often show in the eyes, so regular eye tests may help these problems to be diagnosed early, and treated more effectively. If you do develop an eye disorder, regular eye examinations will allow its progress to be monitored, and help doctors to give you more beneficial treatment and advice.

GLAUCOMA IN THE FAMILY

My elder brother has chronic glaucoma. Should I have my eyes tested?

You should definitely have your eyes tested; and as the relative of someone who suffers from chronic glaucoma, you are entitled to a free test, since you have a one in ten chance

of developing the disease. You are at further risk if you suffer from diabetes, or are very short-sighted. It is vital to detect any sign of glaucoma as early as possible, since with prompt treatment good vision can be preserved, but without it a sufferer may eventually go blind. People over 65 should visit the optician regularly for eye tests. If a glaucoma test is not offered as part of the package, they should ask for one. The optician blows a puff of air against the eye to test the internal pressure, and looks into the eye to see if the optic nerve has been damaged.

Glaucoma affects about one in twenty people aged over 65. It occurs when a build-up of fluid in the eye increases the internal eye pressure and damages the optic nerve. Since the condition is quite often painless, the optic nerve can be damaged without the patient being aware of it, though sufferers may experience a gradual loss of peripheral vision early on.

Treatment is usually supervised by an ophthalmologist, or eye specialist, based at a hospital. It starts with eye drops – which reduce the production of clear fluid within the eye, or allow the fluid to drain away more easily – and may proceed through various medicines to surgery, possibly by laser, to create a tiny hole on the edge of the iris for drainage.

SELF HELP FOR CATARACTS

I have been told that I have cataracts, but I am hesitant about having my eyes operated on. Is there anything else I can try before resorting to surgery?

Cataracts – a painless clouding of the lens of the eye – are so common in the over-60s that they are considered almost a 'normal' part of the ageing process (see panel, top left). Unfortunately, there is no way of curing cataracts other than by surgically removing them – though prescription glasses may help you if the cataracts are causing only minor vision problems. But by no means all cases of cataracts require surgery. In many people, they develop so slowly that it is possible to go through life without ever needing an operation. Moreover, doctors prefer to wait until vision in the eye that is unaffected or less affected by cataracts deteriorates to the point that daily activities – such as working, driving a car, reading, or watching television – become troublesome. Even if you do have to have surgery, the operation is a relatively simple one (see panel, bottom left).

Furthermore, there is plenty that you can do to make living with cataracts more comfortable. Avoid direct sunlight by wearing a hat and sunglasses outdoors, as cataracts can scatter light, causing glare. Use the sunvisor to reduce glare when driving. Do not use bright lights indoors. To reduce the glare from a printed page, try covering it with a sheet of dull black paper that has a slit cut in it large enough to expose a few lines at a time, and move the paper up and down as you read. When you watch television, make sure that there is no light source too close to your line of vision.

WHEN VISION IS BLURRED

I seem to be losing the sight in the centre of my field of vision. Why is this? Can anything be done about it?

You should contact your doctor as soon as possible for a complete eye examination. It sounds as if you may have macular degeneration, one of the principle causes of loss of vision in elderly people. The disease usually affects both eyes, sometimes simultaneously, sometimes one after the other.

The macula is the part of the retina that is responsible for central vision. As a person gets older, the cells making up the macula begin to waste away. Also, the membrane separating the macula from the blood vessels that feed it can break down, allowing fluid to leak through. Abnormal blood vessels form, and bleed into the retina, causing the nerve tissue of the macula to be replaced with scar tissue. This sometimes leads to blurred and distorted eyesight, and a gradual loss of central vision. Straight lines may look wavy, and it may become difficult to read, or to recognise faces. When a sufferer peers out of the corner of his or her eyes, vision may not seem too bad, but when he or she turns to look at something directly, it may appear blurred or grainy.

Unfortunately, there is no way of reversing macular degeneration, but the process can sometimes be slowed or halted by laser treatment to the retina. So early detection and regular follow-up examinations are crucial. Moreover, if one eye has been affected, it may be possible to protect the other. If your doctor suspects that you are suffering from macular degeneration, he should refer you to an eye specialist. The eye specialist can examine your retina with an ophthalmoscope, having first enlarged the pupil by administering eyedrops. If the blood vessels do not lie directly under the centre of the macula, he may decide to perform a fluorescein angiogram – a test in which abnormal blood vessels are outlined with the help of an orange dye, and then photographed.

Even where nothing can be done to stop the progress of macular degeneration, life can be made easier through the use of magnifying devices and bright light.

AN EYE TEST TO TRY AT HOME

The Amsler grid was designed by the Swiss eye specialist Marc Amsler to test for visual distortion and loss of central vision — two signs of macular degeneration (see left). It is reproduced below so that you can test your own eyes.

Hold the page in a good reading light at the distance you normally hold a book. If you wear reading glasses, you should use them for the test. Cover one eye and focus on the dot in the middle of the grid with the other eye. You should be able to see the dot and the entire grid clearly, without any distortion or blurring. The lines should appear parallel and straight, and no part of any line should be missing. Repeat the test with the other eye. If the grid appears broken, with either eye, or if any part of it seems distorted, see your doctor and describe the test results. You should also be wary if you see dark spots, or if the grid appears grainy, as either of these could also be a symptom of problems with your retina. If macular degeneration is diagnosed and treated early enough, it may forestall serious vision problems.

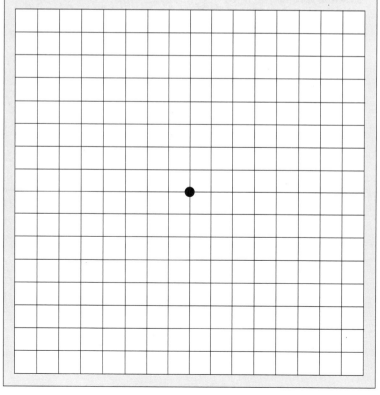

HOW DOES THE WORLD LOOK WHEN VISION IS IMPAIRED?

Most people's eyesight deteriorates to some extent as time passes, so it is important to have regular eye tests, particularly if you have high blood pressure, diabetes or a family history of glaucoma. If detected early enough many eye diseases can be successfully treated. Left too long, there are serious risks of blindness or permanently and severely impaired vision.

Normal vision Healthy eyes show a scene similar to that reproduced by a standard camera lens – in this case traffic and pedestrians bustling along London's busy Regent Street.

Macular degeneration Degenerative changes in the central part of the retina – the macula – cause a blind spot in the centre of the visual field. Early treatment is essential.

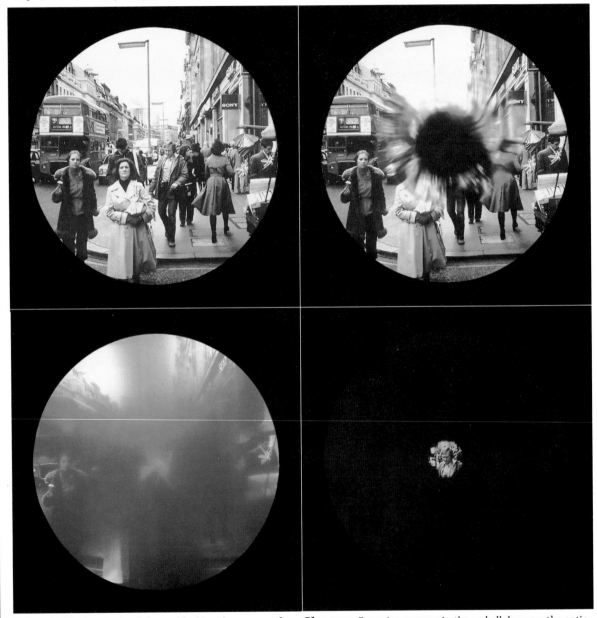

Cataracts The lens is clouded over, blocking the passage of light to the retina. The photographic clarity of normal vision is lost, and the world appears hazy, as if viewed through a frosted window. Simple procedures can rectify the problem.

Glaucoma Excessive pressure in the eyeball damages the optic nerve and destroys peripheral vision as the nerve sends the brain only a partial image. Eventually just a small central spot remains. Regular screening is recommended for everyone.

Help with hearing problems

VANISHING HIGH PITCH

I have started having difficulty hearing women's voices, but not men's. What is happening to my hearing?

It seems that you are suffering from presbycusis – a progressive loss of hearing that occurs with age. About one person in three suffers some degree of hearing loss with age – the result of gradual wear and tear on the nerve fibres of the inner ear, often caused by a lifetime's exposure to loud noises. At first only the high frequencies, or treble sounds, are lost, so that women's voices and high-pitched musical instruments become harder to hear. You may also find that although speech may sound loud, it is difficult to distinguish what people are saying. In a noisy atmosphere, it may be difficult to hear the speech of someone close to you over the noises in the background.

There is, unfortunately, no actual cure for this kind of age-related hearing loss, but there is help. Special high-frequency hearing aids are available and make the condition much easier to live with.

OBTAINING A HEARING AID

I am gradually losing my hearing. How do I go about getting a hearing aid?

The first thing you should do is see your doctor – the problem may well be treatable. If medication, wax removal or other simple treatments do not work, your doctor may refer you to an ear, nose and throat specialist at the local hospital.

The specialist will examine your ears and arrange for a hearing test, conducted by an audiologist. The test will show whether or not a hearing aid would help. If so, you will be sent to the hospital's hearing-aid department, which will help you to find the best type for your needs. Hearing aids can be really successful only if they are fitted with a made-to-measure ear mould for each person, so a technician will need to take an impression of your ear.

The NHS supplies hearing aids free, but if you do not want to wait for an appointment with the ear, nose and throat specialist – a wait which can last up to six months – or if you want a special hearing aid that the NHS does not supply, or even if you simply want an extra hearing aid, you can buy one from a registered hearing-aid dispensing business.

You can either go to their premises or ask them to send someone to your home. In either case, try to find one that has been recommended by a friend and preferably one with a permanent office in your area, so that you can easily go back to them, should you need to, after the purchase. Make sure that the dispenser offers a money-back guarantee with at least a 30-day trial period, since it can be very difficult to get a refund. Always try out a hearing aid before you sign any agreement or hand over any money, particularly if you are buying for the first time.

When you buy a hearing aid, you will have to sign an agreement to purchase the aid. This is a legal contract, and is extremely hard to break, so read it carefully before signing. The agreement should cover the terms of the guarantee, the servicing arrangements, and the price. If you are unhappy with any of these conditions, do not sign the agreement.

Dispensers are not allowed to make unsolicited visits to your home, but if you do buy a hearing aid during such a visit, you have seven days in which to reconsider. If you cancel within that time, you are entitled to a full refund. Some dispensers enforce the seven-day deadline rigidly, so make sure you decide promptly.

AIDS FOR THE FRAIL

My grandmother is 95 years old, and cannot cope with a hearing aid. Is there anything else she could try?

People who are very old and frail often find it difficult to use modern electronic hearing aids, as the controls are small and the batteries fiddly to insert. As an alternative, your grandmother could try an old-style ear trumpet or a conversation tube. These are simple devices that have no controls to fiddle with and do not need batteries. Both are available through the NHS.

If your grandmother suffers from only moderate hearing loss, there are a number of battery-operated devices with headphones. They have larger controls that can sit on a table or hang around the neck, are fairly easy to operate and generate an adequate amount of amplification.

FACT
—— OR ——
FALLACY?

'Commercial hearing aids are better than NHS ones.'

Fallacy NHS aids are just as good as the equivalent commercial models and are, in fact, generally made by the same companies. Commercial dispensers can, however, supply a wider variety of types of hearing aid; for example, in-the-ear hearing aids, digitally programmable hearing aids – some with remote control – and spectacle aids.

DO'S
—— AND ——
DON'TS

for living with the hard of hearing

Do reduce background noises in order to avoid a confusion of sound.
Do explain the problem to friends and relatives.
Do face the person when you are speaking.
Do try to ensure that any light falls on your face, and does not come from behind you.
Do speak slowly.
Do rephrase sentences if you are misunderstood.

Don't shout.
Don't mumble. Always speak clearly.
Don't exaggerate your facial movements when speaking. This will only add to the confusion.

CONSUMER PROTECTION

I have heard of people having problems with hearing-aid sellers. Is there any way to check a retailer's credentials before I buy a hearing aid, and anyone I can complain to if I am unhappy with the service?

If you wish to check the credentials of, or complain about, a hearing-aid dispenser, you should contact the Hearing Aid Council, First Floor, Moorgate House, 201 Silbury Boulevard, Central Milton Keynes MK9 1LZ. The Council's function is to control the conduct of hearing-aid dispensers, and it has drawn up a code of practice which goes some way to safeguarding the interests of buyers. According to this code of practice, a hearing aid can be sold to you only if you have been examined by or in the presence of a Registered Hearing Aid Dispenser.

All dispensers must abide by the code of practice, which amongst other things specifies the conditions under which a patient must be referred to a doctor. A copy of this code of practice must always be available for inspection by any prospective client.

All hearing-aid dispensers must pass a Hearing Aid Council examination. They can then apply to join the British Society of Hearing Aid Audiologists (BSHAA) and to use the initials MSHAA after their name.

CHOOSING THE RIGHT HEARING AID FOR YOU

It takes time to get used to a new hearing aid. Distinguishing sounds can be tricky at first, so practise at home for a few hours each day – the first week is usually the hardest. To insert a behind-the-ear aid, push the ear mould into the ear first, making sure that the top point goes behind the ridge of skin. Then lift the body of the aid over the ear. Some hearing aids are turned on and off by means of the volume control, but many models have a separate switch marked O, T and M. The O setting is off; switch to M for normal use. The T setting is for use with equipment such as loop systems and special telephones. To ensure that your hearing aid lasts the four or five years it should, and gives the best possible results, keep it away from high temperatures and chemical products, including hairspray, and keep your ears free of wax. When you take your aid out at night, turn it off, disengage the batteries to extend their life, and wipe the exterior with a dry cloth.

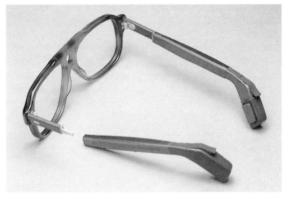

Sight and sound Spectacle aids are glasses with hearing-aid parts housed in the arm. They are expensive as they require the expertise of an optician and a hearing-aid specialist.

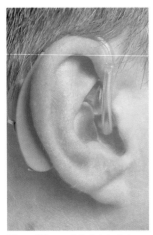

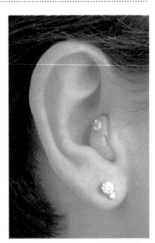

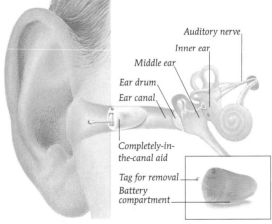

Versatile model Behind-the-ear aids are comfortable to wear. There are various models available to suit people with most types of hearing loss.

Neat fit In-the-canal aids fit into the opening of the ear canal. They are very discrete but generally suit only those with mild hearing loss.

Invisible aid The smallest type of hearing aid is a new development known as the completely-in-the-canal aid. The instrument is worn entirely within the ear canal and is completely concealed from sight. The battery compartment incorporates the on/off switch and volume control.

Looking after your teeth

PRESERVING A FULL SET

I am 65 years old and still have all my own teeth. What can I do to keep them as long as possible?

There is no reason why you should not keep your teeth for the rest of your life, as long as you look after them well. Older people need to be particularly diligent about their dental care, as the plaque which causes tooth decay and gum disease builds up more quickly on teeth than when they were younger. The reason is that gums tend to recede with age, exposing more of the root surfaces – which are not as smooth as enamel – of your teeth.

This problem can be made more serious by a decline in saliva production, either because of malfunctioning saliva glands or because drugs are causing the mouth to dry up. Saliva acts as a natural mouth rinse, diluting and neutralising the acid in plaque that eats away at tooth enamel. Chewing sugar-free gum helps to stimulate saliva, as does eating citrus fruits. You should also be sure to have regular dental check-ups – many dentists suggest that people have their teeth examined every six months.

GETTING USED TO DENTURES

My grandmother complains that her new dentures are very uncomfortable. Should she persevere with them, or go back to the dentist to have them adjusted?

It always takes a little while for the mouth to adapt to new dentures, so your grandmother should give her dentures a few weeks to 'run in'. In fact, dentists often recommend that people with new dentures wear them 24 hours a day for a few days to get used to them. The muscles of the cheeks and lips need to adjust to the dentures, sometimes making eating awkward. If, however, your grandmother has developed any sore spots in her mouth, she should visit her dentist again, so that he can make the necessary adjustments. He may have to check the fit of the dentures several times before they are as comfortable as they should be.

Precise fit is very important because your grandmother should be able to wear them all day long without having to think about them. If they are uncomfortable, she will be self-conscious and miserable. If she does not use them regularly, her mouth may change shape, and they will not fit properly when she next puts them in.

If your grandmother's dentures are still causing her pain after several weeks, she should see her dentist. Occasionally, small fragments of tooth may be lying just under the surface, and that may be what is causing her gums to feel sore.

DENTURES THAT DON'T FIT

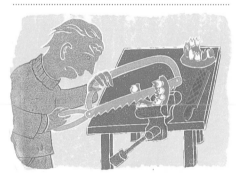

My dentures do not seem to fit in my mouth as well as they once did, and they are beginning to bother me. What could be causing this?

It is not unusual for dentures to become uncomfortable after being worn for months or years. Once you have lost most or all of your teeth, the shape of your mouth is likely to change. Changes in the gums and in the bones supporting them can make dentures feel distinctly uncomfortable.

If the fit of your dentures changes, see your dentist right away so that he can adapt or reline them. You should, in any case, see your dentist regularly, so that he can check that everything is in order. Poorly fitting dentures can irritate your gums, tongue and cheeks, possibly causing mouth ulcers and infections, and even bone loss. Eventually the ridges can shrink to such a degree that it becomes almost impossible to fit them with a new set of dentures.

Don't try to fix your dentures yourself, as you might damage them. If necessary, use a denture adhesive to secure them until you can see your dentist. If you continue to have trouble with the fit of your dentures, speak to your dentist about the possibility of a modern alternative – tooth implants.

Trouble cleaning your teeth?

There are a number of devices to help those who struggle to clean their teeth. They can be bought at pharmacies or through catalogues of aids for handicapped people. Your local community dental service or branch of Age Concern should be able to tell you where you can get the catalogues.

If you struggle to hold a toothbrush, you can buy special wide-handled models, or modify an ordinary toothbrush by fixing a sponge round the handle. Wrapping sticking plaster round the handle can make gripping easier. Some people find that an electric toothbrush is easier to manipulate than a regular one.

Pharmacies carry special dental-floss holders that make flossing a little easier. If you still have problems try interdental cleaners – small brushes that can be pushed between the teeth. Don't use toothpicks, as they do not clean below the gum line, and can damage sensitive gum tissue. If all else fails, rinsing thoroughly after every meal, with water or a mouthwash, will help to dislodge food, and is certainly better than doing nothing.

Dental treatment in your home

If you are housebound and unable to visit a dentist, you can ask your dentist to treat you at home. Dentists don't have to oblige but most will try. If your dentist is unwilling, contact the Community Dental Service through the local health authority, to see if there is a domiciliary service or mobile unit.

CARING FOR YOUR DENTURES

I have recently been fitted with dentures. How should I clean them? Must they be cleaned as often as natural teeth?

Dentures collect plaque just as natural teeth do, and should be cleaned daily. The best way to do this is to take them out of your mouth and rinse them. Then, using a soft brush designed for dentures (or a soft toothbrush), brush thoroughly but gently with baking soda, hand soap, a mild dishwashing liquid, or denture-cleaning paste – check with your dentist which is the best method for your particular dentures. Be careful around metal clasps, or you might bend them. To remove tartar, soak your dentures in a solution of one tablespoon of white vinegar to eight fluid ounces of water, or better still, take them to your dentist, or a dental laboratory, and have them cleaned professionally.

It is also important to keep your mouth clean, in order to prevent mouth odour and infection under the dentures – with time, the plastic base becomes porous and soaks up saliva and food residues. While your dentures are out, brush your gums, your tongue and the roof of your mouth with toothpaste and a soft-bristled toothbrush to remove food debris and bacteria and to stimulate blood circulation.

If you wear a partial denture, take good care of your remaining teeth (see page 132). When you brush and floss each day, pay particular attention to the teeth where denture clasps are connected, as plaque tends to collect abundantly in these places.

For the first few days, wear your new dentures day and night, to get used to them. After that, you can remove them at night. Since they need to be kept moist to hold their shape, place them in a container of cool water or denture-cleaning solution (ask your dentist for advice). If your dentures have metal parts, do check that the cleaning solution is safe for them, and don't soak them any longer than recommended, or the metal may discolour. Never put dentures in hot water; heat can warp them.

FACT
— OR —
FALLACY?

'Older people should take smaller dosages of medicines than younger people.'

Fact The body's sensitivity to drugs increases with age, so older people can suffer serious side effects from drug dosages that would be harmless to younger people. Elderly people are often particularly sensitive to psychoactive drugs, such as sleeping pills. Unfortunately, overdoses of these drugs can go unrecognised. The symptoms – dizziness, fatigue, and confusion – are often interpreted as simply being part of ageing.

Good medical care

REGULAR CHECK-UPS

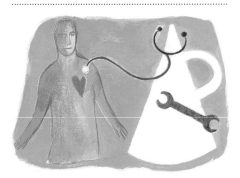

Now that I am getting on a bit, I wonder if I should see my doctor for an occasional check-up? He is always so busy, and I do not like to bother him unnecessarily.

Under the terms of their NHS contract, all family doctors are obliged to offer an annual check-up to any patient aged 75 or over, either in the surgery, or in the patient's own home – the choice is the patient's. However, if you want to be seen at home, the doctor may send a colleague instead. The check-ups enable doctors to monitor their patients' general health, and diagnose and treat problems before they become serious. The tests include measuring the height and weight of the patient, testing the blood pressure and urine, and checking the heart, lungs, and mobility of the joints, as well as checking for any commonly occurring diseases. Routine tests apart, never hesitate to consult your doctor if you have a problem that is worrying you. Your doctor's job is to look after you – and that includes setting your mind at rest. Doctors far prefer to see a patient who is well than one who has left it too late.

Do not let your doctor brush aside any of your physical complaints by replying 'What do you expect at your age?' A patient's age is no excuse for a doctor not making a proper diagnosis and giving effective treatment. Older people can respond to treatment just as well as the younger generation, and they deserve the same care and attention. When one great-grandmother went to visit her doctor, to complain of a sore shoulder, she was told: 'Well, you know, that shoulder is 83.' 'So is the other one,' she snapped back, 'but it doesn't hurt a bit.' On further examination, it turned out that she was suffering a severe sprain.

In addition to seeing your family doctor every year or so, you should continue having your eyes and teeth examined regularly.

SEEING A CHIROPODIST

I have heard that elderly people need to be particularly careful about their feet. Should I be visiting a chiropodist regularly? How should I look after my feet?

There is no need for you to see a chiropodist if your feet are not troubling you and you are able to take care of them easily yourself. If, however, you are unable to cut your toenails, or have problems such as painful feet, corns, or poor circulation, then you should see a chiropodist regularly for foot care. People who suffer from diabetes, or some other ailment that impairs the nerve supply to the feet, should also see a chiropodist regularly, as they may not feel minor chafing, cuts or bruises. These may develop into ulcers if not treated – a problem which could eventually become serious enough to necessitate a visit to the doctor.

To take proper care of your feet, wear well-fitting shoes that offer firm support. Avoid high heels, as these cause your toes to be compressed into the front of your shoes and may lead to bunions. Wash and dry your feet carefully every day, and keep them warm by wearing wool or cotton socks, stockings or tights. Avoid sitting with your legs crossed. If you wish to keep your feet raised, rest them instead on a footstool. When trimming your toenails, cut straight across the nail – never down the edges, as that could result in ingrown toenails and infection. Check your feet regularly for athlete's foot and corns (see page 147).

To maintain or improve circulation in your feet and legs, make a point of taking regular exercise. If your circulation is poor, and you smoke, you are at increased risk of ulcers, infections or gangrene. You should stop smoking immediately.

TOO MANY MEDICINES?

At the moment I am taking several different drugs for different ailments. Is there any danger that they could interact with each other and do more harm to me than good?

The risk of side effects produced by drugs increases with age. Not only do older people react more sensitively to a drug than younger people do; they are also often taking two or three medicines at once, which can combine in unfriendly ways. Not always, mind you: some drugs interact to the patient's advantage, one counteracting the unpleasant side-effect of another. Doctors are aware of the risks in combining drugs, and your doctor should regularly review the medicines you are taking and monitor their side effects, so that he can stop any particular treatment as soon as the risks outweigh the benefits. If he does not do this, you should ask him to. And you should in any case be on the lookout for side effects yourself.

Be careful when buying drugs over the counter, as they could react with various prescription medicines that you are taking. Check with your pharmacist for any possible clashes. If you remain worried, carry all your medications – including over-the-counter medicines and vitamins – to your doctor, so that he can advise you as to which ones you should keep taking and which ones you can do without.

KEEPING TRACK OF PILLS

My 75-year-old aunt has to take a number of different drugs to combat her various ailments, and gets very confused as to which ones she should take when. How can this problem be overcome?

Pharmacists are mindful of this problem, and will discuss it with a patient or relative of a patient when the prescription is being made up. Various pill-containers are available, with compartments clearly marked for the day and the time when medication has to be taken. You should be able to buy one of these from your local pharmacy. A pill or capsule is put into each compartment at the start of each round, and the patient simply follows the directions until all the compartments are empty.

Many drug companies are now packaging drugs in 'calendar packs'. These contain a complete course of a drug, with each pill in a separate compartment for the day when it should be taken.

Alternatively, your aunt could simply keep a record on a chart, where she ticks off each pill as she takes it.

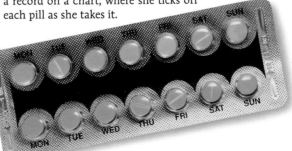

Pill of the day   Labelled packs of pills enable you to check how many you have taken.

Lids to make life easy

If you find it a struggle to remove childproof lids from medicine bottles, tell your pharmacist when you take a prescription in to be made up. He or she will then put your medicines in a container which can be opened more easily.

TURNING TO SLEEPING PILLS

I have noticed that I do not get as good a night's sleep as I used to, and that I sometimes 'drop off' during the day. Should I ask my doctor for sleeping pills?

It is quite natural for people's sleeping patterns to change as they reach old age. Elderly people find it harder to get to sleep at night, wake up more frequently at night, and spend less time in non-REM sleep (see page 158) – without which people will not waken feeling refreshed. Taking cat naps during the day is one way of making up for sleep lost at night, so don't worry if you tend to drop off to sleep during the day.

Before you ask your doctor for sleeping pills, try more natural methods of combatting insomnia (see page 159). Sleeping pills can sometimes be habit-forming, and may have nasty side effects or interact dangerously with other medications. They may also mask rather than solve the problems behind sleeplessness. Also, since older people have slower metabolisms, drowsiness brought on by a sleeping pill often continues into the next day, increasing the risk of accidents.

What symptoms mean

Signs of diabetes

One form of diabetes tends to afflict people only when they are at a fairly advanced age. It is usually manageable without insulin, being controlled by diet, or a combination of diet and drugs. The symptoms may be nothing more than a vague deterioration in general health, but there are some other indicators that might alert you.

● Continual feelings of thirst, which are not relieved by drinking.
● Passing excessive amounts of urine.
● Persistent itching of the vulva in women, or of the penis in men.
● Constant tiredness and irritability.
● A tendency to suffer from boils, skin infections and infections of the vulva or penis.
● Disturbances of vision, including difficulties with focusing.
● Ulcers on the feet.
● Pins and needles, or numbness of the feet and hands.

WALKING WITH A SHUFFLE

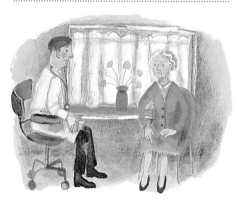

My grandmother's walk has become increasingly stiff and shuffling. Is this just a sign that she is getting older, or is it a symptom of disease?

It could be either. It could even be the effect of medications your grandmother may be taking, or simply the result of a sedentary way of life. Arthritis can produce a shuffling gait, as can a number of diseases affecting the mind, such as Alzheimer's disease (see page 441).

If, however, your grandmother shuffles along with bent knees, is bent at the waist and keeps her arms bent and motionless at her sides, she may well be suffering from Parkinson's disease. Other symptoms that you should look for are a slight tremor in her hand or arm when it is at rest, a frozen facial expression, dribbling, less blinking, and difficulty in swallowing.

Your grandmother should see her doctor as soon as possible about her shuffling gait, particularly if she exhibits some of the other symptoms of Parkinson's disease. Treatment for the disease involves a combination of antiparkinsonism drugs and physiotherapy, and is aimed at alleviating the symptoms of the disease and maintaining and improving the patient's mobility.

NIGHT-TIME CRAMPS

I sometimes suffer from cramps in my feet, or a creeping sensation in my legs at night. What can be causing this?

Night cramps in the feet are a common problem among elderly people, and often occur either after a lot of physical activity during the day, or after very little. Unfortunately, doctors are not sure what causes them. The cramp can be relieved by stretching the muscle which has gone into spasm. For prevention, there is a gentle stretching exercise that is worth trying. Stand facing a wall from a distance of one pace, and place your hands flat against it. Keeping your legs straight and your heels on the floor, lean slowly forward until the muscles in your calves feel stretched, but are not painful. Hold the stretch for ten seconds, straighten up and relax for five seconds, then stretch again. Repeat this exercise three times a day.

Some people are helped by lying on their backs and raising their feet in the air. Alternatively, quinine sulphate tablets, taken at night, may give relief.

The creeping sensation is called restless legs and can be very tiresome. Once again, doctors are not sure what causes the condition, but it is harmless. Most people are helped by moving or massaging their legs, or by getting out of bed and walking about.

LEG PAIN WHEN WALKING

I have recently experienced a cramp-like pain in my calf muscle when out walking. It subsides if I rest for a while and massage the muscle, but tends to strike again, sometimes extending right up to the buttock. What causes this?

It is important that you see your doctor as soon as possible, as your cramp-like pain sounds very much like a condition known as intermittent claudication. This is caused by narrowing arteries impeding the supply of blood to the leg muscles during exercise. If you use your arms a lot, you may find similar symptoms occurring. If you do not have the condition seen to, you will find that the symptoms occur more and more quickly each time you do any exercise.

Your doctor may refer you to a specialist for an assessment. In the meantime, he or she may suggest that you keep walking, stopping when the pain occurs and starting again once it has subsided. This will force the blood through smaller blood vessels, causing them to open, and thereby improving the blood supply to your leg. To tackle the root of the problem, take all the recommended precautions against adding to fatty deposits in the arteries (see pages 364–365). Most importantly, if you smoke, stop.

Drugs have proved disappointing in treating this condition, and drugs for other medical conditions may even make it worse. If the condition becomes serious, an arterial bypass operation can be done to improve the flow of blood to the leg.

LOSING YOUR BALANCE

My sister, who is in her 70s, has started having dizzy spells, and is afraid of falling and injuring herself. What is behind this problem and what can be done to treat it?

Dizzy spells occur frequently among elderly people, and can be caused by a variety of problems. Most doctors distinguish between light-headedness, or feeling faint, and vertigo, which is more of a spinning sensation.

Slight unsteadiness or light-headedness is often nothing more than a sign of tiredness, stress or depression, though it can also be brought on by anaemia, low blood pressure, arthritis in the neck, an under-active thyroid gland, or heart or circulation problems.

Vertigo, on the other hand, is normally related to disorders of the inner ear, where the balance centres are located. It is only rarely a sign of disease – such as viral infection – and even then it is usually severe and accompanied by other symptoms.

Severe attacks of vertigo on moving the head in a certain way, or changing position, may be a sign of positional vertigo, a mild condition that usually subsides with time. On the other hand, it could indicate arthritis of the neck, which causes pressure on veins in the neck, restricting the supply of blood, when the head is turned.

If the dizzy spells happen on sitting or standing up rapidly, the cause may be postural hypotension, a sudden drop in blood pressure caused by a change in position.

Your sister should see her doctor, so that checks can be made on her ears, blood pressure, and any drugs she is taking. If she experiences a dizzy spell, she should sit or lie down quietly until the spell passes.

SHORTNESS OF BREATH

I get very short of breath when I climb the stairs nowadays, and I have heard this might be an indication of heart trouble. Is this true?

Finding yourself more out of breath than normal may be a symptom of heart disease, though it is more likely to be the result of a lung disease. The most common cause of breathlessness is chronic bronchitis, which may in turn bring on emphysema.

If, however, breathlessness brought on by exertion – such as climbing stairs – is accompanied by breathlessness while you are in bed, and swelling in both ankles, it may well be a symptom of heart trouble.

What underlies these symptoms? The two sides of the heart act as a pump, the right side taking blood from the body and feeding it to the lungs, and the left side taking blood from the lungs and pumping it back into the body. As the pumping action of the heart becomes weaker – for example, if a valve is faulty, or after a severe heart attack – either side may pump less well – or both. If it is the right side of the heart that is failing, the blood in the body backs up, and the back pressure squeezes blood out into the legs and abdomen, causing swelling. If the left side fails, the fluid is pushed into the lungs, causing breathlessness. Often both sides fail, resulting in both symptoms.

Heart failure can be treated by various drugs. These include Angiotensin Converting Enzyme (ACE) inhibitors, which inhibit one of the enzymes that raises blood pressure – though sometimes at the risk of harming the kidneys – and diuretics, which increase the amount of fluid that the body excretes as urine.

Don't hesitate to see your doctor if you are suffering from abnormal breathlessness. If it turns out to be a symptom of heart trouble, the sooner it is treated the better.

UNEXPLAINED COLLAPSE

A few days ago my mother collapsed, and for a few hours afterwards struggled to speak. She seems fine now, but should she see her doctor? What caused the collapse?

It sounds as if your mother's collapse was brought on by a transient ischaemic attack, or TIA. A TIA is a brief interruption of the blood supply to the brain – due to either a blockage or a narrowing of the arteries. TIAs cause temporary strokelike symptoms, and are a common problem in people over 65. The effects last no more than a day – often only a few seconds or minutes – and may be imperceptible or no more alarming than a brief dizziness or numbness. Nevertheless, TIAs should be taken seriously, as they can be a prelude to a full-blown stroke.

A suspected TIA should be brought to your doctor's attention without delay. He or she can rule out other possible causes of the symptoms, and begin to look for evidence of high blood pressure or narrowed arteries. Treatment, often with aspirin or anticoagulant drugs, is aimed at preventing a major stroke. Patients with a more than 70 per cent blockage of one of the large carotid arteries supplying the brain may need an operation to remove the inner layer of the artery and the fatty deposits attached to it.

TROUBLE WITH URINATION

Although I feel the need to urinate frequently, it's always a struggle to start, and the urine flows slowly. Why is this?

There are several possible causes – such as diabetes, or some prescription drugs – for this symptom in men, and it is important for you to see a doctor, to get a definite diagnosis. The most likely cause of your problem is an enlarged prostate, a problem encountered by many men over the age of 60. The prostate is a gland lying at the neck of the bladder and in front of the rectum in men, which is responsible for producing part of the semen. It is the size of a plum and surrounds and feeds into the urethra – the canal through which urine is discharged. If the prostate becomes enlarged, it may press on the bladder at the same time as constricting the urethra, leading to the symptoms that you are describing. An enlarged prostate is usually benign, but in this case it will require treatment to allow you to pass urine normally again. There is a small risk that the operation may cause impotence.

However, your problem may have a more serious cause – prostate cancer. This condition – one of the most common cancers in men – gives rise to the same symptoms as an enlarged prostate. Doctors are aware of this, and will take it into account when examining patients. It is sometimes possible to make a diagnosis by feeling the prostate in a rectal examination. A blood test may also help. Whatever condition your doctor suspects, he will probably refer you to a consultant urologist for specialist advice, and, if necessary, treatment.

Overcoming illness

TREATING PROSTATE TROUBLE

Can cancer of the prostate be detected early enough for treatment to be successful?

It is sometimes possible to detect prostate cancer early enough to treat it, though not always. Cancer of the prostate is the third most common cancer among men – after lung cancer and bowel cancer – affecting nearly 14 000 people each year in Britain. It is mainly a disease of elderly men, and rarely strikes before the age of 50. Its behaviour is inconsistent: sometimes it spreads rapidly

causing death within a year of diagnosis; sometimes it progresses very slowly and can be kept under control; sometimes it produces no symptoms at all, and comes to light only after the patient has already died from some other cause.

Provided the cancer has not spread beyond the prostate by the time it has been detected, there are two options for treatment. The prostate gland can be removed surgically, which may cure the cancer, though it can lead to impotence and incontinence afterwards. Alternatively, drugs, usually including hormones, may be used to shrink the cancer.

This is the preferred treatment for patients suffering from more advanced cancers, and for patients who are not really fit enough to risk surgery.

It may not always be a good idea to have treatment, however, as, in some cases, the side effects of the treatment outweigh the benefits. In Britain, about half of all men aged between 70 and 80 develop localised prostatic cancers which never become life-threatening. In many cases, the best treatment is no treatment at all.

Since national screening programmes for cancer are expensive, it is unlikely that one will be set up for prostate cancer in Britain until there are better ways to identify which cases would most benefit from treatment.

AN END TO OSTEOPOROSIS?

Can I do anything about my osteoporosis now that I am in my 60s, or have I left it too late?

Osteoporosis is a loss of density in the bone, which makes it porous and weak, and easily broken. It is usually painless, but it explains why people over the age of 65 so often fracture their hips when they fall. It occurs in women more often than men. Caucasian women living to the age of 90 have a 30 per cent risk of fracturing a hip, and osteoporosis is usually a contributory factor.

The reason for this loss of bone mass is that, with age, the body becomes less efficient at gathering the calcium necessary to maintain bone density. Up to the age of about 30, a person's bone mass increases steadily, but after that it slowly decreases. In women, this decline accelerates at the onset of menopause. Certain women are at greater risk than others: white rather than black, those who are small and fair, or smoke and drink heavily, or take little exercise, and those who have had several children.

Unfortunately, there is no cure for osteoporosis, but its progress can be slowed by a diet rich in calcium and vitamin D, and a programme of weight-bearing exercises – such as weight training, jogging or walking. Non-weight-bearing exercises, such as swimming, have less effect on bone loss, but they will help you to maintain your flexibility and balance so that you are less likely to fall.

A proven preventive measure for women is hormone replacement therapy (HRT) (see page 394). It cannot restore lost bone mass, but it will dramatically reduce future losses, and it is never too late to start. Some doctors also recommend calcium supplements.

TREATING PARKINSON'S DISEASE

A friend of mine was recently told that she has Parkinson's disease. Is there any cure for the disease?

Unfortunately there is no cure for Parkinson's disease. However, there is a lot that can be done to treat the symptoms. Exercises can help maintain mobility and improve the patient's morale, while drugs can help to slow the progress of the disease.

Drug treatment can be complex, as several kinds of drugs may have to be administered in a variety of combinations. The disease is caused by a degeneration of the nerve cells situated at the base of the brain which produce dopamine, a chemical that helps to control muscle action by damping the messages sent from the brain. If the amount of dopamine produced is reduced, the characteristic tremors and muscle rigidity begin. The most effective drugs given to a Parkinson's sufferer are those, such as levodopa, which boost the level of dopamine in the brain. In a few cases, a brain operation may be performed to try to reduce the muscle tremor and rigidity cause by the condition.

Though the disease will worsen over time, these treatments can do much to improve the quality of life of a Parkinson's sufferer.

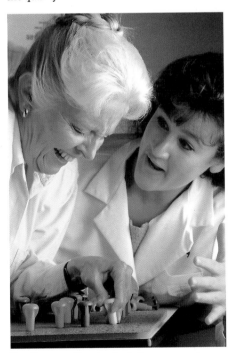

Peg therapy Simple physiotherapy exercises such as fitting pegs into holes can help to promote dexterity in patients coming to terms with arthritis or Parkinson's disease.

Treating high blood pressure in older people

Until recently, high blood pressure was thought to be a natural part of the ageing process, the body's way of compensating for the hardening of the arteries. And because the drugs used to lower blood pressure can produce unpleasant side effects (see page 362), particularly among elderly people, doctors sometimes resisted prescribing them.

Now things are changing. Recent studies have shown that medication can reduce the risk of a stroke in certain older patients with high blood pressure, even when in their 80s.

Still, the best way of getting and keeping blood pressure down remains regular exercise and a healthy diet.

How much treatment do you want?

All medical treatment involves some trade-offs of pros and cons, and older people in particular need to be certain that treatment will improve the quality of life, especially if it involves strong drugs or major surgery. Never feel pressured to start or to continue a course of treatment you are not sure about. Discuss any doubts with your doctor and don't go ahead until they are laid to rest.

RECOVERY FROM A STROKE

My elderly sister recently had a stroke. What are the chances of making a good recovery late in life? Are there any special types of therapy to help older people?

Strokes have varying effects on people of all ages and although age does affect recovery to some extent, many elderly sufferers do make remarkable progress. Certainly, some degree of recovery is the rule rather than the exception. The main factors that determine recovery are how severe the attack is, how swiftly it progressed – those that progress slowly will usually do less damage – and how soon treatment is given after the attack.

Stroke treatment is the same for people of any age. Once the immediate effects of the stroke have been dealt with, the patient is put on a course of physiotherapy, to help regain abilities as much as possible. Patients often suffer from depression after a stroke, and family and friends can be a great help in alleviating it, by offering a sympathetic ear, suggesting practical solutions to problems, and offering encouragement with each step towards recovery. (See also pages 366-367.)

About 95 per cent of all stroke sufferers recover sufficiently to achieve some form of independence, and most learn to walk again. About half recover more or less completely.

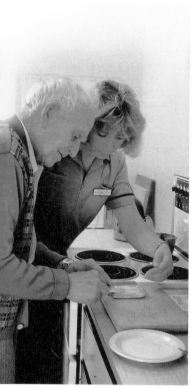

Old tricks Occupational therapy helps stroke patients to relearn everyday tasks, such as buttering toast.

HIP REPLACEMENTS

How successful are hip replacements in older people? Is the operation safe?

The insertion of an artificial hip joint has become a routine operation, having a 90 per cent rate of success. One result is that there are ever-lengthening waiting lists under the NHS. As long as a patient is in reasonably good health, the operation is a safe one, regardless of age. In fact, most operations are done on older people, firstly because they are more likely to suffer from stiff or arthritic hips, and secondly because younger patients, being more active, risk putting too much strain on the artificial joint.

The operation enables people previously crippled to walk again freely and without pain. Although the operation can be painful immediately afterwards, the pain is usually no more than that suffered before the operation. The new joint will be unstable at first, but within a few weeks of surgery nearly all patients report little or no pain, and even find that they are able to resume activities that they had had to give up. An artificial joint lasts for about ten years. It then needs to be replaced, as it starts to come away from the bone.

HOW SAFE IS HEART SURGERY?

I have heard of people being refused heart surgery on the grounds of age. How much riskier is it, and how are decisions made?

Since people over the age of 70 tend to be more frail than younger patients, the risks from cardiac surgery are higher, particularly during post-operative care. However, simple chronological age is never the key factor in making the decision whether to operate. Far more important considerations are the general condition of the patient and the likelihood of success. In turn, the prospects of success vary according to the kind of operation that needs to be performed. Although older patients are seldom considered for heart transplants, because of the difficulties involved in obtaining donated organs, most other heart operations should be possible, to a greater or lesser extent.

A healthy state of mind

TALKING ABOUT THE PAST

My grandfather is always talking about life in the 'good old days'. Is it healthy for him to be so occupied with the past?

Reminiscence is a healthy source of pleasure for older people, and a common way of passing down knowledge and experience from generation to generation within a family. After all, when someone has lived a long and eventful life, it is fun for them to savour again the extraordinary – as well as the ordinary – moments.

It is natural for your grandfather to look back and enjoy his memories. Remembering triumphs, tragedies and lessons learned may help him to come to terms with later life and to put things into perspective.

You could help him in this by expressing an interest. Most older people wish to have their experiences admired and appreciated.

If you are concerned that your grandfather is obsessed with the past, try to interest him more in the present. Keep him up to date with happenings in the family, and make an effort to spend time with him at family gatherings. If he tells the same stories over and over again, divert him by expressing an interest in another aspect of his life. Be patient rather than irritable with him: there may well be a great deal that you can learn from his experiences.

FEARS AND SUSPICIONS

My father is becoming increasingly suspicious in his old age. Is this paranoia, and is there anything I can do about it?

The fact that your father is becoming more and more suspicious does not mean that he is suffering from paranoia. Quite often, older people grow more suspicious for perfectly valid reasons, such as their knowledge of cases of theft or crime against elderly people. Elderly people are no more likely to have paranoid delusions than anyone else. In fact, the diseases which cause paranoia, such as schizophrenia and manic-depressive illness, usually occur when people are in their 20s, 30s or 40s.

Occasionally older people become suspicious because they find it difficult to give up control when younger family members take over their household and financial responsibilities. To some it feels as if the youngsters are trying to usurp their position of authority. If your father has recently had to give up driving, say, or been forced to move in with one of his children, or into a residential or nursing home, the change could leave him feeling angry and helpless.

If your father is suffering from memory lapses or visual problems that cause him to lose things, he may believe that someone is stealing from him rather than acknowledging the real reason. Simply making sure that his glasses are the correct prescription may solve the problem. Similarly, if your father has poor hearing, he may hear his name spoken – or imagine that he does – and think that people are discussing him behind his back. If this is the issue, help him to find a good hearing aid (see page 429).

Remember too that if your father spends much of his time alone, he may feel uncomfortable in the company of other people. What may seem like a suspicious attitude to you may just be loneliness and social awkwardness, and anything you can do to lessen his isolation will help.

'SEEING THINGS'

Recently my mother has started having hallucinations. Is something badly wrong?

Hallucinations are a fairly common experience in later life, and not an indication that a person is going mad. People with visual disorders quite often suffer from hallucinations, and disturbing visions are sometimes a side effect of drugs – for example, those prescribed for Parkinson's disease. They can also occur if someone who is an alcoholic suddenly stops drinking. People suffering from depression may also sometimes hallucinate; as do those who have recently been bereaved. Encourage your mother to see her doctor, so that he can diagnose the problem behind the hallucinations and prescribe the appropriate treatment.

KEEPING SPIRITS UP

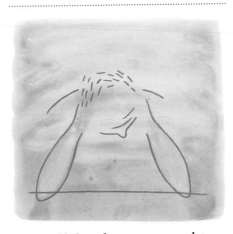

My grandfather often seems very unhappy. Is there anything I can do to cheer him up?

You can do a lot to brighten up your grandfather's life just by visiting him regularly, showing an interest and finding time to talk. Make plans to take him out for a meal. If he likes to play cards or watch films, help him to organise a group of friends for regular card games or trips to the cinema.

But take care not to help out too much. Researchers have found that one reason elderly people seem to slip into depression is that the people who care for them do not allow them enough independence. Elderly people are more likely to flourish when they can keep control of their lives (see page 442).

Encourage your grandfather to decide for himself what he really wants to do. If he does, he will enjoy greater self-esteem, and that will go a long way to cheering him up.

What are the causes of confusion?

Confusion is a state in which the sufferer is unable to make sense of the situation in which he finds himself and therefore feels lost and muddled. He may not be able to recognise well-known people or places or to complete simple tasks, and may respond inappropriately to questions or requests.

The condition has a variety of causes, including dementia, hypothermia, prescribed drugs, head injury, or a mental condition such as depression.

If someone shows signs of confusion, stay calm and call a doctor.

How to deal with depression

Everyone feels depressed at times but if the feeling is prolonged or severe, it needs treatment. It is not uncommon for elderly people to suffer from depression – the loss of health, financial security or friends or loved ones can all be contributing factors. Symptoms include a lack of interest in normal activities, frequent crying, loss of appetite, disturbed sleep and mood variations.

Never ignore such symptoms in yourself or others, and never tell someone depressed to 'pull yourself together'. Proper help is necessary and available from many sources – see pages 197-199, or ask your doctor.

When memory starts to fail

DO'S AND DON'TS

for talking to a dementia sufferer

Do make an effort to speak slowly and clearly.
Do try to use short, simple sentences.
Do maintain eye contact, to help the person focus on what is being said.
Do use physical contact. Holding the person's hand will help to keep their attention.
Do use gestures to reinforce your meaning.
Do use the person's name frequently, to strengthen his or her sense of identity.
Do allow the person plenty of time to respond to what you have said.

Don't raise your voice, as this can be upsetting to the sufferer.
Don't move around too much, or distract the person's attention.
Don't talk over competing noises.
Don't allow yourself to appear tense or agitated.
Don't be condescending to the person.
Don't offer complex choices. Ask one question at a time.

BECOMING FORGETFUL

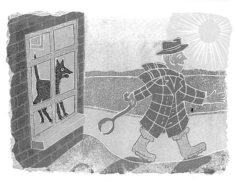

A friend in his late 70s seems to be losing his short-term memory. Is this a symptom of senile dementia, or is it just old age?

It may well be neither. There is no real evidence to suggest that a failing short-term memory is a normal part of old age. Elderly people who have a tendency to forget names or lose their keys were probably just as forgetful when they were younger.

Short-term memory loss could be caused by a number of conditions, few of which are serious. Some of the most common include stress, fatigue, grief, a bad cold and even just trying to remember too much. All of these can affect the ability to concentrate, which may in turn weaken the memory. If one of these is the root of the problem, your friend should find his memory improves as soon as he has a chance to relax or recover. On the other hand, if he just has a bad memory, he could try the techniques on page 177.

If memory loss becomes severe, however – for instance, if your friend gets lost in an area he knows well – and if it becomes progressively worse your concern may be well-founded. If this is the case, encourage your friend to see a doctor for proper diagnosis.

LIVING WITH DEMENTIA

My father has been diagnosed as having dementia, and I am now taking care of him. What can I do to lessen the problems caused by his condition?

The main problem for someone suffering from dementia is the fear and confusion that occur when he or she loses track of time and place, and the anger felt at no longer being able to do simple tasks. Fortunately, there are many simple things you can do to help your father to stay in touch.

● Keep a large, easy-to-read clock in the living room, and one with a bright digital face next to his bed in case he wakes up during the night.
● Buy a tear-off day-by-day calendar, and make sure to keep it up to date so that your father always knows which day it is.
● Label doors 'bedroom', 'bathroom' and so on, or put pictures on them to help your father find his way about the house.
● Keep photographs of family members and close friends on view.
● Remind your father about events shortly before they happen, and keep providing clues about what is going on. If you have a visitor, introduce his or her name into the conversation tactfully from time to time.
● Break tasks down into smaller ones, and it will then be easier for your father to manage. Instead of telling him to get ready for bed, say, work through the list: brushing teeth and so on.
● Have your father's vision and hearing checked regularly. Poor eyesight and hearing will rob him of sensory information, adding to his confusion.

PREVENTING WANDERING

Why do people with dementia sometimes take to wandering? What can family members do to help?

The reasons for wandering vary – and they also give the best clue to preventing this worrying behaviour. Some people who wander are simply bored or restless, in which case mental stimulation and exercise will usually solve the problem. Others search for things they have lost, so keeping their personal possessions on display can help.

Often sufferers wander after they have visited a strange place, or a routine in their lives has changed. Carers and relatives can help by making any such changes as smooth and stress-free as possible.

It is not a good idea to give medication such as sedatives, as anything strong enough to prevent wandering may well make the person drowsy and perhaps incontinent. If there is no apparent reason for wandering, it may be necessary to take special measures in order to prevent the person from leaving the house unattended.

● Hide all keys to outside doors. Make sure, however, that other members of the household know where they are, in case there is a fire.
● Try to find the time to go out with the person as often as you can. Do not leave him or her unaccompanied.
● People with dementia should carry some form of identification – an identity bracelet, for instance – in case they get lost.
● Tell neighbours and local shopkeepers about the problem. Ask them to contact you if they see the person wandering off.

If a person with dementia does get lost, there is no need for panic. He or she is unlikely to come to any harm. However, if the person cannot be found in the neighbourhood, the police should be contacted. Once the person has been found, try not to get angry, as he or she will probably already be confused and frightened. Carers should also remember not to blame themselves – or anyone else – if a dementia sufferer gets lost. No one can be expected to keep a 24-hour watch on someone else.

ALZHEIMER'S DISEASE

What is Alzheimer's disease? Is it the same as senile dementia?

Alzheimer's disease – a progressive degeneration of nerve cells in the brain – is one of the principal types of senile dementia, accounting for more than half of all dementia sufferers. Unfortunately, no one really knows what causes the disease.

Alzheimer's manifests itself differently in different people, although most cases follow a similar progression: from problems with memory and concentration, through trouble with speech and a tendency to get lost in familiar locations, to a state of confusion so severe that sufferers are unable to look after themselves. The disease may take years to run its course, but once the patient becomes bedridden, life expectancy is not long.

If these symptoms become apparent, the sufferer should see a doctor, and if necessary, a psychiatrist, to determine whether the cause really is Alzheimer's disease, or whether it is some other form of dementia – perhaps curable.

Unfortunately, there is no known cure for Alzheimer's disease, though certain symptoms, such as anxiety, depression, psychotic thinking, sleeplessness and behavioural disturbances can be treated with drugs. Also helpful are proper nutrition, guided exercise and physical therapy and the maintenance of a daily routine and social contact.

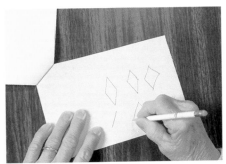

Drawing conclusions One of many tests to check the progress of Alzheimer's disease is to see if the patient can still copy simple shapes.

INHERITED ALZHEIMER'S

My father suffered from Alzheimer's disease. Does this mean I will get it too?

Only a small percentage of Alzheimer's cases are inherited, so you are very unlikely to be affected. Even when the illness runs in a family, only half the members contract it.

Unfortunately, there is as yet no way of genetically screening for Alzheimer's disease, so it is impossible to be absolutely certain whether any individual case of the disease is genetically inherited. However, where heredity does play a part, the onset of the disease is usually fairly early – between the ages of 35 and 60. So, unless you know of at least three family members who have developed Alzheimer's at about the same age, and that age was less than 60, it is highly unlikely that there are any genetic risks in your case. Remember that the disease is fairly common among elderly people, so even if two or more family members over 65 do contract it, that does not necessarily indicate the the disease has been genetically passed on.

GETTING HELP

Where can relatives go for help if a family member develops Alzheimer's disease?

Start by seeing the doctor of the person concerned, who can put you in touch with specialist services and community nursing staff. For further advice and support, families may also find it helpful to contact the Alzheimer's Disease Society, 2nd floor, Gordon House, 10 Greencoat Place, London SW1P 1PH.

DO'S AND DON'TS

for looking after a person with dementia

Do allow and encourage as much independence as possible. The more dignity can be preserved the less frustrated and helpless the person will feel and the easier it will be for carers.
Do establish routines so that the person finds it easier to remember what is supposed to happen, thereby easing your task.
Do help the person to maintain their general fitness and health. Physical and mental wellbeing are very closely related.
Do ensure that the home is as safe as possible. People who are confused are more prone to accidents.
Do maintain a sense of humour. Although dementia is a tragic illness, it will help both you and the patient if you can see the funny side of a situation.

Don't suddenly start treating someone as an invalid just because dementia is diagnosed. Try to keep things as normal as possible.
Don't argue if you can avoid it. If the person is reluctant to do something necessary, such as change dirty clothing, try introducing a distraction. Patients soon forget that they don't want to comply.
Don't introduce sudden changes or rush a person with dementia. It will only add to the confusion they feel.

Caring for others - and for yourself

Finding information about benefits

Information on benefits for carers and those they care for is available from the Carers National Association, 29 Chilworth Mews, London W2 3RG, and from the Disablement Information and Advice Line (01302) 31 0123.

Local branches of Age Concern and Help the Aged can also help, as can organisations for specific illnesses.

If you have a social worker, he or she should be a good source of information too. In addition, you can contact your local social security office or Citizens Advice Bureau.

HOW MUCH SHOULD YOU DO?

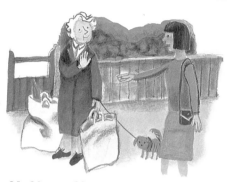

My 80-year-old mother is determined to be independent and never asks for help, even when it is clearly needed. How much should I insist on doing for her?

It is best to let elderly people do as much as they feel they can. In fact, they should be encouraged to be independent, even to the point of taking risks. Only if your mother is placing herself at risk of serious physical injury should you attempt to intervene.

HELPING WITH HYGIENE

I have noticed that an old friend of mine has begun to lose interest in her appearance, becoming untidy and even sometimes forgetting to wash. How can I get her to take care of herself again?

The problem of explaining to people that their hygiene is deteriorating is never an easy one. Your friend may welcome your help, or she may resent what she sees as intrusion. You will need to speak to her in a forthright way, and try to determine the cause of her lapse in hygiene if you can.

Sometimes depression is the root of the problem. People suffering from depression can become apathetic and bored with daily rituals such as washing. If you suspect this is the cause, encourage your friend to see her doctor, as in most cases depression can be successfully treated.

Alternatively, she may have an alcohol problem (see page 206). Older people sometimes feel that alcohol is their only solace when they are lonely and depressed, and can easily become addicted, losing interest in everything else. If your friend is neglecting her hygiene simply because she is too weak to take proper care of herself, try to arrange help for her. Social services can provide care assistants who will help with bathing, and home helps too can make a great difference.

ALLOWANCES AND BENEFITS

I gave up my job to take care of my father after his stroke. Now we are finding it increasingly difficult to cope financially. What financial assistance am I entitled to?

Both you and your father are entitled to benefits from the Department of Social Security and your local authority. These may be paid weekly, or as a one-off grant, or over a limited period. Apply for benefits as soon as you can, as most are payable only from the date of application. If you are not happy with the benefits you receive you can appeal, but do so quickly as there is often only a short time permitted for lodging an appeal.

Some of the allowances and benefits listed below may be applicable to you:

● Income support – for those working less than 16 hours a week – is intended to ensure that you have enough to live on. It is means-tested.

● Unemployment Benefit is paid for the first 12 months after you have become unemployed, as long as you have paid National Insurance contributions.

● Council Tax Benefit is paid to relieve you from some or all of your council tax. It is means-tested.

● Housing Benefit will help to pay the rent if you are on a low income. It is means-tested.

● Home Responsibilities Protection protects the pension rights of a carer who is looking after someone 35 hours a week for 48 weeks a year, and cannot contribute to his or her own pension. The person being cared for must be receiving Attendance Allowance.

● Invalid Care Allowance is given to those of working age who are looking after a disabled person for more than 35 hours a week and earning less than £50 a week.

● Attendance allowance is paid to people over 65 who are severely disabled and need looking after at home.

If you are in any doubt as to whether or not you are eligible for a particular benefit, do still apply.

WHEN YOU CANNOT MANAGE

My husband has started to need round-the-clock care, and I can no longer cope alone at home. What are my options?

As a carer you have a right to receive support in the valuable job that you are doing. The first person you should speak to if you are struggling to cope is your doctor. He can refer you to a range of professional people with special skills. A district nurse can visit your husband to change dressings, and may help with bathing and toileting. A night nurse can provide nursing care if your husband is very ill or has long-term needs, and give you a break. A range of professional people – such as occupational therapists, chiropodists dieticians and psychiatrists – can help with specific medical problems. Your doctor may also be able to organise short hospital stays for your husband, to give you a few days' rest.

It is also possible to get social services help via your local authority. Respite care – in which either someone comes to your home or your father goes to a day centre or to a respite home – will allow you some time off, whether this is for a few hours a day or, pehaps, for a week's holiday. There are also adult placement schemes, which will allow your father to stay with a local family every other day, and sometimes for longer periods.

Be persistent when asking for help. Don't give up if it is refused; keep on repeating what you want. On the other hand, don't refuse assistance simply because it is not exactly what you were looking for. You may not get another offer.

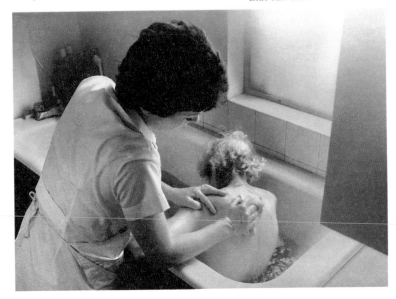

Washing aid District nurses or care assistants will make home visits to help with washing and other tasks that can cause trouble.

Facing the end without fear

PREVENTING PAIN

I am not afraid of death, because I have a strong religious faith, but I am afraid of the pain and suffering that may precede it. Is death usually a painful experience?

In most cases, the days, weeks or months before death can be made peaceful and free from pain. The easiest deaths are those that happen suddenly, from a heart attack or stroke, for example. About one in ten people over the age of 50 die peacefully in such ways. Even for those people who die slowly, the final stage is almost always placid rather than pain-ridden.

Good doctors and nurses are immensely compassionate people, and will do all that they can to alleviate the suffering of a dying patient. Methods of pain control have been studied and developed, and the approach now advocated is to give pain-killing drugs at regular intervals, to control the pain at all times. Many nurses take special training courses in caring for the dying, and know how to relieve problems such as vomiting, breathlessness and constipation in a dying patient. They also learn how to support the patient psychologically, so that he or she does not feel isolated, and they can offer emotional support to relatives and friends.

Whether you die in a hospital or at home, well-trained doctors and nurses will make the ending of life as comfortable and dignified as they can.

EXPRESSING YOUR WISHES

How can I make sure that my wishes will be carried out at the end? Can I insist that I am not kept alive artificially if there is no hope of recovery?

The freedom to decide what medical treatment you get is the right of every competent person. However, if you become so ill that you can no longer make or communicate your own decisions, relatives, friends and

Talking about death

Always be sensitive when talking to someone facing death, and let yourself be guided by their needs. It is natural to be optimistic about recovery, and no purpose is served by insisting on brutal realism to someone still hoping to get better.

That said, there may come a time when a dying person wants to talk about the end and perhaps to say goodbye or set things aright. Make sure there are chances to do so, and to be alone with those who are close, but leave it to the dying person to raise the matter. Don't avoid the subject either or give false comfort – listening and honesty are what's needed most.

doctors must make them for you. This may mean that you are kept alive for far longer than you would wish, as these people may well feel that they cannot claim the right to let you die.

A possible solution is to draw up a living will. This is a document that comes into operation only if the person loses the mental competence or power of communication to instruct the doctor directly, and it states in advance the person's express wish not to be kept alive by treatment if the quality of life would then be unacceptable. Living wills are now fairly widely permitted and regulated in the United States, but in Great Britain the medical, ethical and legal issues continue to be debated, and legislation still lies ahead.

It is possible to get a living-will form from stationers in Britain, though it is not a legally binding document. Nevertheless, it will allow you to let family, friends and doctors know your wishes, and it should influence their decisions.

HOSPICE CARE

I believe there is something called hospice care, which helps people to die in peace and with dignity. What exactly is a hospice, and how do I find out if there is one near me?

A hospice is a place where those who are dying can be tended by medical staff with special skills in that area. The hospice movement was started in 1967 by Dame Cicely Saunders, who believed passionately that the

care given to dying patients was inadequate. The principles of the movement are that pain should be kept under control by regular administration of drugs, that staff should be expert in controlling pain and other distressing symptoms, and that patients and their relatives should be given all the psychological, emotional and spiritual support they may need.

Patients are often discharged and returned home when their symptoms have been controlled, and hospice nurses visit them to give what nursing care they require, so allowing them to stay at home for as long as possible.

Hospices tend to be financed by independent charities, often with a supporting grant from the NHS. The best way to find out if there is one in your area is to ask your doctor or your local health authority.

NEAR-DEATH EXPERIENCES

Do scientists know anything about what it is like to die? I have heard that people who have been near death but have been revived have talked about this experience. What have they said?

The near-death experience has often been described both in national newspapers and medical journals, mainly by people who have been resuscitated while in coronary care or intensive care units. The descriptions have been remarkably similar – of time being distorted to let you view your life as a whole, of leaving your body and floating above it while watching the doctors and nurses trying frantically to bring you back to life, of the disappearance of pain and discomfort, of a feeling of peace and joy, of a sensation of warmth and light, and of a sense of moving, often through a dark tunnel, towards welcoming figures, perhaps loved ones already dead. And there is a reluctance to return, which is overcome only by conscious effort and by thoughts of friends and family left behind.

Scientists have speculated on the causes of such experiences. The usual theory seems to be that a sudden drop in blood pressure or loss of oxygen to the brain affects various mental faculties – the visual sense, notably – and produces hallucinations of bright light, floating and so on. But some researchers remain unconvinced, and are investigating the phenomenon by taking it at face value. By hiding marked objects in intensive care units – on top of cupboards, for instance, where they could be seen only from ceiling level – they are hoping to test any reported out-of-body experiences.

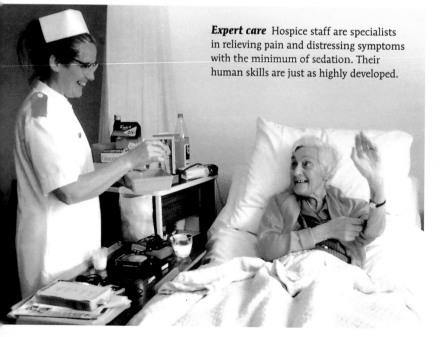

Expert care Hospice staff are specialists in relieving pain and distressing symptoms with the minimum of sedation. Their human skills are just as highly developed.

COPING WITH EMERGENCIES

Lives are saved every day by people with basic first-aid training. To be useful in an emergency, you must stay calm and think before you act. You must know how to tell when injury is serious and when it's not, when to go for help and what to try yourself.

Could you cope in an emergency?

When accidents and emergencies happen, following a few simple steps can save lives and prevent serious injury, so it is important to have a sound knowledge of the basics of first aid. Try this test to find out how well you would react in an emergency. Tick the right answer to each question and check your score below.

1 *You have found someone unconscious and holding a power drill. You suspect that he may have had an electric shock. What would you do first?*

a) Telephone for an ambulance. ☐
b) Pull the person clear of the drill. ☐
c) Attempt to turn off the electricity. ☐

2 *A man has fainted and is lying on the floor. Which of the following actions should you take, once you have made sure he is breathing?*

a) Raise his feet above the level of his head. ☐
b) Put a pillow under his head. ☐
c) Give him a sip of brandy. ☐

3 *A little girl has a piece of broken glass embedded in her forearm and is bleeding heavily. After you have summoned medical help, what should you do next?*

a) Attempt gently to remove the glass from her arm. ☐
b) Press down on either side of the wound to staunch the bleeding. ☐
c) Tie a tourniquet around the upper arm to stop the blood flow. ☐

4 *You suspect a child has swallowed some sleeping pills, thinking they were sweets. After calling an ambulance, what should you do?*

a) Give the child large quantities of water to drink. ☐
b) Put a finger down the child's throat to induce vomiting. ☐
c) Get the child to lie down and keep him or her warm. ☐

5 *A friend has accidentally poured boiling water over her hand and scalded it. What should she do?*

a) Hold her hand under cold running water. ☐
b) Put a sticking plaster over the scalded area. ☐
c) Smear cold butter on the site of the scald. ☐

6 *An elderly woman is weak and confused, and complains of feeling cold. You suspect hypothermia. You call an ambulance and wrap her in a blanket. What do you do next?*

a) Give her a glass of brandy or whisky. ☐
b) Give her a hot, sweet drink such as tea or chocolate. ☐
c) Get her to walk around to warm up. ☐

7 *You witness a young man having an epileptic fit. What should you do?*

a) Put something in his mouth to stop him biting his tongue. ☐
b) Move furniture and other sharp objects out of the way. ☐
c) Try to restrain him. ☐

SCORING

Score 1 point for each of these answers: 1(c), 2(a), 3(b), 4(c), 5(a), 6(b) and 7(b). Add up your score.

5-7: You would be a useful person to have around in most emergencies.

4 or less: Your common sense may help you in some situations, but if anything serious happened you might find yourself out of your depth.

Whatever your score, consider enrolling for a first-aid course or for refresher training.

The Principles of First Aid

BEFORE EMERGENCY STRIKES

A basic understanding of first aid should be part of everyone's general knowledge. Even if you never have to use the advice in these pages, reading them should leave you feeling confident and capable of dealing with most situations that call for urgent action. And if you are ever faced with a real emergency, knowing what to do and staying calm can help to prevent serious injuries, comfort any casualties and even save lives.

BE PREPARED
Don't put it off, but get organised now. Just a few hours is enough for the basics.

● Consider taking a first-aid course or at least learning the basic life-saving techniques of artificial respiration and cardiopulmonary resuscitation (CPR). The British Red Cross, St John Ambulance, St Andrew's Ambulance and the Royal Life Saving Society all run courses, some lasting as little as two hours.
● Keep an up-to-date list of emergency numbers by the telephone. Include your doctor, dentist, local hospital, police station, and gas, electricity and water helplines.
● Work out the best route to your nearest hospital accident and emergency department. Practise it from time to time if it is out of your normal way.
● Assemble or buy good first-aid kits (see page 167) for your home and car. Make sure to replace used items straight away and don't let any use-by dates expire.
● Install fire extinguishers and smoke alarms at home and test them regularly.

ASSESSING A DANGEROUS SITUATION

Whenever an accident or emergency occurs, it is important to take stock of the situation before going into action.

● Get your feelings under control. Take a few deep breaths if necessary.
● Think before you act. On no account do anything that places your own life in danger.
● Call for help if you are alone and someone may hear you.

● Deal with any continuing threats before giving first aid.
● Determine the number of casualties and the seriousness of their injuries.
● Consider who is available to help and whether specialist help should be summoned by dialling 999.

CHECKING A CASUALTY'S CONDITION

Before giving first aid, evaluate the severity of the casualty's injuries. Ask yourself the following questions:

IS THE PERSON CONSCIOUS?
To find out, ask a loud, clear question such as 'Can you hear me?'. Gently shake the person's shoulders. If there is no response at all, the casualty is unconscious. If the eyelids flicker or the person groans or utters a sound, he or she is probably semiconscious.

HAS BREATHING STOPPED?
Watch the chest to see if it rises and falls and listen for sounds of breathing. Clear the airway (see page 450) and feel with your cheek for air movement from the mouth.

IS THERE A PULSE?
A strong pulse means that the heart is beating well. Take the pulse at the carotid artery in the neck (see page 449). In babies under a year, you can also try at the brachial point halfway up the inside of the upper arm.

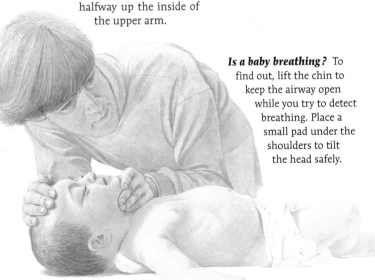

Is a baby breathing? To find out, lift the chin to keep the airway open while you try to detect breathing. Place a small pad under the shoulders to tilt the head safely.

447

When you dial 999

Follow this procedure in any situation where there are casualties.

1 Dial 999 and ask for the ambulance service.

2 Have the following information ready:

- Your exact location.
- Any local landmarks.
- The type of accident.
- The number, sex and ages of casualties.
- The suspected nature and severity of injuries.
- Any continuing hazards in the area.

3 Ask about giving first aid while you wait for help to arrive.

4 Wait for the emergency control officer to clear the line before hanging up.

TAKING ACTION

In any situation where you suspect serious injury, the procedure depends on how many people are available to help at the scene.

IF OTHERS ARE PRESENT

Send someone to telephone 999 for the emergency services while whoever is most qualified gives first aid.

IF YOU ARE ALONE

Take action according to the condition of the casualty:

UNCONSCIOUS, NO PULSE, NOT BREATHING
The chance of resuscitation is slight, so telephone 999 for an ambulance, then administer artificial respiration (see pages 449-452) including, if trained, chest compression.

UNCONSCIOUS, NOT BREATHING, PULSE PRESENT
First give ten mouth-to-mouth ventilations (see pages 450-451), then telephone 999 for an ambulance, then continue ventilation.

UNCONSCIOUS, BREATHING, PULSE PRESENT
Treat any serious injuries, place casualty in the recovery position (see panel below) and then go for help.

CONSCIOUS, BREATHING, PULSE PRESENT
Treat any injuries as appropriate, then go for help if needed.

WHEN HELP ARRIVES

Be ready to give as much information as you can to the doctor or ambulance personnel. Mention all of the symptoms you have observed, any hazards in the area and any possible clues to what may have happened – signs of poisoning or pill-taking, for example. Then ask what more you can do to help and follow any instructions scrupulously.

PLACING A CASUALTY IN THE RECOVERY POSITION

Once any immediate threats to life have been attended to and help is on its way, casualties who are unconscious but still breathing should be placed in the recovery position. The position is designed to keep the windpipe clear and to prevent choking or swallowing the tongue. Only when the casualty is in the recovery position is it safe to tend to other wounds.

CAUTION Casualties with suspected back or neck injuries of any sort should not be moved at all, even to place them in the recovery position. They need expert help.

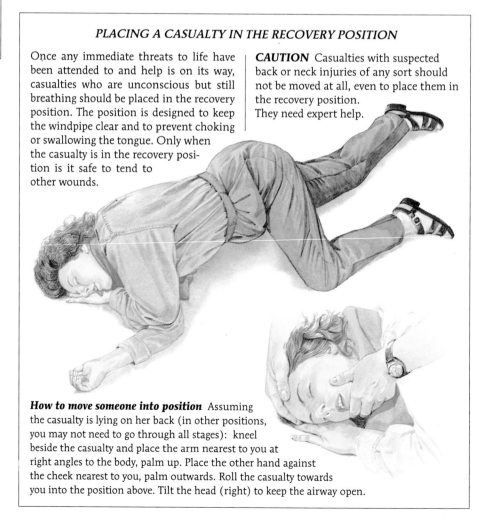

How to move someone into position Assuming the casualty is lying on her back (in other positions, you may not need to go through all stages): kneel beside the casualty and place the arm nearest to you at right angles to the body, palm up. Place the other hand against the cheek nearest to you, palm outwards. Roll the casualty towards you into the position above. Tilt the head (right) to keep the airway open.

Emergencies A-Z

ALLERGIC REACTION

A massive allergic reaction to a sting, drug or food can give rise to a condition known as anaphylactic shock. It can occur within seconds or be delayed 30 minutes or more. If not treated immediately, the casualty may lose consciousness, and stop breathing.

WARNING SIGNS
- Feeling very weak and sick.
- Tight chest, wheezing, difficult breathing.
- Swollen face or throat.

ACTION
Call for emergency medical help at once. While you are waiting, lay the person on his back. Raise his feet on a cushion or folded coat or blanket. Keep the head low and turn it to one side in case of vomiting. Keep the airway open and if necessary give mouth-to-mouth resuscitation (see pages 450-451).

Apply a cold compress to the stung area if symptoms follow a sting, but do not place ice directly on the skin (it might cause frostbite). Keep the casualty warm with a blanket or rug. Loosen tight clothing around the neck and waist to make breathing easier. Don't give anything to eat or drink, and do not allow smoking.

Give an adrenaline injection – some sufferers of severe allergic reactions keep one in the refrigerator – or antihistamine if possible. If the casualty becomes unconscious or breathing becomes difficult, put him in the recovery position (see panel, facing page).

ARTIFICIAL RESPIRATION

Artificial respiration, properly administered, can save lives, and should be applied if a casualty is not breathing on his own. Always take time to establish the casualty's condition before proceeding.

ASSESSING THE CASUALTY
First check that the airway is clear and then check to see if the casualty is still breathing. Kneel down next to the casualty with your ear just above the mouth and nose. Look along the chest. If the person is breathing, you should hear and feel air movement and see the chest rising and falling.

If breathing is laboured, clear the airway and then, if necessary, give mouth-to-mouth resuscitation. If breathing has stopped, the next step is to check for a pulse. The carotid artery in the neck is the best place for adults and older children (the wrist pulse is not a good indicator.) For babies under a year, feel the pulse on the inside of the upper arm.

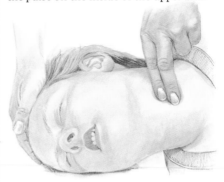

Feeling for a pulse To feel the neck pulse, place two fingers gently in the hollow of the neck between the Adam's apple and the large neck muscle.

WHEN THERE IS A PULSE BUT NO BREATHING
Brain damage and death can occur within minutes, so it is essential to get air into the lungs as quickly as possible. First clear the airway (see page 450) – this alone may be enough to start breathing in some cases. If not, give mouth-to-mouth resuscitation (see pages 450-451). If you are alone, give ten puffs of air and then telephone 999 and ask for an ambulance. If help is available, one person should telephone while the other attempts resuscitation without interruption.

NO BREATHING AND NO PULSE
Resuscitation is always much more difficult in these circumstances. It requires a combination of mouth-to-mouth ventilation and chest compression – also known as cardio-pulmonary resuscitation (CPR). In this situation, contacting the emergency services is the first priority. Once help is on its way, you may begin chest compression (see pages 451-452) provided you have been trained.

Remember, however, that chest compression can be dangerous. If the heart is compressed while it is still beating, even faintly, it may stop completely. Damage to the lungs, liver, spleen and ribs can also occur. You can administer chest compression safely only after establishing conclusively that the casualty's heartbeat has stopped completely (signalled by a lack of pulse). Administering chest compression requires understanding, skill and practice. Attempt it only if you have been formally trained. The instructions that appear on pages 451-452 are intended only as a memory aid for trained first aiders, and as an encouragement for others to learn.

CLEARING THE AIRWAY

Opening up the windpipe is the first stage of resuscitation. It is safe provided there is no neck or back injury.

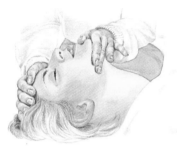

1 Lift the chin with one hand and press down on the forehead with the other. This extends and opens the windpipe.

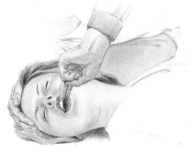

2 If breathing does not begin, turn the casualty's head to the side and with your fingers clear the mouth of any foreign matter.

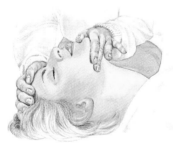

3 Listen for breathing. See if the chest rises and falls. Place your ear close to the nose and mouth and feel for exhaled air. If regular breathing resumes, put the casualty in the recovery position (see page 448) until medical help arrives. If opening the airway doesn't restore breathing, start artificial respiration.

MOUTH-TO-MOUTH VENTILATION

If clearing the airway alone does not restore breathing, you will need to try mouth-to-mouth resuscitation. This is a simple but vital skill, best learned at a first-aid course. Get someone to call an ambulance while you lay the casualty face up on a firm surface.

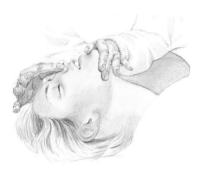

1 After clearing the airway, pinch the nostrils together with one hand to close the nose. Take a deep breath.

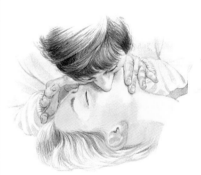

2 Seal your lips around the casualty's open mouth and breathe out for 1 to 1½ seconds. Then remove your mouth. The casualty's chest should rise and fall. If it does not, check for choking (see page 456).

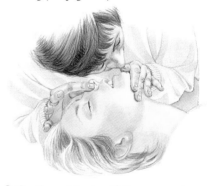

3 Continue giving ventilations every six seconds until the casualty breathes alone, or until expert help comes. Remove your mouth after every breath and observe closely for signs of breathing – chest movement, air movement or sounds of breathing.

VENTILATING A BABY OR SMALL CHILD

1 After clearing the airway, seal your lips around both mouth and nose.

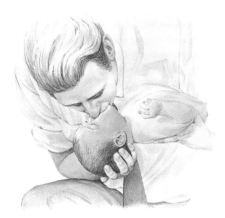

2 Administer gentle puffs of air so that the infant's chest rises visibly. Give one puff every three seconds for a baby and one every four seconds for a child of one year or older. Check carefully for any signs of breathing after you give each breath.

IF MOUTH-TO-MOUTH IS IMPOSSIBLE

Occasionally a mouth injury or a case of suspected poisoning may prevent mouth-to-mouth resuscitation, or make it inadvisable. In such cases, hold the mouth shut with your hand and breathe into the nose using the same technique as for mouth-to-mouth.

Check the pulse regularly. If it stops, a trained person should begin chest compression immediately.

CHEST COMPRESSION ON AN ADULT

Chest compression is used when both heart and breathing have failed – signalled by a complete lack of pulse (see page 449). Only trained first-aiders should administer it, and only once help has been sent for.

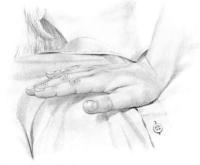

1 Kneel beside the casualty and place the heel of one hand on the chest, two finger-widths up from the bottom of the breastbone. Keep your thumb and fingers raised, so that they do not press on the ribs.

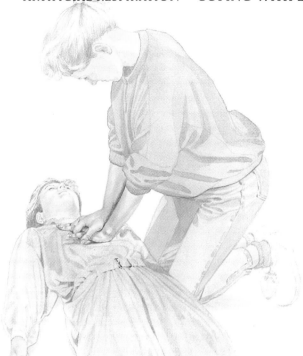

2 Clench your second hand over the first and apply pressure with the heel of the hand. Press down 1½-2 in (4-5 cm), keeping thumbs and fingers raised. Let the chest rise again. Give 15 compressions at normal pulse rate (80 beats a minute), then inflate the lungs twice by mouth-to-mouth ventilation. Repeat four times a minute, checking for a pulse every minute. Watch closely for signs of returning circulation, such as improved colour in the lips or earlobes. If they occur, check the pulse and stop if beating has resumed.

COMPRESSION ON A BABY

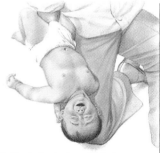
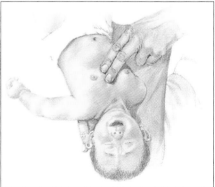

1 Begin by laying the baby down on a firm surface, such as a table, or hold him on your arm, cradling his head in your hand. Put your index finger on the breastbone at the level of the nipples, then move your index finger one finger width below this point. This is the area of chest compression.

2 Use two fingers only to administer chest compression to a baby – the index and middle finger of one hand. The depth of compression must be no more than 1 in (2.5 cm) and the rate about 100 times a minute. Pause to give one breath of mouth-to-mouth resuscitation after every five compressions.

COMPRESSION ON A CHILD

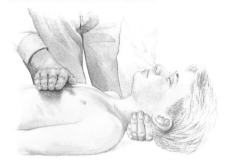

Giving compressions Using only the heel of one hand, press down on the lower breastbone 1-1½ in (2.5-4 cm) about 100 times a minute. Give a breath of artificial ventilation after every five compressions.

ASPHYXIATION

Many conditions can lead to asphyxiation, a state of dangerously reduced oxygen levels in the blood. The commonest causes include a blockage or constriction of the airway by food or drink, or by the tongue falling back in the throat. A heavy weight on the chest can have a similar effect, as can smoke or gas inhalation, suffocation and fluid entering or accumulating in the lungs. Strangulation can also be a cause. Children are particularly at risk of suffocation from plastic bags.

WARNING SIGNS
● Difficult or noisy breathing. Without help, breathing may eventually stop.
● Face turns blue and becomes congested. Nails may turn blue.
● Loss of consciousness and possibly fits.

ACTION
Deal first with any ongoing danger such as smoke or escaped gas. Once the area is safe, clear the casualty's airway by turning the head to one side and removing any debris from the mouth. Take care not to push any obstruction farther back towards the throat. Check for breathing and pulse and, if necessary, give artificial respiration (see pages 449-452). Treat for choking (see page 456) if you suspect this is the problem.

Once the casualty's breathing has been stabilised, place him or her in the recovery position (see page 448). Summon medical attention urgently, but try not to leave the person unattended for any length of time. Observe breathing closely and be prepared to resume artificial respiration if you find it faltering at any stage.

Stings in the mouth or throat

The danger of a sting in the mouth or throat is that the throat may swell rapidly and block the airway to the lungs. Give the victim an ice cube to suck or cold water to rinse the mouth and then spit out. If the casualty has difficulty breathing, start mouth-to-mouth resuscitation immediately (see pages 450-451). Telephone 999 for an ambulance.

ASTHMA ATTACK

A serious asthma attack can be extremely frightening and distressing for all those concerned. The muscles of the patient's air passages contract, making breathing difficult. Attacks can be triggered by an allergy, by nervous tension, respiratory infections, changes in temperature or exercise. Sometimes there is no obvious cause. Night time seems to be more common, but the reason is not known.

WARNING SIGNS
● Difficulty in breathing, especially in breathing out.
● Wheezing on breathing out.
● Distress and anxiety.
● Speaking in a whisper.
● Lips and finger nails turning blue.
● Exhaustion owing to struggling for breath.
● In extreme cases, unconsciousness.

ACTION
Offer reassurance and help the casualty to sit down, leaning forward and resting on his arms. Ensure that the air supply is unobstructed. Assist in finding and using medication if it is available. If the casualty is not carrying an inhaler, a pharmacist or doctor may provide one in an emergency.

Dial 999 for an ambulance in the case of a first attack, an attack that does not respond to medication or an attack that causes severe breathing difficulty.

After an asthma attack, it is always advisable to inform the doctor, who may be able to alter medication to prevent future attacks.

BITES AND STINGS

MAMMAL BITES
Bites from dogs, cats, rabbits, gerbils and other mammals – including human beings – are dangerous because germs from the animal's mouth enter the wound, and can cause infection. Keep your antitetanus injections up to date – you should have one every ten years as a preventive measure.

Any bite should be washed thoroughly, and if the skin has been broken the casualty should see a doctor. Serious wounds need treatment at a hospital accident and emergency department.

INSECT STINGS AND BITES
Stings and bites from bees, wasps and ants may be very painful, but they are not usually dangerous unless they are multiple, you are

bitten in the throat or mouth, or you have a serious allergic reaction – in which case they can be life-threatening.

BEE STINGS

If you have been stung by a bee, the sting will usually be embedded in the skin. Remove it by gently scraping the skin with a clean knife blade. Don't squeeze the sting with tweezers. By compressing the sting, you may force more venom into the body. Wasps and ants do not leave a sting behind.

SHOCK REACTION

A very small number of people have severe allergic reactions to certain types of bite or sting. Seek urgent medical assistance and treat as for allergic reaction (see page 449) if any of the following symptoms appear:

- Sudden weakness and sick feeling.
- Tight chest, difficult breathing or wheezing from the chest.
- Swollen face.

SNAKEBITE

Being bitten by a snake is generally more frightening than dangerous. In Britain, the only poisonous snake is the adder, whose bite is seldom serious and almost never fatal. Travellers abroad, however, can be exposed to more venomous reptiles. Consult a good guide book and take sensible precautions such as thick shoes in risky areas.

WARNING SIGNS
- Puncture marks, usually a pair.
- Severe pain at site of bite.
- Redness and swelling around the bite.
- Nausea and vomiting.
- Disturbed vision.
- Increased salivation and sweating.
- Laboured breathing or, in very extreme cases, breathing may stop.

ACTION

Lay the casualty down and instruct him to stay calm and keep still. Keep the affected part of the body immobilised and below the level of the heart. Wash the area thoroughly with soap and water but be careful not to apply any pressure and this will increase blood circulation and spread the venom.

Call an ambulance or doctor. If possible, note down a description of the snake for antivenom treatment.

CAUTION Despite the common belief that it is the right thing to do, do not apply a tourniquet to a snakebite casualty. Don't incise the bite or try to suck out the poison.

BLEEDING

Although bleeding can be alarming and dramatic, most cases are not fatal, provided the injury is treated promptly.

Bleeding can usually be stopped by pressing down on the wound, which slows the flow of blood and helps it to clot. The flow of blood can also be slowed by raising the injured area above the heart, but this is safe only if no fracture is involved.

CAUTION If severe bleeding is left untreated it can lead to potentially fatal shock.

SEVERE BLEEDING

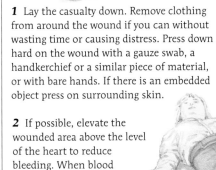

1 Lay the casualty down. Remove clothing from around the wound if you can without wasting time or causing distress. Press down hard on the wound with a gauze swab, a handkerchief or a similar piece of material, or with bare hands. If there is an embedded object press on surrounding skin.

2 If possible, elevate the wounded area above the level of the heart to reduce bleeding. When blood flow stops, apply a sterile dressing or a clean handkerchief.

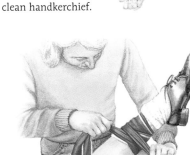

3 If bleeding continues, apply another dressing on top of the first. Tie it in place with a bandage or strip of material. Keep the casualty still. Give sips of fluid, but no food.

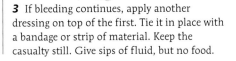

LARGE WOUNDS

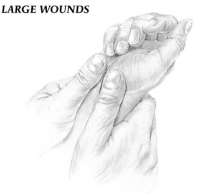

To staunch blood flow Squeeze the sides of a large wound together gently but firmly, and maintain the pressure for up to ten minutes. Treat as on page 453 and call an ambulance.

FOREIGN OBJECT IN A WOUND

Do not try to remove a piece of glass or any other object embedded in a large wound – you could do further damage to tissue or increase bleeding.

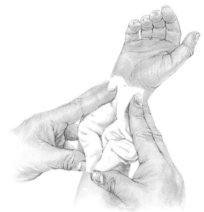

1 Applying pressure to the sides of the wound reduces bleeding. If you can, bind up the wound using pads on either side.

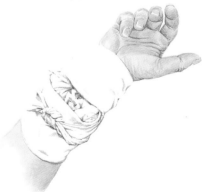

2 Bandage up the pads to hold them in position. Take care not to pass the bandage over the embedded object.

Is a bandage too tight?

Undo a bandage and retie it more loosely if you notice any of the following signs in the bandaged limb.

- Tingling in the fingers or toes.
- Extremely cold fingers or toes.
- Inability to move the fingers or toes.
- Nails that turn blue or white.
- A pulse reading that is weaker.

BURST VARICOSE VEIN

If a varicose vein bursts or is injured, severe blood loss can occur rapidly. Lay the victim down and press on the wound with a dressing. If no dressing is available to hand press the wound with your bare fingers.

Raise the leg above the level of the heart and maintain the pressure for up to ten minutes to stop the bleeding.

Put a clean dressing on the wound and tie it firmly in place with some sort of a bandage. If bleeding continues, place additional dressings and bandages over the first.

Let the patient rest, and prop up the leg with pillows or on a chair seat. If the bleeding is severe and does not stop with elevation and application of pressure, call an ambulance.

BLEEDING FROM NOSE, MOUTH OR EAR

An injured person who is bleeding from the nose, mouth or ear may be suffering from a severe injury to the head, the chest or the abdominal region.

A fractured skull may cause a trickle of blood from the nose or ears. An injury to the lungs, such as a puncture caused by a fractured rib, may result in pink frothy blood dribbling from the mouth and nose.

First, dial 999 for an ambulance. Then, if the patient is unconscious, check the airway, breathing and circulation, and start artificial respiration if necessary (see pages 449-452). If conscious, the patient should be placed in a half-sitting position with the head tilted toward the side from which the blood is coming. Cover the bleeding point with a pad of material, but don't apply pressure. Don't give the patient anything to eat or drink. Treat as for shock (see page 465).

BLEEDING SCALP

An injury to the scalp may look more threatening than it actually is because the scalp has a rich supply of blood and bleeds profusely, even from small cuts. And because the skin of the scalp is stretched tight over the head, a wound may also gape open, giving the impression of a much larger and more serious injury than might be the case.

However, if the injury has been severe, or if the person has been unconscious, or is drowsy or vomiting, they should be examined by a doctor as soon as possible. In the meantime, don't clean the wound or remove any foreign matter; as long as there are no bone fragments or a skull depression, try to control the bleeding by holding your hand or a compress, such as the inside of a clean, folded handkerchief, on the wound.

STOPPING BLOOD FLOW AT A PRESSURE POINT

If severe bleeding from an injured arm or leg cannot be stopped by elevation and direct pressure on the wound, it may be possible to do so using one of the body's two main arterial pressure points. These are places where an artery can be pressed against an underlying bone to stop the flow of blood. This technique should be used only to reduce severe bleeding, only as a last resort, and only with great care. Reduce the pressure after ten minutes to restore circulation. If bleeding resumes, continue pressure as long as necessary.

THE FEMORAL PRESSURE POINT

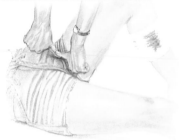

High inside the thigh, the femoral artery can be pressed against the pelvis to stop blood flow. Lay the casualty down, bending the injured leg up at the knee. Press firmly in the centre of the crease of the groin, one thumb above the other, pushing against the rim of the pelvis. Do not press hard for more than ten minutes.

THE BRACHIAL PRESSURE POINT

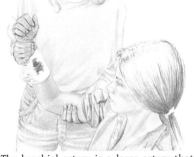

The brachial artery is a large artery that runs along the inner side of the upper arm. To staunch bleeding from the lower arm, it needs to be pressed against the humerus, or upper arm bone. When such an injury occurs, hold the casualty's arm at right angles to the body as shown. Then put one hand under the upper arm and press your fingers firmly against the bone.

BREATHING, LACK OF

Cessation of breathing, for whatever reason, is an urgent and life-threatening emergency. Check the casualty's respiration by feeling with your cheek over the mouth and nose. Watch the chest to see if there is any rising and falling motion and listen for any sound of inhalation or exhalation. If breathing has stopped or is very laboured, clear the airway and administer mouth-to-mouth resuscitation as described on pages 450-451.

BROKEN BONES
See FRACTURES, page 461.

BRUISES

A bruise is a visible sign of bleeding beneath the skin. Before treating a minor bruise, check that there are no other injuries, especially fractures (see page 461). Applying a cold compress to a bruised area helps to limit the swelling. The compress can be a small towel, a piece of cloth soaked in cold water and wrung out, or a plastic bag of crushed ice or frozen peas wrapped in a towel or cloth. Apply the compress as soon as possible and keep it on for at least 30 minutes. Alternatively, hold the bruised area under cold running water. If a serious bruise develops on an arm or a leg, elevate the limb above heart level to reduce swelling.

BURNS AND SCALDS

First-degree burns redden the skin and are painful, but affect only the surface. Second-degree burns cause blisters and deeper damage. Third-degree burns destroy the skin completely; the burned area will look charred or white. All but minor burns and scalds are potentially serious and should be seen by a doctor.

MINOR BURNS

When a burn is extremely painful, it is usually superficial. Hold it under a slowly running cold tap or put it in cold water for at least ten minutes. If no water is available, use some other cold liquid, such as milk or juice. Gently remove any rings or jewellery. Cover with a piece of clean, non-fluffy material, or clingfilm.

For minor burns and scalds in the mouth, give the casualty cold water and tell him or her to rinse and spit.

Is a bruise serious?

A bruise requires consultation with your doctor under the following circumstances:

● If it is around the eyes or behind the ears after a head injury.

● If it has not started to fade within a few days.

● If the pain is severe or there is difficulty in moving the bruised area 24 hours later.

● If there is a large bruise near the abdomen or on the back.

● If there is no apparent reason for bruising.

● If the lower leg is bruised and the casualty is elderly or has poor circulation.

● If vision is disturbed as the result of a black eye (see page 460).

Burns a doctor should see

Any burn or scald that does not heal naturally or that is larger than a 50p piece should be seen by a doctor. Burns and scalds of the mouth and throat are especially dangerous, as swelling of the airway may obstruct breathing. Don't hesitate to call an ambulance if in doubt.

DEEP BURNS

If a burned area of skin appears grey or is peeling or charred, the burn may be deep. It may not be painful because the nerves in the area may have been destroyed. Whatever the size of a deep burn, cool the area down first by running cold water over it, then cover with clean, non-fluffy material or clingfilm. Treat for shock (see page 465) and get medical help immediately; there is a strong risk of serious infection.

WIDESPREAD BURNS

Burns covering a large area of the body, such as an arm, a thigh or the chest, are medical emergencies that must be treated in a hospital as quickly as possible and with minimum interference to the damaged skin.

Cool the burned area down by running cold water over it. Remove rings, watches or tight clothing before the area starts to swell. However, do not try to remove any material clinging to the skin. Cover the burn with clean, non-fluffy material or clingfilm. If the casualty is unconscious but breathing, place in the recovery position (see page 448) and then call for an ambulance. If breathing suddenly stops, administer artificial respiration (see pages 449-452).

CHEMICAL BURNS

If the burn is caused by a chemical, such as caustic soda, dry lime or acid, irrigate the affected area copiously with cold water. Wear gloves to protect your own hands while you help the burn victim. Check that the casualty is not lying in the chemical.

CARDIOPULMONARY RESUSCITATION
See ARTIFICIAL RESPIRATION, page 449.

CHOKING

When a piece of food or some other object gets caught in your windpipe, your breath is either partially or fully cut off and you choke. If the blockage is partial, you may be able to take in enough air to cough out the object yourself. If the blockage is complete, you can die of suffocation within minutes if nothing is done.

Not chewing food properly or laughing while you eat can cause choking; so can drinking too much alcohol, which dulls the nerves that control swallowing. Peanuts and hard sweets are a common cause of choking in very young children and should not be given to under-fives. Children can also choke on small toys or pieces of toys that become detached, and adults sometimes choke on dentures that have come loose in the mouth.

Instant action is vital if you are to save someone who is choking. The first signal is cessation of breathing and inability to speak. As oxygen deprivation takes effect, the skin, lips, tongue, beds of the fingernails and the earlobes may start to turn blue and veins on the head and neck stand out. People who are choking instinctively clutch at the throat.

TREATING A CONSCIOUS ADULT

Encourage the person to cough; this may be enough to expel the obstruction. If coughing or speaking is impossible, bend the casualty over so that the head is lower than the chest. Give five hard slaps between the shoulder blades. This may be sufficient to dislodge the object. Check the mouth. If the obstruction is visible but not coughed out, remove it with your fingers. If it does not come out, apply the Heimlich manoeuvre as shown in the panel on the facing page.

For very obese people or pregnant women, the Heimlich manoeuvre is best performed higher on the torso. Clench your fist and hold it at the base of the breastbone just above the place where the bottom ribs are joined. Grasp your fist with the other hand and thrust upwards into the chest.

TREATING YOURSELF

Choking is extremely alarming when you are on your own, but don't panic. There are two ways of performing the Heimlich manoeuvre on yourself.

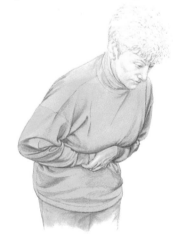

Fist method The first and most important step is to try to stay calm. Clench one fist and place it against your stomach, thumb side towards you and positioned slightly above the navel. With the other hand, jerk the fist firmly inward and upward. Repeat the thrust until the obstruction is dislodged and expelled.

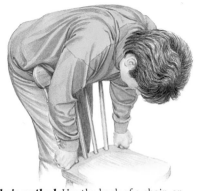

Chair method Use the back of a chair, or stand at a railing, and press your abdomen right above the navel firmly against the hard edge. Thrust yourself downwards and forwards.

TREATING AN UNCONSCIOUS PERSON

First, get someone to call for an ambulance while you attend to the casualty. Make the call yourself if no one else is around.

Put a choking casualty who has passed out on his or her back immediately, and try to open the blocked airway by tilting the head back and lifting the chin (see page 450). Check for breathing. If there is still none, attempt a finger sweep of the mouth. With your thumb on the tongue and your fingers under the chin, lift the person's lower jaw with one hand while you perform a sweeping movement with the index finger of your other hand along the cheeks and deep into the throat. Try to hook round and remove the obstruction but be careful not to push it deeper into the throat. Don't use this mouth sweep with infants or small children unless you can clearly see the obstruction.

If breathing still is not restored, position the casualty's head for mouth-to-mouth ventilation (see pages 450-451). If artificial ventilation is not possible, roll the person onto one side and perform four back-slaps. Check the mouth. If you can see the object, remove it with your fingers. If the casualty still does not breathe, perform the Heimlich manoeuvre with the person lying on his back. Kneel astride the hips and put the heel of one hand slightly above the navel and well below the bottom of the breastbone. Cover this hand with the other and, with arms straight, give a quick, upward thrust. Repeat five times.

After the first five thrusts, check the mouth again. If the obstruction has not been expelled, try artificial respiration again. If the lungs don't expand after two breaths, repeat the sequence of thrusts, finger sweeping the mouth and giving artificial respiration. Continue as long as necessary.

CAUTION Anyone who has been revived by the Heimlich manoeuvre should see a doctor afterwards.

THE HEIMLICH MANOEUVRE

When an adult is choking and neither coughing nor back-slapping dislodges the obstruction, it may be necessary to resort to the Heimlich manoeuvre. This involves applying a series of sudden, sharp thrusts to the abdomen to jerk the diaphragm upwards, compress the lungs and force air out of the windpipe, simultaneously expelling the obstruction.

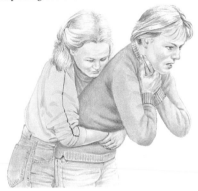

1 Tell the choking person what you are going to do. Stand behind the casualty, who can be standing or sitting, and put both your arms around the waist. Make a fist with one hand and place the thumb side against the casualty's abdomen, just above the navel but below the breastbone.

2 Grasp the fist with the other hand and press it forcefully into the casualty's abdomen with a quick inward-and-upward thrust. You are trying to push the upper abdomen against the bottom of the lungs to force out the remaining air and with it the obstruction.

3 Repeat five times, pausing briefly between each thrust to see if the obstruction has been dislodged. Check the casualty's mouth and remove anything that has come up.

4 After the obstruction is dislodged, the casualty may be winded and unable to breathe for a few moments.

5 When breathing begins again, encourage the person to sit quietly. If requested to, give a sip of water to drink. When fully recovered, the casualty should make an appointment to see his or her doctor to make sure no damage has been done by the vigorous thrusts.

TREATING CHILDREN AND INFANTS

Watch closely but don't interfere – except, perhaps, to tell the child to cough harder – as long as the youngster can breathe, speak or make sounds and is coughing. These are all signs that the child is getting some air in through the windpipe and may be able to expel whatever is causing the partial blockage. Be ready, however, to act quickly the minute he or she stops breathing or making sounds. Lie the child head-down on your knee, and give vigorous shoulder slaps. If necessary, commence artificial respiration (see pages 449-452).

For babies under a year old, use the following technique:

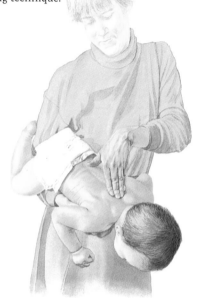

1 Hold the baby face down along one forearm and tilt your arm so that the baby's head is lower than the body. If you find it easier, sit down and rest your forearm along one thigh. Support the baby's chest and neck firmly with your hand.

2 Slap rapidly but firmly on the baby's back between the shoulder blades with the fingers of your free hand. Do this up to five times. Apply much less force than you would for a choking adult, and use the top section of the fingers only – never the whole palm or the heel of the hand.

CAUTION Be very careful when trying to remove anything from a baby's mouth. Put your finger into the mouth only if you can actually see the object that is causing the obstruction. Take care not to push it farther down the throat. Do not attempt to use the Heimlich manoeuvre on a child unless you have been trained. Never use it on a baby.

CONCUSSION
See HEAD INJURIES, page 463.

CONVULSIONS

Convulsions, or fits or seizures, are caused by a disturbance in the functioning of the brain, resulting in involuntary contractions of the body's muscles and unconsciousness.

There are many causes for convulsions, including poisoning, drugs, head injury, lack of oxygen and illness. The most common causes, however, are epilepsy and, in young children, a high temperature.

PETIT MAL SEIZURES

Minor epileptic – or petit mal – fits cause nothing more than a momentary blurring of consciousness or a lapse of attention. The person may suddenly 'go blank' or lose track of what was being done or said.

WARNING SIGNS

● Sudden inattention or staring blankly straight ahead.
● Slight twitching of lips, eyelids or head.
● Strange involuntary movements such as lip-smacking, making odd noises or fiddling with clothing.

ACTION

Get the casualty to sit down. Remove any potential dangers such as hot drinks. Talk calmly and reassuringly but avoid asking any unnecessary questions. Stay with the person until completely recovered. Advise reporting the episode to a doctor if the person is not aware of the condition.

GRAND MAL SEIZURES

Major epileptic – or grand mal – fits are much more dramatic and more serious than petit mal. In some cases, the person feels a premonition or 'aura' before they happen, or notices a particular taste or smell.

WARNING SIGNS

● Person falls to the ground, possibly with a cry, and loses consciousness.
● The body becomes rigid; the back arches.
● Breathing may stop, lips and ears turn blue or face and neck become slightly swollen.
● Convulsions (rhythmical, jerky movements), sometimes with clenched jaw, noisy breathing or incontinence.
● After return of muscle control, normal breathing resumes and consciousness returns, usually within minutes.

ACTION

If possible, protect the person when falling. Move any hard or dangerous objects well away. Loosen clothing at the neck and protect the head. Do not attempt to put anything in the mouth.

After convulsions stop, place the casualty in the recovery position (see page 448). Stay until he or she is fully recovered. Dial 999 for an ambulance if this is the first fit, if there are repeated fits or if unconsciousness lasts more than ten minutes.

CAUTION Do not use force or restraint during an epileptic fit. Never attempt to give water or anything else by mouth.

CONVULSIONS IN CHILDREN

Fits are uncommon in babies under 18 months, but not in young children, particularly when there is a very high temperature. Although they can be alarming for parents, such episodes are rarely dangerous if treated sensibly. Nevertheless, any convulsions in a child should be taken seriously. Always consult a doctor even if there is a rapid and dramatic recovery. There may be an underlying problem that needs treatment.

WARNING SIGNS

● A high temperature; hot, flushed skin; sometimes sweating.
● Violent muscle twitching, clenched fists and arched back.
● Fixed or upturned eyes.
● Breath held; face and neck congested.
● Unconsciousness.

ACTION

Remove clothing and bedclothes. Ensure a supply of cool, fresh air but do not make the child too cold. Sponge with lukewarm water from head to toe and place pillows or other soft padding all around the child to prevent accidental injury.

Ensure that the child's airways are open (see page 450) and telephone your doctor for advice or, failing that, call an ambulance.

DIABETIC COMA

People with diabetes may lose consciousness if there is either too much or too little insulin in the blood.

EXCESSIVE INSULIN (low blood sugar)

Diabetics are usually very well aware of the danger of allowing their blood sugar level to fall too low and most are expert at regulating their food intake to prevent it. When it does happen, however, it can lead to unconsciousness, so urgent action is required.

Warning signs include paleness, profuse sweating, a rapid pulse, shallow breathing and trembling. The person may seem confused, even intoxicated. If they do not get sugar fast enough, faintness follows, then rapid loss of consciousness.

INSUFFICIENT INSULIN (high blood sugar)

This condition usually builds up over a few days. Symptoms include thirst; excessive urination; dry skin; rapid pulse; deep, sighing breaths; a smell of acetone on the breath. Eventually unconsciousness may occur.

ACTION

If the casualty is unconscious, place him or her in the recovery position (see page 448) and summon help. If conscious, give a little sugar, honey or jam and watch the response. A rapid improvement in condition indicates low blood sugar, in which case more sugar can safely be given.

DISLOCATED JOINT

A bone that is wrenched out of place at a joint is said to be dislocated. The shoulders, elbows, fingers, hips, kneecaps and toes are most often affected. Dislocation is usually accompanied by torn ligaments (a sprain) and sometimes by a break in the bone.

Symptoms of dislocation include severe pain, swelling and bruising, deformity of the joint and difficulty in moving it.

If you suspect dislocation, treat as for fracture (see page 461) and get the casualty to hospital urgently.

CAUTION Never try to push a dislocated bone back into place.

DROWNING

Assume that anyone you see in the water fully clothed is a possible victim, and be prepared to help. A swimmer who develops a cramp or becomes exhausted is less easy to recognise, however, and a swimmer who is having breathing problems may not be able to draw attention by shouting.

Suspect a problem if you notice a swimmer's body tending to sink until it is vertical with only the head showing above water. Other signs include erratic strokes and movements that appear jerky or simply stop.

Don't become a victim yourself

Never go into the water to rescue someone unless you are trained in life saving and there is no alternative. It is easy to get into difficulties, and a panicky victim can drag an inexperienced would-be rescuer under.

Removing an insect from the ear

Calm and comfort the person and prevent the response of pushing a finger into the ear, which comes naturally to most people. Put a few drops of vegetable oil into the ear to kill the insect. Hold the casualty's head still with the affected ear angled toward the ground. The insect's body should float out on the oil.

If attempts to remove the insect fail get medical help.

Treating a black eye

A blow to the forehead, eye or cheek often causes blood to collect in soft tissues around the eyeball, which colours the skin dark blue or black and produces swelling.

Put a cold compress over the eye to limit the swelling and relieve the pain. To make the compress, put crushed ice, ice cubes, or frozen peas into a plastic bag, seal the bag, and wrap it in a cloth. Or soak a small towel in iced water and wring it out.

Cool the eye for at least 30 minutes, replacing the compress as it becomes warm.

If the black eye develops soon after an injury, take the victim to a doctor or hospital as soon as possible. A blow that is violent enough to blacken the eye socket could fracture the skull or cause serious damage to the eye itself.

The face may become congested, and the lips and ears turn bluish.

REVIVAL TECHNIQUES

If the drowning person has stopped breathing, start artificial respiration as quickly as possible (see pages 449-452).

Victims of drowning sometimes swallow water, which may be brought up with food during artificial respiration. Turn the head to one side and regularly clear the mouth. Once breathing resumes, place the casualty in the recovery position (see page 448) and treat any injuries while you wait for help. Even a casualty who appears to have recovered fully should be examined by a doctor.

EAR INJURIES

Damage to the middle or inner ear can be caused by injuries to the head, a very loud noise, diving into water or probing in the ear – to remove a foreign object, for example.

Although a perforated eardrum is not necessarily serious, bleeding from the ear or discharge of watery, straw-coloured fluid after a head injury can be a sign of a fractured skull and should be checked without delay.

Symptoms of an ear injury include severe earache, dizziness and loss of balance, deafness, and discharge of blood or fluid.

Stop the casualty of an ear injury from hitting the side of the head to try to restore hearing; this will only make the damage worse. Cover the injured ear with a piece of clean cotton or gauze as protection. Bandage it lightly. Don't try to plug the ear canal; this can cause a buildup of blood or pus. Sit the victim up with the head tilted over on the injured side so that blood or fluid can drain out. If the casualty is unconscious but breathing, put him in the recovery position (see page 448) with the injured ear downward and a clean pad underneath it to absorb fluids. If breathing stops at any stage, begin administering artificial respiration as a matter of urgency (see pages 449-452).

FOREIGN OBJECT IN THE EAR

Children often stick things into their ears harmlessly, but when an object is pushed hard and deep into the ear canal, the canal may be blocked, or the eardrum perforated. The symptoms are variable and sometimes there are no signs at all. More usually, there is discharge, pain, buzzing or deafness.

Apart from insects (see panel, left), never attempt to remove a foreign object yourself. Always try to get medical help.

ELECTRIC SHOCK

Electricity can kill or produce a wide range of very dangerous injuries, including severe burns and cardiac arrest.

RESCUE METHODS

Never touch the casualty of an electric accident until you are sure that you are not risking a shock yourself. If the person is still touching the source of electricity, cut off the power at the main fuse box or circuit-breaker panel. If the person is in contact with an electrical source and you cannot turn off the power, do not touch any part of the body. Instead, push the person away with a piece of wood that you know to be completely dry, such as a broom handle. If you can, stand on an insulating material while you do so, such as a rubber mat or a wad of newspapers.

Once an unconscious person is away from the electrical source, check for pulse and breathing, and give artificial respiration if necessary (see pages 449-452). Put a casualty who is still breathing in the recovery position (see page 448). Then, whatever the circumstances, telephone 999 for an ambulance. Treat burns as described on page 455.

CAUTION Remember that water conducts electricity. If you touch the victim with anything that may be even slightly moist, you can electrocute yourself.

EPILEPTIC FIT
See CONVULSIONS, page 458.

EYE INJURIES

Getting an eyelash or a piece of grit lodged in your eye is the most common mishap that eyes suffer. More serious injuries are caused by corrosive chemicals or sharp objects, such as flying fragments of glass or metal.

Injury can also occur if contact lenses get displaced or stuck to the eyeball. If you have any difficulty with a contact lens, get help from your optician or doctor rather than risk hurting your eye.

FOREIGN OBJECT IN THE EYE

Don't let the casualty rub the eye. Turn his or her face up to the light. With your thumb and forefinger, push the eyelids away from the eyeball. Ask the casualty to look left, right, up and down while you look for the foreign matter on the exposed eyeball. If you can see the foreign object, try to wash it out.

Tilt the person's head to the injured side, and gently run cool or lukewarm water over the eye from a tap or jug. Alternatively, encourage the casualty to blink underwater.

If flushing fails, try to lift the object off the eye with a moistened piece of clean gauze or the corner of a clean handkerchief.

CHEMICAL BURNS

If chemicals – either liquid or solid – get into the eye, tilt the head, injured eye downward, over the sink. Flood the open eye with gently running water from a tap or jug for at least ten minutes. You may need to force the eyelids open if they are shut tight in a spasm of pain. When you have thoroughly flushed the chemical from the eye, dry the face and put a clean dressing lightly over the eye. Get the casualty to hospital immediately.

OBJECT IMPALED IN THE EYE

Do not try to remove foreign matter embedded in an eye yourself. Doing so could cause irreparable damage. Protect an injured eye by covering it with a clean paper or plastic cup, taking great care not to touch or apply any pressure to the eye itself. Put a bandage over the cup to keep the eyes from moving, then take the casualty to hospital immediately or telephone for an ambulance.

FAINTING

If the blood supply to the brain is suddenly reduced, fainting may result. Any powerful emotional stimulus such as bad news or a fright can cause fainting. So can a stuffy room, a drop in blood sugar due to missed meals or dieting, standing still for a long time, or standing up suddenly. If fainting is caused by illness or injury, if it occurs often, or if the fainter is old or has a cardiac problem, a doctor should be consulted.

WARNING SIGNS

A person who is about to faint becomes pale or a greenish white. Frequent yawning may indicate a lack of oxygen. The skin becomes cold and clammy. Beads of sweat appear on the face, neck and hands. The casualty may complain of feeling very warm or hot, and may experience blurred vision, dizziness, nausea, or general weakness.

ACTION

Get the person to sit down at the first signs of faintness. Loosen tight clothing at the neck and waist, and place the head down on the knees. Alternatively, stretch the casualty out flat on his back and prop up his legs at a height of 8-12 in (20-30 cm).

If the person actually faints, first check for breathing. Then raise the feet above the level of the head to increase blood circulation to the brain.

FRACTURES

A fracture is a crack or break in a bone. There are three main types:

CLOSED FRACTURES

The bone is broken but the skin over it remains intact.

OPEN FRACTURES

These occur where a piece of broken bone protrudes through the skin or there is a cut over the area where the break occurred. In either case, germs may enter the wound, and there is a risk of serious infection resulting.

GREENSTICK FRACTURES

The bone is bent or torn but not completely broken. Greenstick fractures occur in children, whose bones are still soft and pliable.

WARNING SIGNS

Often a casualty will actually hear or feel the bone snap and be aware of the sensation of broken bone ends grating together, which sometimes makes a definite sound.

The casualty will probably not be able to use the injured part of the body and will feel pain when attempting to do so. Only occasionally can a broken bone still be moved, and then awkwardly.

A broken limb may lie in an unnatural position, or look deformed when compared with the uninjured side of the body. The area around the break will be tender to the touch, swollen or bruised.

ACTION

To be on the safe side, all doubtful cases of injured bones should be treated as fractures. The principles of treatment are the same in all cases:

● Don't move the casualty unless he or she is in imminent danger.
● Deal with any difficulty in breathing, unconsciousness or any severe bleeding before treating the fracture.
● Make the casualty as comfortable as possible and provide support for the injured limb with a rolled-up blanket or coat, or with pillows or cushions.

DO'S
AND
DON'TS

for treating a faint

Do get medical help if the casualty doesn't recover in minutes.
Do check for any injury that may have occurred during the fall. Anyone whose head receives a bang hard enough to cause a cut or wound, for example, should be examined by a doctor for possible concussion.

Don't give anything to eat or drink until full consciousness returns, and then only sips of cold water. In particular, avoid alcohol which acts as a depressant and may worsen whatever condition caused the fainting spell in the first place.
Don't put a pillow under the head; it could obstruct breathing.
Don't pour water over the head of someone who has fainted. If smelling salts are available, try waving them under the nose.

461

- Don't move the fractured bone unnecessarily and never try to push a displaced bone back into position.
- Take action to limit shock (see page 465).
- If it is essential to move the casualty – and if time allows – try to immobilise the injured limb first.

BROKEN ARM

IF THE ELBOW WILL BEND

Place the arm across the chest and get the casualty to support it with his good hand. Using a triangular bandage, scarf or piece of cloth, make a sling with the apex of the triangle protruding well beyond the elbow and the upper corner going over the shoulder on the uninjured side and round the back of the neck. Take the lower corner up and over the injured limb and tie it to the upper corner in the hollow just above the collarbone on the injured side. Pin or tuck in the loose material at the elbow.

IF THE ELBOW CANNOT BEND

Lay the casualty down in the most comfortable position. Place some padding between the injury and the body, and strap the arm to the body with three pieces of wide material spaced apart to avoid the immediate area of the fracture.

BROKEN LOWER LEG

If medical help is on the way, ease the limb into a natural position, provided this does not cause excessive pain. Keep the leg supported and as comfortable as possible.

If you have to move the casualty or expect some delay before help arrives, make the casualty as comfortable as possible and then follow these steps.

1 Carefully remove clothing from the area if there is an open wound over the break. If the patient becomes unconscious, check airway, breathing and circulation, and give artificial respiration if needed (see pages 449-452).

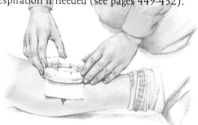

2 Cover the wound with a clean piece of non-fluffy cloth, and place a built-up dressing around any protruding bone. Alternatively, protect it with a matchbox or cigarette packet.

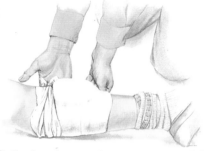

3 Bandage the wound, supporting it carefully. Do not tie the bandages too tightly or you risk restricting the circulation in the limb.

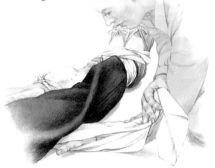

4 To immobilise the broken leg, place padding between the knees and ankles and tie the feet together with a bandage or scarf in a figure-of-eight pattern. Knot the ends together on the outer edge of the foot on the uninjured side. Tie the knees together with material.

BROKEN KNEE

A fractured knee is extremely painful and may be bent in an unnatural way. Do not try to straighten it forcibly, but lay the casualty down with the leg in the most comfortable position possible.

Support the knee – without changing its position – by placing a cushion or a rolled-up piece of clothing underneath it. To give the knee further support, place rolled-up coats or rugs around the leg. Do not tie a splint over the break.

BROKEN JAW

A person who has suffered a broken jaw will often have a wound inside the mouth. The casualty may have difficulty speaking, and there may be an excessive flow of saliva, often tinged with blood and broken teeth.

On the way to the hospital, the casualty can support his jaw by cupping it with his hands. In order to allow him to clear secretions effectively from his mouth or to vomit if he has to, it's better not to support the jaw by tying a bandage around the head. Watch the patient to make sure he is not having difficulty with breathing.

DO'S
— AND —
DON'TS

for treating frostbite

Do remove clothing from the frostbitten part of the body.
Do take off jewellery from an affected hand.
Do cover affected ears, nose or cheeks with warm hands.
Do exercise affected fingers and toes.
Do raise the affected area above heart level to restore circulation.
Do place sterile gauze or cloth between fingers and toes to keep them separated.
Do immerse the frostbitten part in a basin of lukewarm water.

Don't thaw a frostbite if there is any danger of further injury from cold.
Don't apply direct heat or try to warm up the area too fast.
Don't rub or massage the frostbitten area.
Don't break any blisters.
Don't apply medication.
Don't walk on a foot affected by frostbite.

RIB FRACTURES

A severe blow to the chest or a bad fall can fracture a rib, causing a sharp chest pain when the casualty breathes deeply or coughs. A person who appears to have only a simple rib fracture can be taken to a hospital in a car. However, call an ambulance at once if you notice any of the following signs of a more serious chest injury:

● The casualty cannot breathe properly and seems to be suffocating.
● Red frothy blood issues from the mouth.
● The casualty becomes restless and complains of thirst.

FROSTBITE

Exposed parts of the body, such as the nose, ears, cheeks and chin, can be susceptible to frostbite in freezing weather. Frostbite occurs when crystals of ice form in the skin and underlying tissues, constricting blood vessels and thereby cutting off the blood supply. Damage or death to the affected area follows. The hands and feet can become frostbitten even when they are enclosed in warm gloves and boots. Treatment is essential as unless a frostbitten area is warmed up and circulation to it is restored, it may have to be amputated because of gangrene.

WARNING SIGNS

The frostbitten part of the body first feels cold and stiff, with an aching, sharp pain. The skin becomes hard, then turns a white or greyish blue colour in fair-skinned people, or becomes lighter in people with dark complexions. The affected area finally becomes numb, and the pain misleadingly disappears.

ACTION

If possible, get the victim into a building for shelter. Warm the exposed area with body contact but don't apply direct heat. When colour and feeling return, wrap a towel or cloth around it, then cover with a blanket or sleeping bag. Follow the advice in the panel, on the facing page. Seek medical attention if feeling does not return or if there is obvious damage to the tissue.

HEAD INJURIES

Traffic accidents and falls are among the most common causes of bad head injuries; sports such as cycling, hockey and boxing are also a frequent source of damage. A blow to the head can damage the brain. Especially in the elderly, a knock to the head may cause internal bleeding which, if not recognised and treated promptly, can result in permanent damage.

Anyone who has been unconscious, or is confused or drowsy after receiving a head injury, should be taken to a doctor or to the accident and emergency department of a hospital for examination – even if the injury does not appear to be serious.

CONCUSSION

Since the brain is free to move within the skull, a blow to the head can shake and disturb it. This causes a widespread, though usually temporary, disturbance of the brain, a condition known as concussion. Symptoms may include confusion, slurred speach, vomiting, unsteadiness, inability to follow commands, loss of memory about events at the time of the injury, and loss of consciousness. The loss of consciousness is brief, and is always followed by a complete recovery. Concussion can be accurately and safely diagnosed only after recovery.

HEART ATTACK

Many conditions other than a heart attack can cause chest troubles (see pages 350-354). But because early intervention can save lives and lessen damage to the heart, report chest pains to your doctor at once.

The classic sign of a heart attack is a crushing pain in the chest that often radiates to the jaw, neck and arm. The person may also become breathless, sweat profusely and feel weak, nauseated, restless and anxious. For some days or weeks before a heart attack, many people report experiencing unaccustomed indigestion, chest pain, fatigue, shortness of breath and nausea.

ACTION

Call for a paramedic ambulance, making it clear that you suspect a heart attack. If you know of a history of heart disease with the victim, tell the paramedics immediately they arrive. While waiting for the ambulance, help the patient, if conscious, into a comfortable half-sitting position, with the head and shoulders supported by pillows and the knees bent. Loosen any tight clothing around the neck, chest and waist to help circulation and breathing.

Give the person an aspirin to chew slowly, if available, but nothing else to eat or drink. Don't allow any unnecessary movement as it

---

After a blow to the head

Report any of these symptoms to a doctor.

● Confusion or drowsiness, which may or may not be followed by unconsciousness.
● Headache.
● Loss of memory about events just before or at the time of the accident.
● Weak pulse and unusually shallow or noisy breathing.
● Clear fluids or blood flowing from the nose or ears; blood coming from the mouth.
● Vomiting, convulsions, or a change in pulse rate.
● The pupils of the eyes are unequal in size.

can put an extra strain on the heart. If the patient becomes unconscious, check airway, breathing and circulation, and give artificial respiration (see pages 449-452) if necessary.

HEART STOPPAGE

If someone's heart stops beating – signalled by a lack of pulse, call the emergency services immediately and, if a trained person is present, begin artificial resuscitation using chest compression (see pages 449-452).

HEAT EXHAUSTION AND HEATSTROKE

People who exercise or otherwise exert themselves too much during hot, humid weather may suffer from heat exhaustion or from even more serious heatstroke. Both conditions can lead to unconsciousness, and both require medical treatment.

Profuse sweating on a hot day depletes the body of vital fluids and minerals. If they are not replaced, muscles will cramp and the sufferer will feel a general weakness.

The symptoms of heat exhaustion include dizziness, headache, fatigue and nausea. The casualty's body temperature stays normal or rises very slightly. The skin feels moist; the face looks pale. Breathing is fast and shallow and the pulse is fast and weak. The condition is made worse if the person has recently suffered diarrhoea or vomiting, causing the body to lose even greater amounts of fluid.

Those most vulnerable to the effects of extreme heat include the very young and the very old, the chronically ill, the overweight, and patients on certain drugs.

Heatstroke occurs suddenly and dramatically, with body temperature rising to 40°C (104°F) or higher, often with a rapid, strong pulse. The skin feels hot and may also be dry. At first, the casualty may complain of headache, dizziness or nausea; later, as the condition becomes worse, there may be confusion and irritability. Some people have a seizure or lose consciousness.

TREATING HEAT EXHAUSTION
Place the person in a cool area, preferably indoors, and give a drink of cold (not iced) salted water (¼ teaspoon of salt to a cup of water), juice or a sports or glucose drink. If the victim passes out, check airway, breathing and circulation, and begin artificial respiration if necessary (see pages 449-452). Also call for medical help.

TREATING HEATSTROKE
Call for medical help immediately you notice any symptoms of heatstroke. Without quick treatment, a heatstroke casualty may die. In the meantime, move the sufferer to a cool place. Remove as much clothing as possible, sponge the face and cover the body with a wet sheet or spray it with cool water.

Keep the person wet and cool with cold water and by fanning until the body temperature comes down to normal. Do not induce shivering. If the casualty loses consciousness, check the airway, breathing and circulation and, if necessary, begin to administer artificial respiration (see pages 449-452). Continue to give cooling treatment.

HYPOTHERMIA (exposure)

Hypothermia is a serious condition in which body temperature drops from the normal level of 37°C (98.6°F) to 35°C (95°F) or lower. Babies, young children, and elderly people are the most at risk. Alcoholics and people suffering from malnutrition and heart disease are also vulnerable. Anyone in these categories who complains of feeling cold should always be taken seriously. If it is not treated, hypothermia may worsen and cause symptoms such as mental confusion, fatigue, muscular stiffness, uncontrollable shivering and slurred speech. Without help, any hypothermia victim – young or old – will eventually pass out; suffer heart, lung and brain failure; and eventually die.

WARNING SIGNS
Symptoms include shivering in the early stages, cold, pale, dry skin, lethargy and irrational behaviour. As the condition worsens, the pulse and breathing slow, and the person may lose consciousness.

ACTION
If you suspect that someone is suffering from hypothermia, check for drowsiness, low body temperature, numb body parts and a glassy stare. Call for medical help without delay and follow the advice in the panel.

POISONING

Many poisonings occur when a person – often a child – drinks some household or garden chemical. Adult gardeners have been known accidentally to drink insecticides and weed killers that they themselves had stored in soft drink bottles. Some common plants

DO'S
— AND —
DON'TS
for treating exposure

Do remove wet clothing.
Do wrap a dry blanket or rug around the person, covering the body but not the face, and put a warm hat on his head.
Do lay the victim down.
Do check the airway, breathing and circulation of an unconscious casualty. Begin artificial respiration as necessary (see pages 449-452).
Do lie down beside the person, to keep him or her warm.
Do wrap a hot-water bottle in a towel or cloth and put it on the victim's trunk – not on the arms or legs.
Do increase the room temperature if possible, or move the person to a warmer room.
Do give conscious patients hot, sweet drinks such as milk, tea, or hot chocolate.

Don't give alcohol.
Don't massage the person's limbs or suggest taking exercise.
Don't apply any sort of heating device directly to the skin.

can be toxic if ingested (see pages 326-327). Almost any nonfood substance is poisonous if taken in large doses. Few cases are fatal but as many as 37 000 children are taken to hospital with suspected poisoning every year. To reduce the risks, keep all medications and dangerous chemicals well out of reach of children, and never store weed killers or insecticides in unmarked bottles.

WARNING SIGNS

- Stomach pain.
- Vomiting and nausea.
- Diarrhoea.
- Erratic behaviour or excessive sleepiness.
- Burns around the mouth if the poison is corrosive, and severe pain throughout the mouth, throat and stomach.
- Unusual breath or body odour.
- Difficulty in breathing.
- Unconsciousness.

ACTION

If the casualty is conscious, try to find out what substance was swallowed. Remember that the person may lose consciousness at any time. Look around for a container or the remains of a poisonous plant that might be a clue to what has been taken. If the casualty has vomited, collect samples.

Call 999 and ask for an ambulance. If the person is unconscious, check airway, breathing and circulation, and begin artificial respiration as necessary (see pages 449-452). Take care not to get poison on your mouth and avoid inhaling the casualty's breath. If the casualty has to be taken to hospital, be sure to give the ambulance crew anything that may help to identify the poison, such as pill containers or a sample of vomit.

DRUG OVERDOSE

Anyone who has taken an overdose of a drug requires immediate medical attention. This applies to an overdose of a prescribed medicine or an over-the-counter drug such as aspirin or ibuprofen as much as it does to an illegal drug such as heroin.

WARNING SIGNS

Symptoms depend on the size of the overdose and the type of drug, but they can include any of the following:

- Vomiting.
- Difficulty in breathing.
- Unconsciousness.
- Sweating.
- Hallucinations.
- Dilation or contraction of the pupils.

- Excessive and abnormal sleepiness, a state of confusion, or bizarre outbursts of speech.

ACTION

Call 999 for an ambulance. Ask for advice on what to do while waiting for help. Generally, don't induce vomiting unless a doctor or the ambulance personnel suggest it.

Don't try to keep a person who may have overdosed awake with strong black coffee or by walking about. Physical activity will only help to speed up absorption of the drug. If the person loses consciousness, place him or her in the recovery position (see page 448).

GAS POISONING

Many gases are toxic, including fumes from burning polyurethane, ammonia – used in refrigeration plants, cleaning products and fertilisers – and carbon monoxide from car exhaust fumes.

WARNING SIGNS

Casualties of gas poisoning often demonstrate unsound judgment and are difficult and uncooperative. Some become confused or stupefied, or lose consciousness.

ACTION

AMMONIA

The strong, acrid smell will alert you. Poisoning usually occurs only when trapped in an enclosed area. Do not enter without a mask. The gas disperses very slowly.

BURNING POLYURETHANE FOAM

These fumes can kill in minutes. Call the fire brigade and allow experts to handle the situation. Do not try anything yourself.

CARBON MONOXIDE

If you suspect that a car or garage is filled with carbon monoxide, open the doors and get any occupants into the open air.

In all cases of suspected gas poisoning, from whatever cause, make sure you check the airway, breathing and circulation as on page 448. If necessary, dial 999 for an ambulance and administer artificial respiration as advised on pages 449-452.

SHOCK

Severe injury or illness may produce clinical shock – a dangerous reduction in the flow of blood throughout the body which, if not treated, can cause the victim to collapse, fall

---

Alcohol poisoning

People who drink excessively may lapse into a stupefied state, leading to coma. In extreme cases, breathing may stop altogether.

Don't assume that someone who seems intoxicated has necessarily had alcohol, however. Various other conditions – including head injury, stroke and diabetes – can produce similar symptoms, as can certain drugs.

Treating an overdose

If the victim stops breathing, administer artificial respiration (see pages 449-452).

If the victim is unconscious but still breathing, use your finger to clear any obstruction from the mouth and throat. Do not try to induce vomiting.

Put the victim in the recovery position (see page 448), loosen clothing at the neck and waist, and check that the airway is still clear.

Call an ambulance if the victim remains unconscious or cannot be roused, or if there is an uneven or weak pulse, difficulty in breathing, persistent vomiting, seizure or continued state of excitement or agitation.

Also call for emergency help if the casualty is a diabetic or if you suspect drugs have been taken with alcohol.

into a coma or even die. Serious bleeding, heavy vomiting or diarrhoea, and widespread burns can all reduce the blood or body fluid volume sufficiently to cause shock. Clinical shock is not the same as emotional shock or fear which comes on after an injury or other unpleasant experience. This usually requires only calming and comforting although in cases of deep distress a doctor may administer a sedative.

WARNING SIGNS

The body reacts to a diminished blood supply by concentrating blood in vital organs such as the heart, brain and kidneys. Less important areas, such as the muscles and skin, are drained of blood, and the victim weakens and becomes pale. Symptoms include:

- Fainting.
- Anxiousness and restlessness.
- Nausea and perhaps vomiting.
- Pallor.
- Thirst.
- Sweating.
- Shallow, rapid breathing with yawning and sighing.
- A weak, fast pulse, sometimes irregular.

ACTION

Call for an ambulance. Reassure the casualty, lay him down with the head low, and follow the instructions in the panel on the left. Treat any injuries. If the person has difficulty breathing, vomits or becomes unconscious, put him in the recovery position (see page 448). If breathing stops, begin artificial respiration (see pages 449-452).

ANAPHYLACTIC SHOCK

Severe allergic reaction (see page 449) can cause a general response known as anaphylactic shock. If this occurs, seek medical help as a matter of urgency.

SPRAINS

A sprain is a stretching or tearing of the ligaments that hold a joint together. Sprains are often difficult to distinguish from fractures, which involves actual damage to the bone. The symptoms of both include immediate, often severe, pain, swelling or bruising of the joint; pain when the ankle is moved; and inability to stand on the injured leg. If in any doubt, treat as for fracture (see page 461).

SPRAINED ANKLE

Although the wrist, elbow, knee, hip and shoulder can all suffer sprains, the ankle is the joint that people most often sprain. A fall or stumble that makes the ankle bend or twist excessively can sprain (or break) it.

If you think you have sustained a fracture or a sprain, remove the shoe and raise the foot above the heart. If you are near a source of ice or cold water, limit the swelling by applying a cold compress to the ankle for 20 to 30 minutes. Then bandage the ankle firmly and see a doctor as soon as possible.

A cold compress helps to decrease swelling of the soft tissue surrounding the injury. Once started, it should be applied several times a day for 15 to 20 minutes at a time during the first 48 hours after the injury.

Don't apply heat to the ankle or soak it in hot water for the first 48 hours after the injury. Don't put weight on a sprained or fractured ankle if you can help it. If you're a long way from help, support the ankle (see below) before using it.

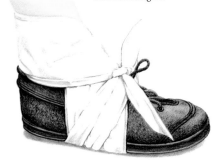

Support for a sprained ankle If you injure your ankle out on a hike or away from help, leave your shoe and sock on for support and cool the foot if possible, for example, by immersing in water. If you can find a strip of bandage or cloth, bind it in a figure-of-eight pattern under and over the instep and heel as shown. As soon as you can, give proper treatment as described above.

OTHER SPRAINS

If you sprain your wrist, elbow, or shoulder, apply ice and compresses to the joint and bandage it firmly. Then support it – above the level of the heart, if possible – with a sling. Have the injury checked as soon as possible by a doctor to make certain there is no fracture.

To make a sling, you will need a triangular bandage or a square of strong fabric measuring about 3 ft x 3 ft (1 m x 1 m) folded diagonally into a triangular shape.

Get the casualty to sit down if possible and support the injured arm by holding it across the chest and, if possible, slightly raised. Apply the sling as follows.

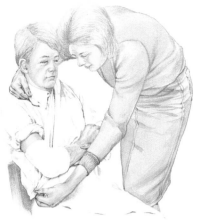

1 While the casualty continues to support the injured arm with his hand, place the sling between the chest and forearm.

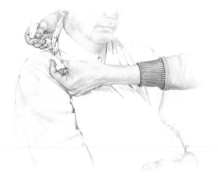

2 Take the upper end of the bandage over the shoulder on the uninjured side, around the back of the neck, and tie it to the lower end.

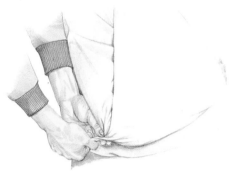

3 Pin the point near the elbow, or twist or tuck it in. Check that any other bandages on the arm are not too tight.

STROKE

The signs that someone may be experiencing a stroke include difficulty in speaking or swallowing, weakness or paralysis on one side of the body, impaired vision, sudden headache, confusion, drowsiness, involuntary urination and loss of bowel control. Some of the symptoms can resemble drunkenness. A severe stroke may sometimes cause loss of consciousness.

ACTION

Call your doctor or an ambulance immediately if you suspect a stroke. While waiting for help, and if the casualty is conscious, lay him down with head and shoulders slightly raised on pillows or cushions. Tilt the head to one side – the weaker, if possible – so that saliva can drain from the mouth. Loosen tight clothing at the neck, chest and waist. Assure the person that help is on the way, but don't offer anything to eat or drink.

If the casualty loses consciousness, check for breathing and pulse, and give artificial respiration if necessary (see pages 449-452). When breathing is stable, place in the recovery position (see page 448).

UNCONSCIOUSNESS

There are many degrees of unconsciousness, and a person who has suffered illness or injury may be at any level of alertness from being wide awake to being deeply comatose. Patients who are becoming more and more deeply unconscious are obviously in greater danger than those who are waking up. Test for unconsciousness by seeing if the casualty will respond to your voice or being gently shaken on the shoulder.

A person who becomes unconscious needs to be checked immediately for any obstruction to the airway. If breathing has stopped, begin artificial respiration (see pages 449-452). If breathing is normal, make sure the airway stays unblocked while you are waiting for the ambulance by placing the casualty in the recovery position. Vomit, blood or saliva may block the windpipe, or the tongue may slide back and close it.

If the cause of unconsciousness is not at first apparent, always suspect a head, neck or back injury. In such circumstances, take great care not to move the neck. If an unconscious person is breathing normally and is in a safe place, it is best not to disturb him at all. Moving someone with a back or neck injury can cause serious, even fatal, damage.

Handle any serious wound gently. Treat any injuries that can be treated and do what you can to staunch bleeding without moving the casualty, while you wait for the ambulance to arrive.

CAUTION Don't leave an unconscious person alone at any time, and don't give anything to eat or drink, even if consciousness returns. Anyone who has been unconscious, if only for a short time, should see a doctor.

INDEX

Page references in *italic* indicate text accompanied by an illustration.
Entries in *italic* are titles of institutions or associations to whom further enquiries
can be directed, and whose address or telephone number is given in the text.

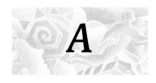

A

Abdominoplasty (removal of loose
  abdominal skin) 388
ACCEPT 206
Access to Medical Records
  Act 1988 245
Accidents at work 242
Acid rain 309
Acne 141, 348
Activities in retirement 413-15
Acupressure for motion-sickness
  relief 169-70
Acupuncture 226
*Acupuncture and Traditional Chinese
  Medicine, London School of* 349
Acupuncture, The Council for 226
Addiction
  to drugs 207-11
  to exercise 96
  and personality 208
  smoking 156-7
Additives in food 56
Adfam 211
Aerobic exercise
  and blood cholesterol 99
  for increasing metabolism 94-95
  workout at home *86-87*
Aerobics
  choosing a class 115-16
  definition 115
Aerophobia (fear of flying) *201*
Affairs
  effect on marriage 182
  in middle age 395
Ageing
  and appearance 422-3
  attitudes to 410
  different rates 409
  disproportionate effect on
    women 383
  of population 410
  reaching middle age 381
  sleep patterns 158
  slowed by antioxidants 411
Age spots 387
Aggressive behaviour in
  children 292-3
Agoraphobia (fear of open
  spaces) 200
AIDS (acquired immune
  deficiency syndrome) 259

Aids
  for the disabled 375
  hearing 429
  mobility 421
  teeth cleaning 431
  walking 422
Air bags *338*
Aircraft emissions 306
Air
  decreasing moisture 309
  increasing moisture 307
  pollution 303-7
  quality in home 307
Al-Anon 206
Alcohol
  advantages 155
  before and after exercise 94
  dependence 206-7
  effects on mind 207
  leading to liver damage 357
  in old age 425
  poisoning 465
  risks 404
  safe levels 154-5
  tolerance 155
  units 155
Alcohol Concern 206
Alcoholics Anonymous 206
Alcoholism 206-7
Allergies *346*
  anaphylactic shock 449, 453
  cause of asthma 350-1
  immune response 124
  medication for relief 347
  triggered by respiratory
    sensitisers 338
All-night surgeries 219
Allowances for carers 442
Alternative medicine 230
Alzheimer's disease *441*
  aluminium salts in
    antiperspirants 141
  aluminium saucepans 321
  shuffling gait 434
Alzheimer's Disease Society 441
Amalgam fillings 130-1
Amarant Trust, The 394
Amenorrhea (lack of periods) 67
Amino acid supplements 44
Amniocentesis 268
Amsler grid (eye test) *427*
Anaemia 48
Anaesthesia 238
  legal responsibility under 247
Anaesthetics
  in dentistry 240
  epidural in childbirth 275

in surgery 273, 278
Analgesics (painkillers) 165-6
Anaphylactic shock 449
  response to stings or bites 453
Angina 363
  and heart attacks 364
  surgical intervention 365-6
Angiography (scanning of
  blood vessels) *233*
Angioplasty 365
Animal deaths, reporting to
  authorities 340
Anisakis parasites in fish 33
Ankle sprains *466*
Ankylosing spondylitis (fused
  vertebrae) 373
Annual check-ups for the
  elderly 432
Anorexia nervosa 205
Antacids 150
  see also histamine (H$_2$) blockers
Antenatal classes 271
Antibiotics 224-5
  treatment for peptic ulcers 354-5
Anti-flu inoculations 134-5
Anti-inflammatory drugs 165-6
Antioxidants 40-41
  slower ageing process 411
Antiperspirants 141
Ants in the house 332
Anxiety 200-2
  before surgery 237-8
  cause of nail-biting 138
  speaking in public 186
  underlying anorexia and
    bulimia 205
Aphrodisiacs 256
Apnoea, sleep 158
Appendicitis 286
Appetite
  decreased with age 424
  drugs to suppress 153
  increased by exercise 95
Appointments system in general
  practice 217
Arguments between
  partners 182
Arm fractures 462
Aromatherapy *229*
Arteriosclerosis 363
Arthritis 372-4
  aids for the disabled 375
  copper therapy 320
Artificial insemination 265
Artificial respiration
  assessing the casualty 449
  chest compression 451

clearing the airway and
  ventilation *450*
ventilating babies and small
  children 451
Artificial sweeteners 18
Asbestos 322
Ascorbic acid *see* Vitamin C
Aspartame (artificial
  sweetener) 18
Asphyxiation 452
Aspirin
  against heart attacks 365, 389
  groups at risk from 365
  not suitable for children 288
  properties of 165-6
Assaults in the street 340
Assertiveness training 177
Asthma 350-3
  attacks 452
  causes *350-1*
  first aid 452
  identification 287
  pollution 351
  prevention of attacks 352-3
  relief through drugs 351
  safe exercise 101
  triggers 338, 350-1
Astigmatism *127*
Athlete's foot 147
Attendance allowance 442

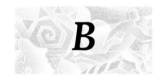

B

Babies
  choice of gender 265
  choking 458
  chubby 13
  cot death 285
  crying *279*
  dogs jealous of 332
  examination after birth 275
  feeding 278-9, 283
  first year of life 280-1
  massage *282*
  new-born held by mother 275
  overweight 13
  passive smoking 306
  premature or late 274
  reflex reactions 275
  sharing bed with parents 284-5
  sleeping through night 284

468

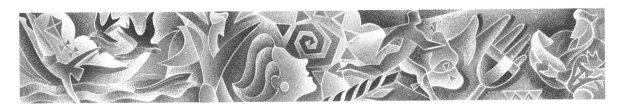

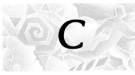

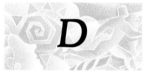

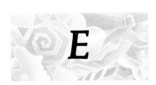
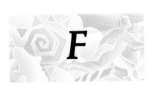

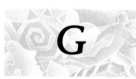

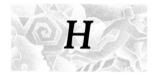

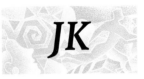

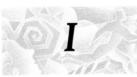

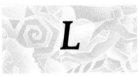

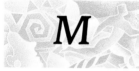
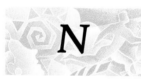
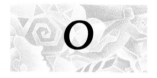

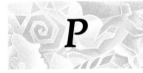
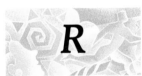

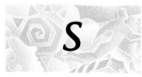

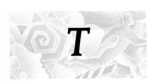

T'ai Chi Ch'uan 119
Talking
    to babies 289
    about cancer 376
    to children 295-6
    about death 444

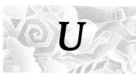
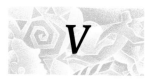
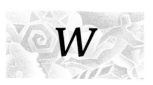
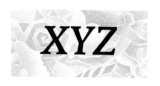

ACKNOWLEDGMENTS

PICTURE CREDITS
The sources of the illustrations in the *Good Health Fact Book* are listed below.

Abbreviations: T = Top; B = Bottom; L = Left; C = Centre; R = Right.

11 (BR) Telegraph Colour Library/ R. Chapple. **12** (BL) Collections/Anthea Sieveking. **13** (TR) The Bridgeman Art Library/Christopher Wood Gallery, London. **16** (BR) ET Archive. **18** (TL) Telegraph Colour Library/S.Wheeler. **22** (BL) The Ronald Grant Archive/King Features. **24** (CL) Comstock. **28** (TR) Tessa Traeger. **30** (TR) Collections/Sandra Lousada. **38** (BL) Telegraph Colour Library/K. Evans. **39** (CL) The Anthony Blake Photo Library. **45** ET Archive/Bibliotheque Nationale, Paris. **46** (Tomato and mackerel) The Anthony Blake Photo Library. (Margarine) Science Photo Library/Sheila Terry. (Brown rice) Tessa Traeger. (Cheese) The Anthony Blake Photo Library/Eleanor Bell. (Peas) The Anthony Blake Photo Library/Rosenfeld. **47** (Steak) Holt Studios Ltd/Nigel Cattlin. (Oranges, watercress and almonds) The Anthony Blake Photo Library. (Potatoes) Holt Studios Ltd/Nigel Cattlin. (Oyster) John Heseltine. **50** (T) Robert Harding Picture Library/Adam Woolfitt. (CR) The Anthony Blake Photo Library. (BL) Robert Harding Picture Library/Adam Woolfitt. **52** (CL) Tony Stone Photo Library, London/Andre Perlstein. **57** (CR) (TR) Science Photo Library/Barry Dowsett. **64** (L) The Image Bank/Steve Dunwell. (TR) Split Second. (CR) Action Plus/R. Francis. **65** (TL) Telegraph Colour Library. **65** (TL) Action Images Sports Photography. **66** (L) Mary Evans Picture Library/Roger Mayne. (R) The Image Bank/Infocus Int'l. **67** (B) (R) (L) Camp Beaumont. **68** (T) (B) Collections/Anthea Sieveking. **69** (T) The Image Bank/Larry Pierce. **71** (CR) The Image Bank/William Sallaz. **74** (CR) Science Photo Library/James King-Holmes. **84** (L) Split Second. (R) Action Plus/Glyn Kirk. **85** (BR) John Walmsley. **88** Ace Photo Agency. **93** (CL) The Image Bank. **97** (L) Lupe Cunha Photos. (R) The Image Bank/William Sallaz. **101** (Background) Network. **102** (B) Collections/Anthea Sieveking. **104** (T) The Image Bank/Benn Mitchell. (B) Colorsport/Jeff Thorner. **105** (T) The Image Bank/Walter Bibikow. (B) Action Plus/Mike Hewitt. **112** (L) All-Sport (UK)/Vandystadt/Sylvain Gazenave. (R) All-Sport (UK)/Bob Martin. **113** (TR) Sporting Pictures (UK) Ltd. **114** (CL) Ace Photo Agency/Fotopic. **117** (B) Hulton Deutsch. **118** (L) The Kobal Collection/Rank. (R) The Kobal Collection/Robbie Robinson. **119** (BR) Network/Barry Lewis. **124** (T) Science Photo Library/Biology Media. (C) Science Photo Library/Biology Media. (B) Chauvin Pharmaceuticals. **125** Science Photo Library/Adam Hart-Davis. **126** (BR) The Image Bank/Jay Freis. **128** (L) Science Photo Library/Will & Deni McIntyre. (R) The Image Bank. **132** (T) British Dental Health Foundation. **134** (C) (Background) Ann Ronan at Image Select. **137** (L) Science Photo Library/CNRI. (R) Science Photo Library/Dr Tony Brain. **138** (Top to bottom) Science Photo Library. National Medical Slide Bank. National Medical Slide Bank. National Medical Slide Bank. Science Photo Library/John Radcliffe Hospital. **140** (T) (C) Science Photo Library/Dr P. Marazzi. (B) Science Photo Library/James Stevenson. **148** (T) (B) Clarks Shoes. **157** (TR) Science Photo Library/Jim Selby. **158** (L) Rainbow/Dan McCoy. (C) Science Photo Library/James Holmes. (R) Science Photo Library/James Holmes. **159** (CR) Science Photo Library. (L) (C) (R) Science Photo Library/James Holmes. **164** (BL) Polartechnics Limited. **168** (TL) Science Photo Library/BSIP, Cortier. (R) Science Photo Library/Chris Priest & Mark Clarke. (CL) Science Photo Library/James Stevenson. **169** (BL) Science Photo Library/Van Bucher. (BR) The Boots Company. **175** (BR) Impact/Mark Cator. **176** (BR) The Bridgeman Art Library/British Museum. **183** (BR) Impact/Brian Harris. **185** (L) Camera Press/F. Fischbeck. (R) Colorific. **187** (L) (R) Richard and Sally Greenhill. (C) Ace Photo Agency/Kevin Phillips. **188** (L) Ace Photo Agency/Dave Bruce. (R) The Image Bank/Steve Dunwell. **189** (BL) Colorific/Penny Tweedie. **193** (T) Science Photo Library/Martin Dorhn. **194** (TL) Images Colour Library. (TR) (BL) Split Second/Leo Mason. (BR) Telegraph Colour Library/Masterfile. **195** (TL) (BR) Images Colour Library. (TR) Richard and Sally Greenhill. (CL) Split Second/Leo Mason. (CR) John Walmsley. (BL) The Image Bank/David W. Hamilton. **196** (L) Impact/Simon Shepheard. (R) Ace Photo Agency/Beryl Bidwell. **198** (T) Science Photo Library/National Institute of Health. (B) Camera Press/Karsh of Ottawa. **199** (BL) (BC) (BR) South West News Service. (Background) Network. **200** (BL) The Kobal Collection. **201** (C) (CR) (BR) Aviators/Rob Judges. **202** (C) The Press Association Ltd. **203** (TL) John Walmsley. **208** (BL) The Fotomas Index. **209** (Background) Telegraph Colour Library. **211** (C) Science Photo Library/National Institute of Health. **213** (B) The Image Bank/Stan Flint. **219** (BR) Lupe Cunha Photos. **220** (C) Science Photo Library/Chris Priest and Mark Clarke. **221** (L) (R) Science Photo Library/Simon Fraser. **222** (BR) John Walmsley. **224** (BR) Science Photo Library/CNRI. **226** (L) Science Photo Library. (R) Bubbles Photo Library/Loisjoy Thurston. **227** (TL) (R) John Walmsley. (B) Science Photo Library. **228** (L) Telegraph Colour Library. (TR) Science Photo Library/Francoise Sauze. (B) Richard and Sally Greenhill. **229** (TR) Collections. (BL) The Image Bank/Patti McConville. (BR) Bubbles Photo Library/Loisjoy Thurston. **231** (BR) Science Photo Library. **232** (L) Science Photo Library. (TR) Colorific/GE Medical Systems. (BR) Science Photo Library/Manfred Kage. **233** (TL) Science Photo Library/Custom Medical Stock Photo. (BL) Ace Photo Agency/Phototake. (TR) Science Photo Library/GJLP/CNRI. (BR) Science Photo Library/CNRI. **235** (C) John Walmsley. **238** (BR) Science Photo Library/Royal Shrewsbury Hospital/Simon Fraser. **240** (T) (B) Eastman Dental Hospital (Orthodontic Dept). **241** (CR) Science Photo Library/Adam Hart-Davis. **244** (TR) Tony Stone Photo Library, London/Andy Sacks. **250** (L) Science Photo Library/Jerry Mason. (R) Science Photo Library/Matt Meadows. **265** (BR) Science Photo Library/Richard Rawlins/Custom Medical Stock Photo. **266** (CL) (CR) Rex Features Ltd. (Background) Network. **269** (T) Science Photo Library. (C) Science Photo Library/St Bartholomew's Hospital. **271** (C) Collections. **274** (T) Richard and Sally Greenhill. (B) Science Photo Library/Ron Sutherland. **277** (BR) Bubbles Photo Library/L.J. Thurston. **279** (BR) Collections/Sandra Lousada. **279** (BR) Lupe Cunha Photos. **280** (C) Bubbles Photo Library/Loisjoy Thurston. (B) Tony Stone Photo Library, London. **281** (TL) (BL) Collections/Anthea Sieveking. (TR) Richard and Sally Greenhill. (CL) Collections/Sandra Lousada. (BR) Bubbles Photo Library/Loisjoy Thurston. **282** (L) Collections/Anthea Sieveking. **283** (R) Richard and Sally Greenhill. **285** (TR) Bubbles Photo Library/Ian West. **290** (BL) The Image Bank/Schmid/Langsfeld. **291** (BR) Bubbles Photo Library/ P. Cutler. **292** (BR) Bubbles Photo Library/John Garrett. **297** (C) Telegraph Colour Library/Barbara Peacock. **299** (R) Henri Cartier-Bresson/Magnum. **303** (BR) Format/Melanie Friend. **304** (T) (B) Popperfoto. **306** (B) Science Photo Library/Dr Jeremy Burgess. **308** (L) The Bridgeman Art Library/By courtesy of the Board of Trustees of the V & A. **310** (T) Images Colour Library. **311** (BR) Tim Woodcock. **314** (BL) NHPA/David Woodfall. (Background) Network. **318** Science Photo Library **321** (BL) Ace Photo Agency/Jason Burns. **322** (CR) (BR) National Medical Slide Bank. **324** (T) John Walmsley. **326** (TR) The Garden Picture Library/Vaughan Fleming. (CR) Bruce Coleman Ltd/Hans Reinhard. (BL) The Garden Picture Library/Rowan Isaac. (BR) The Garden Picture Library/John Glover. **327** (TL) The Garden Picture Library/Roger Hyam. (TC) John Buckingham. (TR) NHPA/Vicente Garcia Canseco. (CL) NHPA/Laurie Campbell. (C) NHPA/Kevin Schafer. (CR) The Garden Picture Library/J.S. Sira. (BL) Bruce Coleman Ltd/Dr Eckart Pott. (BC) The Garden Picture Library. (BR) Bruce Coleman Ltd/Neville Fox-Davies. **328** (L) (R) By courtesy of Consumers' Association/Steve Bielschowsky. **331** (TR) The Garden Picture Library/Vaughan Fleming. (CR) Holt Studios Ltd./Duncan Smith. **335** (BR) Ace Photo Agency/Peter Adams. **336** (L) (CL) John Frost Historical Newspaper Service. (BL) Popperfoto. **338** (BR) Tony Stone Photo Library, London/Donald Johnston. **339** (L) Mothercare. (R) Bubbles Photo Library/Ian West. **346** (BL) Science Photo Library/David Sharf. **349** Colorific/Steve Benbow. **350** (TL) Ace Photo Agency/Auschromes. (TR) Bubbles Photo Library. (BL) Robert Harding Picture Library. (BR) Science Photo Library/Alex Bartel. **352** (TL) Action Plus/Chris Barry. (Background) Network. **353** (BR) Science Photo Library/GCa-CNRI. **354** (L) Science Photo Library. **355** (T) (B) Dr Peter Howdle/St. James's University Hospital, Leeds. **359** (L) Science Photo Library/Chris Priest. (R) Collections/Anthea Sieveking. **360** (L) British Diabetic Association. **363** (R) Science Photo Library/Mehau Kulyk. **365** (R) Science Photo Library. **367** (R) The Image Bank/Barros & Barros. **372** (L) Network/Alain Soldeville/Rapho. **373** (T) (B) William MacQuitty. **374** (L) Science Photo Library/Princess Margaret Rose Orthopaedic Hospital. (R) Science Photo Library/Mike Devlin. **375** (R) Richard and Sally Greenhill. **382** (L) Camera Press/Roustan/L'Express. (Background) Network. **385** (L) Retna Pictures/George Lange. (R) Sygma/B. Nation. **386** (B) Camera Press/S. Rud/Alfa. **389** (L) (R) Robert Harding Picture Library/Richard Waite/Woman's Journal. **390** (C) (B) Science Photo Library/Professor P. Motta/University 'La Sapienza', Rome. **397** (R) Telegraph Colour Library/Carola

ACKNOWLEDGMENTS

Bayer. (L) Robert Harding Picture Library/Tim Megarry. **400** (L) Richard and Sally Greenhill. (R) Network/John Sturrock. **401** (T) The Image Bank/Lou Jones. (R) Impact/Peter Arkell. **402** (L) Lupe Cunha Photos. **403** (L) Impact. (R) Collections/Anthea Sieveking. **411** (L) ET Archive. (R) The Mansell Collection. **413** (B) John Walmsley. **414** (TL) (BL) Impact/Caroline Penn. (CR) Richard and Sally Greenhill. (BR) Impact. **415** (C) Format/Mo Wilson. (BR) Format/Brenda Prince. **416** (L) Photo of Grandma Moses by Otto Kallir 1946/Courtesy Grandma Moses Properties Co., New York. (Background) Network. **418** (L) Tim Woodcock. (R) Arcaid. **419** (TL) Arcaid/Ian Bruce. (TR) Arcaid/Joe Low. (BL) The Image Bank/Kay Chernush. (BR) Robert Harding Picture Library/Larsen-Collinge. **420** (L) Impact/Peter Arkell. (R) Format/Brenda Prince. **430** (C) (BL) (BC) (BR) A & M Hearing Ltd. **433** Science Photo Library/Adam Hart-Davis. **437** (B) The Image Bank/Barros & Barros. **438** (C) Science Photo Library/Hattie Young. **441** (L) Science Photo Library. **443** (R) Collections/Anthea Sieveking. **444** (B) Richard and Sally Greenhill.

....

The publishers of the *Good Health Fact Book* would like to acknowledge substantial assistance from the following sources:

Alcohol Concern

Arthritis Care

British Diabetic Association

British Heart Foundation

British Society of Experimental and Clinical Hypnosis

Child Accident Prevention Trust

Wendy Coles
Amateur Swimming Association

Eating Disorders Association

Olive Elderton and Eddie Foulds
Publishers of 'Dance Diary'

Electricity Association

Gas Consumers Council

Dr D J Gawkrodger, MD, FRCP, FRCPE
Consultant Dermatologist,
Royal Hallamshire Hospital
Author of 'Dermatology: An Illustrated
Colour Text'

Jonathan Goh, DO(Hons), MRO
Registered Osteopath

Institute for the Study of Drug Dependence

National Asthma Campaign

The National Back Pain Association

National Poisons Unit, Guy's and St Thomas' Hospital Trust

National Radiological Protection Board

National Rivers Authority

National Society for Epilepsy

St John Ambulance

S A N E

The Stroke Association

Len Unwin
British Cycling Federation

Many other people and organisations contributed to the production of this book. The publishers would particularly like to thank: Camping and Outdoor Centre (41 Ludgate Hill, London), Friends of the Earth, The Keep Fit Association, Thomas H Loveday Ltd, Marie Stopes International, Robert Dyas Ltd (167 Fleet Street, London), Nike, Ramblers' Association, Reebok UK Ltd, Thames Water, Women's Environmental Network.

....

The sources of the illustrations on the dust jacket of the UK edition of *Good Health Fact Book* are as follows:

Front: (TL) The Anthony Blake Photo Library. (CL) Telegraph Colour Library. (CR) Science Photo Library/A.B. Dowsett. (R) Britstock-Ifa Limited/Amadeus. (BL) Art Directors Photo Library. (BR) Science Photo Library. **Back:** (TL) Science Photo Library/Custom Medical Stock Photo. (C) Science Photo Library. (TR) Science Photo Library/Royal Shrewsbury Hospital/Simon Fraser. (BR) Science Photo Library.

Separations Dot Gradations Ltd, South Woodham Ferrers, UK
Printing and binding Milanostampa SPA, Farigliano, Italy
Paper Smurfit Townsend Hook Ltd, Snodland, UK
Cloth Van Heek Textiles B.V. Losser, Netherlands